1983
Medical
and
Health Annual

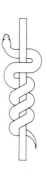

Encyclopædia Britannica, Inc.

CHICAGO

AUCKLAND • GENEVA • LONDON • MANILA • PARIS • ROME • SEOUL • SYDNEY • TOKYO • TORONTO

1983 Medical and Health Annual

Editor	Ellen Bernstein
Associate Editor	Anita Wolff
Contributing Editor	Charles Cegielski
Medical Editor	Drummond Rennie, M.D. Chairman of Medicine West Suburban Hospital, Oak Park; Associate Professor of Medicine Rush Medical College, Chicago
Art Director	Cynthia Peterson
Design Supervisor	Ron Villani
Picture Editors	Holly Harrington, *senior picture editor;* LaBravia Jones
Layout Artist	Richard Batchelor
Illustrators	John L. Draves, Richard A. Roiniotis
Art Staff	Patricia Henle, William Karpa, Lillian Simcox, Paul Rios
Copy Director	J. Thomas Beatty
Senior Copy Editor	Barbara Whitney
Copy Staff	Marsha Check, Anne B. Hedblom, Stephen Isaacs, Cheryl Lapham, Paul Mendelson, Kay Skvorc
Copy Control	Mary C. Srodon, *supervisor* Mayme R. Cussen
Director, Composition/Indexing	Robert Dehmer
Editorial Typesetting Manager	Melvin Stagner
Computer System Manager	Ronald Laugeman
Typesetting Staff	Duangnetra Debhavalya, Griselda Chaidez, Dora Jeffers, Judith Kobylecky, John Krom, Jr., Thomas Mulligan, Arnell Reed, Gwen Rosenberg, Van Smith
Index Manager	Frances E. Latham
Index Supervisor	Rosa E. Casas
Index Staff	Mansur G. Abdullah, *senior indexer;* Katherine M. Arneson
Librarian	Terry Miller
Associate Librarian	Shantha Channabasappa
Administrative Secretary	Ines Baptist

Editorial Administration

Editor-in-Chief
Philip W. Goetz

Executive Editor
Margaret Sutton

Director of Budgets and Control
Verne Pore

Encyclopædia Britannica, Inc.

Chairman of the Board	Robert P. Gwinn
President	Charles E. Swanson
Vice-President/Editorial	Charles Van Doren

Foreword

The summer of 1982 saw millions around the world join together to proclaim their opposition to the mounting nuclear arms race. The most poignant voices in this vast chorus crying for an end to the making of nuclear weapons were the Japanese survivors of the atomic bombs that were dropped in August 1945 on Hiroshima and Nagasaki. In many countries groups of physicians stood in the forefront of the movement. Their message was simple: Nuclear war today would be the most significant threat to human health and survival the world has ever known. Despite its immense sophistication, modern medicine would not be able to cope.

The full extent of the suffering and destruction caused by the relatively primitive weapons dropped on Japan has recently come to light. An accounting of the physical, medical, and social effects of the bombs, compiled in Japan, has summarized 35 years of research and statistical analysis. In the feature article that opens this volume, ''Reaping the Whirlwind: The Scars of Hiroshima and Nagasaki,'' two Japanese physicians who were instrumental in issuing that comprehensive report present a vivid picture of the nightmare that is nuclear war.

* * *

In the 1980s many individuals are searching for relief from their anxieties, unhappinesses, fears, sexual difficulties, sleep disorders, weight-control battles, and other coping problems through various forms of therapy. Some see psychoanalysts four times a week for 50-minute, on-the-couch sessions (often for years). Others seek briefer, more direct psychotherapies to overcome their immediate life problems. Still others are turning to ''vogue'' treatments: screaming, immersion in water, acupuncture, biofeedback, running, adopting pets, and taking megadoses of vitamins, to name just a few. The most desperate souls may simply pour out their hearts anonymously to advice columnists: ''Dear Anybody: I am depressed. I cry all the time and eat too much. People at work gossip about me. My husband calls me a wet blanket. My children can't understand what ails me. I need help!''

The bewilderment of those who search for mental health is not surprising considering the complexities of modern-day life. The dubious effectiveness of traditional means of treating emotional ills certainly creates a climate in which these hit-or-miss approaches thrive. As *Time* magazine recently put it, psychiatry itself is ''on the couch.''

For centuries emotional disorders of all sorts were lumped together, and sufferers were more often than not viewed with a combination of fear and revulsion. Today mental illnesses can be attributed to specific genetic, biologic, developmental, environmental, psychological, and social factors. The advent of psychoactive drugs in the 1950s meant that, for the first time, the most severe disorders, schizophrenia and some forms of depression, could be effectively treated (though not necessarily cured). Some mental illnesses are now seen as medical problems linked to specific neurochemical and hormonal imbalances, and precise and highly reliable methods of diagnosing and treating them are emerging. Moreover, today various forms of psychotherapy are on scientific trial—*i.e.,* they are being standardized and tested in reproducible studies.

This year the *Medical and Health Annual* offers seven feature articles that focus on the broad areas of mental health and illness. The distinguished contributors to this symposium shed light on several topics: the history of institutional care of the insane; the diagnosis, treatment, and prevention of the specific problems of addictions, phobias, depressions, and schizophrenia; the rationale behind various ''talking'' therapies; and the relationship of physical exercise to that most elusive state, mental well-being.

* * *

The other feature articles in this volume examine the new field of diagnosing and treating disorders in unborn children; the challenges and controversies in contemporary epidemiology; and, finally, the tragic neurologic disorder Huntington's chorea.

* * *

The 1983 *Medical and Health Annual* also includes *The World of Medicine*—alphabetized entries (including 11 Special Reports) that highlight major developments in medicine and health; *Health Education Units* that provide reliable and practical information on common illnesses, medical procedures, and other important matters of health and wellness; and a *First Aid Handbook,* with easy-to-follow, illustrated instructions for coping with medical emergencies. All the articles in the *Annual* have been prepared in the manner of *Encyclopædia Britannica*—by outstanding authorities in their respective fields. We hope their efforts will help readers keep pace with the exciting developments in medicine today.

Ellen Bernstein

—Editor

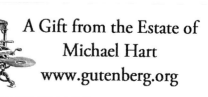

Contents

Reaping the Whirlwind: The Scars of Hiroshima and Nagasaki

by Sōichi Iijma, M.D., and Eisei Ishikawa, M.D.

In the early morning of Aug. 6, 1945, a U.S. Army plane, the "Enola Gay," invaded the skies of Hiroshima at an altitude of 9,600 meters (31,500 feet). This plane carried the first atomic weapon ever to be wielded in anger in a global war. The bomb was dropped; 43 seconds later, at 8:15 AM, the bomb exploded at an altitude of about 580 meters (1,900 feet).

This bomb was one of the three that had been produced after careful preparation of more than three years under the Manhattan Project. Prior to the attack on Hiroshima, one of the three bombs, a plutonium bomb, was exploded in an experiment carried out on July 16 at the Alamogordo testing grounds in the desert of New Mexico. The bomb that was dropped on Hiroshima, nicknamed "Little Boy" (in reference to Franklin D. Roosevelt), was a uranium bomb measuring 3 meters (10 feet) in length by 0.7 meters (2.29 feet) in diameter and weighing 4.4 (U.S.) tons. The energy released by "Little Boy" was estimated to be the equivalent of about 12.5 kilotons of conventional high-explosive trinitrotoluene (TNT). The energy released by 20 kilotons of TNT is equivalent to the energy released at the time of complete nuclear fission of one kilogram of uranium 235.

The third A-bomb was a plutonium bomb of the type exploded at Alamogordo; it was dropped on the city of Nagasaki at 11:02 AM on August 9, and it exploded at an altitude of 503 meters (1,650 feet). This bomb, named "Fat Man" (in reference to Winston Churchill), measured 3.5 meters (11.5 feet) in length by 1.5 meters (4.9 feet) in diameter and weighed nearly 5 tons. The energy released by "Fat Man" was equivalent to about 22 kilotons of TNT.

The target cities

Hiroshima is located on the northern bank of the Inland Sea of western Japan, on the island of Honshū. The city, founded in the 16th century, was built on a delta at the mouth of the Ota River, which flows into the Inland Sea from the Chūgoku Mountains. Hiroshima covers an area of about 33 square kilometers (12.7 square miles), and at the time of the bombing there were about 76,000 houses and a population of 320,000. With military personnel

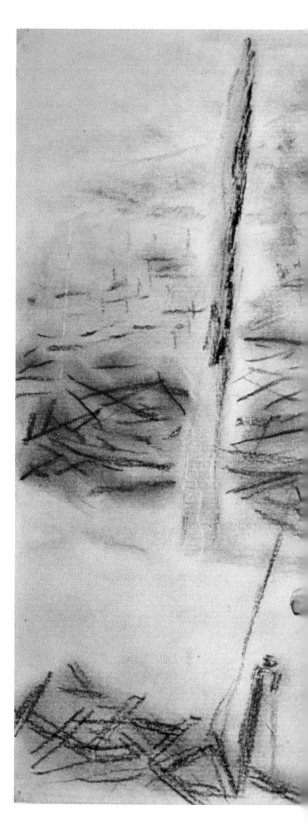

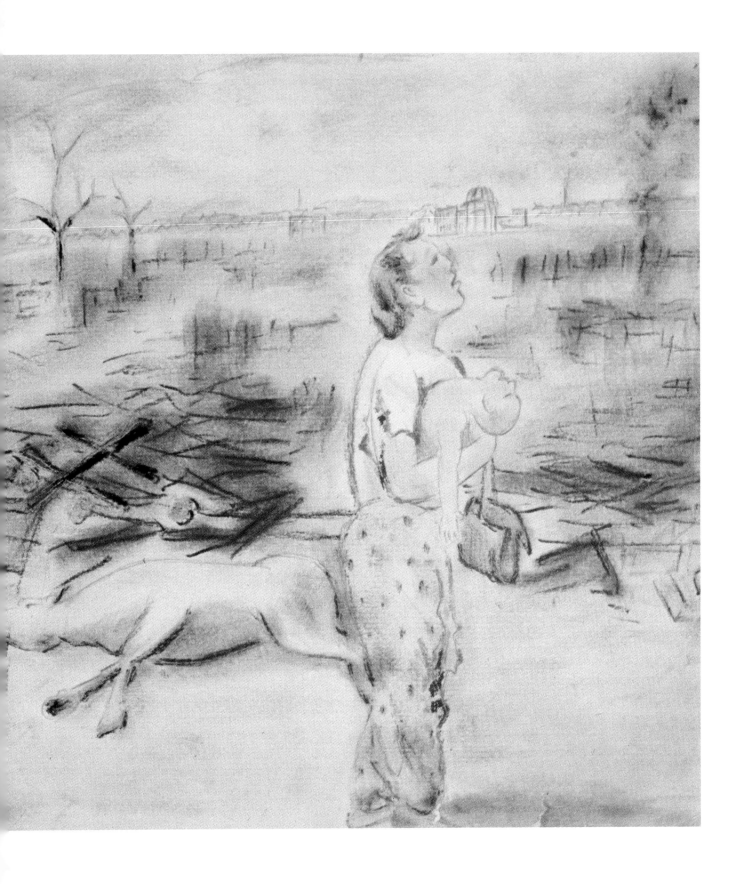

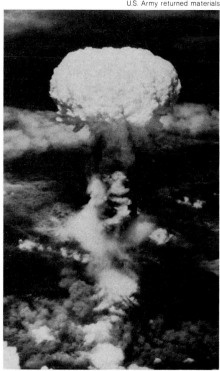

Sōichi Iijima, M.D., *is President of Nagoya University and Professor of Pathology at Nagoya University School of Medicine, Nagoya, Japan.* **Eisei Ishikawa, M.D.,** *is Professor of Pathology at Jikei University School of Medicine, Tokyo. Dr. Iijima was a member of the editorial committee that produced* Hiroshima and Nagasaki: The Physical, Medical, and Social Effects of the Atomic Bombings *(English edition, New York: Basic Books, 1981). Dr. Ishikawa translated the natural science sections of the book for the English edition.*

Drawings in this article are from Unforgettable Fire: Pictures Drawn by Atomic Bomb Survivors, *edited by Nippon Hoso Shuppan Kyokai (The Japanese Broadcasting Corporation), Tokyo, 1977.*

Photographs are from Hiroshima-Nagasaki: A Pictorial Record of the Atomic Destruction, *edited by Hiroshima-Nagasaki Publishing Committee, Tokyo, 1978.*

(Overleaf) Drawing by Yuji Ichida

and other additions there were between 353,000 and 363,000 people in Hiroshima on August 6.

This city had flourished as a castle town of the Asano feudal clan during the Edo era (1603–1868). As the seat of Hiroshima's Prefectural Office from the Meiji era (1868–1912), it had been the center of administration, economics, education, culture, and military affairs of the Chūgoku district. At the time of the bombing, the district's population was augmented by the presence of the Chūgoku Military Headquarters, branch offices of various central government agencies, Hiroshima University of Literature and Science, Hiroshima Higher Normal School, Hiroshima Higher School, Hiroshima Technical College, other schools, and the Second Army Headquarters and its attached corps.

The A-bomb exploded at the center of Hiroshima. Over 60% of the houses were completely destroyed and burned down, 5% were completely destroyed, and 24% were either half destroyed, greatly damaged, or half burned, while a mere 10% escaped damage. The burned-out district covered 40% of the entire city and the destroyed district about 92% of the city. Of the people present within 500 meters (1,640 feet) of the hypocenter, the point directly over which the bomb exploded, 90.4% died instantaneously. The death rate was 59.4% at distances between 0.6 and I kilometer (0.4–0.6 mile) and 39.8% within 2 kilometers. There have been widely varying estimates of the death total at Hiroshima, but it is agreed that at least 78,000, and perhaps as many as 130,000, soldiers, civilians, and foreign residents died in the bombing.

Nagasaki is a harbor city facing the China Sea on the west side of the island of Kyushu. It was the only open port and thus the center of foreign trade in Japan during the Edo era. Vestiges of the cultural exchange and foreign trade of that era between Japan and Spain, Portugal, England, China, Holland, and Southeast Asia can be found in Deshima, a reclaimed island where the foreign trading post had been established and where foreigners were kept isolated after 1639.

After the Meiji era Nagasaki city was the administrative center and seat of government for Nagasaki Prefecture. The population at the time of the bombing was about 270,000. Educational facilities included the Nagasaki Medical University and Nagasaki Commercial College. Nagasaki was a heavily industrialized city; it was the headquarters for the Mitsubishi Heavy Industries Nagasaki Shipyard, the Mitsubishi Steel Manufacturing Co., and the Mitsubishi Electric Corp.

The city was divided into two districts, Nakajima and Urakami, along the Nakajima and Urakami rivers; a hill separates the two districts. The Mitsubishi factories lined the Urakami River from the west bank of Nagasaki Bay, and from the slopes of the hills to the interior stood the educational facilities (Nagasaki Medical University and other schools), Urakami Roman Catholic Cathedral, and residential areas. The A-bomb exploded above the center of the Urakami district. Because of the shielding hills of the area, only about 36% of the houses and buildings in the city were damaged, but those in the Urakami district were almost totally destroyed and burned down. About 6.7 square kilometers (2.6 square miles) of the city was utterly destroyed. Casu-

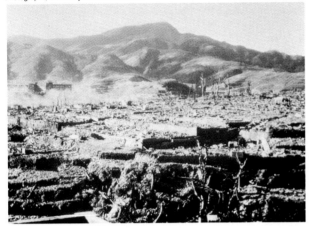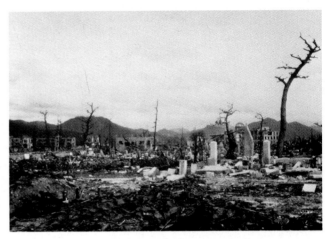

alties from A-bomb injury in Nagasaki numbered nearly 74,000 killed and as many injured by the end of 1945.

The bombs' deadly effects

The explosion of an atomic bomb releases an enormous amount of energy in the form of heat (thermal) rays, blast and shock waves, and ionizing radiation. The release takes place in a fraction of a second and in a confined space. Since it was impossible to carry out a survey of the effects of the bomb at the time of the explosions in Hiroshima and Nagasaki, the following data were obtained from the tests carried out in the United States in the 1940s and 1950s with bombs of approximately 20 kilotons and from information gathered in Hiroshima and Nagasaki after the explosions.

Thermal rays. More than a third of the energy of nuclear fission is released as thermal (heat) rays. The maximum temperature at the bursting point immediately rises to several million degrees Celcius, and all elements composing the A-bomb vaporize into an ionizing gas. Electromagnetic waves of short wavelength are immediately absorbed by the surrounding air, forming a fireball about 15 meters in diameter, with a temperature of about 300,000° C. The front of the shock wave coincides with the surface of the fireball. A sharp pressure wall is formed on the shock front. The fireball expands rapidly, while the shock wave moves even more rapidly. The fireball grows in size and reaches its maximum size; these events are concluded within one second after the explosion.

After reaching a temperature of about 7,700° C (0.2 second after the explosion), the surface temperature of the fireball gradually drops, with loss of brightness, after about ten seconds. The thermal rays emitted by the fireball are ultraviolet rays, near-ultraviolet rays, visible rays, and infrared rays. Since the ultraviolet rays and near-ultraviolet rays were almost completely emitted within 15 milliseconds (thousandths of a second) after the explosion and were absorbed in air, the total energy of these rays reaching the ground in Hiroshima and Nagasaki was assumed to be extremely small. It was probably the infrared rays, which were emitted in vast amounts 0.2 to 3 seconds after the explosion, that caused the thermal burns.

At the time of the explosion the energy released by the thermal rays was

(Opposite page) At 11:02 AM on Aug. 9, 1945, a 22-kiloton plutonium bomb was dropped on the city of Nagasaki. By the end of 1945 nearly 74,000 persons had died as a result of the bombing, and an equal number had suffered injuries. (Above) The ruins of Nagasaki (left) and Hiroshima (right) at the hypocenters—the points over which the bombs exploded. The desolation was caused by the immensely powerful heat and blast energy released by the bomb and also by the fire storms that engulfed both cities.

9

Eiichi Matsumoto

Adapted from Hiroshima Shiyakusho, *Hiroshima genbaku sensaishi* ("Record of the Hiroshima A-bomb War Disaster"), Hiroshima, 1971, vol. 1

Total number of casualties due to the atomic bomb, Hiroshima, Aug. 10, 1946*

distance from hypocenter (km)	killed	severely injured	slightly injured	missing
under 0.5	19,329	478	338	593
0.5–1.0	42,271	3,046	1,919	1,366
1.0–1.5	37,689	7,732	9,522	1,188
1.5–2.0	13,422	7,627	11,516	227
2.0–2.5	4,513	7,830	14,149	98
2.5–3.0	1,139	2,923	6,795	32
3.0–3.5	117	474	1,934	2
3.5–4.0	100	295	1,768	3
4.0–4.5	8	64	373	
4.5–5.0	31	36	156	1
over 5.0	42	19	136	167
total	118,661	30,524	48,606	3,677

*Military personnel not included.

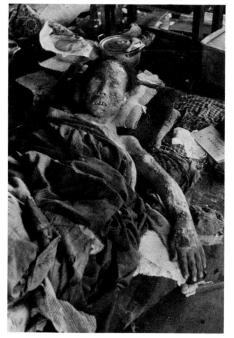

A mortally injured woman, severely burned and suffering from radiation sickness, awaits death at a relief station set up in an elementary school in Hiroshima. The table (right) gives the total number of casualties in Hiroshima. Within 500 meters of the hypocenter more than 90% of the residents were killed instantaneously.

estimated to be about 35% of the total potential energy of the bomb. Since the amount of heat escaping by conduction is small when a vast amount of thermal rays are emitted within a short time, the absorbed heat energy is confined to the surface of the material contacted, causing a tremendous rise in surface temperature. The ground surface temperature at the hypocenter in Hiroshima and Nagasaki has been estimated to have reached 3,000° C to 4,000° C—the melting point of iron is 1,538° C (2,800° F).

Shock wave and blast. When an atomic bomb explodes in air, the expansion of intensely hot gases causes the emanation of a shock wave. The air after the passage of the shock front becomes very dense and hot and moves in the same direction as the shock wave but at a somewhat slower speed. The velocity of this scorching wind depends on the maximum pressure of the shock wave and drops as it travels away from the burst point. When the distance from the hypocenter becomes greater than the height of the burst point, the primary wave, caused by the explosion in air, and the wave front, reflected from the ground surface, fuse and form a new shock front (Mach stem). Its pressure is, in general, greater than the primary wave. This pressure is great enough to crumple buildings into rubble and to hurl people and heavy objects considerable distances.

About half of the latent energy of the A-bomb is released as energy of blast; the pressure this blast exerted on the ground at the hypocenter was estimated to be 5 to 7.4 tons per square meter in Hiroshima and 7.4 to 11 tons per square meter in Nagasaki. The duration of blast pressure was assumed to be about 0.4 second.

Radiation. The radiation released by the atomic bomb consists of initial radiation, emitted immediately after the explosion, and residual radiation, which can be detected for some time later. The initial radiation comprises alpha particles, beta particles, gamma rays, and neutrons. Alpha particles are emitted from uranium and plutonium which have escaped complete fission, while beta particles are emitted from fission products. Since the ranges in air of alpha and beta particles are short, they fail to reach the ground; gamma rays and neutrons are responsible for the injurious effects on humans, animals, and plants.

10

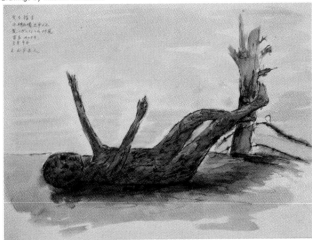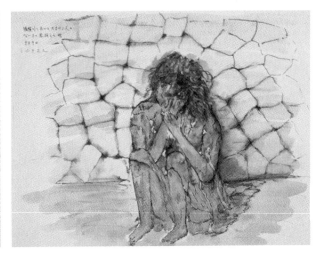

There were many studies on the estimated in-air doses of initial radiation in Hiroshima and Nagasaki. The most reliable study calculates dosages by what is termed the tentative 1965 dose (T65D), reported by the Oak Ridge National Laboratory in 1966. This estimated value was obtained from the theoretical calculation of the structure and nature of the A-bombs used on Hiroshima and Nagasaki, from the analysis of radiation effects in both cities, and from the enormous data of the nuclear tests carried out in the United States beginning in 1955.

These figures are expressed in rads, an acronym for radiation absorbed dose. Total body irradiation of 1,000 rads is almost certain to be fatal. Five hundred rads will cause acute radiation sickness and possibly death. A person receiving 4,000 rads would live only three days at most and would experience symptoms such as vomiting and diarrhea within an hour. Mild radiation sickness results from a total-body dose of about 100 rads.

According to the T65D the in-air dose of gamma rays in Hiroshima was 10,300 rads at the hypocenter and that of neutrons 14,100 rads. These values varied with distance from the hypocenter: 2,790 rads and 3,150 rads at 500 meters, 255 rads and 191 rads at 1,000 meters, and 21.6 rads and 10.1 rads at 1,500 meters.

At the hypocenter in Nagasaki the in-air dose of gamma rays was 25,100 rads and that of neutrons 3,900 rads. These values were 7,090 rads and 703 rads at 500 meters, 888 rads and 35.9 rads at 1,000 meters, and 119 rads and 1.7 rads at 1,500 meters. Recently, however, it has been pointed out that the in-air dose of neutrons in both cities may have been overestimated; these values are being restudied.

Figuring of the actual in-air dose of the initial radiation to which the human body was exposed should include the effects of shielding by houses, soil, and other barriers. Since the actual conditions of individual exposure differed greatly, it is necessary to consider each condition separately and estimate the exposure dose as affected by various shields. In Hiroshima and Nagasaki the individual exposure doses were actually estimated by this procedure. When the shielding conditions were not clear, the average penetration coefficient was used, taking into account the Japanese style of construction.

In May 1974 an elderly man visited the Japanese Broadcasting Corporation's studio in Hiroshima. He brought with him a drawing entitled "At about 4 PM, August 6, 1945, near Yorozuyo Bridge," depicting a scene he had witnessed as he was searching for his missing son. In June the station broadcast an appeal for additional drawings from the bomb's survivors. There was a flood of responses. In all, 975 drawings were received; 104 of these were collected into a book entitled Unforgettable Fire: Pictures Drawn by Atomic Bomb Survivors. *The drawings above are both by Masato Yamashita, and both depict events of August 9. (Left) "On the west embankment of a military training field was a young boy four or five years old. He was burned black, lying on his back, with his arms pointing toward heaven." (Right) "With no one to help her, a girl died leaning on the bank of the Enko River."*

11

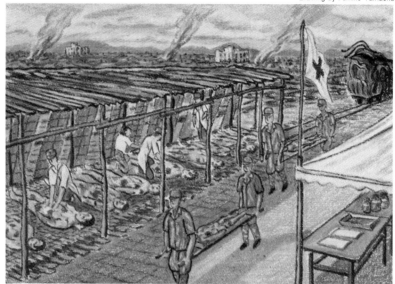

Relief and first-aid stations were improvised in structures that remained standing or in the open air. Persons suffering from burns and blast injuries were the first to seek treatment. They were soon followed by those with acute radiation sickness.

Whole-body doses of radiation and their acute effects

dose (roentgen)*	biological effects
less than 1	No detectable effect.
10	Barely detectable qualitative changes in lymphocytes.
100	Mild acute radiation illness in some. Slight diminution in white cell counts. Possible nausea and vomiting. Possible transient suppression of hemopoietic activity.
1,000	Depression of blood cell and platelet formation. Damage to gastrointestinal mucosa. Severe acute radiation illness. Death within 30 days.
10,000	Immediate disorientation or coma. Death within hours.
100,000	Death of some microorganisms.
1,000,000	Death of some bacteria.
10,000,000	Death of all living organisms. Some denaturation of proteins.

*A roentgen is equivalent to 0.9 rad.

Adapted from S. Warren, *The Pathology of Ionizing Radiation,* Springfield, Ill., Charles C. Thomas, 1961

Though public buildings were constructed of stone, brick, and concrete, most of the housing consisted of light frame buildings.

A dosage estimate based on these considerations indicates the radiation dose acting on the skin surface only. In order to study injuries caused by radiation, one needs to know the dose absorbed by various organs of the body, the organ dose. According to the data obtained in both cities, when a person outdoors is exposed to radiation from one direction, the gamma rays and neutrons received by the center of the body diminish to about one-half and one-tenth, respectively, of those acting on the skin surface. Organs with rapid cell division (bone marrow, ovaries, testes, and gastrointestinal tract) suffer the greatest damage from radiation.

Residual radiation includes the induced radioactivity imparted to objects on the ground by the bomb's explosion and the radioactivity of fallout. The intensity of induced radioactivity was the highest at the hypocenter in both cities. According to meteorological conditions at the time of the bombing, the radioactivity of fallout tended to be concentrated from the north to the west of the hypocenter in Hiroshima and in the vicinity of Nishiyama reservoir, located about 3 kilometers (1.8 miles) to the east of the hypocenter in Nagasaki. The intensity of induced radioactivity in Hiroshima was estimated to be about 20 rads for those entering the city near the hypocenter one hour after the explosion and staying there for five hours, becoming less than 10 rads for eight hours on the following day. The exposure dose in Nagasaki was presumed to be about 40% of that in Hiroshima. The main source of fallout was nuclear fission products (gamma rays), which have accumulated to 4–40 rads in Hiroshima and 50–285 rads in Nagasaki (Nishiyama district) up to the present.

The toll of human suffering

Injuries to the human body in those exposed to the A-bombs in Hiroshima and Nagasaki can be classified into three phases. These are: initial phase injuries (the acute phase of A-bomb injury), delayed effects of these injuries, and aftereffects, including genetic effects.

The acute phase of A-bomb injury. This stage includes direct injuries from the A-bomb and secondary symptoms observed from immediately after the explosion to the end of four months. The acute phase can further be subdivided into three stages.

Stage 1, the early stage, was the time immediately after the explosion up to the end of two weeks. The enormous energy released by the explosion of the A-bomb, especially the compounded action of intense heat and blast, was the primary cause of death and injury. It was at stage 1 that about nine-tenths of the total fatalities from exposure to the bomb occurred. The vast majority (about 90%) of the wounded treated by the medical relief teams after the explosion were suffering from thermal burns.

Stage 2, the intermediate stage, extended from the beginning of the third week to the end of the eighth week after the bombing. During this time there were many cases of moderate injuries caused by radioactivity. About one-tenth of the remaining fatal cases died at this stage.

Stage 3, the late stage, extended from the beginning of the third month to the end of the fourth month after the bombing. Although this was the stage when symptoms frequently showed improvement, some victims suffered from complications and died during the period. At the end of the fourth month (December 1945) the majority of the victims in both cities had apparently recovered from their injuries. It can be said that the acute phase of A-bomb injury had come to an end by late December. The conditions that were seen in the acute phase were the complex result of the heat rays, blast, and ionizing radiation. The injuries can be classified according to their main causal mechanism.

Thermal injury. Thermal injuries included flash burns (primary thermal burns), which were directly caused by thermal rays emitted by the A-bomb, and scorch burns, contact burns, and flame burns (secondary thermal burns), which resulted from fires caused by the A-bomb's thermal rays. The intense heat of the bombs set buildings and rubble afire; fire storms raged through both cities. The record of thermal injuries seen in the victims 20 days after the explosion in Hiroshima revealed that 83.2% were suffering from primary thermal burns, 1.9% from secondary thermal burns, and 14.9% suffering from both primary and secondary burns. In Nagasaki the respective figures were 90.9%, 3.4%, and 5.7%.

Flash burns were characterized by uniform, shallow lesions on exposed skin, which were well demarcated from the normal deeper tissue. In the mild cases there was only erythema (reddening of the skin, or red burn), while with increased severity the skin suffered coagulation necrosis and became white (spotted or diffuse white burn). Blisters then formed (blebbed white burn), and in the most severe cases carbonization took place (charred burn). The energy of thermal rays was extreme, and in exposed persons the charring extended through all thicknesses of the skin and into the underlying muscles and other organs. Many persons near the hypocenter were instantly and totally charred.

The victims with marked thermal injury had their clothing burned, and they

Adapted from A. W. Oughterson and S. Warren, *Medical Effects of the Atomic Bomb in Japan,* New York, McGraw Hill, 1956, p. 30

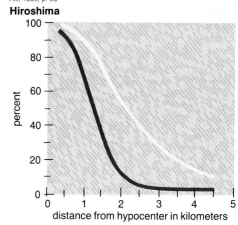

Hiroshima

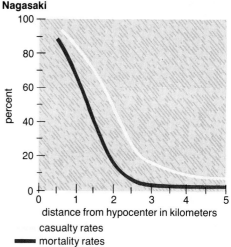

Nagasaki

casualty rates
━━━ mortality rates

The tables above show the relationship of the percentage of fatalities to distance from the hypocenter in both cities. The table below indicates that nearly half of the total number of deaths occurred more than a week after the bombings, as victims succumbed to the effects of their injuries.

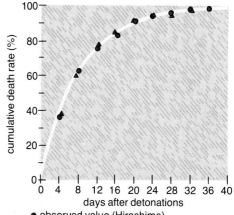

● observed value (Hiroshima)
▲ observed value (Nagasaki)
calculated value

Adapted from M. Masuyama, "Statistical Study of Human Casualties of the Atomic Bomb, . . ." CRIABC, Science Council of Japan, 1953, vol. 1, p. 510

13

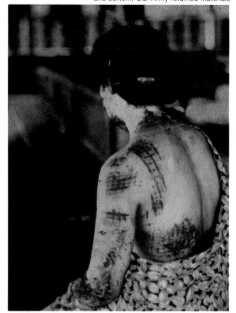

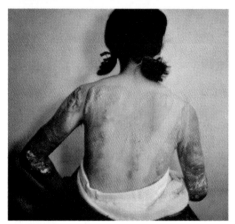

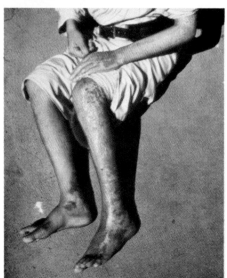

were hurled through the air by the blast; they sustained trauma and radiation injury as well as burns. Their exposed skin became immediately inflamed and peeling—in many cases the skin dropped down in flaps. The horrifying sight of victims in this condition was reported by many eyewitnesses. The effects of ionizing radiation caused delayed healing and pus formation in the wounds due to lowered resistance to infection. In relatively mild flash burns the injured epidermis became covered by an eschar (dry scab), which then dropped off to reveal a reddish or black-brown, shiny surface. Keloids developed at a high rate later in some of these victims (*see* below).

Trauma. Trauma consisted of primary injury, which was caused directly by the blast, and secondary injury (buried injury, compression injury, fragment injury), which occurred indirectly. Although not a few of the victims were killed instantaneously by blast injuries, most of the victims in both cities suffered from secondary injuries, especially fractures, contusions, and fragment wounds. Glass splinters, chips of wood, branches, and other small bits of flying debris caused lacerations or cuts, with some fragments embedded deep in tissue near the bone. Thermal injuries and traumas also caused hemorrhage and shock. Malnutrition (caused by subsequent food shortages) and lowered resistance to infection led to delayed healing and gangrenous changes in wounds.

Radiation injury. In the four-month acute phase after the bombing, injuries caused by radioactivity were the gravest. The enormous amount of gamma rays and neutrons emitted by the A-bomb and the radioactive materials and induced radioactivity formed by the explosion penetrated deep into the body and destroyed cells and tissues, especially those having great capacity for regeneration and proliferation. From 3 to 120 days after the bombings Japanese pathologists carried out autopsies on 213 fatal cases in Hiroshima and Nagasaki. The main pathologic findings encountered in the victims during the early and intermediate stages consisted of necrosis (tissue death) of intestinal mucosa, devastation of bone marrow, depletion of lymphocytes (blood cells important in countering infection) in lymph nodes and spleen, and changes in testicles resulting in absent or decreased sperm production.

The following phenomena were seen as results of radiation injury: (1) drop in red blood cell count, with marked anemia; (2) destruction of blood platelets, altered blood coagulation, tendency to bleed easily, and difficulty in stopping hemorrhage; (3) loss of hair and lack of regeneration of hair; (4) lowered resistance to infection and delayed healing due to decrease in number of leukocytes (white blood cells) and lymphocytes; (5) diarrhea and bloody stool caused by destruction of intestinal mucosa, the lining of the intestines; and (6) nausea, vomiting, and fever. These conditions constitute what is called acute radiation illness. It occurs when the radiation dose exceeds 100 rads, and a critical condition and death may follow a dose of over 1,000 rads. It is assumed that the victims within 1,300 meters (l,420 yards) of the hypocenter in Hiroshima and within 1,500 meters (1,640 yards) of the hypocenter in Nagasaki were exposed to over 100 rads (gamma rays and neutrons combined). A few days after the explosion in both cities, a great number of victims were suffering from nausea, vomiting, purpura of skin (areas of reddening due to superficial bleeding under the skin), mucosal

14

hemorrhage, diarrhea, bloody stool, and marked anemia.

Symptoms of acute radiation illness appeared in even those without thermal burns or trauma, and many were in critical condition. In the victims who also had thermal burns and trauma, lowered resistance to infection and altered healing process led to poor repair of wounds and delayed healing. The above injuries were mainly encountered in the intermediate stage of the acute phase.

The main pathological changes seen between the end of the intermediate stage and the late stage were gangrenous tonsillitis, gangrenous and hemorrhagic infection of the oral mucosa and throat, intestinal ulcers, skin ulcers, pneumonia, pulmonary edema (fluid in the lungs), and septicemia (blood poisoning). These were considered to have been caused by the drop in vital defense mechanisms following exposure to the A-bomb. A specific type of generalized wasting and malnutrition was also found in some cases.

Delayed effects. The acute stage of A-bomb injury passed its peak after about four months. By this time many of the victims had recovered to a certain degree. This, however, was not the end of the injury. Sterility, cessation of menstruation, abortion, blood disorders, developmental disturbances of children, keloid formation, A-bomb cataract, microcephaly following exposure *in utero,* and psychoneurological disorders appeared after more than four months as delayed effects and aftereffects. The latter four delayed effects are discussed below.

Keloid. As the trauma wounds and thermal burns began to heal, many wounds formed extensive scars that caused deformity and contracture, a common occurrence after severe burns. Many of the victims also developed keloids. Keloids are overgrowths of scar tissue on the wound surface that form during the repair process following thermal burns. In this condition the tissue forms, on the skin surface, an irregular-shaped protrusion resembling the shell and legs of a crab.

The vast majority of the flash burns occurring in the victims exposed to the A-bomb between 2,000 and 3,000 meters (2,190 to 3,280 yards) from the hypocenter healed within a short period. Initially, the scars were composed of simple, thin tissue; presumably the victims were at a significant distance from the hypocenter and their exposure was of short duration and low intensity of temperature, and they absorbed low doses of radioactivity. These mild flash-burn scars, however, developed into conspicuous keloids after three to four months or later.

The development of keloids in Hiroshima and Nagasaki reached its peak 61 to 90 days after the bombing and gradually declined after 150 days. Although the keloids tended to become smaller in size with the lapse of time, the severe ones required repeated plastic surgeries and the scars remained thereafter in many of the cases. Young girls with keloids and fibrous scar contracture on their faces, heads, arms, and legs suffered greatly. They were called the atomic bomb maidens and later underwent extensive plastic surgery in U.S. hospitals.

A-bomb cataract. A-bomb cataract was first discovered among the victims in Hiroshima in 1948 and in the following year in Nagasaki. This is a condition in which the lens of the eye becomes opaque. A-bomb cataracts developed

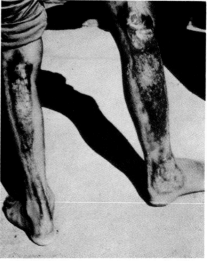

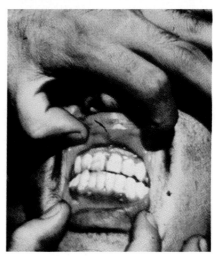

Many of the injured in both cities sustained burns caused by the thermal energy emitted by the bomb itself and by subsequent fires. (Opposite page, top) The pattern of this woman's kimono was seared onto her skin. A strap protected a strip of skin across another woman's back (center); other burned areas show formation of keloids, overgrowths of scar tissue. (Above) Bleeding gums and mouth ulcers appeared as the effects of radiation sickness began to take hold.

15

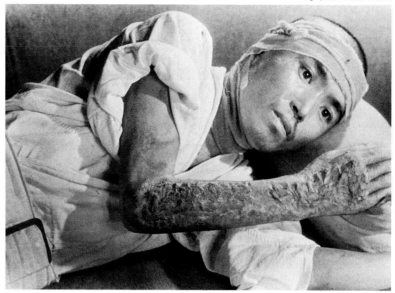

The pattern of burns indicated the direction in which the patients were facing when they were struck by the heat rays from the bombs. In both cities most of the hospitals were destroyed. There were severe shortages of antiseptics and other medical supplies; the injured suffered in agony without medication to ease their pain. Most faced repeated skin grafts and operations to reduce scar tissue.

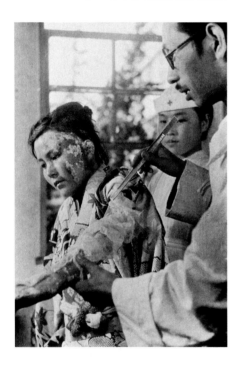

from several months to several years after the explosion, with the serious cases occurring earlier. The incidence and severity of this condition was proportional to radiation doses and age at the time of exposure.

Between 1953 and 1954 a total of 116 cases of A-bomb cataract were found among 435 adult survivors at the clinic of the Hiroshima Red Cross Hospital, an incidence of 26.6%. The incidence in those exposed within 2 kilometers (1.25 miles) of the hypocenter was 54.7%. A survey on those exposed during infancy was made by the department of ophthalmology of Hiroshima University between 1958 and 1959. The incidence of A-bomb cataract in this group was 13.5%, and for those within two kilometers of the hypocenter about 18%.

Exposure in utero *and microcephaly.* The casualties of the bombings included not only those already born but also fetuses carried by exposed pregnant women. Their condition is designated as exposure *in utero.* In the fetal stage there is active multiplication and proliferation of cells, and since these cells are extremely radiosensitive, there was a high incidence of fetal death, developmental disturbance, or anomaly.

According to a survey of 30 mothers who had been exposed within two kilometers of the hypocenter and who had suffered from acute radiation illness, there were 7 fetal deaths (spontaneous abortion and stillbirth, 23.3%) and 6 neonatal and infant deaths (26.1%), and 4 among the 16 living infants revealed mental retardation (25%). In all, 60% of the infants born to the mothers in this survey were either injured or soon died.

Children exposed *in utero* tended to show developmental disturbances after birth, and the most pathetic cases were those with microcephaly, a condition in which the cranium is poorly developed and the head circumference abnormally small. Microcephaly is frequently accompanied by mental retardation. According to a 1956 survey of 169 cases exposed *in utero* in Hiroshima, there were 33 cases with microcephaly, among whom 15 revealed mental retardation and 13 microcephaly of severe degree. Up to

16

1965, members of the department of obstetrics and gynecology of Hiroshima University confirmed 44 living cases with microcephaly. Although the *Kinoko-Kai* (Mushroom Club) has been organized to give help and encouragement to these children, they reached the age of 35 in 1980, and the number with both parents living to look after them was gradually decreasing.

Psychoneurological effects. Since the actuality of the A-bomb catastrophe was something that mankind could not have foreseen, the psychoneurological shock inflicted upon the people in Hiroshima and Nagasaki was immeasurable. Not only the shock sustained at the time of the explosion and immediately after but also the sufferings following injury, the grief over losing one's family, the complete destruction of local society, and loss of the means of day-to-day living bore down heavily upon the people.

As physical disorders passed into a chronic stage, their healing slowed by radiation injury and the postwar shortage of food, the strain was reflected in the mental and emotional state of the survivors. When the disturbance of the body caused by exposure to the A-bomb had been great, it affected the autonomic nervous system, leading to complaints or symptoms of encephalopathy, or diencephalic syndrome, a reflection of the utter disruption of ordinary functioning caused by the massive assault to the body—and mind—of having been caught up in the horrors of the bombing and its aftermath. These complaints covered a broad range of bodily functions, including disturbed digestion, circulatory problems, emotional upsets, skin problems, insomnia, sexual malfunctions, and a host of others—all greatly disturbing to the sufferers. When the survivors began to learn about the conditions known to be caused by exposure to the bombing, the majority of the victims could not get over the fear of impending cancer, leukemia, or even genetic damage that could be passed on to their children.

In a survey carried out five years after the bombings, it was found that psychoneurological delayed effects still remained in those who had experienced marked symptoms of radiation illness. The main complaints were fatigability, loss of vigor, tendency to become introverted, and poor memory. The full scope of the psychological and psychoneural damage caused by the bombings is incalculable.

Aftereffects. Among the aftereffects of exposure to the A-bomb, leukemia and other malignancies require special attention. Previous studies had shown that radiation injury could lead to carcinogenesis in human subjects as well as in experimental animals. Long-term surveys, including analysis of exposed and nonexposed groups in Hiroshima and Nagasaki, have documented a higher prevalence of malignancies in the exposed group.

Leukemia. The first leukemia detected after the bombing was in a 19-year-old male who was exposed to the A-bomb at a distance of one kilometer from the hypocenter in Nagasaki. A diagnosis of acute monocytic leukemia was made in November 1945, three months after the bombing. Soon after, doctors in Hiroshima also started to pay attention to the relation between exposure and leukemia, and records on the annual occurrence of leukemia have since then accumulated. The incidence of leukemia in Hiroshima and Nagasaki has increased gradually since 1947, reaching a peak between 1950 and 1954, and has tended to decline since then. At present the preva-

Shunkichi Kikuchi

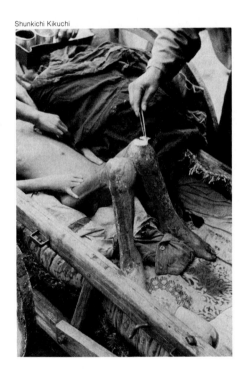

A boy receives treatment at an aid station in October 1945. His legs have become wasted. For many months after the bombing there were shortages of food, water, medical supplies, clothing, and housing. Both cities had to be rebuilt from the ground up. Society had been utterly disrupted.

17

(Top) Ittetsu Morishita; (bottom) Nagasaki Branch of the
Japan Association of Realist Photographers

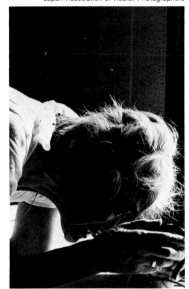

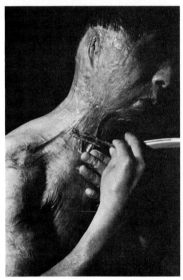

For the hibakusha, *those who sustained
injuries from the atomic bombs, there is
no end to suffering. Hatsue Tominaga
(top) lost her sight from atomic bomb
cataracts in 1977. Senji Yamaguchi
(above) was 14 years old in 1945. In
addition to their injuries, the survivors
must battle fears of the appearance of
delayed malignancies and genetic damage.*

lence of leukemia among the exposed is still significantly higher than that among the nonexposed population. The crude annual incidence of leukemia among the nonexposed in both cities is 1.04–2.82 per 100,000 population, while that among those exposed to more than 100 rads of T65D radiation was 94.85 between 1950 and 1955, 53.26 between 1955 and 1960, 26.13 between 1960 and 1965, and 25.35 between 1965 and 1971.

Up to 1975 a total of 1,838 cases of leukemia had been diagnosed in Hiroshima and Nagasaki. The victims exposed within 10 kilometers (6.2 miles) from the hypocenter totaled 512, and those considered to have been exposed to over one rad of radiation numbered 256. When comparing the incidence of leukemia among the victims exposed to over one rad of radiation in both cities, the number of leukemias in Hiroshima was twice that in Nagasaki. In Hiroshima the incidence of chronic myeloid leukemia was the highest, followed in order by acute myeloid leukemia, acute lymphocytic leukemia, and other types of leukemia. In Nagasaki the most common types, in order, were acute myeloid leukemia, chronic myeloid leukemia, and acute lymphocytic leukemia. The life expectancy after diagnosis of chronic leukemia is usually greater than for acute leukemia. Myeloid leukemia indicates an irregularity in granulocytes, white blood cells that attack invading bacteria; in lymphocytic leukemia the lymphocytes, the cells that mediate the body's immune response, are affected.

Other malignancies. Other malignancies besides leukemia have had a higher incidence among those exposed to the A-bomb. These malignancies, which include thyroid cancer, prostate cancer, salivary gland tumors, lung cancer, breast cancer, stomach cancer, esophageal cancer, cancer of urinary bladder, malignant lymphoma, and myeloma, started to increase between 1955 and 1960 after a latent period of 10 to 15 years.

Among these the high incidence of thyroid cancer, breast cancer, salivary gland tumors, and lung cancer warrant special attention. All of these malignancies have been shown, in studies quite independent of those of A-bomb survivors, to have a higher incidence in persons exposed to high levels of radiation—in uranium miners, for example.

Genetic effects. Since A-bomb radiation is known to injure deoxyribonucleic acid (DNA) within the cell nucleus, not only is there a higher risk of carcinogenesis but there is also a possibility of the occurrence of chromosome aberration and genetic damage. Studies of both plants and animals have proved that irradiation induces genetic mutation. In light of this knowledge there was great concern about possible genetic effects in the offspring of people exposed to the A-bomb, and chromosomal and biochemical genetic studies have been carried out over the years in both cities.

The following items were investigated as indexes for detecting genetic effects of atomic radiation immediately after exposure to the A-bomb: abortions and stillbirths due to lethal mutation, neonatal deaths, decrease in birth weight, growth and development after birth, increased frequency of congenital malformations, and change in sex ratio of offspring. Abnormality of germ cells and accompanying gene mutation can, however, be induced by causes other than radiation, and malformations and congenital abnormalities following injury of the fetus *in utero* are relatively numerous. Compared with

18

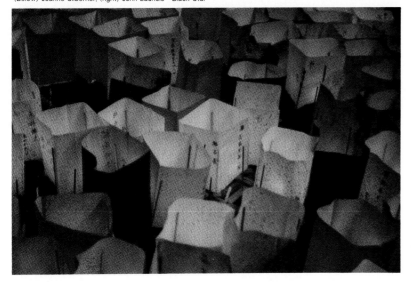

Each year paper lanterns are floated on the Ota River in Hiroshima to memorialize the dead, whose charred bodies "made the river run black." The Peace Memorial Park in Hiroshima (below) is dedicated to those killed in the bombing. The dome visible through the arch is the remains of the only building to survive the blast. It can be seen in the background of the photograph on page 9.

experimental animals, human beings have a longer generation interval, fewer pregnancies and fewer fetuses per pregnancy, and higher rate of spontaneous abortion. These facts, compounded with social and economic factors, make genetic surveys an extremely difficult object of study.

Under these circumstances studies up to the present have yielded no positive correlation between the bombings and genetic defects in the descendants of persons exposed in either city. This, however, does not mean that one can deny the genetic effects of A-bomb radiation in general. Further long-term studies are obviously needed to clarify this difficult problem.

For the future

The atomic bombs dropped on Hiroshima and Nagasaki in the summer of 1945 were primitive bombs compared with the highly destructive nuclear weapons of today—today's weapons are measured in *millions* of tons of TNT, not thousands. Nevertheless, the explosions in Hiroshima and Nagasaki led to the greatest mass devastation and death yet known to mankind. The suffering and agony of this instantaneous incident still remain in the survivors; one cannot neglect this fundamental fact. In a time of escalating nuclear arms acquisition, Hiroshima and Nagasaki have a special lesson to teach to mankind. On the memorial cenotaph in the Peace Park in Hiroshima are engraved the words

"Rest in peace, for the mistake shall not be repeated."

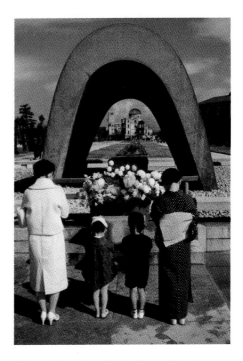

Today it is estimated that the combined atomic weapons held by the U.S. and the U.S.S.R. represent a force one million times more powerful than the "primitive" bomb that unleashed death and destruction on Hiroshima.

FOR ADDITIONAL READING:

The Committee for the Compilation of Materials on Damage Caused by the Atomic Bombs in Hiroshima and Nagasaki. *Hiroshima and Nagasaki: The Physical, Medical, and Social Effects of the Atomic Bombings.* Translated by Eisei Ishikawa, M.D., and D. L. Swain. New York: Basic Books, 1981.

Japan Broadcasting Corporation, ed. *Unforgettable Fire: Pictures Drawn by Atomic Bomb Survivors.* New York: Pantheon Books, 1981.

19

Healing the Unborn
by Mitchell S. Golbus, M.D.

In April 1981 the Fetal Treatment Program at the University of California at San Francisco was called on to try to save a troubled pregnancy. The 18-year-old mother-to-be was in the 20th week, but her uterus had not grown to an appropriate size for this stage. Ultrasound examination revealed serious difficulties: there was very little amniotic fluid cushioning the fetus, which was male. An obstruction in the fetus's urinary tract had stopped the outflow of urine, causing an enlarged bladder and swollen ureters and kidneys as the retained urine backed up in the tract. This also accounted for the lack of amniotic fluid.

In a first attempt to correct the problem, a hollow needle was passed through the mother's abdomen and, guided by ultrasound imaging, into the fetus's bladder; 95 ml (3.2 fl oz) of urine was drawn off. This relieved pressure on the bladder, but the ureters and kidneys did not respond to the procedure, remaining dilated.

The Fetal Treatment team discussed further treatment options with the mother and her family. The needle aspirations of urine could be repeated when the bladder refilled, but this seemed to be having no effect on the kidneys. Each such procedure, of course, carried with it risks to both mother and fetus. More important, the team knew that the fluid pressure was damaging the developing kidneys; if the pressure was not relieved, by the time of birth the kidney function that remained would be so inadequate that the newborn infant would soon die. The team had had success in inserting a catheter into a fetus's bladder in a small but growing number of cases; however, several aspects of this case, including the amniotic-fluid deficiency, all but ruled out trying this procedure.

After much discussion between the mother, her family, bioethicists, and the university-appointed Committee on Human Research, the decision was made to attempt a procedure that had never been tried before: the fetus would be partially removed from the uterus and his problem surgically corrected. The fetus would then be returned to the uterus so that the pregnancy could continue to term.

Surgery was performed when the fetus was in the 21st week of gestation. The mother had general anesthesia and her abdomen and uterus were surgically opened as if for a cesarean section. The lower half of the fetus was lifted out through the incision in the uterus. Small incisions were made on

20

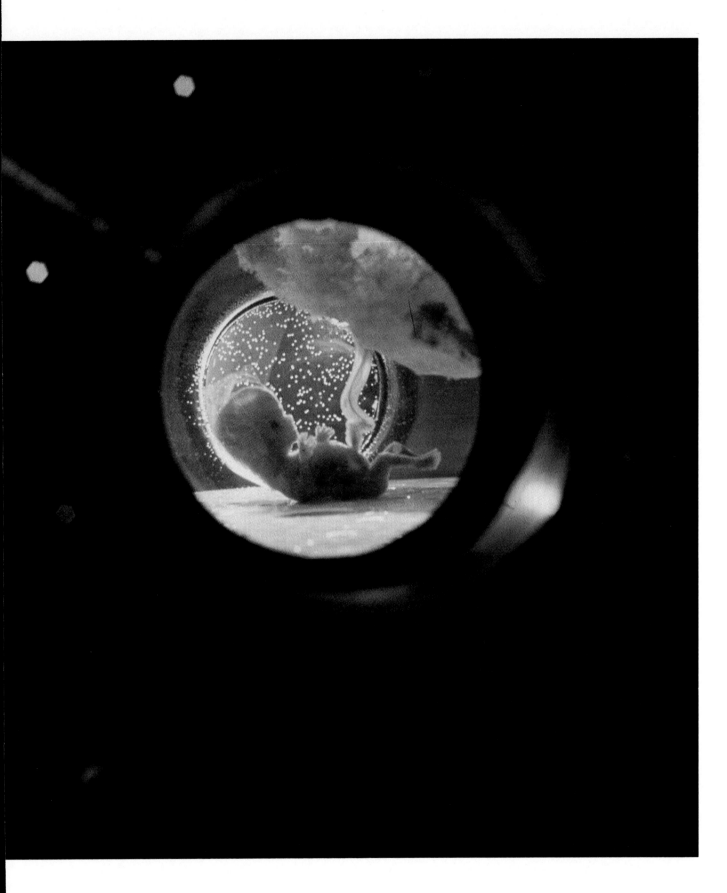

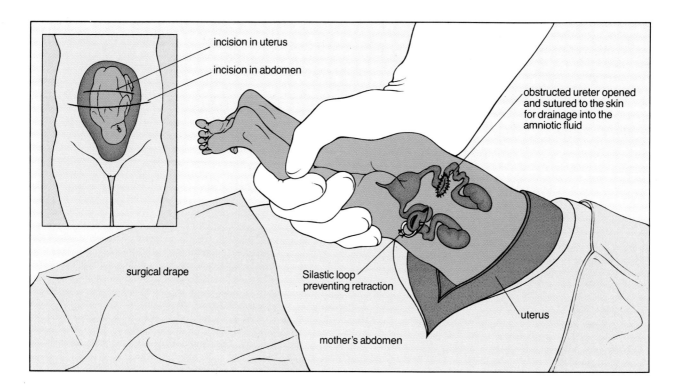

incision in uterus

incision in abdomen

obstructed ureter opened
and sutured to the skin
for drainage into the
amniotic fluid

surgical drape

Silastic loop
preventing retraction

uterus

mother's abdomen

In 1981 a milestone was passed in the progress toward treating the unborn child. A team at the University of California at San Francisco partially removed a fetus from his mother's uterus, performed surgery on the fetus's ureters to relieve a urinary blockage, and replaced the fetus so that the pregnancy could continue to term.

Mitchell S. Golbus, M.D., *is Associate Professor in the Department of Obstetrics, Gynecology, and Reproductive Sciences; Director of the Prenatal Detection Program; and a member of the Fetal Treatment Program at the University of California at San Francisco.*

both the fetus's flanks, and the blocked ureters were opened and fixed to the skin so that they formed pouches that would provide continuous drainage of urine into the amniotic fluid. Within 25 minutes the fetus was replaced in the amniotic sac, and the sac, the uterine wall, and the mother's abdomen were reclosed. Both mother and fetus made uneventful recoveries.

In ten days the mother was discharged from the hospital and returned to full activity and enjoyed an otherwise uncomplicated pregnancy for the next 16 weeks. The fetus's previously massively distended bladder, ureters, and kidneys remained completely decompressed, and the fetus grew normally. However, the amniotic fluid did not increase significantly, and when the fetus was delivered by cesarean section near term, it had insufficient kidney and lung development to sustain life.

In spite of its unhappy outcome, this case is very significant. It represents the first instance in which a fetus was successfully operated on, replaced in the uterus, and carried to term. It is a milestone for a new avenue of medicine, the field of prenatal diagnosis and treatment, an emerging specialty of the 1980s.

Neither the examination, diagnosis, nor the two attempts at treatment would have been possible even ten years ago. Since then, advances in electronics, fiberoptics, instrumentation, and chromosomal and biochemical analysis have fueled an explosion of knowledge about prenatal development, both normal and abnormal. Prenatal medicine is now beginning to be able to intervene, before birth, to alleviate and even cure conditions that previously would have severely compromised the fetus. This promises survival for thousands of threatened lives, but it also raises difficult ethical considerations for both parents and physicians.

(Top) Jean-Loup Charmet, Paris; (bottom) The Bettmann Archive

Beginnings of the science of teratology

The medical approach to a disease or group of disorders routinely has three stages. The first stage is recognition that the disease state exists. The second stage is the development of methods for diagnosing the disorder. The third stage is finding a method of prevention or therapy for the condition.

From more than 3,000 years ago there are records of congenital defects; the Egyptians of that era performed special burial rites for deformed infants. However, advancement from recognition to the second stage, that of considering the fetus as a patient and diagnosing congenital defects before birth, began only 15 years ago in the mid-1960s. And the third stage, treatment of the fetus *in utero,* is beginning only now in the early 1980s.

Modern teratology, the study of abnormal development, is still in the process of determining the effects of nutrition, viral infections, and drugs upon the fetus. Major advances in teratology have resulted from experiments on nutrition in pregnant rats, from examining the effect of maternal rubella (German measles) infection on the fetus, and from knowledge gained from the thalidomide disaster. To provide the embryo and fetus with the best chance of developing normally, physicians must have a full understanding of both normal development and the causes of congenital malformations.

Crucial stages of development

In the human embryo the rudiments of all major external and internal structures have appeared by seven weeks after conception. In this short embryonic period the embryo has grown from a single cell to a well-differentiated, though less than inch-long, form. The early embryonic disk first folded upon itself longitudinally, forming a groove that indicated the position of the future spinal cord, and rolled inward to a cylinder. Along the neural groove, parallel folds arose, curving over until they met and fused to form the neural tube. The fusion began in the middle of the spinal column and progressed both downward and upward to the developing brain. From transverse clefts along the spinal cord pairs of somites, or primitive body segments, arose, from which developed the skeletal, muscular, and nervous systems. On the limbs, which began to bud outward in the fourth week, the future fingers and toes have become discernible. The surface appearance of the seven-week-old embryo now reflects the underlying formation of the brain, heart, liver, somites, limbs, ears, nose, and eyes.

Because the foundations of all essential internal and external structures are formed during the embryonic period, these first weeks constitute the most critical period of development. Developmental disturbances during this period often result in major congenital malformations.

From the 8th week until birth (averaging about the 38th week) is the fetal period, during which tissues and organs that appeared in the embryo enlarge and mature. Only a few new structures appear during the fetal period. From the 12th to the 16th weeks the rate of body growth is greater than it will be at any other time of life. The fetus is far less vulnerable to the teratogenic (birth-defect-causing) effects of drugs, viruses, temperature, and radiation than is the embryo. Nevertheless, in the fetus these agents may interfere with normal functional development, especially of the brain.

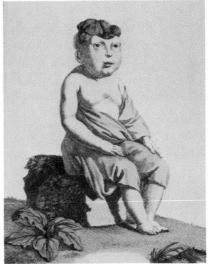

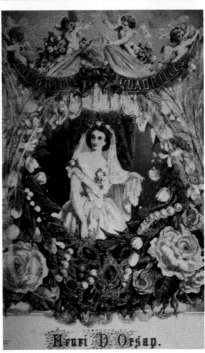

The possibility of birth defects has haunted pregnancies throughout history. The bridal veil was orginally worn to protect the bride against evil spells that might mar her first pregnancy. The early print at top shows an anencephalic child who is suffering from a neural tube defect, one in which the embryonic brain has failed to form properly.

23

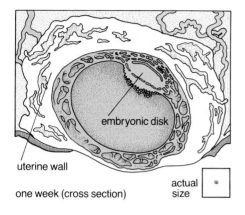

uterine wall

one week (cross section)   actual size

At one week after conception the fertilized egg, now called the embryonic disk (cross section, above), has become imbedded in the wall of the uterus.

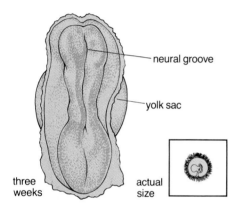

neural groove

yolk sac

three weeks   actual size

By three weeks the embryo has begun to take on a cylindrical shape. The neural groove indicates the position of the future spinal column.

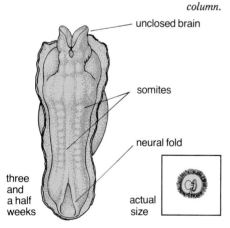

unclosed brain

somites

neural fold

three and a half weeks   actual size

A few days later the neural groove closes to form the neural tube; the brain has begun to form at the upper end. Somites, or primitive body segments, have begun to appear.

Known causes of congenital defects

Congenital malformations are due primarily to genetic or environmental factors, but it is not always possible to separate clearly the causes of various abnormalities. Malformations caused by genetic factors are the result of chromosomal abnormalities or mutant genes in the fetus's genetic makeup. The fact is now well accepted that genes are continually mutating in the process of human reproduction and evolution. Scientists currently believe that 10 to 15% of congenital malformations are due to mutant genes. Chromosomal abnormalities may cause birth defects by producing abnormal proportions of normal genes. Down's (Down) syndrome, which is due to an extra chromosome 21, causes quantitative changes in gene products (proteins), which appear to be as disastrous to development as the qualitative changes caused by mutation.

Environmental influences on embryological and fetal development may be divided into five major categories: drugs and environmental chemicals, maternal metabolic imbalance, infections, radiation, and other factors; *e.g.,* possible effects of heat, magnetic fields, radio waves, and so on. The sum of all documented environmental causes of human congenital malformations explains no more than 10% of anomalies—this figure will undoubtedly rise in the future as new discoveries are made. Interactions between two or more environmental factors also are very likely to be of importance but are very difficult to study.

Prenatal diagnosis

The object of prenatal diagnosis is to determine whether or not a fetus believed to be at risk for a particular birth defect is actually affected. The primary tool of prenatal diagnosis is the chromosomal or biochemical analysis of cells from the fetus that have been shed into the amniotic fluid. The material to be examined is obtained by amniocentesis, the process of inserting a hollow needle through the pregnant woman's abdomen and uterus into the amniotic sac that surrounds the fetus and withdrawing a sample of the amniotic fluid in which the fetus floats. There are presently dozens of amniocentesis programs which have collectively performed over 35,000 amniocenteses.

It is now standard procedure to suggest to prospective parents that amniocentesis be done in the following circumstances: (1) if the mother is 35 years old or older, because of the known relationship between maternal age and the incidence of certain chromosomal abnormalities, such as Down's syndrome, in the fetus; (2) if the mother has had a previous child with Down's syndrome, to allay the parents' fear that the syndrome has occurred again; (3) if the parents are both carriers for a biochemical disorder such as an error of metabolism, in which case each of their offspring is at a 25% risk of having the disorder; and (4) if there has been a previous fetus or newborn with a neural tube defect (anencephaly, in which the brain has failed to develop, or spina bifida, in which the neural tube has failed to close completely). The worldwide experience is that 3.5% of fetuses having prenatal diagnosis for a suspected birth defect have been found to be abnormal.

Much recent activity in the field of prenatal diagnosis has revolved around attempts to obtain, literally, a better picture of what is happening in the fetal world. One method is to use sonography, or ultrasound, high-frequency sound waves which, when they strike any surface, are reflected in such a way as to form a two-dimensional picture. Sonographic machines and techniques now allow visualization of such detail as the individual fingers or the four chambers of the heart of a 20-week fetus. In some cases the physician performing the sonography may be looking for a specific malformation with a known pattern of inheritance in a family at risk (for example, the extra fingers characteristic of Ellis-van Creveld syndrome, which results in severe mental retardation and dwarfism). Many more malformations are identified incidentally during routine sonography done to determine whether twins are present or where the placenta is located.

The usefulness of this technique notwithstanding, the most direct method of examining the patient is still to look at him or her. Direct fetal visualization, or fetoscopy, utilizes a small-bore fiberoptic endoscope, an instrument that can be inserted transabdominally into the uterus under local anesthesia. Isolated parts of the fetus's anatomy can be examined, but visualization of the entire fetus is rarely possible because of the narrow viewing angle (55°) of the fetoscope in the aqueous medium of the uterus.

Fetoscopy has proved most useful in obtaining samples of fetal tissues other than amniotic fluid. Many genetic defects cannot be detected in amniotic fluid constituents but are demonstrable using other fetal tissues or cells. The most readily accessible and easily sampled tissue after birth is blood, and likewise, through a needle attached to the fetoscope, a drop of fetal blood can be obtained from the inner surface of the placenta and umbilical cord. The principal abnormalities which thus far have come under investigation relate to hemoglobin structure and synthesis by red blood cells. It is now possible to detect in the fetus the presence of Mediterranean anemia (β-thalassemia, or Cooley's anemia), a defect causing reduced production of one of the protein components of hemoglobin which is a major contributor to childhood mortality in many countries of the Mediterranean basin. It also is possible to detect structural abnormalities of hemoglobin such as the one that causes sickle-cell anemia.

If fetal red blood cells can be obtained by fetoscopy, it follows that other constituents of the blood are being obtained simultaneously and are available for diagnostic tests. The fetal plasma can be examined for the absence of blood-clotting factors in fetuses at risk for hemophilia. Prenatal diagnosis of disorders involving other serum proteins that are synthesized early in development may be feasible via fetal blood sampling. For example, a deficiency of the plasma protein alpha₁-antitrypsin has been diagnosed. This deficiency, an inherited defect, is associated with liver disease and pulmonary emphysema. Physicians also can use red or white blood cells obtained by fetal blood sampling to identify specific genetic diseases.

Options after diagnosis

Although the ultimate goal for prenatal diagnosis is treatment to correct the defect, for many disorders it is unlikely that effective corrective or preventive therapy will be developed in the foreseeable future. Furthermore, in at least

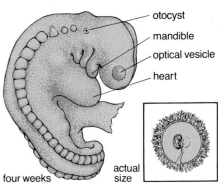

At four weeks the rudiments of the circulatory system and the jaws, as well as the beginnings of the eyes and ears, are present; the embryo takes on a "C" shape.

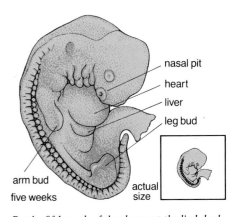

By the fifth week of development the limb buds for the arms and legs are growing rapidly. The liver can be seen under the heart, and there is a distinct nasal opening.

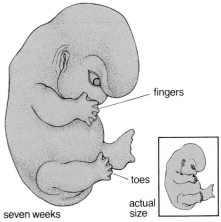

The seven-week-old embryo has begun to look recognizably human. Fingers and toes, though still joined, can be counted. The total length at this stage is about one inch.

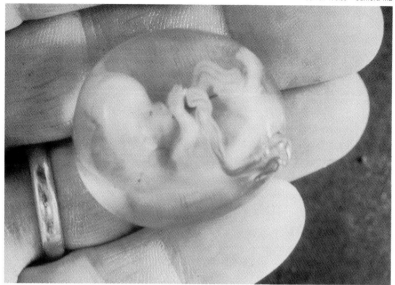

An eight-week human embryo within its amniotic sac. By eight weeks all of the major organ systems in the body have taken their rudimentary form. During the fetal period, the next 30 weeks of gestation, the organs will grow and mature. Only a few new structures appear during the fetal period. From the 12th to the 16th weeks the rate of growth is greater than it will be at any other time of life.

some metabolic disorders, irreversible damage may have occurred by the time the diagnosis is made. Nonetheless, therapeutic alternatives do exist for a number of disorders that can be recognized *in utero.*

Most of the correctable malformations that can be diagnosed *in utero* are best managed by appropriate medical or surgical therapy after the newborn is delivered at term. A full-term infant is better able than a prematurely delivered infant to tolerate surgery and anesthesia. Examples of correctable abnormalities in this category include narrowing or absence of part of the gastrointestinal tract, cleft palate, or a small spina bifida. (When the spinal column fails to close completely, some of the spinal tissues are exposed and may protrude through the skin. This abnormality varies considerably in severity.) Prenatal diagnosis is important because many of these anomalies are associated with an excess of amniotic fluid that may initiate premature labor. Treatment to reduce the excess amniotic fluid or forestall premature labor may allow the fetus to remain *in utero* longer and to be born at term. In addition, the delivery can be planned so that the necessary neonatologists, anesthesiologists, and pediatric surgeons are on hand.

Other fetal anomalies require correction *ex utero* as soon as possible after the diagnosis is made. Premature delivery may be preferable for such disorders as hydrocephalus, in which fluid collects in the brain, or for moderately severe Rh isoimmunization, in which maternal antibodies cross the placenta to the fetus and destroy its red blood cells. In each case continued gestation will have progressive ill effects on the fetus.

Recent advances in the ability to decrease the risk of neonatal respiratory distress syndrome, the main cause of death in preemies, make premature delivery a safer therapeutic tool. The technique is to give the mother certain steroid hormones which will cross the placenta to the fetus and induce the production of lipoproteins in the lung that decrease the risk of respiratory distress after the infant is delivered. This is done three to five days before the planned premature delivery.

26

Another subset of fetal disorders may influence the mode of delivery and require that a cesarean section be performed. This is indicated for an anomaly such that the fetus would not fit through the mother's pelvis during vaginal delivery—examples include conjoined (Siamese) twins or a fetus with a large hydrocephalus. Occasionally, an elective cesarean section may be necessary in the case of a malformation requiring immediate surgical correction in a sterile environment. Examples include a ruptured herniation of the bowel out of the abdominal cavity (omphalocele) or an uncovered meningomyelocele, a consequence of spina bifida in which a portion of the spinal cord, spinal nerves, and their covering membranes protrudes through the back of the infant. Occasionally, infants are delivered who are at risk for a severe immunodeficiency state which causes them to be unable to withstand infections. Such infants may be delivered by elective cesarean section to protect their sterility.

In utero intervention

One area of great potential is the prenatal treatment of fetuses with deficiency states. These are conditions in which some substance vital to life and well-being is not present in sufficient quantity in the fetus. The simplest method of supplying the missing element is to give it to the mother and allow it to be transported across the placenta to the fetus.

Two fetuses diagnosed *in utero* as having vitamin-dependent enzyme deficiencies recently were treated before birth. Vitamins often act as co-enzymes, compounds necessary for proper enzyme functioning. In the absence of the co-enzymes, the metabolic process is disrupted, with severe consequences for the fetus. The first fetus had a vitamin B_{12}-responsive enzyme disorder (methylmalonic acidemia), and the second had a biotin-dependent disorder (multiple carboxylase deficiency). Each was treated by giving the mother massive doses of the required vitamin. Both of these children have developed normally after birth, although they must take huge daily supplements of the necessary vitamin.

Another recent example of medicating the fetus via the mother was the successful treatment of heart rhythm irregularities in a fetus by giving the mother digitalis. The digitalis crossed the placenta to the fetus and returned the fetal heart rate to a normal pattern.

Some substances, however, do not cross the placenta and cannot be delivered to the fetus through the mother. In order to treat deficiencies of these substances the necessary element must be placed in the amniotic sac so that the fetus, who continually swallows the amniotic fluid, will ingest it. Another option is to give the fetus an injection in the buttocks, much as is done with an *ex utero* patient. Thyroid hormone does not cross the placenta but has been given via the amniotic fluid in one instance to treat congenital hypothyroidism and goiter.

Even more complicated is the task of delivering cells, such as red blood cells, to the fetus. In Rh isoimmunization, antibodies from the mother's blood destroy the fetus's red blood cells, sometimes causing the fetus to die of profound anemia. At present it is accepted practice to treat severe cases by transfusing the fetus *in utero*. This is accomplished by inserting a needle into

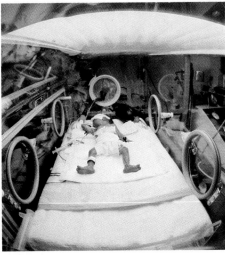

The premature infant faces an immediate battle to cling to life. However, there are some conditions for which premature delivery may be preferable to continued gestation during which damage is being done. Until the 30th week of gestation, the fetus's skin is thin. This and the absence of the subcutaneous fat that develops during the last six to eight weeks account for the reddish, wizened appearance of the premature infant.

27

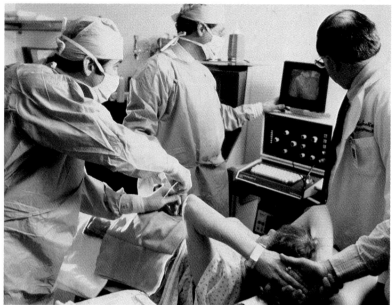 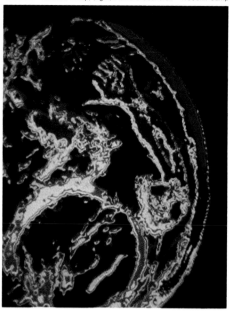

Ultrasound imaging has proved to be an extremely valuable tool in prenatal diagnosis and in the monitoring of pregnancies. In the ultrasound image at right the fetus's arm and hand are clearly visible.

the fetal abdominal cavity and transferring the needed blood cells directly to the cavity. The fetus's lymphatic system absorbs the cells and delivers them to the circulatory system to correct the anemia. In a few instances fetuses who were too sick or too young to receive intra-abdominal transfusions were transfused by injecting the blood cells into an umbilical cord vessel by means of a fetoscope.

The list of substances that can be given therapeutically to the *in utero* fetus is certain to grow. In theory, it may be possible to treat intrauterine growth retardation, in which a normal fetus is not receiving sufficient nutrition, by instilling nutrients into the amniotic fluid. Scientists are also investigating enzyme therapy for enzyme-deficient fetuses.

The potential for surgical therapy

The complement of medical therapy is surgical therapy. The prenatally diagnosable anatomic malformations that warrant consideration for surgical therapy are those which interfere with the development of the fetus's organs but which, if alleviated, would allow normal development to proceed. Treatable malformations of this type are hydronephrosis caused by a urinary-tract obstruction, diaphragmatic hernia, and hydrocephalus.

Urinary tract obstruction. Obstructive fetal urinary tract malformations are being recognized with increasing frequency because fluid-filled masses are particularly easy to detect by sonography. By the third month after conception, the fetus's kidneys are capable of secreting urine. The urine is carried by the ureters to the bladder and ultimately voided into the amniotic fluid. If the urine is prevented from freely flowing along this route, it is retained and backs up in the urinary tract, causing a large distended bladder (megacystis), fluid-filled ureters (hydroureters), and fluid accumulation in the kidneys (hydronephrosis). The increased fluid and back pressure interfere with the development of the kidneys and may cause life-threatening, irreversible

28

damage. Uremia, the buildup of toxic waste products, does not occur *in utero* because the placenta performs the same waste-removal tasks as the kidneys, compensating for the decreased kidney function. The small amount of fetal urine excreted also causes a decrease in the volume of amniotic fluid; insufficient amniotic fluid is associated with underdevelopment of the lungs, apparently because the ebb and flow of amniotic fluid in the fetal tracheae aid lung growth. The fetus also may sustain skeletal and facial deformities caused by its being compressed by the uterine walls in the absence of the buffering amniotic fluid.

Failure to take action to alleviate urinary tract obstruction often leads to the delivery at term of an infant who has neither sufficient functioning kidney tissue nor sufficient lung capacity to survive. Early relief of the obstruction may allow development that will be adequate to support postnatal life and allow catch-up development during early childhood.

There are several methods for decompressing an obstructed fetal urinary tract. Fluid can be removed from the bladder or kidney with a needle under sonographic guidance, but this offers only temporary relief. What is needed is continuous drainage of the urine from the bladder into the amniotic sac.

A catheter has been developed that can be placed to provide continuing drainage. It is made of polyethylene that has a "memory"; it has a curl like a pig's tail at each end but it can be straightened out onto a needle for placement and will resume its original shape when it is pushed off the needle. The catheter has multiple side perforations along its length to allow easy drainage of the urine. This 12-cm (4.7-in)-long catheter can be put into place by slipping it on a long needle with a separate length of tubing above it to act as a "pusher." The needle, guided sonographically, is directed through the mother's abdominal wall, the uterus, the amniotic sac, the fetus's abdominal wall, and into the fetus's bladder. Once the catheter tip is

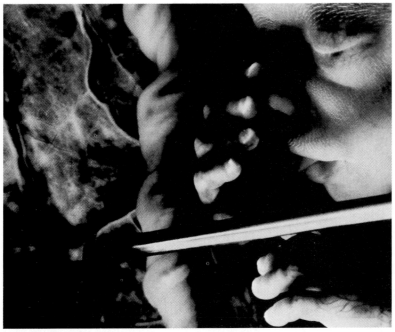

Ingemar Nilsson, Lund University

Through the fetoscope, a tubular instrument that can be inserted into the pregnant uterus, blood and other tissues can be sampled to aid in diagnosis. With a viewing light and fiberoptic endoscope, the physician can look at portions of the fetus to check for abnormalities. Through a hollow needle a sample of blood can be removed from a blood vessel in the placenta.

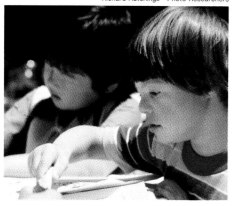

Down's syndrome can now be reliably diagnosed before birth; this is one of the primary reasons for performing amniocentesis in high-risk mothers. Spina bifida (below), failure of the spinal column to close properly, is a common birth defect that varies in severity. In some cases the spinal nerves and membranes protrude through the skin (center). While some children with this defect have lower-body paralysis, others can be helped by surgery and rehabilitation to be mobile.

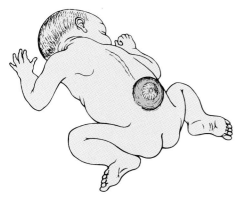

advanced into the fetus's bladder, pressure readings are obtained; the catheter is then advanced off the needle until one pig's-tail loop can be seen sonographically in the bladder. The needle is then withdrawn, holding the catheter steady, so that the second loop will be outside the fetus's body in the amniotic cavity. The loops keep the catheter in place so that it is not dislodged when the fetus changes position.

After the procedure the mother is given intravenous medications to prevent labor, and the fetus and mother are carefully monitored for complications. A series of sonograms over the next few days usually show complete drainage of the bladder and partial to complete drainage of the upper urinary tract (ureters and kidneys). The quantity of fluid in the amniotic sac is also carefully monitored. Unfortunately, there is no way to test fetal kidney function and to know how much reserve remains or whether irreversible damage already has occurred. The destruction of kidney tissue may be so great at the time of the procedure that no amount of successful drainage can help.

The placement of a catheter in this manner is a new procedure which, by early 1982, had been tried fewer than a dozen times. Therefore, it is important to stress that although it is biologically logical that it should work, the procedure should be viewed as unproved. Only when medicine can compare the outcome of a series of treated fetuses with a series of untreated fetuses will it be possible to evaluate the potential of the procedure. The surgery described at the beginning of this article is the next logical course for treating urinary blockage, and for other surgically correctable conditions as well.

Diaphragmatic hernia. Congenital diaphragmatic hernia is usually an isolated anomaly in an otherwise normal full-term infant. This abnormality is a failure of the muscles of the diaphragm to form and separate the abdominal and chest cavities, so that the bowel and other abdominal contents herniate into the chest, pressing on the lungs and preventing them from growing. Surgical correction consists of placing the bowel back in the abdomen and closing the defect in the diaphragm. However, 50–80% of these infants die of lung underdevelopment caused by lung compression during the last half of gestation. Despite marked advances in anesthetic, surgical, and respiratory care over the last two decades, the mortality rate for newborns with this anomaly has not changed.

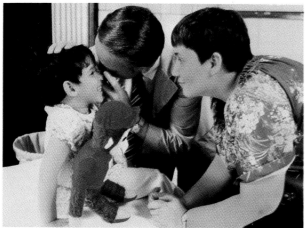

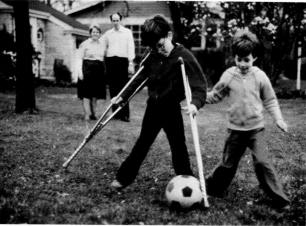

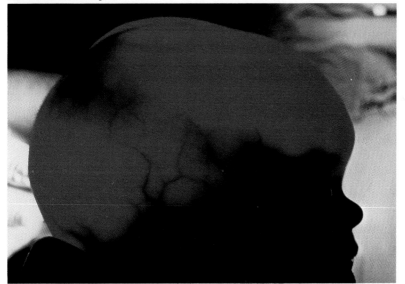

An infant with prenatal hydrocephalus has a faulty circulation of cerebrospinal fluid.The fluid collects in the ventricles, the spaces between the lobes of the brain. This causes swelling of the head and severe brain damage. Physicians have recently succeeded in inserting a shunt to carry off the excess fluid in the head of a fetus, shown below with the shunt still in place after birth.

Diaphragmatic hernias have been created in fetal lambs and rabbits and have demonstrated the changes which lead to death in the newborn. A more sophisticated model was developed by pediatric surgeon Michael Harrison and other members of the Fetal Treatment Program at the University of California at San Francisco. A balloon was inserted into the left chest cavity of a fetal lamb. The balloon was progressively inflated during gestation, simulating the expanding bowel, and produced a clinical and pathologic picture identical to that seen in congenital diaphragmatic hernia. Harrison and colleagues further showed that if later in gestation they deflated the balloon in the chest, the lung grew normally and the lamb survived. The next step is to produce surgically an actual diaphragmatic hernia early in gestation in a lamb or monkey, then to correct the defect later in gestation and to evaluate the outcome. Much experimental work remains to be done, but preliminary experiments show promise of future application for human fetuses.

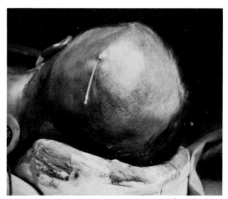

From "A Surgical Approach to Fetal Hydrocephalus," William H. Clewell *et al, The New England Journal of Medicine,* vol. 306, no. 22, p. 1,324, June 3, 1982

Hydrocephalus. Hydrocephalus of prenatal origin occurs in 0.2% of all births. It represents a failure of the normal dynamics of cerebrospinal fluid. When its circulation is impaired, this fluid accumulates in the ventricles, the four spaces between the lobes of the brain. The engorged ventricles swell greatly, pressing on the brain and causing the brain tissues to atrophy. Between one-half and two-thirds of affected fetuses are stillborn, and only one-quarter of liveborn hydrocephalic newborns survive infancy untreated. The primary treatment for hydrocephalus is the insertion after birth of a drainage shunt to carry off the excess fluid from the ventricles and reduce the swelling. Yet of those babies having ventricular drainage for decompression, fewer than half survive, and only one-third have normal intelligence. This contrasts sharply with the outlook for hydrocephalus that develops after birth, in which cases shunting produces 80% survival rates with 70% of survivors having IQ's over 75.

The first attempts at prenatal correction of hydrocephalus in monkeys were recently reported. The ventricles of affected fetuses were drained with

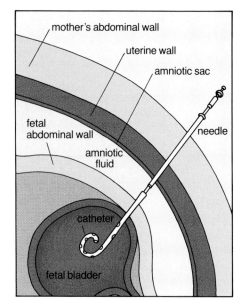

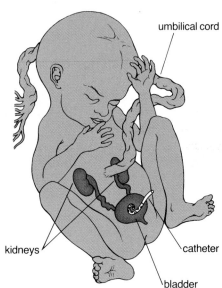

Urinary tract obstruction in a fetus can now be detected through the use of ultrasound imaging. In some cases it has been treated before birth by inserting a tube through the mother's abdominal wall and uterus into the fetus's bladder to carry off the fetal urine and protect the developing kidneys from damage.

Using monkeys (right) and other animals, researchers are perfecting techniques for surgical intervention to correct developmental defects before birth.

a stainless steel valve that allowed the one-way flow of fluid from the ventricles to the amniotic cavity. Researchers noted improved survival and neurologic function in the treated animals.

These experiments with animals are being done because it is clear that progressive prenatal hydrocephalus will often require *in utero* drainage of the ventricles for optimal treatment. Waiting until after a term delivery to treat the condition may critically delay therapy. Two approaches to solving this problem have been tried recently. One group of researchers performed six weekly needle aspirations of the dilated ventricles of a fetus with hydrocephalus. There were no complications of the procedures, but after delivery the infant was found to have other unrelated brain malformations and at two years of age was profoundly retarded. A second group treated two fetuses with prenatal hydrocephalus by implanting a polyethylene shunt to drain ventricular cerebrospinal fluid into the amniotic sac. The first of these fetuses was delivered and manifested a considerable degree of residual brain damage from the hydrocephalus. The second infant was developing normally at two months of age, despite the fact that the shunt had to be placed three times after it became dislodged after the first two attempts. This area of endeavor is just beginning, and much more work must be done. In addition, it remains to be determined whether in some instances uncorrectable brain damage has occurred by the time the prenatal diagnosis is made.

Further considerations

The potential for *in utero* correction of birth defects gives an added dimension to the rapidly expanding field of prenatal diagnosis. Following the first diagnosis, however, any fetus being considered for prenatal therapy for a malformation must be evaluated thoroughly. Because it is known that malformations often occur as part of a syndrome, the medical team must search for associated abnormalities to avoid delivering a newborn with one corrected

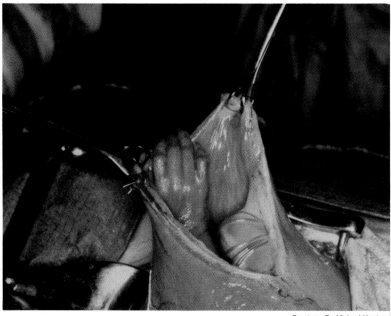

Courtesy, Dr. Michael Harrison

anomaly but with other unrecognized disabling or lethal abnormalities.

For each case the benefits and risks of fetal diagnosis and therapy will have to be carefully weighed. For the fetus they are relatively straightforward: the risk of the procedure and medication versus the benefit of correction or amelioration of the abnormality. The degree of risk deemed acceptable will depend on the severity of the condition and its predictable consequences on survival and quality of life. For the mother the issue is more complicated. Her health will not usually be affected by the fetal disorder, but she will have to bear some risk from the therapy attempt. Risk to her is negligible if the therapy requires only ingesting vitamins, but it is more significant if therapy involves major surgery to gain access to the fetus.

Fetal therapy has begun to raise complex ethical issues. One positive aspect is that prenatal diagnosis of certain conditions may lead to treatment rather than selective abortion. The possibility of diagnosing and treating fetal disorders raises important questions about the rights of mothers and fetuses as patients. Who has the right to make decisions for the fetus? How will we weigh the risk of intervention against the burden of the disorder itself? What if the therapy merely converts a lethal condition into a chronically disabling one? If one of a set of twins has a disorder, what risk may be imposed on the normal twin for the sake of treating the sibling's disorder? These and many more questions will continue to arise, and medicine and society must join forces to answer them.

Our ability to diagnose fetal birth defects has achieved considerable sophistication. Treatment of several fetal conditions is now feasible, and treatment of more complicated defects will expand as techniques for fetal intervention improve. The concept that the fetus is a patient, an individual whose disorders are a proper subject for medical therapy, has been established. A new discipline, "fetology," has been born.

FOR ADDITIONAL READING:

Hilton, Bruce, *et al.,* eds. *Ethical Issues in Human Genetics: Genetic Counseling and the Use of Genetic Knowledge.* New York: Plenum Press, 1973.

Kaback, M. M., and Valenti, C., eds. *Intrauterine Fetal Visualization: A Multidisciplinary Approach.* Amsterdam: Excerpta Medica, 1976.

Milunsky, Aubrey, ed. *Genetic Disorders and the Fetus.* New York: Plenum Press, 1979.

Smith, D. W., and Wilson, A. A. *The Child with Down's Syndrome (Mongolism).* Philadelphia: W. B. Saunders, 1973.

Thompson, J. S., and Thompson, M. W. *Genetics in Medicine.* 2nd ed. Philadelphia: W. B. Saunders, 1973.

U.S. Department of Health, Education, and Welfare, Public Health Service, NIH. *Antenatal Diagnosis.* NIH Publication no. 79-1973, April 1979.

———. *Prenatal Approaches to the Diagnosis of Fetal Hemoglobinopathies.* NIH Publication no. 80-1529, May 1980.

Emily Pinion, here aged five months, underwent surgery while still inside her mother's womb to remove fluid that was causing her lungs to collapse. She was born in September 1981 "pink and pretty as she could be." Only a few years ago, little Emily would not have survived.

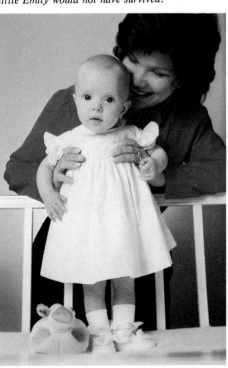

John Marmaras—Woodfin Camp

A Symposium

MENTAL HEALTH AND ILLNESS

insane asylums
depression
schizophrenia
phobias
addictions
psychotherapy
exercise

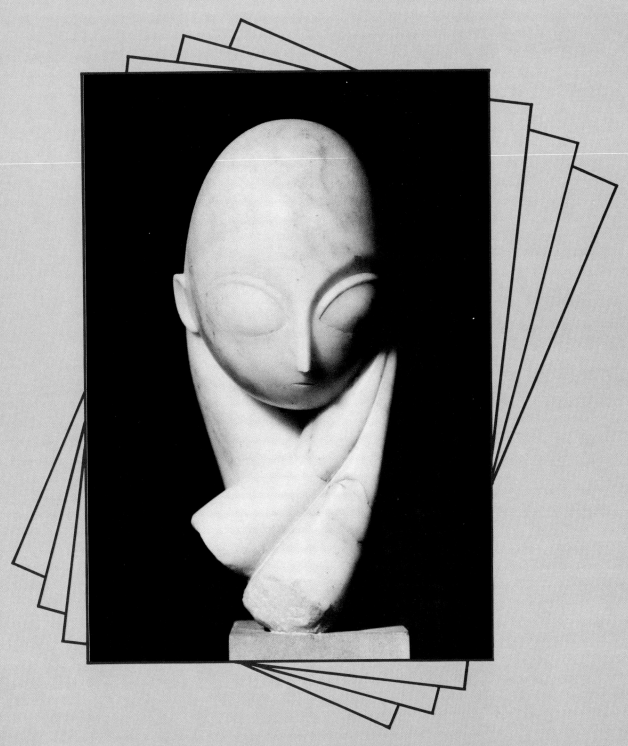

"Mademoiselle Pogany" by Constantin Brancusi, 1913,
Philadelphia Museum of Art, given by Mrs. Rodolphe M. Schauenese

Housing the Insane:
A History
by Grace Goldin

Grace Goldin, *who lives in Swarthmore, Pennsylvania, is a medical historian who has visited and photographed insane asylums in Europe and the United States. She is co-author of* The Hospital: A Social and Architectural History, *Yale University Press, 1975.*

(Opposite page) Several weeks after Vincent van Gogh had a mental breakdown and cut off a portion of his left ear, he had himself committed to the asylum at Saint-Rémy-de-Provence. He stayed there for 12 months, painting intermittently between attacks of insanity. During this time he created some of his boldest and most imaginative works. The view of Saint-Rémy's stark interior has a hauntingly archetypal quality; the scene is one that has repeated itself in housing for the insane in all ages and in all lands. "Hospital Corridor at Saint-Rémy" by Vincent van Gogh, 1889, gouache and watercolor, 24⅛ × 18⅝ in. (61.3 × 47.3 cm). Collection, The Museum of Modern Art, New York, Abby Aldrich Rockefeller Bequest

Asylum. A benevolent institution affording shelter and support to some class of the afflicted, the unfortunate, or destitute; *e.g.,* a "lunatic asylum," to which the term is sometimes popularly restricted.

—*Oxford English Dictionary*

During the first three days of her eighth admission to the ward for disturbed women at Creedmoor Psychiatric Center, Queens Village, New York, in 1978, a 34-year-old schizophrenic given the name Sylvia Frumkin, did, among other things, the following: she verbally abused, struck, kicked, and tried to bite workers and patients; painted her face with lipstick; took off her T-shirt (she was wearing no bra) and made advances to male patients; floated cigarette butts in another patient's leftover Coke and drank the mixture with gusto; filthied herself and the seclusion room on her unit; talked nonsense at high speed, nonstop, for hours at a time; and threw her liquid medication Thorazine into a therapy aide's eyes. Several overworked, physically hostile employees were then needed to give Ms. Frumkin an injection of Thorazine in an attempt to quiet her. But she did not respond to it. That was the trouble. Not only was Sylvia Frumkin the most disturbed patient on the ward (fellow inmates called her "the greatest show on earth"; doctors called her "a genius at being insane"); she required an extraordinarily high dosage of this major tranquilizing drug to gain temporary relief from her deep sickness. The state of her health, as measured by assaultive and infantile behavior, was even worse during her tenth admission to Creedmoor a year later.

Author Susan Sheehan traced the odyssey of chronic schizophrenic patient Sylvia Frumkin in and out of Creedmoor from her first admission in 1964 to her tenth in 1980. In Sheehan's account Sylvia's treatment at Creedmoor is characterized by misdiagnosis, improper medication, abuse, and absolutely no continuity of care. Sylvia herself describes the "torture" of being "sent through the revolving door again and again."

Creedmoor is a huge mental hospital with 70 buildings over 300 acres. It is in many ways typical of the crowded, understaffed, dirty, dingy, sometimes

36

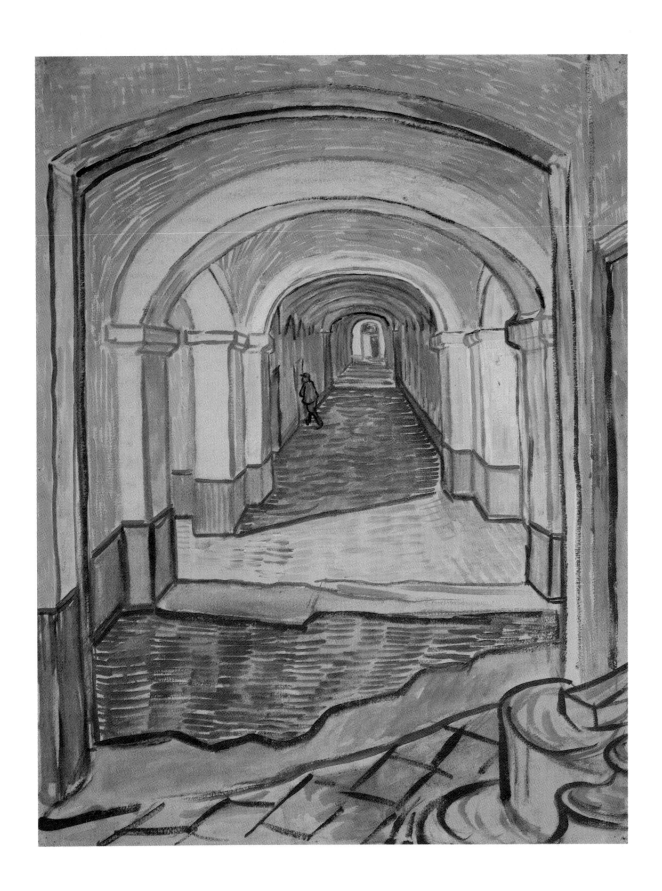

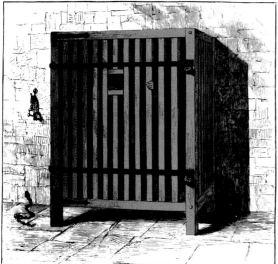

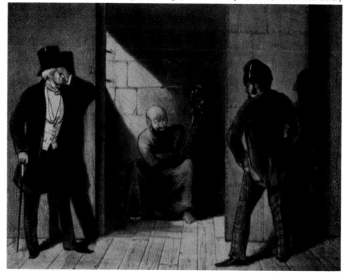

The history of caring for the insane is one in which, more often than not, the mentally ill have been viewed with fear and revulsion. An endless variety of harsh and cruel methods have been used to control patients; they have been chained and put in dungeons, leprosaria, and cages, such as the one above in Belgium.

dangerous, institutions, sorely lacking in competent and compassionate care, that house the chronically disturbed in the United States—this, despite so-called wonder drugs and major mental health system reforms. Sylvia's tale is not an uncommon one.

In considering the history of the institutions that have housed the insane, it is helpful to keep in mind Sylvia Frumkin's excesses of behavior—her most florid symptoms—for throughout history the first thought has been to control the patient, and only secondarily to attempt in whatever manner to control his or her disease. Today drugs usually work to quiet symptoms, but huge doses needed for a drug-resistant patient have serious side effects. Patients before 1952 were not medicated, save in what would seem to us to be weird and inappropriate ways.

A capricious course

No one yet knows the cause of insanity. Thus the history of caring for the insane is an extremely spotty and uneven one punctuated by many dubious, wild, often cruel, and only occasionally compassionate "treatments." It is a history in which human lives have been at the mercy of the theories about insanity and its causes—however preposterous or irrational—then in vogue.

More often than not the mentally disturbed have been viewed with a mixture of fear and revulsion. Humane attitudes have been interspersed with much socially sanctioned cruelty. Even reformers have employed harsh methods of treatment. Benjamin Rush, physician-signer of the Declaration of Independence and a renowned crusader for protecting the rights of the insane, restrained mental sufferers in his notorious "tranquilising chair."

Patients might be restrained "in dark Closets, or cold Garrets, of private Houses, uttering execrations against their relations, and the Almighty" (England, 1815). A cage might be built for them in a cellar (New York, 1736). They might be shut up in empty towers of the old city walls (Germany, 16th century), preferably near some hospital. Patients were lodged in leprosaria (Finland, 1687) or in "eighteen strong boxes under which a brook flows"

38

(Germany, 16th century)—these at least were heated. In the south of England (1811) they were "chained in the cellar or garret of a workhouse, fastened to the leg of a table, tied to a post in an outhouse, or perhaps shut up in an uninhabited ruin." Everywhere the strong walls and barred doors of jails came in handy. In Colonial America makeshift measures gave way to a specific institution (poorhouse or almshouse with rooms for the insane) when a town's population reached about 5,000.

The *harmless* deranged were more widely accepted in former centuries than now. If their liberty was in any degree tolerable, it was tolerated; madmen of nearly every kind and degree were to be found freely wandering the roads in Elizabethan England. Shakespeare's plays have many of the best known madmen and fools in literature, all of whom could in fact have been drawn from life. When the quieter insane were taken into custody, it would probably be into a medieval Christian charity hospital, where the only qualifications for admission were to be poor and in need. There they were tumbled together with paupers, epileptics, the aged, lame, and blind, and those acutely or chronically ill with physical diseases (leprosy and plague were usually excluded, as was syphilis after it was introduced into Europe in the late 15th century).

In Colonial America the insane—all but the truly intractable—were put up at auction by towns responsible for their support and boarded out to citizens who charged least for the service and worked the madman hardest. Thus the mentally ill, who were essentially quite helpless to protect their rights, fared better under the church than under a mercantile system. In other respects religious patronage was not much to their advantage, for the church saw the insane as possessed by devils, and exorcism of devils involved not only the laying on of hands but the plying of whips. There are countless artistic depictions of a devil emerging from the mouth of a patient in response to vigorous applications by the clergy.

Geel: accepting the insane. For centuries the shrine of St. Dymphna in Geel, Belgium, attracted the mentally ill. As the reputed burial place of a saint who had been beheaded on that spot by her father, Geel became known as a place of healing for illnesses of the head. There "treatment" consisted partially of a novena. Three times a day for nine days, patients were led barefoot around the church, each time crawling on their knees through a passage under a reliquary supposed to contain the bones of St. Dymphna. The violent (in chains and behind bars in a "sickhouse" attached to the church) had the holy relics and the service brought to them. By the 19th century, however, such faith had been lost. In 1841 the American asylum physician Pliny Earle, who served as superintendent of the Bloomingdale Hospital in New York, wrote, "The charm [of Geel] is broken, the number of cures is but small, and the place has become rather an asylum for incurables." Even as asylum, however, Geel remained unique. Patients, many awaiting their novena or to make sure they were "cured," were lodged in early years with the priest; subsequently the priest's friends also provided lodging, and in later years patients were taken into homes of residents of Geel. Families in town got used to having the insane around, and though there was a heavy iron ring beside the chimney or attached to a bed where the insane member

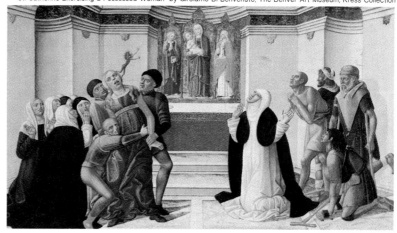

In earlier centuries exorcisms and whippings were the church's method of dealing with the insane; lunatics were thought to be possessed by devils.

might be chained at need, mainly, the mad roamed at large, helping the family, working in the area. They did small harm and met with remarkably few accidents for half a millennium. Twelve hundred insane are today domiciled in the town of Geel, and in the last century or so there has been much interest the world over in the Geel "model."

A painting that remains in Geel today depicts a popular genre of "cure" at the time: treatments direct to the head. The painting shows several patients, one having a substance brushed over his shaved scalp; a woman with one eye closed appears to be reacting to a liquid on her head that stings. Sources are copious on "head-treatments," many literally hair-raising. The ancients had been known simply to remove the hair to give "grosse vapours" a chance to "fume out," but by the 16th century it was thought more effective to apply substances that actually caused inflammation. In the 1820s it was recommended that a long cut on the scalp be filled with a string of peas, which in due time would be sure to suppurate. About 1841 a red-hot iron was applied to the neck in cases of fury, by Jean-Étienne-Dominique Esquirol, the great French psychiatrist, "sometimes with success." This kind of treatment was reluctantly relinquished in 1883 by the physician superintendent of Bethlem (Bethlehem Royal Hospital) in London, on the grounds that "there was a general feeling against it, and it did not look ornamental."

Parisian asylums: a nadir. In Paris in 1656 the insane abruptly ceased to be homogenized in the general population or confined within small institutions. A decree of Louis XIV united the hospitals of Paris under a common administration (the Hôpital Général), in large part to deal with society's less acceptable elements—including the insane. Vagabonds, loafers, paupers, and deviants of every kind were to be swept into one of its component institutions, out of the sight of decent citizens. The king confiscated the funds of small charitable foundations, promising that resources for the new umbrella institution would be taken from the first taxes of the town and that he would himself stand as its protector. Within a few years under the king's strong monarchy an estimated 1% of the general population had been removed from the streets of Paris and dumped into hospitals.

Among the component hospitals housing the insane, the two largest were

40

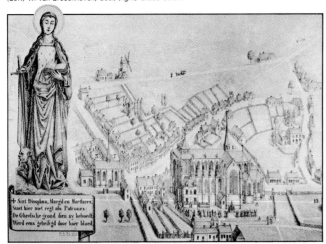

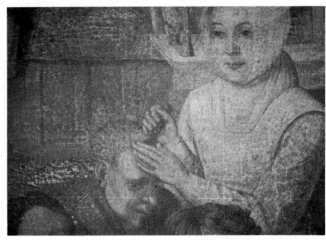

Bicêtre for men and the Salpêtrière for women. The acutely ill continued to be nursed at the huge Paris hospital Hôtel-Dieu, and only when pronounced incurable were they transferred to these vast receptacles, which also contained prisons for condemned criminals and political detainees. By the 18th century there were 3,000 sick and pensioners each year in Bicêtre; the Salpêtrière was even fuller. It received pregnant women and girls, male children between the ages of eight months and five years, geriatric patients, epileptics, paralytics, the blind, cripples, and ringworm cases, as well as prisoners and madwomen, collected each in some distinct section of a tremendous area. The Salpêtrière, "this vast asylum for the poor, this pauper village," as Pliny Earle called it, had 4,000 "patients" in 1656 and 7,800 by the mid-18th century, making it the largest hospital in Paris and probably in all of Europe.

The first "loges" for the insane were built at the Salpêtrière at the end of the 17th century, on marshy ground a little above the Seine. Just at sewer level, it was prey to flooding. There was no attempt to separate kinds of insanity: madwomen in chains mingled with the peaceable and quiet, the fairly tranquil and the imbeciles slept two to a bed in unclean, stuffy quarters.

Bicêtre was divided into *quartiers*—actually into sevenths: the first for the prison, the next three for the "good poor" and the beggars, the fifth for men with venereal disease, the sixth for idiots, imbeciles, epileptics, sick children, and patients with skin diseases. The seventh *quartier,* that of St. Prix, was for the raving mad; 111 loges were arranged along five alleys—one called the Street of Hell. Those brought here might well abandon hope; they would not leave again. They were fettered hand and foot in a cell not six feet square, receiving light and air only by the door with its single wicket scarcely big enough to pass food through. The cots were boards that were always wet, covered with green mold, and glacially cold. (Cells at the Salpêtrière were similar; there, in addition, large rats came up through the sewers and bit the women patients' hands, feet, and faces.) Nurses at Bicêtre were recruited from the prison. For a small coin they would open the door for individual spectators and throw patients subject to delusions of persecution into fits.

In the 7th century an Irish princess named Dymphna was beheaded in Geel, Belgium, by her pagan father. According to legend, extraordinary cures, especially of the deranged, started to occur at the site of the slaying. Dymphna was made a patron saint of the mentally ill, and Geel became known as a place for healing illnesses of the head. A portion of a 17th-century painting (right) shows a man with shaved scalp receiving a "head-treatment." For centuries the mentally sick flocked to the shrine of St. Dymphna, where they were accepted and treated kindly; many were taken in as boarders by clergy and residents of the area, while some stayed in "sickhouses" surrounding the shrine. Geel became a model the world over for incorporating the mentally ill into communities. Even today more than a thousand incurable and feeble-minded mental patients reside in Geel with "foster families."

41

Before vastly improved loges were built by Louis XVI's architect, Charles François Viel, after 1786, Bicêtre and the Salpêtrière represented a nadir in the care of the insane. (Perhaps only an asylum in Cairo could be ranked lower, where there were no provisions to feed patients and their nourishment depended entirely on the charitable gifts of chance visitors.) Small wonder a Frenchman, used to conditions at the Parisian hospitals, was overwhelmed with admiration in 1788 when he visited the hospital of Bethlem in London:

Their doors are open, their rooms wainscoted, and long airy corridors give them a chance of exercise. A cleanliness, hardly conceivable unless seen, reigns in this hospital. Five or six men maintain this cleanliness, assisted by the patients themselves, when they begin to come to themselves, who are rewarded by small presents.

Bedlam: like visiting a zoo. But Bethlem was no monument to humanitarian treatment of the insane. (Indeed, this London asylum was known as Bedlam and gave us the word that commonly denotes a place of uproar and confusion.) There lunatic-watching was raised to the status of a sport; for twopence apiece a hundred people were let in. In 1694 crowds rollicked "from one Apartment to the other." Fruit, nuts, and cheesecake were sold up and down the galleries; professional thieves mingled with the crowd to steal patients' food, clothes, or money. Only in 1770 was the show closed and visitors required permit and escort.

It was in Bedlam that the celebrated inmate William Norris was confined to a dungeon for 14 years with iron rings about his neck and body that slid upward or downward on a bar in the wall behind him. A dungeon approach to housing the mad found dramatic architectural embodiment in 1784 in the Narrenturm, the "Fools' Tower," of Vienna, built round like the impregnable towers of city walls, with 28 cells on each of five stories. The thick walls of the cells were curved at the ceiling for extra strength, and within each cell one or two patients lived in fetters. The doors were massive oak with a small wicket. Thus did the city of Vienna protect itself from its insane. Any attempt in subsequent years to introduce new and bettered treatment in this building was out of the question; it would not adapt.

The Salpêtrière for women was the largest hospital in 17th-century Paris; under Louis XIV's reign it became a "vast asylum for the poor," a "receptacle" for madwomen as well as pregnant girls, prostitutes, geriatric patients, epileptics, paralytics, cripples, and prisoners. Conditions were deplorable in the first "loges" for the insane, which were built on marshland above the Seine. The stuffy quarters were often flooded, and rats from the sewers often bit inmates who slept two to a bed. Under Louis XVI, a century later, vastly improved loges, designed by Charles François Viel (architectural plan, opposite page, top), were built. Only then was an attempt made to separate kinds of insanity. The 1824 painting at right depicts the cours des paisibles—*central courtyard for quiet melancholics. Two of Viel's loges survive to this day. The photograph (opposite page, bottom) is a contemporary view of the entrance and chapel at the Salpêtrière.*

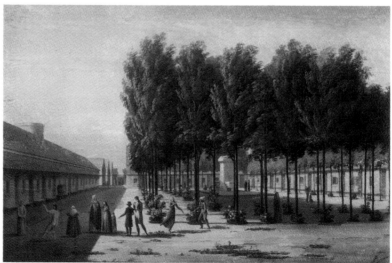

Gouache by Bertin, Museè Carnavalet; photograph, Jean-Loup Charmet, Paris

Private madhouses in England: no lack of abuses. Not all the English mad could be taken into Bedlam or into St. Luke's, the other major hospital for the insane in London, built in the 18th century in an attempt to correct the evils of Bedlam (but hardly a shining example of progress). A flourishing trade in private madhouses thus filled the gap, beginning with doctors taking patients into their own homes, which proved most lucrative. But private institutions, too, were subject to infinite abuses. It was possible for a husband who wanted to enjoy his wife's money to commit her, perfectly sane, to a madhouse, where, as reported in 1740, "he took care that she was so ill used, that she, after a while, was made really mad in good earnest." Madhouses were the nightmare of all classes in the 18th century. Yet they served one useful purpose: since they were passed from father to son, the "mad-doctors," if at all sober and interested, built up a store of practical techniques for managing the insane.

A "dynasty" of madhouse keepers, the Willises—father, sons, and grandson—had principal care of George III of England during his attacks of insanity (presumably caused by porphyria, a rare hereditary disease in which an excess of pigments in the blood intoxicates all parts of the nervous system, producing pain, overactivity, paralysis, and acute delirium). In the mid-1800s Francis Willis, a clergyman, had been taking mentally ill persons into his home in Lincolnshire. These became so numerous they had to be quartered in farms around the small village. William Pitt, the Younger, the prime minister, summoned Willis to London to attend the king, since Willis claimed to have treated 30 private patients a year and to have "cured" 9 out of 10 within three months. Willis took charge and oversaw the management of the patient. To the king's equerry he boasted that he could break in patients like horses. The king was clapped into a "winding sheet," or restraint chair, which he bitterly dubbed his "coronation chair." He was put through the regulation purges, bleedings, cuppings, application of leeches, and induced vomitings and given medicines of bark and saline. And indeed the king did recover from his first attack.

There were five attacks in all. The king regarded his principal physician

Adapted from *La Salpêtrière sous l'ancien régime,* Marthe Henry, Paris; Librairie le François, 1922

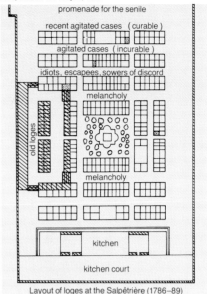

promenade for the senile

recent agitated cases (curable)

agitated cases (incurable)

idiots, escapees, sowers of discord

melancholy

old loges

melancholy

kitchen

kitchen court

Layout of loges at the Salpêtrière (1786–89)

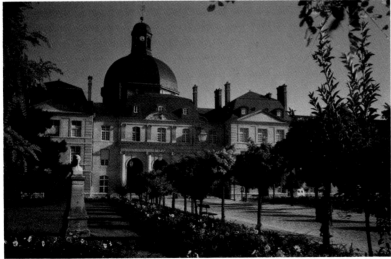

Grace Goldin

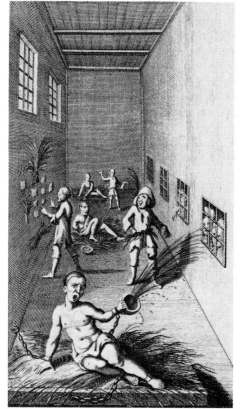

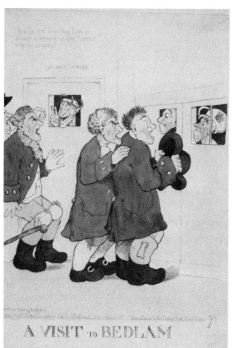

A VISIT TO BEDLAM

with horror and pleaded with Francis's son Thomas Willis, "For God's sake, keep me from your father." He was held in solitary confinement over the protests of his other doctors, who suspected that a mind, however insane, could only deteriorate when restrained from diversions—treatment "far better calculated to drive away the reason of a sane man, than to restore a madman to his senses." During the 32 years of George's intermittent illness, his physicians repeatedly were cross-examined before Parliament about insanity and its treatment. Questions arose in the public mind: Was it indeed desirable to isolate the mad? If a king could go mad, could madness then be "respectable"?

In 1791 (about the midpoint of George's insanity) a Quaker patient named Hannah Mills was locked up for insanity in the York Lunatic Asylum, a charitable institution founded for patients of the middle class. Since Hannah's family lived some distance from the institution, they asked local members of the Society of Friends to visit her. But visitors were barred admittance; it was said that the patient was in no condition to be seen. That was true, for after only a few weeks Hannah Mills died.

An inquiry was attempted but without success. When the York Asylum was founded, its physician offered his services free, but by the time of Hannah Mills's commitment 30 years later, he had the rules changed to admit private paying patients; soon, to the alarm of subscribers to the charity, it had become "an hotel for the reception of persons of condition only."

At last: reform

As a consequence of the case of Hannah Mills, William Tuke, a Quaker from York, along with his son Henry and his grandson Samuel became involved in treatment of the mentally ill. Quakers believed that in every man is a "divine principle" and that nothing could prevent a man from obeying that principle. Insanity was viewed as merely another obstacle, like slavery or poverty, which could be overcome in order to achieve inward enlightenment. In 1792 William Tuke visited St. Luke's in London, where he saw insane patients lying on straw and in chains. "He was distressed with the scene," his son wrote later, "and could not help believing that there was a more excellent way." Reform of the York Asylum proving impossible, the Tukes decided to create their own institution. Henry's wife gave it the name "Retreat," to express what such an institution should be, "a refuge; a quiet haven in which the shattered bark might find the means of reparation or of safety."

The York Retreat was built for 30 patients and later extended to take in 120, not all of them Quakers. It reminded a visiting Frenchman of a large rural farm surrounded by a garden. He particularly remarked that there was nothing prisonlike about it. The Tukes did away with window bars by using sash windows with small panes of glass and subdivisions of iron painted to look like wood. Even though an eight-foot stone wall enclosed the garden, its height was evident only when standing at its base because the ground sloped downward.

The Tukes saw their patients as members of a family—as children who could be violent and dangerous. The power of authority had to be brought to bear upon them. Until then authorities had been afraid of the insane. The in-

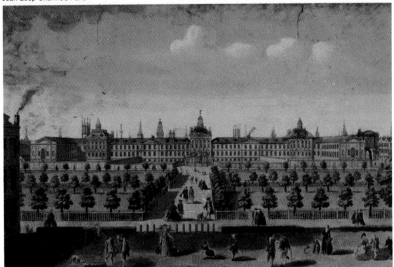

At the Hospital of Bethlem, founded in London in 1247 and shown here in a 1747 engraving, lunatic watching was a sport. Inside the asylum (better known as Bedlam) a circuslike atmosphere prevailed (opposite page, top and bottom).

sane, the Tukes professed, must now be made afraid of authority. Restraint, however, was kept to a minimum; not more than 5% of the patients were restrained by straps or straitjackets or put into seclusion—this at a time when in most asylums every patient was chained all night to the bed.

Once patients "behaved," every effort was made to improve the quality of their lives. Amenities they had been accustomed to—Quaker patients were very unlikely to be paupers—were allowed: tea parties, pets , and pretty furnishings. Food and drink were liberally served. Observing that a full stomach tends to induce calm states and even sleep, the Tukes plied maniacal patients at bedtime with meat, cheese, bread, and good porter—with excellent results. (In other institutions at the time patients were kept on meager diets and put to sleep with opium.) At the York Retreat rooms were warmed; patients got plenty of exercise, and they were encouraged to work; thus problems of "mortification of the feet" that resulted when patients were chained were avoided. Tuke did away with most of the treatments beloved by his age, such as bleeding and purging. He claimed good results from giving patients—especially melancholy ones—warm baths.

The layout and regimen of this Quaker institution were written up in 1813 by 28-year-old Samuel Tuke in a small volume entitled *Description of the Retreat.* The incident of Hannah Mills was referred to as the germ from which the Retreat had sprung, the York Asylum identified only as "an establishment for insane persons, in the vicinity of the City of York." In contrast to "mild" treatment at the "Retreat," that of the "Other Place" was branded "terrific." The reaction of the physician of the York Asylum was ferocious, but the public appeared delighted with the Retreat's reforms.

A bitter squabble ensued as newspapers published attack and counterattack. One of the problems at the York Asylum and elsewhere was that even when "authorities" presumably "inspected," they did not really inspect:

This is something like the watchman's night-call, which obligingly gives the robber notice to stay his hand till the round is finished. . . . Dr. A. insists Dr. B. shall enter first. Dr. B. can't think of it. Whilst they are bowing at each other on the steps, half a dozen

45

manoeuvres are practised to screen the patients from view. The apothecary, perhaps, detains them five minutes in the lobby . . . offers Dr. C. a pinch of his snuff, and accepts the doctor's box in return. . . . At the first landing, Dr. B. is asked how Lady Betty goes on; stops to detail her case, and hears Lord John's in return. At last the gallery is attained. The doors fly open. Dr. A. peeps his head over his shoulder to the right. Dr. B. adopts the same measure to the left. They see nothing wrong, for they scarce see anything at all.

In the same length of time, it was remarked, an able-bodied lad who knew what to look for—an apothecary's apprentice, say—if given the keys to the house, could have judged the whole, "from the garret to the cellar; dayrooms, airing courts, chains, cribs, infirmaries; all the doctors ever did see, and all that they were doomed never to get a sight of." Godfrey Higgins, Justice of the Peace for York, his suspicions aroused by a filthy, neglected patient, forced such an inspection. He turned up himself on the steps of the York Asylum at eight o'clock one morning, determined to go over every inch of it. He forced his way into four cells about eight feet square, the straw saturated with urine, the walls and air holes daubed with excrement. These were the night quarters of 13 women. He demanded to be shown the women and found them upstairs, all together, in a room less than 8 feet by 12. Higgins became very sick and could not remain longer in the room. As a result of that morning's visitation, Higgins had every servant in the house fired; the physician was permitted to resign.

Reform of prisons and of institutions serving the poor, as well as of madhouses, was finally in the air in much of Europe at the end of the 18th century. Quite independently of the Tukes, the French psychiatrist Philippe Pinel unchained the mad at Bicêtre in Paris. A man named Jean-Baptiste Poussin had entered Bicêtre at age 25 to be treated for scrofula (a form of tuberculosis); later, when well again, he was taken on as an employee, as many former patients were. When Pinel arrived in 1792, Poussin had been made governor of the seventh *quartier* for incurable mental patients, the unspeakable St. Prix. Pinel learned a great deal from watching Poussin manage the deranged and often violent inmates. Here is how he disarmed a madman brandishing a knife or cudgel and shouting threats:

As he advances he speaks to him in a firm and menacing tone, and gives his calm advice or issues his threatening summons, in such a manner as to fix the attention of the hero exclusively upon himself . . . until the assistants have had time, by imperceptible advances, to surround the maniac, when, upon a certain signal being given, he finds himself in instant and unexpected confinement.

With 300 madmen to control, Poussin categorically stated that he "never used anything but repressive measures without mistreatment, and never permitted that they be beaten in any way." Poussin employed as attendants many former patients, who knew what it was to be ill-treated.

The first 12 madmen Pinel set free at Bicêtre were put into heavy waistcoats, with extra long sleeves that could be tied behind the back. The first was an English captain who had been in chains for 40 years. With one blow of his manacles he had once killed a keeper. Pinel walked unattended into the man's cell and calmly announced, "Captain, I will order your chains to be taken off, and give you liberty to walk in the court if you will promise me to

46

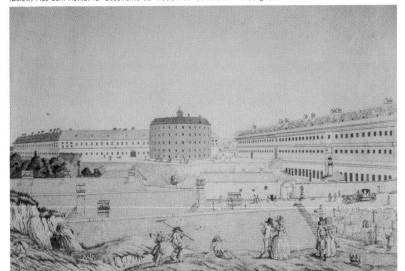

The Narrenturm, which still stands in Vienna, was specially designed and constructed in the late 1700s to protect the city from its mad people. They were housed in a round "Fool's Tower" in thick-walled cells with massive oak doors.

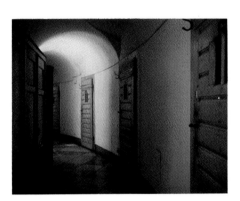

behave well, and injure no one." The astounded patient agreed to don a straightjacket instead.

His chains were removed and the keepers retired, leaving the door open. He raised himself many times from his seat, but fell again on it, for he had been in a sitting posture so long, that he had lost the use of his legs. In a quarter of an hour he . . . came to the door of his dark cell. His first look was at the sky, and he cried out enthusiastically, "How beautiful!" During the rest of the day he was constantly in motion, walking up and down the staircases, and uttering short exclamations of delight. In the evening he returned of his own accord into his cell, where a better bed than he had been accustomed to had been prepared for him.

But other physicians were far from ready to attempt anything so revolutionary. At Bedlam in 1815 a physician defended his timeworn practice of bleeding patients at the end or beginning of May, depending on the weather, then forcing them to vomit once a week for a certain number of weeks, and after that purging them, by saying, "That has been the practice invariably for years, long before my time; it was handed down to me by my father, and I do not know any better practice." Such treatments were routine for acute cases at the Hospice d'Humanité in Paris (the former Hôtel-Dieu). About the practice of bleeding patients Pinel once remarked, "The blood of maniacs is sometimes so lavishly spilled, and with so little discernment, as to render it doubtful whether the patient or his physician has the best claim to the appellation of a madman."

Vomiting was for centuries a trusted standby of European "treatments." "Let Vomitives lead the Van!" the physician to Kings James I, Charles I, and Henry IV of France had rapturously exclaimed in 1676. The desired effect was achieved in most British public asylums in the early 1800s by whirling the patient vertically round and round in a chair suspended from the ceiling. Horizontally, in a device known as Cox's swing, a bed affixed to a perpendicular shaft, vomiting was produced immediately and was followed by bleeding from the ears and mouth to the point of unconsciousness, sometimes causing convulsions—a shock treatment intended to "destroy the links of morbid

47

"St. Luke's Hospital" by Thomas Rowlandson and Augustus Pugin, 1809; photograph, Jean-Loup Charmet, Paris

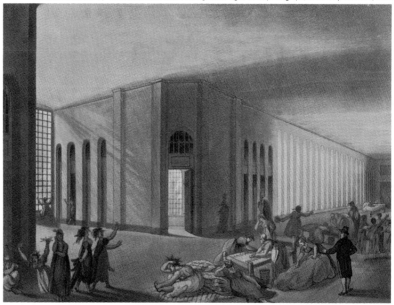

The motivation for opening St. Luke's Hospital for the Insane in the 18th century in London was to correct the evils of Bedlam. Men and women were separated (interior of women's gallery shown here). Incurable patients were housed in the basement apart from acute cases. Some attempt was made to provide purposeful therapeutic activities for the residents. But for the most part, here, too, inmates were subject to abuse and neglect.

Maniacs raved and the melancholy despaired—and little could be said of any real attempt to "treat" mental illness.

association, and break the force and effects of vicious mental habits.''

The use of water to "treat" insanity was also common at many asylums well into the 19th century. There was the bath of immersion: plunge the patient into cold water and withdraw him immediately; repeat up to six times. And the bath of affusion: place the patient in an empty bathing tub and pour cold water on his head, reducing the temperature at each sitting. These methods were recommended by Esquirol as useful to subjects "enfeebled by masturbation" (considered a major cause of insanity throughout the 19th century) "or by long grief, and in whose cases we wish to produce a reaction, by withdrawing from the centre, nervous power, and calling it to the circumference." The douche, a violent drench of water from above, was a most popular treatment:

The douche produces its effects, both by the action of the cold, and the percussion. . . . It causes cardialgia, and desires to vomit. After its action ceases, the patients are pale, and sometimes sallow. It also acts morally, as a means of repression. . . . It is that class of the insane who are young, strong and active, who require the douche.

Even while mad patients in their thousands vomited and bled and came close to drowning, new methods *were* taking hold. There was growing belief that with proper care insanity might be "cured." That conviction revolutionized the care of the insane in the first half of the 19th century. Samuel B. Woodward (1787–1850), one of the founders of the Hartford Retreat in Connecticut, compiled extensive statistical data on patients: color of eyes, occupation, season and phase of the moon on admission, and so forth. Tables of admissions and discharges were drawn up to prove that early treatment often vastly improved the chances for recovery.

New asylums were created during the first half of the 19th century based upon so-called moral treatment: "respect them and they will respect themselves; treat them as reasonable beings, and they will take every possible pain to show you that they are such." There were caveats: Pinel considered certain kinds of patients quite unamenable to moral remedies. He also stressed never disputing with the insane, particularly about their hallucinations. "Persuasion," he insisted, "should be confined to points which affect their liberty or comfort." Systems of rewards and punishments were established: patients were bribed with favorite foods, tobacco, greater degrees of liberty, various amusements, or a better room or clothes. As punishments there were threats of abuse or humiliation: "*Vous passerez aux incurables!*" thundered Esquirol at a rebellious patient.

At Friends' Hospital in Philadelphia it was reported that a male patient continually offended fellow inmates by not disposing of his wastes in the proper receptacles. The patient was forced to wear a petticoat until he learned to control his bowels.

Designing insane asylums

Once the insane were seen as "treatable," it followed that the housing for them had to be reformed as well as the therapies. The asylum itself came to be regarded as an instrument of treatment, part of the cure. Thus every architectural detail received close scrutiny. In building new hospitals designed for "curable" insanity, subdivision became the essential principle. Men and women were kept apart—a precaution that had long been neglected in many insane asylums and which had led to many pregnancies.

Those considered curable were separated from "incurables." In Germany separate "healing" and "nursing" establishments were set up, sometimes located at considerable distances from one another. Patients were separated too by degree and kind of illness. Esquirol pioneered an almost infinitely subdivisible hospital in the form of symetrically arranged one-story square structures, each of four wings around a courtyard. Milder cases were housed toward the center of the complex, the screaming mad at its far ends. Esquirol was very insistent on buildings being only one-story high—to prevent patients from serious falls and to allow for passage of adequate fresh air into the courts. The great French hospital, Charenton, which took nearly 50 years to build (from 1838 to 1885), was laid out on two levels in 18 squares—of two stories; economically single stories proved unfeasible. It was built on the Seine outside Paris, where recovering patients were able to benefit from walks in the wooded and garden areas by the river.

Thomas Kirkbride (1809–83), superintendent of the Pennsylvania Hospital, was considered a guiding spirit of "model" hospital building. He recommended that asylums for the mentally ill should begin with the indispensable minimum: single cells for the violent. If funds were insufficient, construction should then start at the far ends with these and build toward the center. They might be wainscoted with wood so patients would not hurt themselves; in Kirkbride's Philadelphia establishment sharp corners were curved. In England walls of the cell were padded with straw mattresses. At the Salpêtrière detached cottages were put up, one to a patient, but this layout rendered heating and surveillance during the night almost impossible.

Grounds were generally surrounded by sunken walls. A seemingly ordinary fence enclosed Friends' Hospital in Philadelphia. The top of the fence

George III of England suffered five bouts of "insanity." His treatment, which consisted largely of purges and bleedings, was described as "far better calculated to drive away the reason of a sane man, than to restore a madman to his senses." In this caricature poor King George is shown idling away the day toasting muffins.

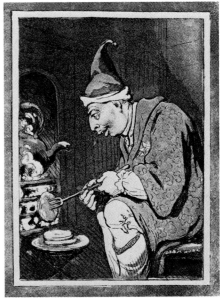

49

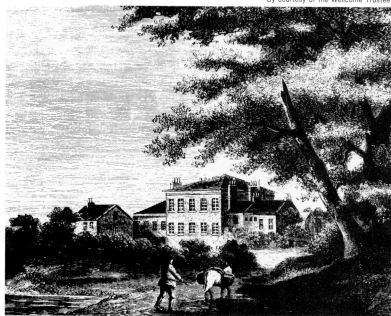

In 1792 William Tuke, a Quaker, visited St. Luke's in London. He was distressed with the conditions and believed there must be "a more excellent way" to care for the insane. The Tuke family created its own institution in York, a quiet country "retreat" with nothing prisonlike about it (save the eight-foot stone wall enclosing the garden).

was pivoted, however, so that anyone attempting to climb it from the inside would be gently dropped back upon the hospital grounds, while a bell rang to inform the attendants. Courtyards must not look like prisonyards. Pliny Earle reported that those in an Antwerp asylum in 1841, "like almost everything connected with lunatic asylums in general have, within the last few years, been made to blossom as the rose."

Stairs were to be broad enough to admit three persons abreast; a patient, if struggling, and two attendants to restrain him. Wickets in doors made it possible to see in and out. Walls were to be painted some deep color, often green. It was even proposed to give walls different colors according to the different forms of illness, a concept comparable to the system of identification of patients in an asylum in Venice in 1841, where patients wore a strip of cloth as an epaulet: mania, red; monomania, deep blue; melancholy, green; idiocy, orange; "stupiditá," light blue; and the demented went in yellow.

After centuries of belief that the insane were insensitive to cold, it was now thought patients should not be exposed even to cold feet, "which might become fatal to them, because of their tendency to congestion of the brain." Therefore floors were to be of wood and treated with linseed oil, and often the floor was given a slope toward the door to let water run off.

Beds, too, required special attention. In Berlin at the end of the 19th century the incontinent slept on moss mattresses. In Utrecht in 1841 cribs described by Pliny Earle had a concave bottom descending toward an aperture for the escape of urine.

Generally, the insane, throughout the greater part of history, were not considered up to partaking in spiritual matters. Where there were chapels, in Roman Catholic countries more than others, these might have separate compartments for men and women, so arranged that all might witness the ceremonies before the altar. The Nuncio Hospital in Toledo, Spain, was built

50

in 1783 with a central chapel at the head of a splendid ceremonial flight of stairs leading straight to it from the front entrance. The two patient compartments are to either side of the altar, but barred.

Throughout history there has been nothing if not differential treatment of the rich and the poor. In insane asylums this has been particularly manifested in the matters of control and privileges. Patients can be controlled in two basic ways: with a sufficient number of attendants or with physical restraints. The wealthy were attended, while the poor were bound. A private institution at Paris-Ivry in the early 19th century provided an attendant for each patient. At the York Retreat the rich insane—men and women—if at all genteel were allowed the privilege of eating with the superintendent. At York there were four economic classes, paying from 4 to 80 shillings per week. At the top price, "superior patients" had access to a flowering lawn gently sloping southward.

At the Royal Lunatic Asylum in Glasgow, pauper patients were put on the first floor, the lowest class of paying patients on the second, the highest on the third. In Bordeaux paying patients ate from earthen dishes, the indigent from tin. At Rennes paying patients were given wine and the paupers cider. In Worcester, Massachusetts, only paying patients were permitted to keep trunks in their own rooms and take personal charge of their possessions. Privilege paid off: at Scottish asylums in 1807 it was estimated that "the board paid for superior accommodation by the rich has been sufficient, and in some cases it has been more than sufficient, to defray the whole charge of the general maintenance and management."

For upper classes amenities included such things as Oriental rugs, oil paintings, aeolian harps, and stuffed peacocks in dayrooms. Then there were the middle-class patients, often well educated, but short on funds—clergymen, artists, governesses, and professors—prone to mental instability but not poor enough (and far too proud) to turn to charity for help, yet not rich enough either for private nursing homes or special subsidies to the asylums. Usually these patients were allowed fewer amenities than wealthy patients but a greater degree of privacy than poor patients.

The Nuncio of Toledo is primarily for the insane of the province who cannot pay. Many distinctions there are based on degree of illness and behavior. On the women's half of the building, in one of the corner towers,

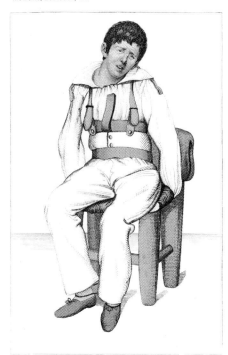

While the Tukes, Quaker reformers of the 18th century, firmly believed that the insane could and should be treated with kindness and compassion, few others of the time were willing to embrace such radical notions. In most European asylums patients continued to be "controlled" with physical restraints. Patients were chained or bound in chairs by day, and at night they were chained to beds or even confined in locked criblike contraptions such as the one pictured here.

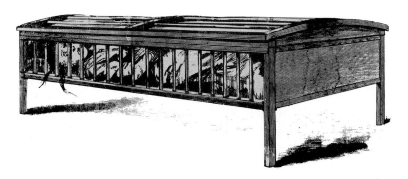

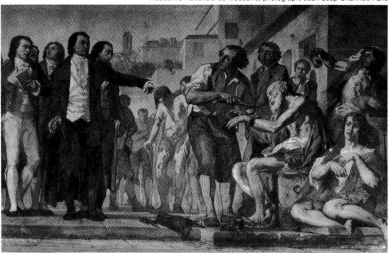

could be found in 1968 a dormitory for some dozen well-behaved women: two tall shuttered windows, flowers in the center of the room, beds arranged around the walls and not crowded together, each with a pretty blue and white bedspread and the patient's individual doll. For badly behaved patients (including the incontinent) there was a crowded, unpleasant smelling dormitory in the basement, reached from a tall and bleak corridor, locked at night by a massive door, lighted by one naked bulb, with walls thick as a dungeon, rows of beds covering the floor space, plain white bedspreads, and scarcely a doll in sight.

Work as therapy

In the 1820s W. C. Ellis, superintendent of the Wakefield County Asylum in York, England, made the revolutionary suggestion that hard work might be a boon to agitated patients; he proposed that patients work on the grounds of the asylums—but not without being chained to a keeper. It was also suggested that patients might be allotted one corner of the garden to dig up over and over all the year round. There was, of course, a fear of putting into the hands of a violent madman a spade or a hoe. But Pliny Earle could report of the Utrecht Asylum in 1841 that "no accident has hitherto occurred from the use of edge tools by the patients." Confinement began to be seen as backward. By 1854 in certain asylums work was considered an honor and a privilege.

Social class determined the kinds of work patients agreed to do. At the asylum in Zaragoza, Spain, most patients were engaged each day "in the soothing and delightful pursuits of agriculture and horticulture," returning each evening "calm and contented, to pass the night in solitary tranquility and sleep." Not so, however, the Spanish grandees, "whose pride of birth and family presents unsurmountable obstacles to a degradation so blessed and salutary." This was the reason, Pinel noted, patients of the upper classes "seldom recover the full and healthy possession of a deranged or lost intellect." Samuel Tuke marveled at the success of a German asylum "in *inducing,* not *compelling,* the *wealthy* patients to labour." Across the Atlantic at Friends' Hospital, Philadelphia, some of the more affluent patients

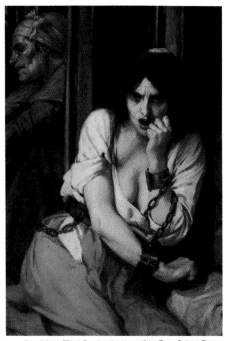

52

who flatly rejected farmwork consented to try their hand at woodworking.

Women's work was for the most part traditional: sewing, washing, ironing, and cooking. In Dublin in 1827, at an asylum with 300 patients, the linen was woven by the female paupers, who produced during the year 140 shirts, 115 bolster cases, 56 pairs of sheets, 53 rollers, 83 bodices, and 80 nightcaps, in addition to keeping all clothing of men and women patients in repair. At Wakefield patients of both sexes were principally responsible for making the beer, bread, and shoes.

The exhilaration of the *privilege* of labor soon wore off as patient manpower came to be exploited by the institutions. In 1841 Pliny Earle reported from Antwerp that it had been found difficult or nearly impossible to induce men and women to work, except by the stimulus of pecuniary reward. At Wakefield, in addition to their regular meals, laboring patients were allowed two extra "drinkings" during the day, each consisting of three-quarters of a pint of beer and four ounces of bread, plus an ounce of tobacco a week.

A fine line has always existed between "therapeutic" and exploitative labor. In 1948 Albert Deutsch, in a provocative report on U.S. state hospitals, reported that he saw patients working 12 to 14 hours a day. The advent of so-called occupational therapy in the 20th century came as a kind of reform, and meant that patients were more likely to participate in what was termed horticultural therapy rather than farming to benefit the asylum. Instead of repairing curtains or mattresses, female patients turned out beaded belts and needlepoint.

It was never suggested that upper-class women busy themselves with useful activities. They were guided toward occupational therapies typical of the society from which they came: walking, riding on horseback, dancing, playing cards, and playing musical instruments. In 1838 the matron at Hanwell Asylum, a large 19th-century institution in England, organized some 50 fine needlewomen to prick out fancy items for a bazaar. A 19th-century lithograph pictures female patients skipping rope and playing shuttlecock on the grounds of "Mrs. Bradbury's Establishment for the Reception of Ladies Nervously Affected" near London. Distractions in the cure-minded asylum were legion. An extremely popular circular railway on the front lawn of Friends' Hospital—a small car operated by means of a crank—proved an ideal outlet for the energies of Quaker women as well as men.

Optimism abounds

The ultimate achievement of the asylum for "curable" insane—as indeed of the whole history of insane asylums—must be considered the abolition of physical restraints. By 1838 it was widely accepted that, as Robert Gardiner Hill, resident medical officer at the Lincoln Asylum, in England, said: "In a properly constructed building, with a sufficient number of suitable attendants, restraint is never necessary, never justifiable, and always injurious, in all cases of Lunacy whatever." John Conolly was also quite outspoken on the matter. He visited Hill just before becoming physician superintendent to the County Lunatic Asylum at Hanwell, which had nearly a thousand patients. Within three years Conolly had abolished every mechanical restraint in the house. He kept it restraint-free for 16 years. Restraint, Conolly wrote,

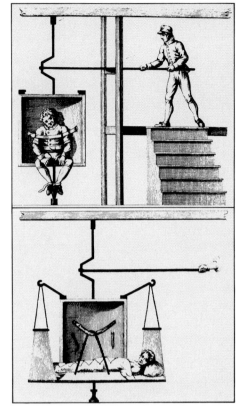

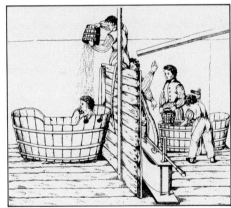

While Pinel was unshackling inmates at Bicêtre, most physicians of his day stuck with traditional methods of treatment, such as whirling patients around in various contraptions suspended from the ceiling to induce vomiting (top and center) and employing specially contrived douches (bottom) that enabled the drenching of patients with icy water from above.

(Top and center) *Traité sur l'aliénation mentale et sur les hospices des aliénés*, Joseph Guislain, Amsterdam, J. van der Hey & Sons, 1826; photograph, The Francis A. Countway Library of Medicine, Boston; (bottom) *Oeffentliche Rechenschaft über meine zwölfjährige Dienstführung*, Ernst Horn, Berlin, Realschulbuchhandlung, 1818; photograph, Yale Medical Library

in his *Construction and Government of Lunatic Asylums and Hospitals for the Insane* (1847), "was the grand substitute for inspection, superintendence, cleanliness, and every kind of attention."

Hill was deeply impressed. Around that time he reacted strongly upon viewing a patient at his Lincoln institution with poultices on his wrists; an attendant was standing by to prevent him from eating these poultices, which, Hill learned, were for injuries produced by the use of handcuffs. So he, too, instituted a no-restraint policy. These achievements were so lastingly influential that at Creedmoor today when a Sylvia Frumkin becomes violent, she is not bound or handcuffed but locked in a seclusion room for two-hour intervals, a "treatment" imposed and renewed only by a physician's order.

Conolly made his system work with the judicious use of well-paid attendants. The attendants were in fact so favorably impressed by the new method that they were as eager as their superiors to extend its operation. They brought to it what Samuel Tuke described as the necessary attitude for effectively attending the insane—that is, it is necessary to think of patients as, at the same time, both brothers and mere automata. "To applaud all they do right; and pity, without censuring, whatever they do wrong, requires such a habit of philosophical reflection, and Christian charity, as is certainly difficult to attain."

County asylums like Hanwell were founded to rescue the British insane from the abuses of private madhouses. In the United States state asylums—some 32 were built between 1841 and 1877—arose in response to a smashing campaign by social reformer and humanitarian Dorothea Lynde Dix against the prevailing "hellholes." But the problem on both sides of the Atlantic was their size. The first concern of Thomas Kirkbride, who was superintendent of the Pennsylvania Hospital's branch for the insane in Philadelphia and who played such a major role in determining the architectural mode of new housing for the mentally ill in the U.S., was to keep an asylum small. Kirkbride shook his head over mid-19th-century British asylums like Colney Hatch, with 2,000 patients. Its facade extended one-third of a mile. Kirkbride

Social class almost always determined the amount of freedom patients had. At private institutions wealthy residents often had amenities, such as open airy rooms and gardens to enjoy. At Mrs. Bradbury's home near London (right) upper-class women engaged in many frivolities such as skipping rope and playing shuttlecock. But even in days of reform, asylums that housed the less well-off remained comparatively prisonlike. In the early 1900s so much as a wicket in a cell door was considered an advance.

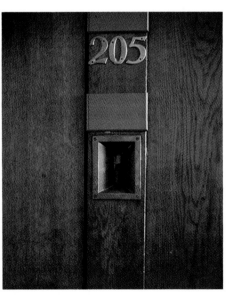

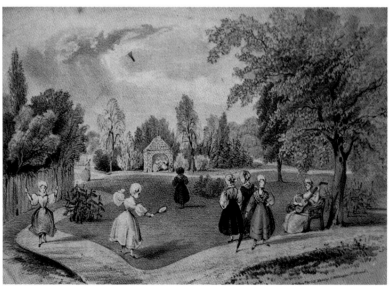

(Left) Grace Goldin; (right) "Mrs. Bradbury's Establishment for the Reception of Ladies Nervously Affected," 19th-century lithograph, by courtesy of the Wellcome Trustees; photograph, Grace Goldin

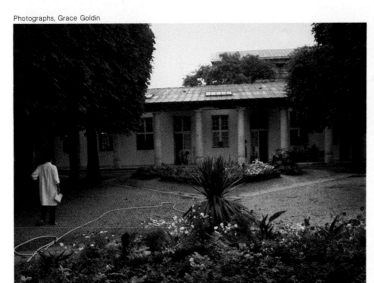
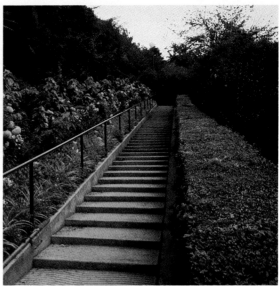

set a limit of 250 patients. If you must take in more, he argued, it was better to build another asylum.

The resurgence of hellholes

It did not prove possible, however, to limit asylums to 250 patients. Moreover, a universal no-restraint system never was arrived at, for lack of both morale and personnel. After Conolly's achievement at Hanwell abolition of restraints could never be said to be humanly impossible. But considering the degree of dedication required, and the high caliber of attendant necessary, it was humanly improbable in most receptacles for the insane the world over.

The fact could no longer be overlooked that most insanity was not curable. The drive engendered by the optimism of Kirkbride, Conolly, Dix, and others faded away as discharged patients broke down again and again and had to return to institutions, as they became "chronic." In the U.S. so-called back wards developed. Repeated stays in the asylum had to be counted as part of one illness. As the British psychiatrist Henry Maudsley put it in 1879:

There are some persons who have been begotten and conceived in an insane spirit, bred in an insane moral atmosphere, and have thought, felt, and acted in an insane way all their lives; these people will remain lunatics as long as they live, will die lunatics, and, unless they have been made new creatures meanwhile, will rise lunatic spirits at the day of judgment.

The back wards filled up with incurables; the dayrooms, hallways, even bathrooms for supposedly calming warm baths were to be given were taken over as sleeping quarters; "treatment" in most instances became impossible. Less and less attempt was made toward any active regimen. By the second half of the 19th century a therapeutic nihilism prevailed; in about 31% of cases recovery was spontaneous, so the average medical superintendent was prone to say, "Oh, let them alone, they will get well by and by."

"Public confidence was greatest when the justification for institutionalization of insane patients was expressed in restorative terms," the historian Gerald N. Grob has observed. "When hospitals became custodial, suspi-

The great Charenton asylum outside Paris, where the Marquis de Sade was confined (1803–14), was a model for more inspired asylum designs that recognized mental patients should not be housed like prisoners but could actually benefit from fresh air, gardens, and attractive surroundings.

55

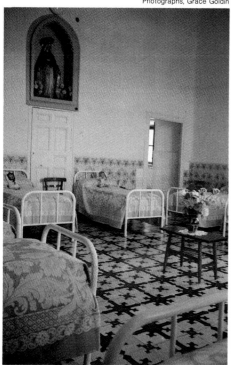

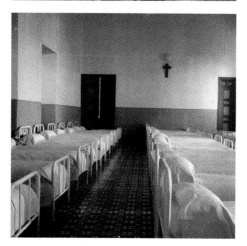

At the Nuncio in Toledo, Spain, where most inmates are nonpaying, distinctions are made on the basis of behavior—for well-behaved women, sunlit and cheerful rooms (top); bleak basement wards (bottom) for the badly behaved.

cions rose." By law, U.S. state asylums were forced to take every patient sent to them. As mandated receptacles for paupers and the criminally insane, they became merely custodial institutions in the public mind. Private hospitals thrived, offering the best treatment available, but, of course, only to a small minority of wealthy patients. Even today most insurance policies cover only 90 days of private hospitalization at certain intervals. As the chief of her unit said, sadly, on one of Sylvia Frumkin's many readmissions, "The ninety-first day is always Creedmoor."

In late-19th-century England magistrates who were generally unwilling to spend money on pauper lunatics were still less willing to spend it on *incurable* pauper lunatics. In New England it was said, "Once christen the disease insanity and the cost of treatment shrinks in the public estimation to less than that of living in health."

Curative treatment has always been more expensive than custodial. During the second half of the 19th century it was earnestly discussed whether "chronics" should not be put into "cheap storage." For a time there was a surge of reinterest in the Geel arrangement—*i.e.,* dispersion of patients rather than their aggregation in ever increasing numbers in the discredited asylums. The idea was to create a freer, more normal life for patients, with the possibility of work and a family to belong to. In Britain such interest led to the boarding-out of patients in licensed houses, particularly in Scottish villages called "Geels of the North," and to a system of trial dismissal from the asylum to the charge of trustworthy cottagers in some English villages. In 1883 a colony, similar to Geel, was proposed for Lierneux in Belgium. The town's burgomaster roundly rejected the idea: "Nothing is so contagious as insanity, and while I am burgomaster, no lunatic shall ever enter Lierneux!" Nevertheless, in 1884 four patients were quietly installed in homes there. Caretakers welcomed the subsidy, and with luck they also acquired a willing worker. Applications for patients soon became more numerous than it was thought prudent to grant.

U.S. interest in Geel took the form of a cottage system—grouping a number of small units around a central building rather than tossing all patients into a congregate custodial asylum. Most U.S. psychiatrists were in favor of the cottage plan, but since it was harder to supervise and would be considerably more expensive to run, it failed to take hold. (Today in the U.S., though there is no "Geel" per se, there is interest in giving mental patients as normal an environment as possible; an estimated 25,000 chronic patients reside with "foster families.")

Today contemporary Geel continues on a small scale with its time-tried alternative to institutionalization. It is universally preferred by the patients assigned by Belgian psychiatrists to its residential program, many of them after long hospitalization. Today these are exclusively severe cases: one-third psychotic and two-thirds retarded—all considered incurable. Periodically they are checked by a district nurse and may be returned to the hospital if things do not work out, but most patients decidedly benefit from Geel's centuries of experience in living with and handling very disturbed patients.

By the beginning of the 20th century the word asylum had been so debased that the institutions were renamed mental hospitals. Around 1902 an

(Top left) Photograph by Snowdon; (top right) Jim Pozarik—Gamma/Liaison; (bottom) photographs, Jerry Cooke

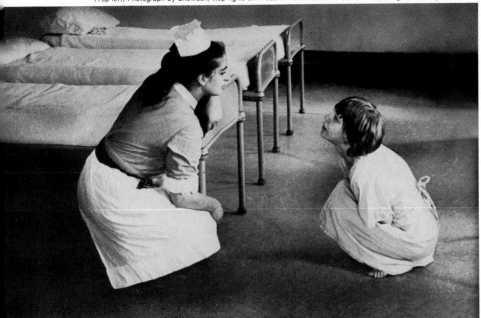
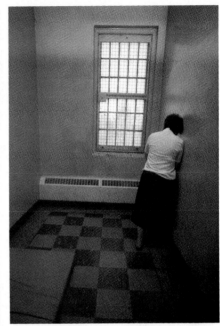
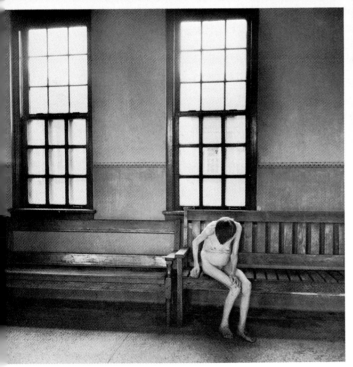
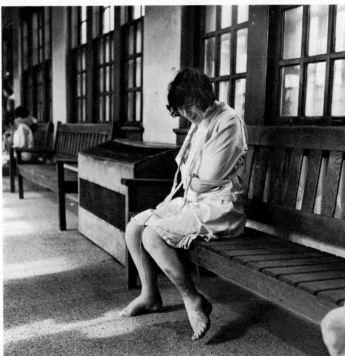

For a time mentally ill patients on both sides of the Atlantic were seen as "curable," and their care was greatly humanized. No-restraint policies took hold beginning in the mid-1800s, and caring staff devoted themselves to patients. But true reforms were not to last into the 20th century, largely owing to lack of funds and dedicated attendants. The scene at a British asylum, 1968 (top left), is a rare one. Many, if not most, public institutions reverted to being receptacles for chronics. In the U.S. custodial care was the rule in state hospitals. (Top right) A patient today at Creedmoor in Queens, N.Y. (Bottom, left and right) Female inmates of Ohio state institutions, 1946.

57

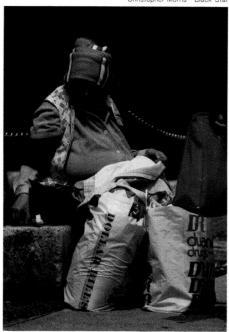

Today many "bag ladies" in big cities are former mental patients—hapless victims of "reforms" of the 1960s when patients were put on tranquilizing drugs and state hospitals were emptied.

important incident occurred. A man named Clifford Beers, a young New Englander from a "good" family, was institutionalized at a state hospital. He was determined to see the worst of the hospital's facilities. He behaved in a way to get himself consigned to the basement, where he himself was tortured by the attendants. Later he reported on actual conditions in *A Mind That Found Itself,* which was read by millions. One attendant who choked a man into insensibility was indignant at being discharged. "They're getting pretty damned strict these days discharging a man simply for *choking* a patient." However, this brutal soul soon found new employment in a similar institution not 20 miles distant. Poorly paid, ill-trained attendants were everywhere. In 1943, at a private mental hospital, an attendant—in fact, a wartime conscientious objector—is said to have slapped a female patient's face very hard while she was held absolutely immobile in a wetpack. The helplessness of insane patients seems to bring out what Pinel called "the savage and murderous cruelty of underlings."

Attendants at U.S. state hospitals were the most underpaid of "underlings." Conditions were likened to those in jails. Per diem allowance for an inmate was often lower. "For years," sighed a weary physician-administrator in 1942, "the state has followed the unwritten policy that the best institution is the one run at the least per capita cost." Only rudimentary medical treatment was possible, and psychotherapy, the most expensive treatment, was out of the question. No accepted psychoanalytic method was ever devised to handle patients en masse. "All we can do is feed them and sleep them while they're with us," said an administrator in Detroit. Conditions in a great many hospitals were so bad that an attendant in Georgia stated, under affidavit, about his own institution: "A patient who could get well here could get well just as easy if he were lost out in the Okefenokee Swamp."

Suddenly, in 1953, new drugs were discovered, among them chlorpromazine (Thorazine) and its derivatives, used for the major chronic illness, schizophrenia, which had long been responsible for overloading mental hospitals. By 1955 state hospitals using the tranquilizers were calling them "a miracle." The wild behavior of schizophrenics could be controlled, except in a very few cases, enabling institutions once considered bedlams to achieve a semblance of order. Plans were made to discharge patients; community mental health centers were established to treat the discharged as outpatients. With this new policy public hospitals were emptied. Between 1965 and 1982 the number of institutionalized mental patients in the state of New York declined from 80,000 to 23,000.

Physician Lewis Thomas, president of the Memorial Sloan-Kettering Cancer Center in New York City, and prolific commentator on contemporary health issues, writing in 1981 "On the Need for Asylums," has described the result of this policy with which we and the insane are living today. "The mentally ill were out of the hospital, but in many cases they were simply out on the streets, less-agitated but lost, still disabled but now uncared for." The drugs, he points out, do not turn off the disease. When they are not in attendance at the mental health centers in the community, many patients may be found on the streets—cold, hungry, and vulnerable to assault or to their own impulse toward suicide. They are sleeping in a row on the floor of the ladies' room in New York City's Pennsylvania Station and the Port-Authority bus terminal—both of which have the haunting appearance of medieval hospitals—indiscriminate receptacles for the poor, the sick, and the mad. They are curled up under public telephones or they pace the waiting rooms at three o'clock in the morning, muttering. This has led Thomas and many others to conclude that even a place that will only feed them and sleep them begins to look good. Of Philadelphia's deplorable Byberry institution it was said in 1942 that there just was not enough privacy to permit a successful suicide attempt.

Indeed the quality of mental-health facilities continues to be variable throughout the world. In the U.S. the present system of housing the mentally ill is not working. Lewis Thomas has suggested that a new era of reform is once again called for. New "asylums" must be established, restoring the word to its original sense: *i.e.,* a secure place of refuge, shelter, and compassion, so that mentally disturbed patients may come in off the streets to live in decency and warmth.

FOR ADDITIONAL READING:

Beers, C. W. *A Mind That Found Itself.* New York: Doubleday, Doran & Co., 1944.

Deutsch, Albert. *The Shame of the States.* New York: Harcourt, Brace, 1948.

Earle, Pliny. *The Curability of Insanity: A Series of Studies.* 1887. Reprint. New York: Arno Press, 1972.

Gilman, S. L. *Seeing the Insane.* New York: John Wiley & Sons, Inc., 1982.

Greenberg, Joanne. *I Never Promised You a Rose Garden.* New York: New American Library, 1964.

Grob, G. N. *The State and the Mentally Ill.* Chapel Hill: University of North Carolina Press, 1966.

Hunter, Richard, and Macalpine, Ida. *Three Hundred Years of Psychiatry, 1535–1860.* London and New York: Oxford University Press, 1963.

Masters, Anthony. *Bedlam.* London: Michael Joseph, 1977.

Pinel, Philippe. *A Treatise on Insanity.* New York: Hafner Publishing Co., 1962.

Roosens, Eugeen. *Mental Patients in Town Life: Geel, Europe's First Therapeutic Community.* Beverly Hills: Sage Publications, 1979.

Scull, Andrew, ed. *Madhouses, Mad-Doctors, and Madmen.* Philadelphia: University of Pennsylvania Press, 1981.

Sheehan, Susan. *Is There No Place on Earth for Me?* New York: Houghton Mifflin, 1982.

Thomas, Lewis. "On the Need for Asylums." *Discover* 2 (1981): 68–71.

Tuke, Samuel. *Description of the Retreat.* Edited by Richard Hunter and Ida Macalpine. London: Dawsons, 1964.

Grace Goldin

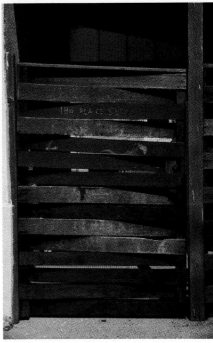

Gate at a Pennsylvania mental hospital, 1982. Clearly it is time for a new era of reform.

Depressive Disorders
by Joseph J. Schildkraut, M.D.

O, that this too too solid flesh would melt,
Thaw, and resolve itself into a dew!
Or that the Everlasting had not fix'd
His cannon 'gainst self-slaughter! O God! God!
How weary, stale, flat, and unprofitable,
Seem to me all the uses of this world!
　　　　　　　　—*Hamlet*, Act I, scene ii.

Descriptions of states of depressions are found throughout written history. The state of depression, which the ancient Greeks believed to be caused by black bile, was known to Hippocrates as melancholia, a term that in the 1980s is undergoing revival in psychiatric practice.

"Depression" may refer to normal unhappiness—grief, mourning, disappointment, or failure. In a psychiatric context "depression" refers to a variety of pathological disorders as well as clinical syndromes (*i.e.,* clusterings of signs and symptoms). It is estimated that throughout the world over 127 million people suffer from pathological depressions. In the United States alone between 8 million and 20 million people are currently suffering from a depressive disorder. Moreover, some reports suggest that up to 25% of the U.S. population may experience at least one major depression during the course of their lives.

Over $10 billion are spent annually for the treatment of depressions, and this figure is compounded by the economic loss resulting from impaired performance at work and time away from the job. The fiscal costs, however, can never be compared with the price exacted in human suffering. The pain of depression is not limited to that experienced by the depressed patient but also greatly affects family members and friends. It has been estimated that the long-term risk of suicide in a patient with a depressive disorder is between 10 and 15%; moreover, a large majority of the 30,000 people who commit suicide in the United States each year are thought to be clinically depressed. Inasmuch as most depressions are treatable conditions, this tragic figure represents a staggeringly high mortality rate.

The many faces of depression

As in all other areas of medicine, an accurate diagnosis is essential for effective treatment of depressive disorders. Despite differences in approach, numerous studies have shown that depressions can be separated into meaningful groupings on the basis of clinical signs, symptoms, and history. However, as in many other areas of medicine, disorders that appear to be

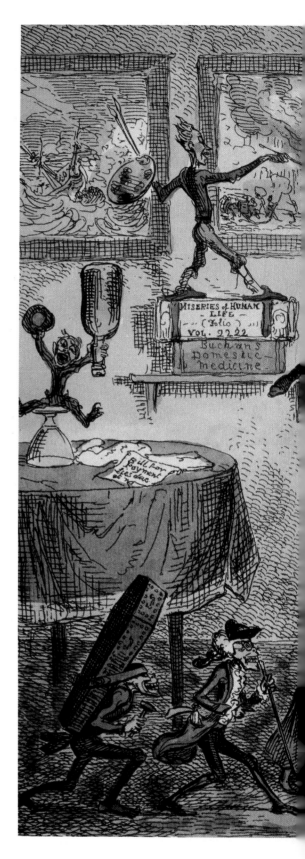

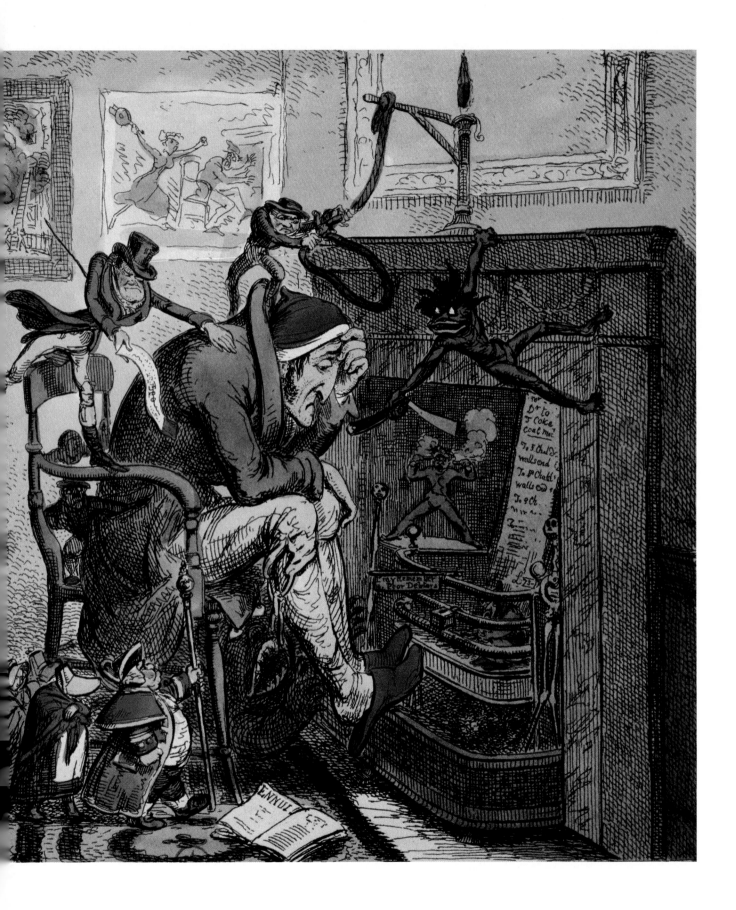

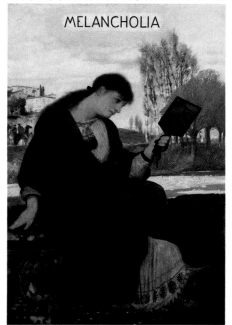

MELANCHOLIA

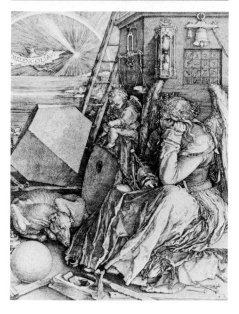

Joseph J. Schildkraut, M.D., *is Professor of Psychiatry at Harvard Medical School; Director of the Neuropsychopharmacology Laboratory at the Massachusetts Mental Health Center; and Director of the Psychiatric Chemistry Laboratory at New England Deaconess Hospital, Boston.*

(Overleaf) "The Blue Devils" by George Cruikshank; photograph, Jean-Loup Charmet, Paris

clinically indistinguishable may, nonetheless, have quite different underlying causes. Conversely, some disorders that manifest themselves very differently may actually have similar causes, many of which are now understood to be biologic in nature. While various clinical criteria, *e.g.,* signs and symptoms, may be of value in determining the appropriate treatment for some patients, recent findings indicate that proper diagnosis may be usefully augmented by various biological criteria. Since depressive syndromes may occur as one of the manifestations of many different medical and neurological disorders, a thorough general medical assessment is an extremely important component of the diagnostic evaluation.

A major breakthrough in the classification of depressions came in the late 19th century when the influential German psychiatrist Emil Kraepelin distinguished what he called manic-depressive psychosis from schizophrenia. Kraepelin defined manic-depressive psychosis broadly, including under this diagnostic rubric not only patients who experienced both manias and depressions (what we now term bipolar affective disorders) but also those patients who experienced only episodes of depression (what we now call unipolar depressive disorders) or only manias. Kraepelin's separation of the manic-depressive disorders from the schizophrenias was based not only on the differing symptoms and overall clinical pictures but on the courses of the illnesses; Kraepelin noted that the schizophrenic patient generally progressed to a state of chronic mental deterioration, while the manic-depressive patient had episodes of illness alternating with periods of apparent well-being and the capacity to function normally.

Since Kraepelin's initial classifications many attempts have been made to subclassify the various depressive disorders. Throughout the 20th century many dichotomous subdivisions have been suggested. These have included the distinctions between psychotic and neurotic depressions, retarded and agitated depressions, endogenous and reactive depressions, primary and secondary depressions, biological and psychological depressions, and bipolar and unipolar depressions. Many of these terms, however, have lacked precision and in some instances produced even more confusion than clarification. Although these dichotomous groupings have had some limited value in the study and treatment of the depressive disorders, it is now recognized that simple dichotomies are not adequate to classify the wide range of disorders into biologically meaningful and therapeutically relevant subgroups. Consequently, more complex classification systems have recently been formulated. The third edition of the *Diagnostic and Statistical Manual of Mental Disorders* (*DSM-III*) in the early 1980s introduced a totally new nomenclature—representing an attempt to provide more systematic and operational criteria for diagnosing all psychiatric illness, including the major depressive disorders and manias.

The term endogenous depression, for example, has often been used inappropriately to refer to a depression occurring in the absence of a precipitating life event, rather than to a depressive syndrome in which the patient's mood is unresponsive to environmental events or interpersonal interactions. Although "endogenous depression" has been replaced in the *DSM-III* classification by the designation of major depressive disorder with melancholia,

62

the term is still widely used by clinical investigators when referring to specific clinical syndromes characterized by some or all of the following: psychic retardation (*i.e.,* slowing of thought and speech); decrease in interest and ambition; loss of energy; loss of initiative; impaired sense of vitality; indecisiveness; the inability to anticipate or attain the usual satisfactions or pleasures customarily obtained from work or recreational activities; and associated feelings of hopelessness, helplessness, worthlessness, and guilt.

Among the other clinical characteristics of endogenous depression are diurnal variations in the intensity of symptoms, typically with a worsening in the morning and a partial remission later in the day. Other commonly occurring symptoms include sleep disturbances (typically insomnia with early morning awakening but sometimes hypersomnia—*i.e.,* increased sleep) and appetite disturbances (usually anorexia with accompanying weight loss but sometimes increased food intake with weight gain). Endogenous depressions, or major depressive disorders with melancholia, are further characterized by the lack of reactivity or responsiveness of the affective state either to alterations in the patient's environment or to social or therapeutic interpersonal interactions, whether or not the depression was initially precipitated by events in the patient's life. While sadness of affect is often present, it is not invariably so; some patients may in fact strongly deny feelings of unhappiness, describing themselves rather as lacking in any feeling and experiencing a sense of dullness or numbness.

Patients with endogenous depressions usually have histories of good previous social adjustment and a prior capacity to function well both occupationally and socially. Recovery is usually complete.

In contrast to the endogenous depressive syndromes are depressive syndromes that are often referred to as chronic characterologic depressions. In these syndromes depressions may be an inherent part of a lifelong personality problem; relatively minor stresses or changes in life patterns may precipitate symptoms such as unhappiness, dissatisfaction, helplessness, dependency, and emotional instability, among others.

The situational depressions (sometimes called reactive depressions) occur as a result of an overwhelming situational stress. These depressions are very common and include pathologic bouts of grief and mourning. In such cases remission usually occurs within a few months. Occasionally, however, a situational depression may evolve into what appears to be a major endogenous depressive syndrome in which the symptoms become autonomous of the initial precipitating stress or subsequent related life events. Such instances provide clear-cut examples of endogenous depressions that indeed are precipitated by external environmental factors.

Emerging evidence of biological causes

Brain chemistry and depression. The brain consists of billions of cells called neurons, which interact with each other through electrical and neurochemical processes. Pharmacologic agents or environmental stimuli ultimately exert their effects in the brain by altering the processes regulating neurotransmission—*i.e.,* the communication within and between the neurons in the brain. When a neuron is stimulated, the nerve impulse causes a

"Melancholia," the title of both works on the opposite page, describes a profound state of depression. It is the term by which Hippocrates knew this emotional condition, which the ancient Greeks presumed was caused by the presence of black bile in the bloodstream. In the 1980s "melancholia" has been revived in the psychiatric nomenclature. Today a major depressive disorder with melancholia is characterized by a lack of response to pleasurable stimuli; it may also include early morning awakening, marked psychomotor slowness or agitation, significant weight loss, and inappropriate guilt. The engraving below of a restrained patient in a 19th-century French asylum depicts the manic phase of manic-depressive illness, a disorder in which episodes of sadness alternate with periods when mood may be elevated, expansive, or irritable.

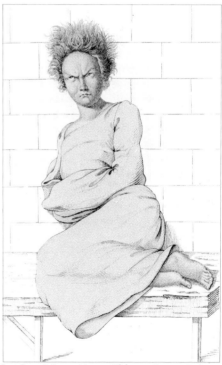

From *Des maladies mentales considérées sous les rapports médical, hygiénique et médico-légal,* E. Esquirol, Paris, J. B. Baillière, 1838; photograph, The National Library of Medicine, Bethesda, Md.

63

release of chemical substances called neurotransmitters from specialized regions at the neuronal ending that is in close proximity to another neuron. The space between the two neurons is called the synaptic cleft; the neuron leading into the synaptic cleft is called the presynaptic neuron, while the neuron leading away from the cleft is called the postsynaptic neuron. Neurotransmitters released into the synaptic cleft from the presynaptic neuron briefly interact with receptors on the postsynaptic neuron resulting in either electrical stimulation or inhibition in the postsynaptic neuron. Many different neurochemical substances act as neurotransmitters; many other chemical substances serve as neuromodulators and neuroregulators, which produce subtle alterations in the processes of neurotransmission.

Approximately 25 years ago two major classes of antidepressant drugs—the monoamine oxidase inhibitors and the tricyclic antidepressants—were first introduced, and shortly thereafter evidence began to suggest that these medications worked at least in part through their effects on brain catecholamines—one of the many groups of chemical substances that function as neurotransmitters. Of these catecholamines norepinephrine appeared to be particularly important in the pathophysiology of certain types of depressive disorders. Monoamine oxidase inhibiting drugs increased brain concentrations of norepinephrine by blocking its metabolism. Shortly thereafter the drug imipramine, a tricyclic antidepressant, was found to enhance the physiological effects of norepinephrine. At about the same time, reserpine (a drug used in the treatment of hypertension) was found to cause clinical depressions in some patients, and reserpine was also noted to deplete catecholamines in the brain.

On the basis of these and other data a hypothesis was proposed: that some depressive disorders may be associated with a deficiency of catecholamines, particularly norepinephrine, at functionally important synapses in the brain. Manias, on the other hand, might be associated with an excess of such catecholamines. From the outset it was recognized that this focus on catecholamine metabolism was at best an oversimplification of extremely complex biological states that undoubtedly involve abnormalities in many other neurochemical systems as well as endocrine changes and other biochemical abnormalities. Nonetheless, the possibility that different subgroups of patients with depressive disorders might be characterized by differences in their metabolism of norepinephrine and by abnormalities in the physiology of their noradrenergic (norepinephrine-containing) neuronal systems, including alterations in receptor sensitivity, was suggested. Studies by many research groups subsequently provided data supporting this possibility.

Since the late 1960s it has been recognized that a chemical compound known as 3-methoxy-4-hydroxyphenylglycol (MHPG), which is excreted in the urine, is a major metabolite (breakdown product) of norepinephrine originating in the brain. While urinary MHPG may also derive from noradrenergic neurons outside of the central nervous system, and the fraction of urinary MHPG deriving from norepinephrine originating in the brain remains uncertain, many investigators have explored the possibility that measurements of urinary MHPG levels might be of value in elucidating the functional changes occurring in depressions and in discriminating among biological subgroups

64

of depressed patients. Many studies of individual patients with bipolar manic-depressive disorders, for example, have shown that levels of urinary MHPG are lower during periods of depression and higher during periods of mania or hypomania (mild mania) than during periods of remission (wellness). But all depressed patients do not excrete comparably low levels of MHPG.

In contrast to the relatively consistent findings showing that patients with bipolar manic-depressive depressions have low urinary MHPG levels, consistent findings have not been obtained in studies of patients with diagnoses of unipolar depressions (made on the basis of the absence of a history of prior manic episodes). The data from these studies further substantiate that so-called unipolar depression is a broad grouping comprising many dissimilar subgroups, with only some showing low MHPG levels (comparable to values in bipolar depressions). MHPG levels in most depressed patients fall within the broad range of values observed in normal control subjects. While urinary MHPG levels may help to differentiate among subtypes of depressive disorders once a clinical diagnosis of depression has been made, these levels are not likely to be of value in making a diagnosis of depression *per se.*

Findings from a number of laboratories have now shown that measurement of urinary MHPG levels in depressed patients prior to treatment may aid in predicting clinical responses to certain antidepressant drugs. Moreover, data from recent studies suggest that measurements of urinary MHPG, particularly when taken in conjunction with urinary measurements of other catecholamine metabolites as well as norepinephrine itself, may aid in identifying patients with bipolar manic-depressive disorders even prior to the first clinical episode of mania.

Major leads concerning the possible underlying biochemical causes of depressive disorders have also come from studies of other neurotransmitters in the brain, such as dopamine (which is also a catecholamine) and serotonin (which is an indoleamine). Of considerable interest, too, are recent studies suggesting an important role for acetylcholine. Drugs that stimulate acetylcholinergic activity have been found to induce depressions in control subjects, to exacerbate depressions in depressed patients, and to decrease the intensity of episodes of mania. In this regard it is of interest to note that many of the commonly prescribed antidepressant drugs have anticholinergic properties (*i.e.,* they antagonize the effects of acetylcholine). These effects have long been recognized to be responsible for some of the side effects of the antidepressant drugs, such as dry mouth and constipation. Recently it has been recognized that anticholinergic effects *per se* may also be of importance for the antidepressant effects.

In addition to groundbreaking studies of specific neurotransmitters that are enhancing understanding of depression and how antidepressant drugs work, recent investigations have shown that the specific receptors upon which neurotransmitters act in order to exert their effects may also be of major importance. These receptors may be involved in the mechanisms of action of many antidepressant drugs. Additionally, alterations in receptors may have a role in the abnormal physiology of some depressive disorders. These possibilities are currently under active investigation in a number of laboratories throughout the world.

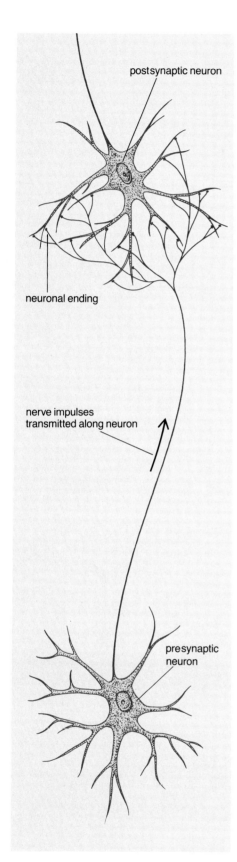

postsynaptic neuron

neuronal ending

nerve impulses
transmitted along neuron

presynaptic
neuron

Hormones and depression. In recent years it has been well documented that many patients with depressive disorders show abnormalities in various endocrine systems. Abnormalities in the secretion of growth hormone have been observed in some depressions.

A major finding, which has been replicated extensively, is that secretion of the adrenal hormone cortisol is significantly increased in certain depressed patients and that the normal circadian (daily) rhythm of cortisol secretion is abnormal in some depressions. In normal subjects administration of the drug dexamethasone suppresses cortisol secretion. These observations form the basis of increasing use by psychiatrists of the dexamethasone suppression test (a test commonly used in the diagnosis of certain endocrine disorders that involve overproduction of cortisone by the body). It has been found that certain depressed patients do not show a normal suppression of cortisol secretion after administration of dexamethasone. Secretion of cortisol by the adrenal gland is controlled, in part, by a hormone secreted by the pituitary gland, which in turn is controlled by a releasing factor that derives from the hypothalamus in the brain. The neurotransmitters norepinephrine, serotonin, and acetylcholine all appear to be involved in the regulation of this hypothalamic-pituitary-adrenocortical endocrine axis.

Thus, it is becoming increasingly clear that the abnormal processes at work are not restricted to brain function. Depressive disorders must be conceptualized as complex neuro-endocrino-metabolic disorders that involve many different organ systems throughout the body.

Sleep studies. One ongoing line of research into depressive disorders involves the study of sleep, since sleep abnormalities are very common in depressed patients. Insomnia with early morning awakening is one of the classic symptoms of endogenous depressions, although, as already noted, some depressed patients may show increased sleep. All-night electroencephalographic (EEG) recordings have shown that sleep occurs in stages that can be differentiated on the basis of EEG patterns. One of these sleep stages, rapid eye movement (REM) sleep, which is characterized by bursts of rapid eye movements, and by dreaming, may be abnormal in some depressions. A decrease in REM latency (the time between sleep onset and the first REM period of the night) has been well documented to occur in certain depressed patients. Recent studies have suggested that acetylcholinergic mechanisms are involved in initiating REM sleep, a finding that supports the notion that alterations in acetylcholinergic neurons may be involved in the abnormal physiology of at least some depressive disorders.

Genetics and family studies. Studies of the families of patients with depressive disorders show an increased prevalence of psychiatric illness among biological relatives. However, this alone does not establish that depressive disorders are genetically transmitted, since many nongenetic factors that may be of importance in predisposing individuals for depression (*e.g.,* poverty, life-style, and child-rearing practices) tend to run in families from generation to generation just as genetic traits do. Studies of depressive disorders in twins have shown that the concordance rate for depression is considerably higher in identical (monozygotic) twins than in fraternal (dizygotic) twins, and these rates are similar whether the twins are raised together or apart. Since

Photographs, John E. Heuser, University of California, San Francisco

monozygotic twins have identical genetic makeups, whereas dizygotic twins do not, these findings are of considerable value for assessing the genetic contribution to depressive disorders.

Evidence for genetic transmission of depressive disorders can also be obtained through adoption studies by studying adoptees separated at birth from their biologic parents and raised by nonrelatives. Several recent adoption studies have provided further support for a genetic factor in depressive disorders. On the basis of currently available data there appears to be good evidence for a genetic factor both in bipolar and unipolar affective illnesses. However, this clearly does not imply that psychosocial or psychological factors do not also play a role, since one of the conclusions that can also be drawn from the twin studies is that all people who share identical genetic vulnerability to depressive disorders do not show similar clinical manifestations of the illness. Thus, nongenetic familial and environmental factors also appear to be of importance.

While it is clear to most people that genetic disorders are expressed biochemically, it is often not realized that environmental or psychosocial factors also may produce long-term biochemical and physiological changes that can alter an individual's vulnerability to depressive episodes. With this awareness it becomes apparent that sharp distinctions cannot be drawn between genetically induced depressions and those that are environmentally induced or between biological depressions and psychological depressions.

The treatment of depression

There are many forms of treatment currently available for depressive disorders. These include many different types of antidepressant drugs, in some specific cases other ancillary pharmacologic agents (*e.g.,* thyroid hormones and lithium), electroconvulsive treatment (ECT), and psychotherapy.

Decisions concerning the use and choice of antidepressant drugs or ECT are generally made on the basis of the patient's signs, symptoms, and history, sometimes aided by specialized clinical laboratory tests. In contrast, decisions concerning the need for psychotherapy and the specific nature of that psychotherapy are based on criteria that include assessments of interpersonal and intrapsychic factors and of the patient's level of social adjustment and functioning prior to the depressive episode.

It is important to emphasize the fact that most depressive disorders are treatable conditions. The goal should be nothing less than complete restitution. All too often clinicians and patients alike settle for something less.

All depressed patients may be suicidal. This risk, therefore, must be recognized and evaluated in every depressed patient and, to the extent possible, minimizing the likelihood of suicide should be the first step in the treatment of depressed patients.

Psychotherapies. There are a number of specific forms of psychotherapy that have been developed for the treatment of depressive disorders. Two of these, interpersonal therapy and cognitive/behavioral therapy, are currently undergoing evaluation (in comparison with drug treatment) in a large-scale collaborative study sponsored by the National Institute of Mental Health (NIMH)—the first such "clinical trial" of its kind. Interpersonal therapy is a

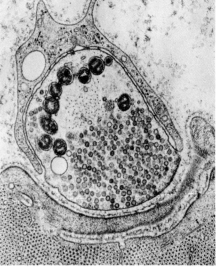

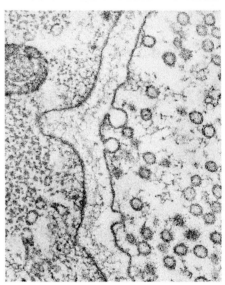

A schematic representation of a neuronal pathway is shown on the opposite page. Neurons communicate impulses by means of a chemical neurotransmitter that is released from the neuronal endings of the presynaptic neuron into the synaptic cleft, where they interact with receptors on the postsynaptic neuron. The photomicrographs above show the neuron ending (top), highly magnified, which is filled with saclike vesicles containing neurotransmitter molecules. On arrival of an impulse these vesicles fuse with the membrane of the neuronal ending and empty their contents into the synaptic cleft between the cells (bottom).

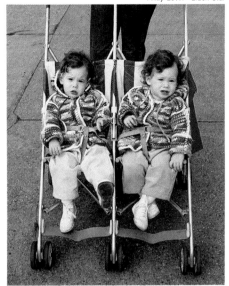

Many recent investigations into possible predisposing factors for the depressive disorders have focused on genetic links and nongenetic environmental and familial influences. Identical twins (who have exactly the same genetic makeup) have shown higher rates of concordance for depressions, even if they are raised apart, than do fraternal twins (whose genes are not identical). Such findings suggest a strong genetic component for at least some depressions.

psychodynamic treatment approach that focuses on the patient's current, rather than past, problems. The goals of therapy are to restore the patient's morale, enhance ability to cope with stress, and help the patient in dealing with the inevitable secondary consequences of illness. Cognitive/behavioral therapy is a short-term intervention that is aimed at correcting the depressed patient's negative view of himself, the world, and the future. To promote behavior and mood changes the patient is encouraged to adopt both positive thinking and more realistic and logical thinking. The goal of this form of therapy is to develop increased mastery of situations that the depressed patient previously considered to be hopeless.

The decision to treat a depressed patient with psychotherapy does not preclude the use of antidepressant drugs any more than treatment with antidepressant drugs precludes psychotherapy. Each form of treatment has its own set of indications (as well as contraindications), and these should be evaluated to determine the optimal therapeutic regimen for each individual.

Drugs. For the past two decades clinically effective antidepressant drugs have been available for the treatment of certain depressions. During the 1960s and 1970s these drugs included tricyclic antidepressants, such as imipramine and amitriptyline, and monoamine oxidase inhibitors, such as phenelzine and tranylcypromine, which, through different mechanisms, were thought to correct suspected chemical imbalances of vital central nervous system substances at critical sites in the brain. More recently, a number of newer types of antidepressant drugs have been introduced, and it is anticipated that during the coming years the range of available pharmacologic agents will increase.

Since many depressive disorders are often episodic in nature, with episodes lasting on average from three to six months, many clinicians will continue treatment with antidepressant drugs for at least six months following remission to minimize the risk of relapse. In some patients long-term maintenance treatment with an antidepressant drug may be needed to prevent the recurrences of depressive episodes. In a minority of cases individuals may not respond to the available antidepressants, and some patients have severe adverse reactions to them.

One of the major treatment advances of the past decade was the use of lithium—in the form of a salt—to prevent the recurrences of both manic and depressive episodes in patients with bipolar manic-depressive disorders. Long-term maintenance and regular dosage monitoring are necessary with this treatment. In some instances, when an acute episode of depression occurs in a manic-depressive patient undergoing preventive treatment with lithium, an antidepressant drug must be given in conjunction with the lithium, which is usually continued at its usual maintenance level.

For many years it has been routine to monitor serum lithium levels in manic-depressive disorders. More recently it has become possible to measure plasma levels of many of the currently prescribed antidepressant drugs. Patients can show marked differences in plasma levels of these drugs at similar doses, largely because of individual variability in drug metabolism. Whether these plasma levels of antidepressants should be monitored routinely is, as yet, an unresolved issue. Some clinical investigators believe that

68

measuring plasma levels may be useful under certain specific conditions, such as the failure to respond to a standard dose of an antidepressant drug or the occurrence of pronounced side effects following small drug doses. Others recommend monitoring routinely (whenever possible) in order to identify those patients who develop very high plasma levels on low doses, to document therapeutic levels at the time of clinical response as a guide to treating future episodes, and to document compliance or possible short-term metabolic changes in patients who respond and then relapse on a given dose. In the case of monoamine oxidase inhibitors measurement of specific plasma levels is not considered to be clinically useful; however, measuring the degree of monoamine oxidase inhibition produced in blood platelets may enable better monitoring of therapy.

Electroconvulsive therapy. A treatment first used in 1938, electroconvulsive therapy remains one of the most effective and safe methods for relieving severe depressions. ECT provides a brief electric shock to the brain, resulting in a seizure. Though no one yet knows precisely how ECT works, there has been a recent resurgence of interest in its use, particularly in cases of depressions recalcitrant to other therapeutic methods and when rapid symptom relief is considered crucial. ECT has been maligned because its initial success led to its overuse and in some cases inappropriate use.

Treatments of choice

Therapy for endogenous depressions. An initial trial of treatment with an antidepressant drug is generally indicated for patients with endogenous depressive disorders. If clinical improvement is not attained after an adequate trial of one antidepressant drug, treatment with another antidepressant with different pharmacologic properties should be considered. In some cases a number of different antidepressant drugs or drug combinations may have to be tried in order to attain the optimal treatment regimen for a given patient. Since a period of one to four weeks is generally required from the time of initial administration of an antidepressant to the onset of definitive clinical improvement, finding the right treatment regimen is sometimes a time-consuming procedure that requires considerable understanding and patience.

The use of ECT should be considered in patients with endogenous depressions who fail to respond to treatment with antidepressant drugs. Owing to the delay in onset of the therapeutic effects of antidepressants, ECT may be selected as the initial form of treatment for some depressed patients, particularly those judged to be highly suicidal.

Although some depressed patients may appear to be relatively unresponsive to interpersonal interactions during the early phase of treatment with antidepressant drugs, the physician's support and optimism are extremely important to both the patient and his family. Moreover, it is important for a physician to provide all concerned individuals with a realistic perception of the patient's prognosis (which is very good in most cases of endogenous depressions) in order to help counteract and attenuate the patient's lingering sense of hopelessness and despair. Attempts to mobilize the patient into purposeful activity at this early stage are often unsuccessful and may only

Depressions are estimated to affect 127 million people across the globe. The high toll of social isolation and emotional pain is of course immeasurable. Staggeringly high suicide rates among the depressed represent an especially tragic outcome since most depressions are treatable conditions.

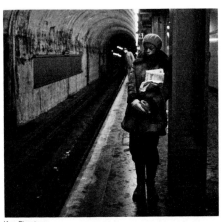

Ken Firestone

69

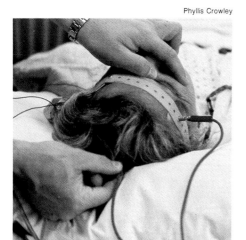

Electroconvulsive therapy (ECT) is a treatment that was first used in Italy in 1938; it remains one of the most effective and safe methods for relieving severe depressions. In the photograph above a mild electric current is about to be delivered into the brain of a patient at the Massachusetts General Hospital in Boston to produce a brief convulsion; throughout the procedure the patient is asleep and receives air and oxygen through a face mask.

reinforce the patient's sense of inadequacy, but support of the patient's self-initiated realistic attempts to maintain activities during this period is crucial.

When a patient with an endogenous depression starts to improve on antidepressant drugs, the effect may be striking. The exact day of onset of clinical improvement can often be identified. The patient may rally in a number of notable ways—his carriage may become more erect, movements more agile, and facial expressions more animated. The patient characteristically becomes more responsive to his surroundings at this time. Whereas decreasing environmental stimulation sometimes serves an important function in the management of manic patients, the reverse may be of value in the treatment of patients with an endogenous depression once clinical improvement has begun. Being in contact with others, participating in everyday activities, and coping with everyday problems can greatly help in restoring a sense of self-worth and can hasten and perpetuate further improvement.

Treating chronic characterologic depressions. Many patients with chronic characterologic depressions show transient improvement with many different forms of therapeutic intervention, including supportive interpersonal therapy. Some of these patients may be stuck in unrewarding life circumstances; thus short-term psychotherapy may help them to make appropriate changes. Since some of these patients will improve when treated with antidepressant drugs, the use of drug therapy is generally indicated for patients who do not respond within a reasonable period of time to psychotherapy alone. More intensive psychodynamically oriented psychotherapy may be required for the long-term treatment of certain chronically depressed individuals.

Therapy for situational depressions. Situational depressions (which include grief reactions and mourning) are generally self-limited conditions; remissions usually occur within a few months. Some patients may require little more than the reassurance that they are experiencing a normal reaction to a loss, although others may benefit from psychotherapy aimed at coping with the loss directly. Antidepressant drugs are generally not required unless the situational depression evolves into a more profound and ongoing endogenous depressive syndrome.

Therapy for drug-induced depressions. In some cases drugs commonly used to treat a wide variety of medical conditions may cause psychiatric symptoms—in particular, depression. The first step in evaluating and treating patients with drug-induced depressions is the identification and discontinuation (if medically feasible) of the drug responsible for the depressive syndrome. Most drug-induced depressions will undergo remission after discontinuation of the offending pharmacologic agent. For those that persist or when it is not feasible to discontinue the drug causing the depression, simultaneous treatment with antidepressant drugs or ECT may be required.

The emerging field of psychiatric chemistry

It is clear that we have already reached a point where the clinical laboratory can be used in psychiatry as it is in other fields of medicine, both to assist the clinician in making more specific diagnoses and to aid him in prescribing more effectively. Recognizing this fact, in 1977 the Harvard Medical School

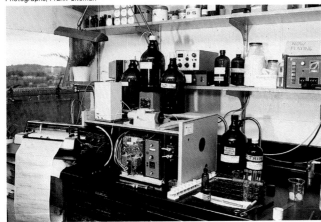 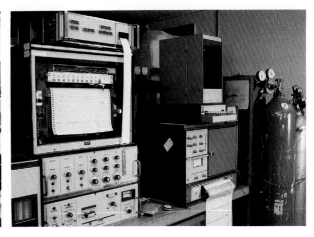

department of psychiatry and the department of pathology at the New England Deaconess Hospital established a psychiatric chemistry laboratory as a model academic facility for the integration and translation of biochemical research into clinical psychiatric practice. In addition to providing specialized lab tests, an explicit aim of the psychiatric chemistry laboratory has been to provide education and consultative services to assist physicians in using and interpreting these tests.

It is now possible and useful to draw an analogy between the pneumonias and the depressions in that both disorders can be diagnosed on the basis of clinical data. In the case of the pneumonias—illnesses caused by a wide variety of agents, mostly bacterial or viral organisms—it is crucial to identify the causative agent for proper treatment. The physician makes a diagnosis based on history and physical examination (including a chest X-ray). After the diagnosis is made, sputum cultures can be obtained from the patient and analyzed in the clinical laboratory to aid in determining the specific type of pneumonia as well as the specific antibiotic or other form of treatment that may be most effective. Similarly, in the case of depressions the physician can make a diagnosis based on clinical history coupled with physical and mental status examinations. He can then use specialized clinical laboratory tests to obtain further information to assist in determining the type of depression the patient has and the forms of treatment most likely to be effective in the care of that patient.

While the biochemical tests we have today do not necessarily enable physicians to select a clinically effective treatment on the first trial, the use of these clinical laboratory tests can increase the probability of their doing so. Considering the time it takes for antidepressant drugs to exert their clinical effects, even a small increase in the percentage of patients who receive an effective drug on the first clinical trial of treatment would represent a major advance in the treatment of patients with depressive disorders.

Today the clinical laboratory can be used in psychiatry as it is in other branches of medicine to assist the physician in making specific diagnoses and to aid in the prescribing of potentially effective medications. The photographs above show two specialized laboratory machines—a liquid chromatograph (left) and a gas chromatograph (right)—which are used in the diagnosis of depressions at Boston's Massachusetts Mental Health Center.

FOR ADDITIONAL READING:
American Psychiatric Association. *Diagnostic and Statistical Manual of Mental Disorders, Third Edition.* Washington, D.C.: American Psychiatric Association, 1980.

Schildkraut, J. J. *Neuropsychopharmacology and the Affective Disorders.* Boston: Little, Brown and Co., 1970.

Teuting, Patricia; Koslow, S. H.; and Hirschfeld, R. M. A. *Special Report on Depression Research.* NIMH Science Reports Series. Washington, D.C.: Government Printing Office, 1981.

Wender, P. H., and Klein, D. F. *Mind, Mood and Medicine: A Guide to the New Biological Psychiatry.* New York: Farrar, Straus and Giroux, 1981.

Winokur, George. *Depression: The Facts.* New York: Oxford University Press, 1981.

Schizophrenia
by Harrison G. Pope, Jr., M.D.

Ask someone off the street for a definition of "schizophrenia," and he may well tell you that it means having a "split personality." Or he may recall that a distant relative was hospitalized with a "nervous breakdown" once when she was in her forties, and that the doctors diagnosed her as "schizophrenic." In fact, neither of these impressions is correct. Schizophrenia is unrelated to multiple personality, and most so-called nervous breakdowns represent cases of manic-depressive illness. What is the correct definition of schizophrenia? Unfortunately, even experienced psychiatrists vary widely in their responses to this question. Perhaps the best way to answer it is to examine the evolution of the term schizophrenia in the 20th century.

The changing definitions of schizophrenia

Emil Kraepelin is usually credited as the person who first defined the syndrome of schizophrenia at the beginning of this century. He did not use the term schizophrenia, however, to name the group of patients being described but rather used *dementia praecox,* because he believed that they suffered from a dementing process in the brain with an onset early in life (hence *praecox,* derived from the Latin, meaning "premature"), which distinguished it from the types of dementia that commonly occur in elderly people. Kraepelin distinguished dementia praecox from manic-depressive illness on the grounds that patients with dementia praecox tended to pursue a chronic course characterized by deterioration in their mental abilities and accompanied by delusions, hallucinations, catatonic symptoms, withdrawal, loss of the capacity to express emotions, loss of social contact, and a gradual decay of many other psychic functions. Patients with manic-depressive illness, on the other hand, displayed a course of illness marked by exacerbations and remissions: they would become periodically manic—euphoric, hyperactive, with racing thoughts, pressured speech, and sleeplessness—and then at other times depressed, with excessive sleep, loss of energy, loss of appetite, hopelessness, guilt, and suicidal feelings. However, in between the manic and depressive episodes, these patients would have periods of complete remission of the symptoms. Unlike dementia praecox patients, manic-depressive patients did not progress to deterioration. These distinctions between dementia praecox and manic-depressive illness constituted a major step forward in psychiatry; it helped to clarify the confusing assortment of

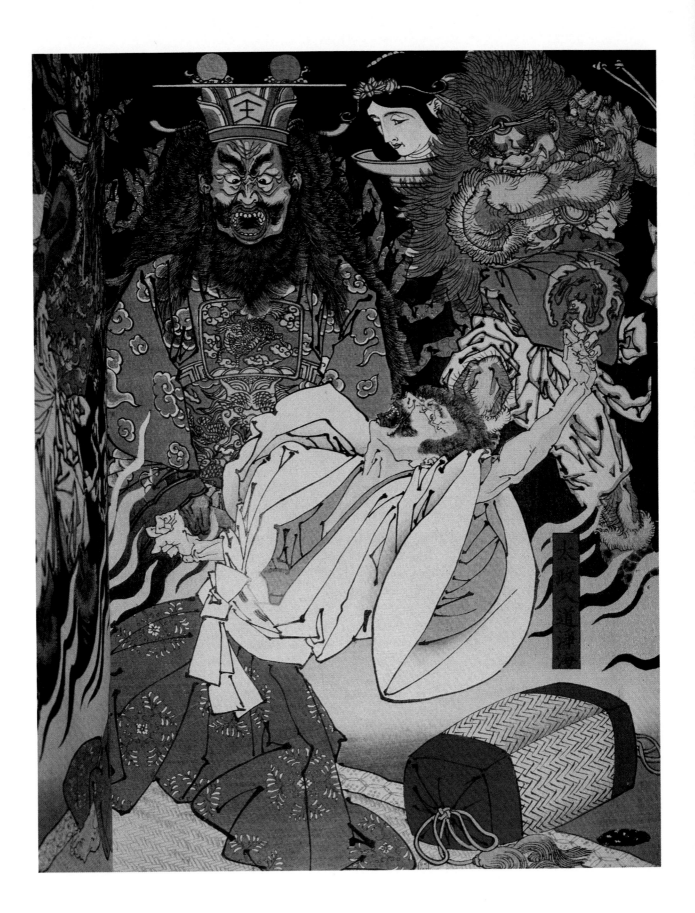

From *Dementia Praecox and Paraphrenia*, Emil Kraepelin, Edinburgh, E. & S. Livingstone, 1919

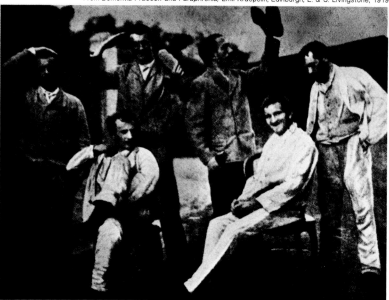

This photograph of schizophrenic patients is from German psychiatrist Emil Kraepelin's Dementia Praecox and Paraphrenia, *published in 1919. Kraepelin was the first to clearly define the syndrome of schizophrenia, which he called dementia praecox. He distinguished the disorder from senile dementia and manic-depressive illness.*

Harrison G. Pope, Jr., M.D., *is Assistant Clinical Professor of Psychiatry at the Mailman Research Center, McLean Hospital, Belmont, Massachusetts, and Instructor in Psychiatry at Harvard Medical School, Boston.*

(Overleaf) 19th-century Japanese print depicting hallucinations, attributed to Yoshi Toshi; photograph, Jean-Loup Charmet, Paris

"psychotic" patients who were in the care of psychiatrists of the day.

As the years passed, Kraepelin's concept was modified in many different ways. The first major figure in this process was Eugen Bleuler, the man who coined the term schizophrenia. Bleuler subscribed to most of the original views of Kraepelin but went on to describe in great detail what he believed to be the fundamental psychic disturbances that caused schizophrenia. At the core of the illness, he hypothesized, was a "splitting" of the psychic functions. This splitting he felt to be manifest in a number of disturbances, which he termed "fundamental symptoms." Among these are the so-called four A's: (1) looseness of *associations,* a tendency for the patient to jump from one subject to another in his thinking and speech without an obvious connection between the subjects; (2) flat or inappropriate *affect,* an inability of the patient to display the normal modulation of mood and expression in response to pleasant or unpleasant subjects or stimuli; (3) *autism,* withdrawal from the world and from social contacts; and (4) *ambivalence,* inability to resolve conflicting ideas. Bleuler considered such symptoms as delusions, hallucinations, and catatonia to be secondary or "accessory" symptoms.

Unfortunately, Bleuler's list of symptoms made it difficult to define precisely the boundaries of schizophrenia. One observer might see flatness of affect or autism where another did not. Furthermore, unlike Kraepelin, Bleuler did not insist on chronicity or deterioration as a necessary part of the clinical picture. As a result patients with briefer, remitting psychotic syndromes came to be diagnosed as schizophrenic, expanding the number of schizophrenic patients over the number Kraepelin would have diagnosed as suffering from dementia praecox.

Over the course of the next several decades the trend continued. Part of this was due to the vague definition, making it possible to apply it to a large spectrum of cases. Another important influence was that of psychoanalytic theory. Psychoanalytic theory tended to regard schizophrenia as the result

of a severe deficit of ego function, and hence the term schizophrenia became, in the hands of many psychiatrists, almost a synonym for "severely
ill." Yet another broadening influence was the suggestion that specific symptoms might be "pathognomonic" for schizophrenia—*i.e.,* these symptoms
were believed to occur exclusively in cases of schizophrenia and not in any
other disorders. The idea of a pathognomonic symptom had great appeal to
many psychiatrists; it meant that if a given patient were found to display one
of the putative pathognomonic symptoms, then the patient definitely had
schizophrenia. One of the greatest exponents of this idea was a German
psychiatrist, Kurt Schneider, who enumerated 11 symptoms which became
known as the Schneiderian first-rank symptoms and were widely used in Europe in the diagnosis of schizophrenia. Among the first-rank symptoms were
certain types of auditory hallucinations, the sensation that others would read
the patient's thoughts ("thought broadcasting"), and the sensation that the
patient was being controlled by outside forces ("experiences of influence").
Recently, many studies have demonstrated that Schneiderian first-rank
symptoms occur in patients with a wide variety of psychiatric disorders other
than schizophrenia. But for years any patient displaying even a single
Schneiderian manifestation was automatically diagnosed as schizophrenic
in many hospitals.

As a result of these influences, schizophrenia became bloated into an
enormous category, embracing a vast group of heterogeneous patients. This
becomes graphically evident when one looks at psychiatric admissions to
various hospitals in the United States. In one study at the New York State
Psychiatric Institute, for example, it was found that in the 1920s about 20%
of patients were diagnosed as having schizophrenia. This figure gradually
rose so that by the 1940s more than half of all admissions to the hospital
were diagnosed as schizophrenic. The trend peaked in the 1950s, at which
point "schizophrenia" accounted for more than 80% of all admission diagnoses. This meant that all other psychiatric disorders combined—manic-depressive illness, alcoholism and other forms of drug abuse, senile demen-
tias, all other organic disorders, all neurotic disorders, all personality
disorders, all sexual deviations, and all other psychiatric disorders—accounted for less than one-fifth of patients. Needless to say, by this point the
term had lost much of its meaning and had become almost useless as a label
that communicated specific diagnostic information about patients.

Finally, starting in the late 1960s and early 1970s, the trend began to be reversed; it was increasingly recognized that "schizophrenia" needed to be
knocked down to size. Two findings were particularly important. First, it was
recognized that many patients diagnosed as schizophrenic were in fact
suffering from various forms of manic-depressive illness. A large percentage
of patients with manic-depressive illness, it was found, display delusions and
hallucinations in the same manner as patients with schizophrenia. Second,
many individuals with odd or eccentric behavior or with personality disturbances that did not respond to psychotherapy, but without actual delusions
or hallucinations, were diagnosed in the '50s and '60s as having "latent
schizophrenia," "pseudoneurotic schizophrenia," or "pseudopsychopathic
schizophrenia." Increasingly it has been acknowledged that these patients

*Des maladies mentales considérées sous les rapports
médical, hygiénique et medico-légal,* E. Esquirol, Paris, J. B.
Baillière, 1838; photograph, The National Library of
Medicine, Bethesda, Md.

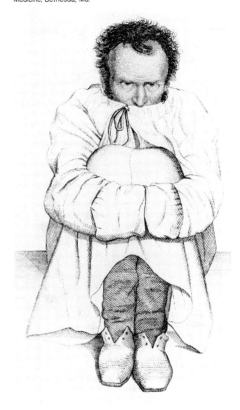

*Delusions, hallucinations, withdrawal, or
loss of social contact often resulted in
the branding of patients as schizophrenic
whether or not the disease showed a
chronic, deteriorating course. Only in
the past 20 years has it come to be
recognized that many "schizophrenics"
were in fact misdiagnosed.*

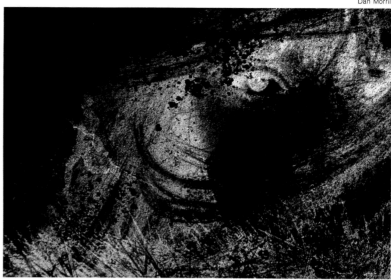

The idea that schizophrenia could be diagnosed by observing any one of a number of "pathognomonic" symptoms— i.e., symptoms thought to be exclusive to this disorder and no other—also served to expand the number of patients categorized as schizophrenic. Among pathognomonic symptoms of the first rank were feelings that others could read the patient's mind and that outside forces were directing the patient's behavior. Recent studies have demonstrated the presence of such symptoms in patients with many other kinds of mental disorders.

do not suffer from schizophrenia either but represent cases of personality disorders. As a result of these changes, the diagnostic category of schizophrenia is now gradually being reduced to its scope of 60 years ago.

In 1980 a significantly revised classification system of all mental illness appeared with the publication of the third edition of the American Psychiatric Association's *Diagnostic and Statistical Manual of Mental Disorders,* commonly known as *DSM-III.* This manual provides a new nomenclature that attempts to bring order to a great deal of the confusion that had long characterized psychiatric diagnoses. *DSM-III*'s definition of schizophrenia is quite elaborate but worth describing in some detail since it represents the "official" definition today.

There are six criteria for the *DSM-III* definition. (1) The patient must display at least *one* symptom from a list of specific symptoms: certain types of delusions; certain types of auditory hallucinations; delusions accompanied by hallucinations or incoherence; illogical thinking or poverty of content of speech associated with flatness of affect; delusions or catatonic behavior. (2) The patient must have deteriorated from a previous level of functioning in such areas as work, social relations, and self-care. (3) The illness must have persisted for at least six months at some time in the person's life with some signs of the illness currently. It is not necessary for the patient to have had active delusions and hallucinations throughout the six-month period, but he must at least have had prodromal symptoms (indicating the onset of illness) or residual symptoms such as social isolation, impairment in role functioning, peculiar behavior, and the like. (4) The patient must not have displayed a syndrome of mania or depression for a long period of time during the course of the illness (this criterion reflects the recent findings, mentioned above, that patients with manic-depressive illness also commonly display delusions or hallucinations). (5) The illness must have begun before the age of 45. (6) The illness must not be attributable to an organic mental disorder (*i.e.,* a neurological disease) or to mental retardation.

76

Adapted from "On Trends in the Diagnosis of Schizophrenia," Judith B. Kuriansky, W. Edwards Deming, and Barry J. Gurland, *American Journal of Psychiatry,* April 1974, pp. 402–408

Patients diagnosed schizophrenic

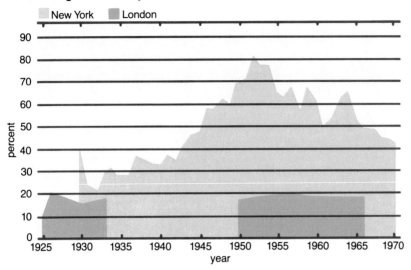

One reason for the far more specific and strict criteria is to make scientific communication possible. If, for example, a psychiatrist in California is studying 50 "schizophrenic" patients, and another individual in Boston conducts a similar study of 50 "schizophrenics," it is crucial that the two workers be sure that they are looking at the same types of patients. Otherwise their findings would be almost impossible to compare.

Another reason for the explicitness of definition is to eliminate from the domain of "schizophrenia" patients who have other well-established psychiatric disorders such as personality disorders and, as already mentioned, manic-depressive illness. This is essential because the treatment of the latter disorders is markedly different from the treatment of schizophrenia.

Experience suggests that the *DSM-III* criteria for defining schizophrenia and other mental disorders will hardly be the last word. In future years further refinements undoubtedly will be made; the current criteria may even be discarded entirely. For the time being, however, the term schizophrenia used here is based on the above six features, since these represent the closest to a "consensus" definition at present.

What causes schizophrenia?

Unlike medical conditions such as pneumonia or diabetes, in which laboratory evidence can be used to confirm or deny a diagnosis, most psychiatric conditions cannot as yet be diagnosed on the basis of objective findings. Hence there are at present no tests to help resolve disputes as to who has schizophrenia and who does not or where the boundaries actually lie. Not surprisingly, therefore, theories on the causes of schizophrenia are as confused and contradictory as the definitions. The etiology, in fact, remains unknown; research in this area has been filled with failures and conflicting findings, in large measure owing to the fact that schizophrenia has been defined in such different ways by so many different individuals that it has been exceedingly difficult for researchers to be sure that they are studying similar

The changing definition of "schizophrenia" in the U.S. over a 40-year span is evident in the dramatic rise and fall in the proportion of patients diagnosed as schizophrenic upon admission to New York State Psychiatric Institute between 1930 and 1970. The most embracing concept of the disorder prevailed in the 1950s, when schizophrenics accounted for more than 80% of all diagnoses at admission. By contrast, at London's Maudsley Hospital schizophrenic admissions remained at a fairly constant level of 20% through the years, suggesting that the concept of schizophrenia in the U.K. remained much more stable and narrowly defined.

77

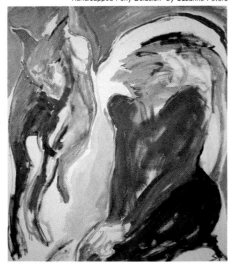

Today certain kinds of delusions and hallucinations may, but need not, constitute one criterion among a total of six that must all be met for a diagnosis of schizophrenia.

(Opposite page) Impulses are passed from neuron to neuron in the brain by means of intimate contacts, called synapses, between nerve endings on one neuron and the body of the next neuron (top). The actual agent of communication is a chemical transmitter, which is released from saclike vesicles in the nerve ending and which diffuses across the synaptic gap to receptor sites on the adjacent neuron (center). Studies suggest that an excess of one such transmitter, dopamine, may be the cause of such psychotic symptoms as delusions and hallucinations. Antipsychotic drugs appear to successfully compete for dopamine receptor sites, thereby blocking access by dopamine (bottom).

populations of patients. The failure of much of the research is attributable then not to the incompetence of researchers but rather to the lack of agreement as to what schizophrenia means.

With these essential caveats in mind, we can summarize the major research on the etiology of schizophrenia. One large body has been concerned with "psychodynamic" forces that might contribute to schizophrenia, such as the behavior of the mother, the father, early childhood experiences, early social experiences, and early environmental influences in development. It is impossible to describe the thousands of studies that have been performed in all of these areas. It often seems, however, that for every six studies suggesting one influence, there are half a dozen other studies supporting an opposite hypothesis. For example, some studies have suggested that schizophrenia is caused in the child by an overly close, binding, and enveloping mother, whereas other studies have suggested that schizophrenia is caused by a distant and cold mother who remains remote from her children during childhood. Still other studies have suggested that schizophrenia is caused by mothers who display a combination of both of these features. And still other studies have suggested that schizophrenia does not have much to do with the mother at all. This is an oversimplification, of course, but it seems fair to say that no *well-replicated,* widely accepted findings have clearly implicated any specific "psychodynamic" factor. This does not prove that psychodynamic factors are of no consequence; it merely suggests that no one factor is likely to be of central importance. It also suggests that it is wrong to "blame" the mother or father or familial situation when schizophrenia appears in a child. It is possible, and even likely, on the basis of what is known thus far, that the mother and father have little influence on the appearance of schizophrenia.

Interpretation of the results of psychodynamic studies is rendered even more difficult by the fact that most were performed in the days before narrow definitions of schizophrenia, such as that of *DSM-III.* Hence, they may have included numbers of patients who would now be considered to have manic-depressive illness and personality disorders, which may partially explain their failure to produce consistent and replicable findings.

So-called biological studies of schizophrenia have risen in prominence in recent years; it is probably fair to say that a majority of researchers now believe that schizophrenia is at least partially a biological disorder. However, these biological studies have fared little better than the psychodynamic ones in achieving consistent or replicable results; for example, putative chemical abnormalities found in the blood or urine of schizophrenics were later found to be due merely to hospital diet, to errors in laboratory technique, or to other external factors.

Two specific biological findings are worth mention because they have so often been cited in conjunction with schizophrenia. A number of different lines of biological evidence suggest that psychotic symptoms—particularly delusions and hallucinations—may be caused by an excess of a substance called dopamine at certain sites in the brain. Dopamine is a neurotransmitter, a substance synthesized at the tip of a nerve cell that diffuses across a very small space to the beginning of the next cell in the chain, causing it in turn to "fire." Antipsychotic drugs appear to block the effects of dopamine, causing delusions and hallucinations to regress. On the other hand, drugs that increase dopamine levels—such as amphetamines—actually cause delusions and hallucinations when taken in large enough doses for long enough periods. Although these important findings provide a clue to the cause of some psychotic symptoms, such symptoms are common to many disorders (manic-depressive illness, depressive psychoses, senile psychoses, and so forth). Understanding the cause of psychotic symptoms alone does not reveal the cause of the underlying disorder, schizophrenia, any more than understanding the cause of "cough" or "fever" reveals the cause of tuberculosis.

A number of other studies have provided impressive evidence of a hereditary component in schizophrenia. Again, though, it is unfortunate that most of the best studies were performed in the 1960s or early 1970s, when the definition of schizophrenia was very broad. There is very strong evidence of a major hereditary component in manic-depressive illness, and a number of studies have demonstrated a genetic component in personality disorders as well—particularly in so-called antisocial personality disorder. Therefore, given that the earlier studies of heredity in schizophrenia may well have included an admixture of cases of other such disorders, these would now have to be factored out. Many recent studies, which have taken care to exclude cases of manic-depressive illness and personality disorders, also have reported a hereditary component in schizophrenia, but a much smaller one.

Currently, a number of biological findings in schizophrenia are the subject of intensive research. For example, upon X-ray examinations of the brain, using computerized axial tomography (the CAT scan), researchers have demonstrated abnormalities in the brains of many schizophrenic patients. In particular the cerebral ventricles—pockets in the center of the brain filled with spinal fluid—appear to be dilated in schizophrenic patients as compared with normal individuals. But other groups, using identical techniques, have been unable to demonstrate this finding in schizophrenic populations. Furthermore, even those groups that have reported positive findings have demonstrated ventricular dilatation in only a fraction of schizophrenic patients. Some patients, who were equally ill and who had comparably severe symptoms, had no dilatation at all. This is typical of the conflicting findings that have emerged from biological studies. At first the temptation might be to assume that, since the results are inconsistent across different studies, they may be of no significance. However, a more likely hypothesis is that schizophrenia is a heterogenous disorder and may perhaps represent a dozen different diseases. Some of these "schizophrenias" may be associated with cerebral ventricular dilatation, whereas others are not.

Similarly, many other biological abnormalities have been demonstrated in certain schizophrenic patients but not in others. Some schizophrenics display a reduced level of an enzyme called monoamine oxidase. Others show a dramatic inability to smoothly track a moving object with their eyes. Others show evidence suggesting that their symptoms might be caused by a "slow virus" with a very long incubation period. Like the CAT scan findings above, all of these findings are positive in a certain number of schizophrenics but

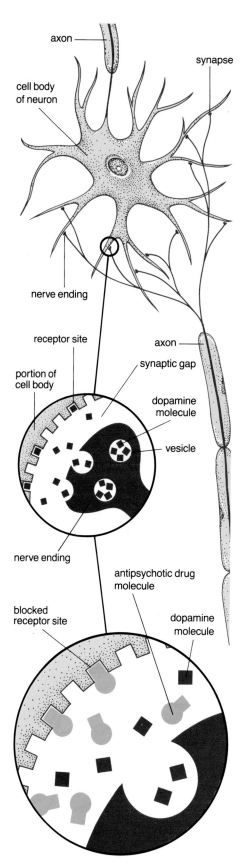

Photographs, Daniel Weinberger and Richard Jed Wyatt, St. Elizabeth's Hospital, Washington, D.C.

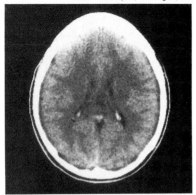

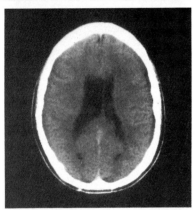

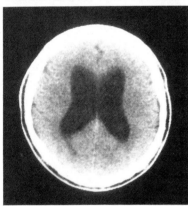

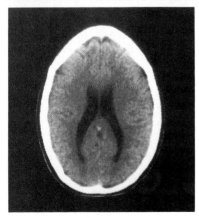

rarely in a majority of cases. Again the most likely explanation seems to be that schizophrenia is a heterogeneous disorder representing several different diseases.

Throughout the years biologically oriented researchers have often pointed to the failure of psychodynamic research as evidence that schizophrenia does not have a psychodynamic origin but is a biological disease. Conversely, psychodynamic researchers have pointed to the failure of biological researchers as evidence that there is no specific biological abnormality in schizophrenia and that schizophrenia is due to psychological or environmental factors. But it seems more likely that neither of these arguments is correct. Schizophrenia, even as narrowly defined as it is in *DSM-III*, may comprise many "schizophrenias," some associated with biological abnormalities and others attributable primarily to psychodynamic factors. Indeed, the question arises as to whether it is even fair to speak of a specific disorder schizophrenia at all. As new research findings emerge, we may be forced to replace the name schizophrenia entirely with several more specific terms.

A paucity of successful treatments

Given the confused state of research on the causes of schizophrenia, it should come as little surprise that treatment approaches have followed comparably contradictory courses. Psychotherapy was for many years the principal method of treatment claiming any success. Although a number of early psychodynamic theorists, including Freud, were skeptical about the efficacy of "talking" therapies for schizophrenia and other psychotic disorders, many volumes were written in subsequent years detailing psychodynamic interpretations for schizophrenics' speech, thought, and actions. The test of these, obviously, is whether psychotherapy actually worked. Again, the literature is filled with anecdotal accounts of schizophrenia successfully treated with psychotherapy, in which the patient apparently emerged with a complete remission of psychotic symptoms. However, as we have seen, earlier definitions of schizophrenia included many patients who would now be diagnosed as cases of manic-depressive illness. Given the fact that manic-depressive illness typically remits by itself, it is possible that the reported successful treatment of some "schizophrenic" patients may have simply represented the spontaneous remission of an illness that would have gotten better regardless of what anyone had done.

More recent and sophisticated studies have placed some schizophrenic patients in psychotherapy and "matched" groups of patients in other treatments. In one of the largest such studies, conducted in California beginning in the early 1970s, patients were assigned to several different groups including some treated with psychotherapy, some treated with drugs, some treated with electroshock therapy, and some given essentially no treatment except for the hospital milieu. These patients were then followed over many years; a long-term follow-up on them was published in 1981. Interestingly, the patients treated with drugs, those treated with shock therapy, and the ones that received no treatment at all (except the standard ward treatment) did about equally well over the long term, whereas patients treated with psychotherapy actually did somewhat worse. Studies such as this, suggesting that psycho-

80

therapy might be ineffective in schizophrenia, naturally have aroused a storm of protest from many quarters. One criticism has been that psychotherapy was performed by inexperienced individuals, suggesting that senior therapists would be more successful. In response, another study was performed in Boston in which one group of schizophrenic patients was treated intensively by well-qualified psychoanalytic therapists and was compared with another group of patients who received no psychotherapy. But again it was found that there were no major differences in the two groups of patients.

These studies suggest that psychotherapy may have little or no effect on schizophrenia at all. However, there are countless other studies of family therapy, occupational and social therapies, group therapy, and other "psychosocial" therapies that have demonstrated *some* beneficial effects in various populations of schizophrenic patients. Again, many of these studies were poorly controlled—they did not have well-matched samples of patients who were used as comparison groups. Also, many of these studies suffered from the old problem of the likely inclusion of manic-depressives.

Nonetheless, it seems fair to say that psychosocial therapies probably do have a modest influence on the outcome of schizophrenia, particularly in helping schizophrenic patients to become reaccustomed to the community and to become involved in better social relationships and in successful employment. But it also appears that such therapies have little effect on delusions, hallucinations, and other psychotic symptoms.

Many readers may be familiar with one or another of the various accounts of schizophrenia that have been written by "schizophrenic" patients; *e.g., The Eden Express* by Mark Vonnegut and *I Never Promised You a Rose Garden* by Hannah Green. Some of these books describe apparent cures of schizophrenia through psychotherapy. An interesting reanalysis of these (and other similar accounts) was performed by Carol North and Remi Cadoret at the University of Iowa School of Medicine. Researchers North and Cadoret found that none of the "first-person" writers appeared to be suffering from bona fide schizophrenia. In fact, most appeared to be suffering from manic-depressive illness, and some, such as patient Blau in *I Never Promised You a Rose Garden*, were diagnosed as probably suffering from hysterical personality, or what *DSM-III* would call "somatoform disorder." Therefore, successful treatments of "schizophrenia," which are described in the popular press, must be regarded with the same skepticism as anecdotal reports in the scientific literature.

Since the discovery of the antipsychotic drugs chlorpromazine (Thorazine) and its derivatives in the early 1950s, pharmacologic treatments for schizophrenia have gradually risen in prominence. Immediately after the introduction of these drugs to the United States and through the "deinstitutionalization" movement of the '60s, there was a dramatic decrease in the number of patients in state hospitals. Unfortunately, rendering a patient capable of being discharged from a hospital does not constitute a cure; although antipsychotic drugs are quite effective in eliminating delusions, hallucinations, and incoherence of speech in many patients, they do little to attack such symptoms as withdrawal, loss of motivation, and loss of appropriate affect. Schizophrenic patients who have responded to antipsychotic drugs may be

John Morihisa, National Institute of Mental Health, and Frank Duffy, Harvard University

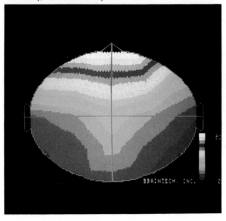

New, noninvasive techniques for imaging the living brain have made it possible to demonstrate abnormalities in the brains of some schizophrenics. A CAT scan of the brain of a normal individual (opposite page, top) is compared with three others taken of schizophrenics; the prominent central dark regions in the latter represent abnormally enlarged cerebral ventricles. Brain electrical activity map (BEAM) of a patient with schizophrenia (above) represents a new color mapping technique based on a computerized analysis of electroencephalographic data.

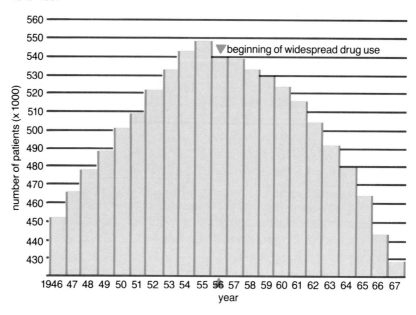

Impact of antipsychotic drugs
1946–1967

Data from the U.S. Public Health Service

number of patients (× 1000)

▼beginning of widespread drug use

560
550
540
530
520
510
500
490
480
470
460
450
440
430

1946 47 48 49 50 51 52 53 54 55 56 57 58 59 60 61 62 63 64 65 66 67
year

The graph illustrates the dramatic change in the population of mental hospitals in the U.S. since the introduction of antipsychotic drugs in the mid-1950s. Although these drugs have eliminated for many patients the bizarre behavior and most florid symptoms of schizophrenia, such as delusions, hallucinations, and incoherence of speech, they appear to have little effect on symptoms of withdrawal, loss of motivation, and the absence of appropriate emotional response to outside stimuli. Hence, schizophrenic patients receiving antipsychotic drugs can still be quite severely handicapped in their ability to function in society.

rational and capable of maintaining coherent conversations, but they may still be visibly withdrawn, lacking in initiative, and lacking in the ability to experience pleasure (a state called anhedonia). Moreover, they are still visibly "mental patients" to even a casual observer. Thus, biological treatments in schizophrenia have a long way to go before they can claim to be "cures."

Aside from the antipsychotic drugs, many other biological treatments have been investigated, but few have been found useful. Drugs such as lithium carbonate and antidepressants or treatments such as electroshock therapy have all been thought effective in *some* schizophrenic patients, but it is possible that most of these patients, once again, were misdiagnosed manic-depressives. Other treatments proposed in recent years include hormones such as the endorphins or thyrotropin releasing hormone (TRH). But whether any of these is truly helpful remains to be established.

In short, then, at the present time it can be said that delusions, hallucinations, and other "positive" psychotic symptoms can usually be controlled pharmacologically with antipsychotic drugs in most patients. Following this, psychosocial therapies appear to have some value in helping to rehabilitate the patient to better social and occupational function. However, neither biological nor psychosocial therapies effectively reverse the "negative" symptoms of schizophrenia; most patients will continue to show withdrawal, impaired social functioning, lack of motivation, and other such features. Most schizophrenics who respond well to drugs still have difficulty in becoming self-sufficient. Those not fortunate enough to live with relatives or in well-staffed halfway houses or group homes often drift into the lowest socioeconomic classes, where they are vulnerable to all of the effects of poverty and often to other medical illnesses. Many of these patients periodically stop taking their medications, are rehospitalized, and are discharged, only to resume the cycle and be readmitted—the revolving-door syndrome.

82

How much is known for certain?

The reader may well be dismayed by the lack of clear or conclusive information about schizophrenia. There continues to be serious disagreement as to what the term means. It even remains unclear whether schizophrenia, however defined, represents a homogeneous group of patients or instead a group with many different disorders that may be totally unrelated. This confusion is further evidenced by the state of research on the etiology and, not surprisingly, even in 1982 treatment remains almost as primitive.

It is difficult to predict the evolution of schizophrenia research, but it may follow a course analagous to studies of other nonspecific syndromes, such as mental retardation. Long ago, mental retardation was considered to be a single broad syndrome. As the years passed, specific types of mental retardation with specific etiologies were discovered, such as Down's syndrome (mongolism) and phenylketonuria. Specific treatments were developed for some of these forms of mental retardation but not for others. However, many cases of mental retardation remain unexplained, and our treatment for them remains unsophisticated. Possibly, schizophrenia will be similarly broken down into smaller diagnosable units, and some of these will prove to be readily treatable. Others may prove to represent irreversible types of brain damage and be virtually untreatable. Still other cases will remain "idiopathic," or unexplained.

This process of breaking down schizophrenia might take several decades, and many of the answers are not likely to come until the early part of the next century. If there is a single conclusion to draw, it is to be wary of any authoritive statements about schizophrenia that claim that its diagnosis, causes, or treatment are well understood. As of 1982 such a statement is likely to be an arrogant overrepresentation of our true knowledge. Years of research will be required before even the most basic questions about the complex psychotic disorder known as schizophrenia are resolved.

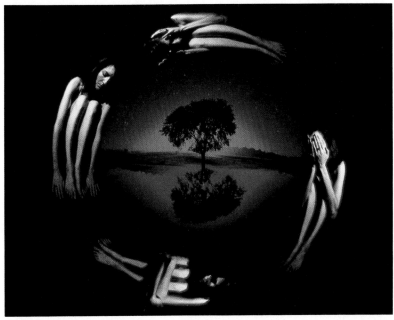

Dan Morrill

FOR ADDITIONAL READING:

Bleuler, P. E. *Dementia Praecox: or, The Group of Schizophrenias.* New York: International Universities Press, 1950.

Brown, G. W., *et al. Schizophrenia and Social Care.* London: Oxford University Press, 1966.

Hirsch, S. R., and Leff, J. P. *Abnormalities in Parents of Schizophrenics: A Review of the Literature and an Investigation of Communication Defects and Deviances.* London: Oxford University Press, 1975.

Kraepelin, Emil. *Dementia Praecox and Paraphrenia.* Edinburgh: E. & S. Livingstone, 1919.

May, P. R. A. *Treatment of Schizophrenia: A Comparative Study of Five Treatment Methods.* New York: Science House, 1968.

May, P. R. A.; Tuma, A. H.; and Dixon, W. J. "Schizophrenia: A Follow-up Study of the Results of Five Forms of Treatment." *Archives of General Psychiatry* 38 (1981): 776–784.

North, Carol, and Cadoret, Remi. "Diagnostic Discrepancy in Personal Accounts of Patients with 'Schizophrenia.'" *Archives of General Psychiatry* 38 (1981): 133–137.

Sheehan, Susan. *Is There No Place on Earth for Me?* New York: Houghton Mifflin, 1982.

Strauss, J. S., and Carpenter W. T., Jr. *Schizophrenia.* New York: Plenum Press, 1981.

Synder, S. H. *Madness and the Brain.* New York: McGraw-Hill, 1974.

Decades of confusion and disagreement over the definition, cause, and treatment of schizophrenia suggest to some investigators that this category of mental illness may comprise many different and possibly totally unrelated disorders. The process of reaching a fuller understanding of schizophrenia could still take many years, but once some of the components are more clearly defined, they may prove to be readily treatable.

Phobias
by Isaac M. Marks, M.D.

Most children are at one time or another afraid of parents abandoning them, of strange noises, and of new or unusual situations. These fears are usually quite volatile and soon outgrown. Adults, too, not uncommonly have fears—of heights, elevators, darkness, flying, spiders, mice, snakes, or taking examinations. Many of us also harbor our share of superstitions: fears of "haunted" houses, of walking under ladders, and so forth. These minor fears, however, do not lead to total avoidance of objects and situations. Fear, in fact, is the *normal* response to realistic danger or threat.

In some people fears can be profound and irrational—indeed sufficiently intense to handicap them in their everyday lives. Such uncontrollable fears are generally referred to as phobias. (The word phobia comes from the Greek *phobos*. In mythology Phobos was a god who instilled enemies with dread.) It would be impossible to list all phobias to which mankind is heir since people can develop exaggerated fears of literally anything and everything. They can even develop a phobia of developing a phobia. Though important-sounding Greek or Latin names are often given to various phobias (*e.g.,* phobophobia), these labels contribute little to knowledge. A phobia is a fear that is clearly out of proportion to the demands of the situation, cannot be explained or reasoned away, is beyond one's voluntary control, and leads to avoidance of the feared situation. Phobics usually recognize that their fears are unrealistic and that other people would not be unduly afraid of the same things.

It should be emphasized that the line between fear and phobia is a fuzzy one; we cannot distinguish precisely, for example, between a marked "fear" and a mild "phobia." Phobias are generally associated with a particular situation or object. The disparity between a phobic object and the reaction to it is obvious when the fear is of something as concrete as moths and butterflies. A woman who was phobic about these creatures had to keep her windows tightly shut at home in summer and several times had to get off buses and trains when she encountered moths or butterflies in them. Her phobia caused her to have several accidents. When she saw a butterfly while bicycle riding, she not only fell off but brought down her friends who were

Isaac M. Marks, M.D., *is Professor of Experimental Psychopathology at the Institute of Psychiatry in London, England.*

(Opposite page) "Phantom of the Castle," 19th-century German engraving by Leo Putz; photograph, Jean-Loup Charmet, Paris

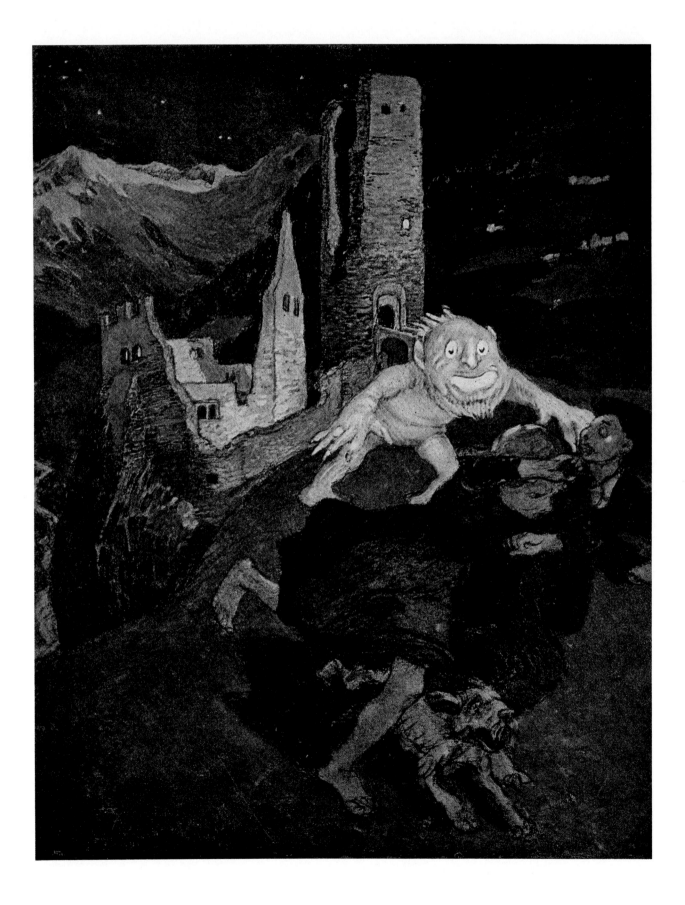

Photographs, Dan Morrill

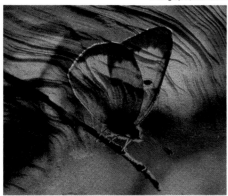

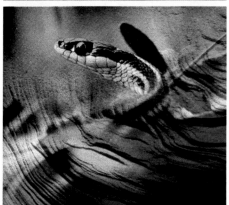

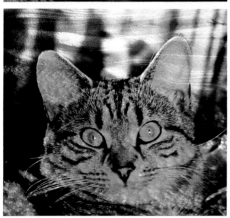

Fears of animals are very common in children between the ages of two and four. Usually these fears disappear. Adults may have very profound and specific animal phobias; a phobic might dread moths and butterflies but have no problem at all with black widow spiders.

riding behind her. Twice she fell backward into a stream when avoiding large butterflies that had flown across her path. On another occasion she was standing on a chair to fix a window drape when she unexpectedly picked up a large dead brown moth; she leaped off the chair and sprained her ankle. This woman always checked for the *absence* of moths before entering any room or closet. Her fear did not extend to "creepy-crawlies." "I'd rather deal with a box full of black widow spiders than one large English moth," she insisted.

There are also more pervasive and complex phobias concerning situations such as leaving one's home or the possibility of having cancer. Such a patient's life was literally crippled by her phobia. She reported:

To go outside to me was fear. If I went outside I couldn't breathe. I had trembly legs so I stayed in. I stayed in for four years and never went out. First I noticed that in crowds I couldn't breathe. Or I got panicky if I went shopping for food and the shop was full; I used to walk out. On a bus, I used to want to get there quicker than a bus generally takes. All these things were gradual at first, but they got worse. I was always crying— because I wanted to go out; I missed going along when my husband took my son out for the day, but I kept the tears back, of course, until my son had left the house. And then I cried. I was so lonely that I used to crawl to bed sometimes; take a drug and crawl to bed and sleep.

Phobics experience overwhelming anxiety when confronted with their phobic situation. Even away from the dreaded situation many also rehearse their frightening experiences in their mind until they are in an agony of fearful anticipation about the next time they will meet it. This fear of fear becomes a fresh source of threat.

To escape their anxiety, patients avoid their phobic situations and restrict their activities and daily functions. They are always on the lookout and become very sensitive to the presence around them of anything connected with their phobia. The phobic patient continually seeks out the phobic object in order to avoid it, finds it in obscure places, and often sees it in his or her peripheral vision. One sign of improvement during treatment is decreased awareness of the phobic object in the surroundings.

Many people develop phobias directed at objects or situations that are commonly encountered and cannot be easily avoided—cats, dogs, and even other people. *Uncommon* events, too, such as thunderstorms in cool countries, can cause much misery to some phobia sufferers. A 48-year-old woman who lived in an area where thunderstorms were infrequent nonetheless had had such a phobia for 28 years: "I sit and wait for it to happen. When and if it does I sit in a darkened cupboard until it's over—all night if necessary. I always listen to every word of the forecast, which I know is silly." Thunderstorm phobics may phone the weather bureau endlessly for forecasts; if storms are predicted they will not leave their home that day. One man became so frightened when he heard a storm was predicted that he went by train 200 miles away to escape the weather.

Phobias can occur either on their own or as part of a whole range of psychiatric disorders. They include such contrasting states as children's ephemeral terrors of darkness, the multiple fears of a housebound housewife, and the vague phobias found in some personality disorders. Phobias may occur as part of a depressive illness, waxing and waning at the same

86

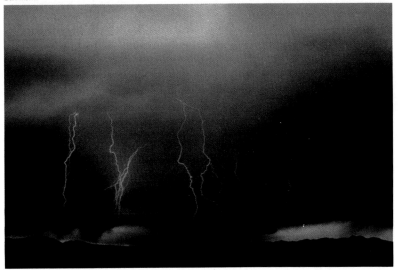

People develop irrational fears of literally anything and everything—of objects or situations they must face every day or of phenomena rarely encountered. A storm phobic might phone the weather bureau for forecasts dozens of times a day or travel great distances to escape violent weather.

time as the more prominent depressive aspects. They may be a feature of a number of personality disorders, of diffuse anxiety states, and even of schizophrenia. In all these conditions treatment of the phobia depends upon management of the major condition. When a phobia occurs as the patient's dominant problem, then it is called a *phobic disorder*.

Phobic disorders are found in about 3% of psychiatric outpatients. There are many phobics in the community who do not go to psychiatrists and never seek any medical aid at all. In a survey in Vermont the total prevalence of phobias was 77 per 1,000 of the normal population, but only 2.2 per 1,000 had severely disabling phobias, and only a quarter of these had been treated for their phobias. In that community survey phobias of injury, illness, and dirt were the most prevalent, but in psychiatric clinics agoraphobia—fear of public places—is the commonest form seen, probably because this phobia produces the greatest handicap.

In general, phobias are commoner in women than in men. This female preponderance is greatest for animal phobias and quite high for agoraphobia (two-thirds of agoraphobics are women), while social phobias occur about equally in men and women.

Why do phobias develop?

Like other species, human beings are preprogrammed to respond to certain situations with anxiety and fear. These emotions have survival value. Someone who is completely fearless is much more likely to enter dangerous situations; survival depends on the judicious blend of courage and caution. We need to steer a path between cowardliness on the one hand and foolhardiness on the other.

In general, fear develops through the interaction of three influences—those that are innate, *i.e.,* present from birth, those that depend on maturation of the nervous system, and those that have developed through learning in the course of individual and social experience. The human infant has a limited range of innate responses. As he matures physically and emotionally,

87

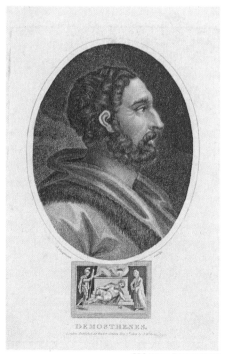

his responses are greatly altered; he develops and learns by his own experience and by what he observes in other people.

Timidity, the lasting tendency to be frightened easily, is one manifestation of fear. Studies have shown that timidity is partly genetically determined. Some animal species are very timid; in some cases this timidity might increase their chances of survival. Rabbits, for example, are more timid than tigers. Some rabbits, however, are more timid than other rabbits. The same applies to human beings. Identical-twin infants tend to resemble each other in the amount of fear they show with strangers in the first year of life; they also tend to exhibit similar degrees of self-confidence or timidity as adults.

Although animals and humans may display fear in almost any situation at some time or another, certain stimuli are much more feared than others. Furthermore, fear of a situation may arise even if there has been little or no previous experience of it.

Some children's fears are modeled on those of their parents. When a parent has a phobia, the child is more likely to develop it too. In a frightening situation children tend to look at any adult who happens to be with them. If the adult shows fear, then the child may pick it up easily. Although the parent's display of fear can precipitate a phobia in a child, only about one-sixth of adults with phobias have close relatives with a similar phobia.

Some stimuli seem to trigger fears that become exaggerated into phobias much more readily than others, and this is especially likely to happen at certain ages. At birth human infants startle readily to noise or to any other intense sudden or novel stimulus that is unexpected. In infancy novelty may provoke fear (though the same novel stimuli can, on other occasions, cause pleasure and be eagerly sought out). That writhing or jerky movements frighten infants is well known. This might be the basis for their early fears of snakes and certain other animals (which are pronounced in most youngsters between ages two and four).

The common fears change as the child grows. Whereas fears of animals are more common between ages two and four, between four and six, as their imaginations develop, fears of the dark and imaginary creatures, like ghosts, are more common. After age 6 children seem resistant to acquiring new phobias of animals; between ages 9 and 11 animal fears diminish rapidly in both boys and girls. Other later fears common in childhood are of storms, thunder and lightning, cars and trains—elements of the outside world, which they encounter as their horizons expand.

There are varying explanations for the rather constant ages at which some fears come and go. The common ages at which many children develop particular fears may partly reflect common changes within the child due to maturation. Experiments with the infants of Rhesus monkeys showed that between the ages of two and four months, they are especially prone to showing fear of threatening stares from another monkey. Similarly, 8- to 20-month-old children commonly develop a fear of strangers once they have learned to tell the difference between strangers and members of their own family.

Some fears start at a given age simply because that is the age at which the child first encounters a particular situation. School phobias are a case in point. When children are exposed to a totally new situation, they generally show anxiety, but this usually soon subsides. Mild fear of school is the rule during the first term or when the child changes to another school; extreme phobias leading to complete avoidance of school are exceptional. In fact, incapacitating phobias of any kind are uncommon in children, despite the proneness of most children to show a wide variety of definite fears.

Just as fears may occur in children for little or no apparent reason, they frequently vanish as mysteriously. During illness children may regress to earlier modes of behavior, during which time forgotten fears may reappear. When the child is well again, the fears disappear once more.

In most cases the origin of the phobia is shrouded in mystery. There is little evidence for the speculation that phobias are symbolic representations of intrapsychic conflict. Trauma, too, is surprisingly rare as the trigger for a phobia. Undoubtedly a dog bite or a car accident can be followed by a phobia of dogs or of cars and driving, but most phobic patients usually give no such history. More often, adult agoraphobics report that their exaggerated fears began during a period of depression—the phobia remaining after the depression cleared up.

Agoraphobia

Agoraphobia is probably the most common and distressing phobic syndrome of which adult patients complain. The word comes from the Greek root *agora,* meaning an assembly or marketplace: the impossibility of walking through certain streets or squares or possibility of so doing only with resultant dread or anxiety. It is also the most pervasive of the phobic disorders. In varying combinations, agoraphobics may fear: going to public places—both open areas such as streets, outdoor markets, and ballparks, and closed spaces such as elevators, shops, theaters, cinemas, and churches and synagogues; travel on underground trains, surface trains, buses, ships, and airplanes (but usually not in automobiles); bridges and tunnels; having haircuts; remaining alone at home; and leaving home.

Agoraphobia usually begins in adults between the ages of 18 and 35; it is rare in childhood. Occasionally children with school phobias go on to show agoraphobia in adolescence. Like many health problems, agoraphobia often develops after some major upheaval in the person's life, *e.g.,* serious illness in oneself or relatives, acute danger or discomfort, leaving home, death of a loved one, divorce, engagement, marriage, pregnancy, miscarriage, or childbirth. It may begin after some unpleasant events in a shop or street or on a bus. Agoraphobics often regard some trivial event as a trigger to the disorder even though such events might previously have occurred dozens of times without any ill effect.

Anxiety, the unpleasant emotion associated with a sense of impending danger, is for most of us a part of the fabric of everyday life; it is impossible to live without some kind of anxiety. For the agoraphobic, however, anxiety may mount to panic—sudden overwhelming upsurges of acute terror. (The word panic is of Greek derivation. Pan, the god of pastures, forests, flocks, and herds, was said to have played on his pipes of reed, producing haunting noises in the still of the night, and striking terror [*panic*] in the hearts of those who encountered his sounds unexpectedly.)

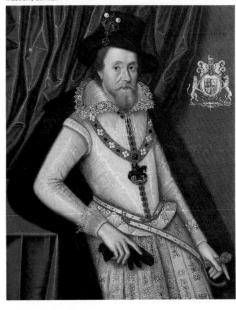

Famous phobics include the first Roman emperor Augustus (63 BC–14 AD), who feared the dark (opposite page, top); the great Athenian orator Demosthenes (c. 384–322 BC), who had acute stage fright (opposite page, bottom); and James I of Great Britain (1566–1625), who was haunted throughout his life by his fears of the devil and the spirit world (above). Father of psychoanalysis Sigmund Freud, depicted below, became apprehensive of traveling when he was in his thirties.

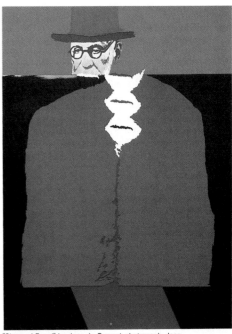

89

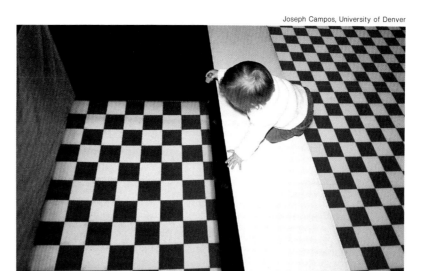

A child's fears arise partly out of innate response and partly from experience. Fears also depend on the developmental process, and they tend to change as the child matures. At the University of Denver's Infancy Laboratory a large glass-covered table (a "visual cliff") was used by researchers to test the emergence of wariness of heights.

The agoraphobic's panic attacks may strike suddenly for no obvious reason. They are usually accompanied by physical symptoms: rapid pulse, pounding heart, chest pain, nausea, difficulty in breathing, and a feeling of having a lump in the throat or of being disoriented and out of control. Many have consulted specialists such as cardiologists and gastroenterologists about these symptoms. The agoraphobic can become so disabled by anxiety that she eventually retreats from life outside her home to become completely housebound.

Not a few agoraphobics develop their problem without any obvious alteration in their life circumstances, however. Many people report brief episodes of agoraphobic symptoms that clear up without special treatment. But once the syndrome has persisted for more than a year, it tends to run a fluctuating course with partial remissions and relapses over many years unless effective treatment is given.

Social phobias

Social phobias are probably the next commonest seen in psychiatric clinics. These take the form of fear of eating, drinking, shaking, blushing, speaking, writing, or vomiting in the presence of other people. At one extreme, social phobias involve only a specific situation, such as eating in restaurants. At the other extreme, a social phobic can be frightened of most forms of social contact and end up shunning all people and living as a recluse. Whereas the agoraphobic's fear of crowds is focused on the mass of people together, a social phobic's fear of crowds is focused on the individuals who make up the crowd. (Some agoraphobics also suffer from social phobia.) Social phobias start most often between puberty and the late twenties.

Social phobics are peculiarly sensitive to being observed. For fear of blushing, sweating, or looking ridiculous they may be unable to sit facing another passenger in a bus or train or to walk past a line of waiting people. They may be terrified of attracting attention by behaving awkwardly or fainting. Some may leave their house early when it is so dark or foggy that they cannot easily be seen. On the job they will avoid talking to superiors. "Stage

90

fright" will prevent them from appearing in front of any kind of group. They may shun swimming for fear of exposing their bodies to the gaze of others.

Social phobics are especially fearful of their hands shaking or trembling in front of others. Thus many will not write checks in the bank; some may even avoid exchanging money. Obviously, this preoccupation would severely limit a person's job opportunities; *e.g.,* work in a large office, restaurant, or factory; sales positions; teaching—all would be out of the question. While generally the fear is that their hands *might* shake—that their writing would be indecipherable, that a coffee cup would rattle in the saucer, that their soup would spill when they raised the spoon to their lips—it is rare for such patients to actually tremble or shake. They make a striking contrast to patients who have brain disorders that cause them to shake vigorously and uncontrollably but usually without self-consciousness. Sufferers from Parkinson's disease, for example, often display prolonged, repeated head nodding and shaking of the hands, yet they have no fear of doing anything in public despite this obviously visible disability.

Specific phobias

Specific or simple phobias are probably the most common type of phobic disorder—though owing to their limited nature many of these may not be seen by professionals. There is an endless list of such phobias that are fo-

Agoraphobia, the most complex and pervasive adult phobia, can cause the sufferer to become so disabled by anxiety that he or she retreats from the outside world altogether. Photographer Jerry Uelsmann has conjured up the haunting world of the agoraphobe who clings to the safety of home in the scene below. The photograph at left is another of Uelsmann's visions of the terror of the outdoors experienced in agoraphobia.

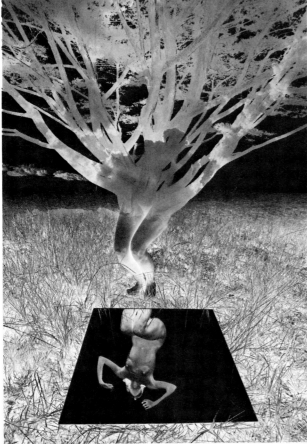

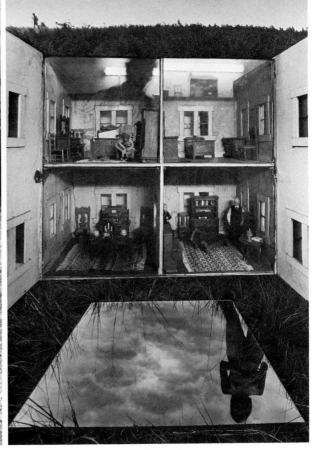

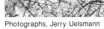

Photographs, Jerry Uelsmann

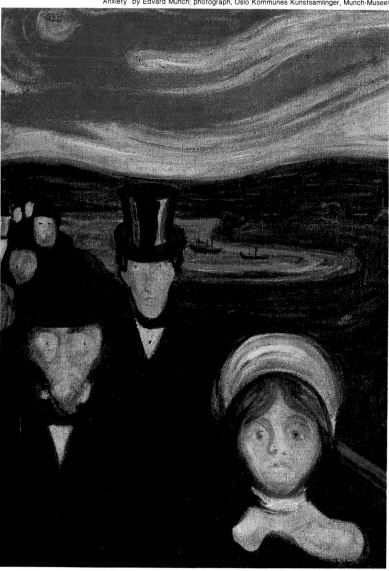

Impending danger and near-hysterical terror are recurring themes in the paintings of Edvard Munch (1863–1944).

cused on specific objects or situations. As already noted, quite frequent are phobias of animals—particularly snakes, insects, mice, and flying creatures. Natural phenomena, too, are common foci; *e.g.,* heights, darkness, thunder and lightning, and open spaces. Flying phobias are not uncommon. Some people are phobic of swallowing, especially solid foods. Another frequent specific phobia is of being far away from toilets; yet another, of urinating or defecating in a public toilet. Many are terrified by dental treatment, injections, or seeing blood; unlike other phobics whose heart rates quicken on contact with the phobic situation, blood phobics frequently faint at the sight of blood, owing to dramatic but transient slowing of their hearts.

Some phobics develop fears of being sick. Fears of illness pass through the minds of most of us at one time or another, but these are usually short-lived, cause no handicap, and require no treatment. Some, however, may be so paralyzed by their illness phobia that they cannot go about their daily lives.

92

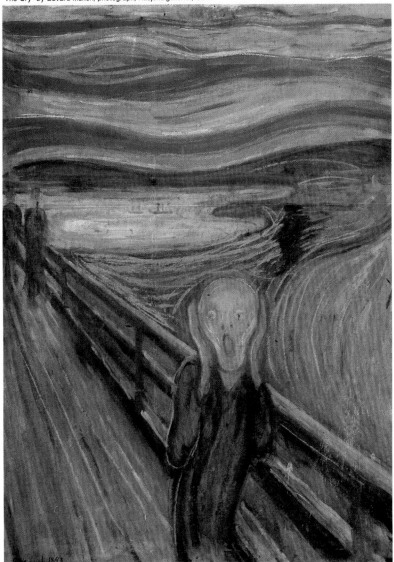

An illness phobic constantly searches his body for evidence of a specific disease; for example, skin cancer. No skin lesion or bodily sensation can be too trivial for his keen senses. He will misinterpret genuine physiological sensations, and his anxiety itself may produce fresh symptoms. The illness phobic's endless quest for reassurance from doctors and other people is a bit like an addiction. Being reassured reduces the anxiety transiently, but the tension soon builds up again to require further comforting within a few weeks, days, or minutes, the intervals between requests for reassurance growing progressively smaller.

Patients with obsessive-compulsive problems may develop obsessive fears about harming other people or worry incessantly about being dirty or untidy. To reduce these fears they may spend many hours a day washing their hands, tidying their homes, or checking that their doors and windows are locked.

93

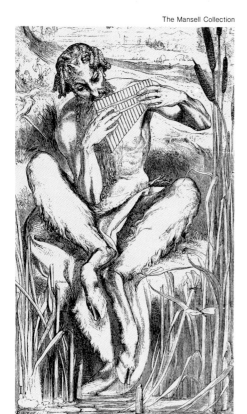

Our word panic is derived from Greek mythology. When the god Pan played haunting tunes on his pipes of reed, he inspired terror in those who encountered him unexpectedly. "Phobia," too, comes from the Greek; the lesser-known god Phobos aroused dread in enemies.

The chart on the opposite page represents four groups of patients treated for phobias: 18 with animal phobias, 12 with situational phobias, 25 with social phobias, and 84 with agoraphobia. The arrows mark the mean ages at which patients sought treatment. An illness phobic can be tortured by never-ending fears of disease and death, as the 19th-century caricature on the opposite page reflects. The sufferer will misinterpret every ache and pain, no matter how trivial; his anxiety itself may produce symptoms, and no amount of reassurance will assuage these fears.

The effects on families

A few phobics manage to conceal their problem without its obviously affecting their own lives or those of people around them. However, as has already been noted, serious work and social problems are seen in many phobics. Severe agoraphobics may have to give up their jobs as they become housebound; social phobics can become total hermits.

The phobic's handicaps will often eventually spill over to involve the family. For example, an agoraphobic mother and housewife may not be able to do the family shopping or to take the children to and from school and other activities; therefore, her husband must take over these roles in addition to holding a full-time job. His dual roles may limit him in his work and mean financial loss for the family.

Obsessive-compulsive patients often drag their families into their rituals. As an example, for reasons that were obscure, a 36-year-old married woman was so frightened of tuberculosis germs that she would not sweep most of her house and left dust to accumulate on the floors because she thought that dust harbored germs and she did not want to go near these germs. She could not feed her two-year-old son because she felt she might give him TB. She kept the child cooped up in a playpen, never allowing him the space or freedom to move about. The child thus grew up as a stranger to the mother and developed many emotional problems of his own. His grandmother was never allowed to see him because of the mother's fear that the grandmother might bring TB germs in. Nor were other visitors allowed in the home because they were potentially "infectious." The woman spent most of her day washing her hands, which became so raw that they bled.

A hopeful outlook with treatment

There are three main classes of treatment for phobic disorders: psychological methods, drugs, and physical methods. At the present time psychological treatments offer the most hope for lasting improvement, except where there is marked coexisting depression, in which case treatment with antidepressant medication is useful.

Psychological management. In the last ten years there has been a revolution in the treatment of phobic disorders. Previously, the most common psychotherapeutic approaches derived from a Freudian model of psychoanalysis. This assumed that phobias usually symbolized other hidden problems that needed to be discovered; when such putatively latent material was revealed through free association and sufficiently worked through, it was thought that the anxieties would disappear. This form of treatment is slow—often taking many years—and costly. Moreover, the psychoanalytic approach has not been shown to be especially helpful for relieving phobias.

In contrast, certain newer behavioral methods are demonstrably effective and lastingly so. (Not all behavioral methods work equally well. Relaxation techniques, for example, do not reduce phobias.) Behavioral approaches that emphasize *exposure* require a few days or weeks, or at most a couple of months of treatment. Moreover, there is now a wealth of research that shows this method works in most cases.

Exposure treatment does not assume that phobias are symbolic transformations of hidden difficulties. It does not delve into the unconscious. Instead, it regards the phobia as the main handicap and tries to eliminate it directly by teaching the sufferer how to face those situations that clearly trigger his discomfort so that he can learn to tolerate them. Even phobias that have been present for as long as 20 years can be overcome in a treatment requiring no more than 3 to 15 hours of therapist time per patient.

Exposure therapies, of which there are several, have in common the principle of direct contact with the feared object or situation. Exposure can be gradual (sometimes called desensitization) or rapid (sometimes known as flooding). Contrary to popular belief, the anxiety that is produced during exposure is not usually harmful. Even if severe panic does strike, it will gradually evaporate and will be less likely to return in the future. Effective exposure treatments developed only as therapists learned to endure the phobic anxiety of their patients, secure in the knowledge that such anxiety is much more likely to lead to their improvement than to be harmful. The important point is to persevere until the phobic anxiety starts to lessen and to be prepared to go on until it does. In general the more rapidly and directly the worst fears are embraced by the patient, the more quickly the monster of terror fades to a tolerable mild tension.

Before severe phobics confront the source of their terrors, it is vital that they first understand what is likely to happen and then structure their exposure so that they can deal properly with the problems that are bound to arise. They must be determined to get the better of their fears and not to run away from them. The fear will not disappear by magic. An agoraphobic cannot simply poke her nose into a dreaded crowded store, feel the surge of panic, and rush out again. She must devote a full afternoon to a shopping trip. She might take a book or knitting or materials to write a letter with her and when the panic strikes sit in a corner of the store and ride out the terror. It may take 30 to 60 minutes for the panic to pass. When she feels better, she can continue her shopping.

Persistence and patience are essential to conquering phobias. Parents

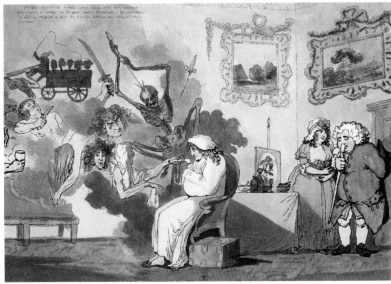

Jean-Loup Charmet, Paris

Adapted from *Fears and Phobias*, I. M. Marks, New York, Academic Press, 1969

Age of onset of four varieties of phobia

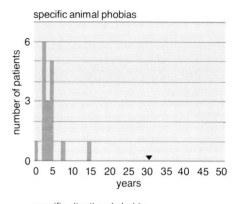

specific animal phobias

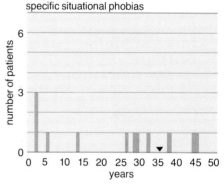

specific situational phobias

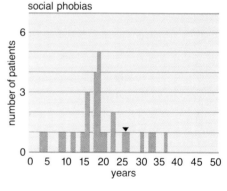

social phobias

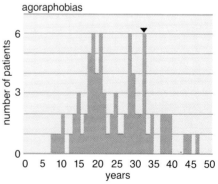

agoraphobias

(Left) TERRAP, Menlo Park, Calif.; (right) CHAANGE, Charlotte, N.C.

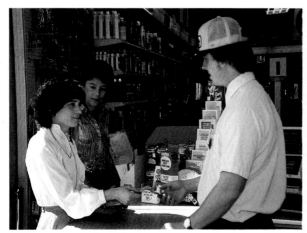

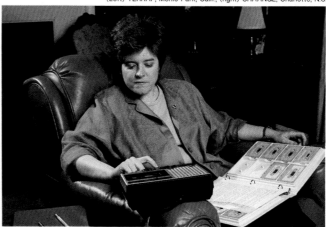

For most phobics the outlook is bright with today's treatments. The agoraphobic patient in the light blouse is confronting her fears of shopping; she is accompanied by a therapist. Perseverence and patience are essential in conquering phobias. The patient at right is following a self-exposure program at home. The figure below shows that over a five-year period untreated *phobias tended to clear up in children, whereas they persisted in adults.*

who want to help a child overcome a school phobia must be prepared to tolerate the child's almost inevitable crying the first few times he or she returns to school. They will need to steel themselves to ignore the complaints of headache or pain in the stomach with which the child will greet them in the morning just before it is time to go to school. Obviously, if the child looks ill, it might be wise to check for fever, but if the temperature is normal for several consecutive mornings, the chances are that this precaution need not be continued. Firm but loving pressure can usually help the school phobic child overcome the problem within a few weeks.

In its simplest form, exposure treatment consists merely of advice to patients to expose themselves every day to a situation they find slightly difficult and to record their daily actions in a diary, which the therapist reviews at the next visit. As they gain confidence, they can set themselves fresh goals to attain from one week to the next. Relatives can aid greatly by helping the patient work out details of his exposure "homework" program, monitoring it, and praising him for any progress achieved.

There is considerable recent evidence that many phobics can treat themselves perfectly adequately by self-exposure without a therapist, using carefully devised self-help manuals. One experiment assigned phobic patients at random to one of three groups. The first treated themselves by following the self-exposure "homework" instructions from the manual *Living with Fear* (*see* Additional Reading list). The second group interacted with a computer, which delivered those same instructions on a video screen and modified them according to progress that was assessed by the information that patients typed into the terminal from week to week. The third group had the usual exposure therapy aided by a therapist. At follow-up, all three groups of patients had improved substantially, and to a similar extent.

Early exposure in some cases may also *prevent* phobias from developing or from becoming full blown. While most phobias do not involve a traumatic precipitating event, there is some evidence that reexposure as soon as possible after a trauma enables the victim to nip a potentially disabling phobia in the bud. Airplane pilots are thus encouraged to fly again soon after a flying accident. Drivers should take the wheel again after an automobile crash. If a rider falls off a horse, it is best to mount it again right away. Once

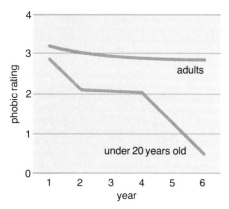

Adapted from "The Natural History of Phobia: Course and Prognosis," W. Agras, N. Chapin, and D. Oliveau, *Archives of General Psychiatry*, vol. 26, pp. 315–317, © 1972

people avoid a frightening situation, they are more likely to steer clear of it again. It is better to face the unpleasantness and anxiety associated with a bad experience than to risk getting into the potentially handicapping habit of continually avoiding it.

Exposure treatment appears to be lastingly effective. Various follow-up studies in Britain, the U.S., The Netherlands, and Greece found that improvements were retained for two to seven years following exposure therapy, depending on the particular study. In some cases brief "booster" treatments may be needed.

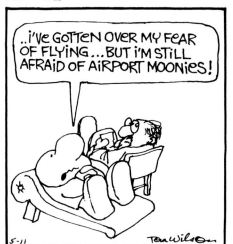

Drug and physical treatments. Sedatives have been widely used as a palliative in the treatment of the anxiety associated with phobias. As long as these drugs are in the body, anxiety is reduced, but the effect disappears when the drug is excreted. In the past, barbiturates were commonly used, but today these have largely been replaced by benzodiazepine derivatives, or minor tranquilizers, like diazepam (Valium). These drugs confer only short-term relief and can lead to addiction. Another class of drugs known as beta-blockers, which diminish physical symptoms like palpitations, have also been tried but are of no proven long-term value for treating phobias.

Similarly, most physical methods are of no lasting help in the management of phobias. Electroconvulsive therapy (ECT) has no part to play in the treatment of phobic disorders except in those few instances where these are complicated by severe, intractable depression. Certain forms of brain surgery (psychosurgery) have helped a tiny number of chronic phobics who have failed to respond to any other method, but these operations are very rarely indicated.

One form of drug therapy is useful under certain circumstances. When phobics are also depressed, as is often the case with agoraphobia, appropriate antidepressant drugs can help; this generally takes a few weeks. The antidepressant drugs of choice are the tricyclics (such as imipramine) and the monoamine oxidase (MAO) inhibitors (*e.g.,* phenelzine). The precise mode of action of these drugs is still uncertain. However, with these drugs, coexisting phobias tend to subside along with the depression. If they do not, exposure therapy can then be undertaken. A problem with antidepressants is that they may need to be taken for months or years to prevent relapse.

Though the mechanism by which treatment produces improvement remains elusive, the outlook for phobics today is good. When relieved of their phobias, they can resume jobs and lead active social lives. The crippling restrictions placed on their families are also alleviated.

FOR ADDITIONAL READING:

Marks, I. M. *Cure and Care of Neuroses.* New York: John Wiley, 1981.
————. *Living with Fear.* New York: McGraw-Hill, 1980.
Mathews, A. M.; Gelder, M. G.; and Johnston, D. W. *Agoraphobia, Nature and Treatment.* New York: Guilford Press, 1981.
Mavissakalian, Matig, and Barlow, D. H., eds. *Phobia: Psychological and Pharmacological Treatment.* New York: Guilford Press, 1981.
West, Margaret. "Disabilities and How to Live with Them: Agoraphobia." *The Lancet,* 7 November 1981, pp.1039–40.

Drug Addictions
by Ray J. Hodgson, Ph.D.

The 84-year-old grandfather who, for 20 years since retirement, every afternoon and evening after a big meal has settled in his old leather chair in the parlor and enjoyed his special blend of tobacco in his favorite briarwood pipe is a drug addict. So is the chief hospital resident "on call" every third night, sometimes working round the clock, who writes himself a prescription for dexedrine to stay alert (just as he would penicillin for a bacterial infection). His schedule does not let up, nor does his use of amphetamines.

Indeed, millions of highly respected, law-abiding citizens throughout the world are well and truly hooked on pipes, stimulants, cigarettes, alcohol, sleeping pills, and tranquilizers. Yet to most people the terms drug dependence or drug addiction evoke the stereotype of a junkie in a big city hustling for his next fix and injecting heroin through a dirty syringe until he succumbs to a fatal dosage or a lethal mixture of alcohol and opiates. Part of this image has to do with society's attitude. Heroin use is illegal; it is connected with crime and the underworld; and, above all, drug addicts are thought to be strange and deviant characters.

A more realistic definition of "drug dependence" was proposed by the World Health Organization (WHO) in 1965: "a state, psychic and sometimes also physical, resulting from the interaction between a living organism and a drug, characterised by behavioural and other responses that always include a compulsion to take the drug on a continuous or periodic basis in order to experience its psychic effects, and sometimes to avoid the discomfort of its absence." Clearly, socially acceptable drugs such as alcohol and tobacco have to be included under this definition.

WHO further attempted to categorize all the drugs that can lead to dependence on the basis of similarities in effects and similarities in the behavioral patterns that develop with excessive use. The following nine categories, or classes of dependence-producing substances, were proposed: (1) the alcohol-barbiturate group: drugs that lower the level of arousal of the central nervous system, leading to sedation and sleep; (2) amphetamines and amphetaminelike substances: drugs that stimulate the central nervous system, reducing fatigue and the need for sleep; (3) cannabis (marijuana, hashish): drugs that produce a "high" in regular users that is generally pleasurable and associated with unusually vivid sensations; (4) cocaine: a natural extract from the leaves of the South American coca shrub, which is both a stimulant

Ray J. Hodgson, Ph.D., *is a Senior Lecturer in Clinical Psychology at the Addiction Research Unit of the Institute of Psychiatry, in London, England.*

(Opposite) "Fumar," by Ed Paschke; photograph, William Bengston

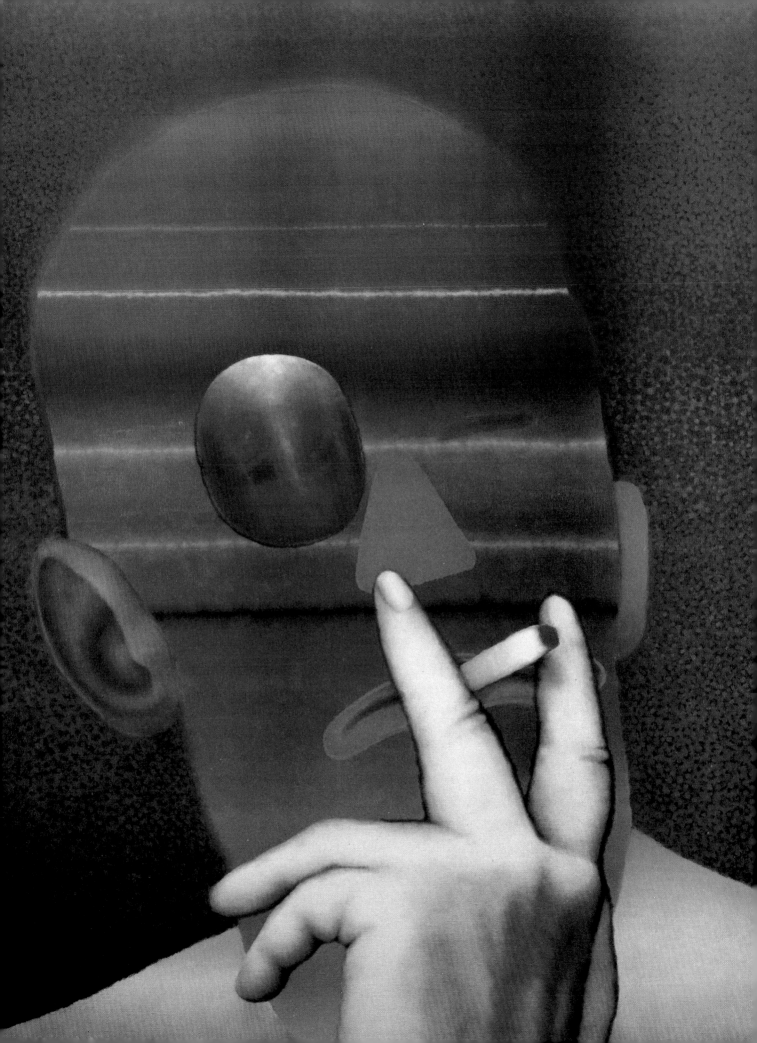

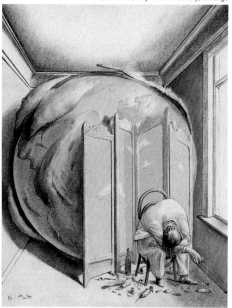

The stereotype of a drug addict is an unsavory junkie living from fix to fix. In fact, there are just as many highly regarded and decent citizens throughout the world who are genuinely hooked on drugs.

and a euphoria-producing drug; (5) hallucinogens (LSD and related substances): drugs that produce perceptual distortions, a sense of ecstatic detachment, and euphoria; (6) khat: a stimulant used primarily in Yemen and Ethiopia; (7) opiates or opioids: a wide variety of natural and totally synthetic substances that have morphinelike effects, relieving pain and inducing a state of indifference to threatening situations; (8) volatile solvents: glue, gasoline, and cleaning fluids, which, when inhaled or sniffed, produce a state of intoxication similar to alcoholic drunkenness but which sometimes result in hallucinogenic ''trips''; and (9) tobacco: a plant used for smoking, sniffing, or chewing, associated with both stimulating and relaxing effects.

Uppers and downers

The amphetamines are a family of drugs that produce an elevation of mood, a decrease in fatigue, and a lowering of appetite. There is also reduced need for sleep. For some people a typical dose leads to hyperactivity—therefore, the term uppers—and sometimes to irritability.

Amphetamines were first synthesized in 1887 but not introduced to the public until 1932, when they were marketed under the trade name Benzedrine in nasal inhalers because they produced constriction of the blood vessels and relieved a stuffy nose. But the public soon discovered their stimulating effects. During World War II amphetamines were given to pilots and soldiers to reduce their need for sleep. At the end of the war the Japanese had produced huge quantities of amphetamines and stockpiled them for wartime use. This led to widespread availability of the drugs and a postwar epidemic of amphetamine use that swept Japan.

Several patterns of amphetamine use have been described. In one, relatively small amounts are used to lift mood and reduce fatigue. This pattern is characteristic of college students burning the midnight oil, long-distance truck drivers, housewives who discover the stimulating effects of their prescribed diet pills, and busy executives who want to keep going without sleep. The main danger of this pattern is a tendency to keep using the drug to avoid the low feeling that occurs when drug use is stopped.

A second, more dangerous pattern is typical of the ''speed freak'' who injects large amounts of amphetamine intravenously for several days. He will remain awake for up to six days and sometimes longer, becoming increasingly tense, tremulous, and paranoid. After the end of a ''run,'' he ''crashes'' into a deep sleep lasting as long as 48 hours. He then repeats the cycle. When experimental rats with implanted intravenous catheters are given access to amphetamines, they behave much like speed freaks. They will repeatedly press a lever to obtain more of the drug; they also appear to be hallucinating. Often they stop eating; they generally continue pressing the lever until death supervenes after a few weeks.

Cocaine also has stimulant properties, but unlike the amphetamines, cocaine is a naturally occurring stimulant. In 1860 it was extracted from the South American coca shrub and was very quickly taken up by the medical profession and purveyors of patent medicines. It was added to many tonic wines, and for about ten years (until 1903) it was an ingredient of a new soft drink produced in the United States which was given the name Coca-Cola.

100

The class of drugs derived from barbituric acid and called barbiturates has roughly the opposite effect of amphetamines; thus these drugs are often called "downers." Depending on the dose, this large family of drugs produces sedation and relaxation, decreased anxiety, sleep, and an inhibition of epileptic seizures. There is no doubt that barbiturates can also lead to severe dependence. This has been known since 1927, but it is only in the last 20 years that physicians have started to prescribe them less frequently. Even today in the United States they are manufactured in vast quantities—enough to supply every citizen with 30 pills per year. Many are shipped legally into Mexico and then brought back into the United States and trafficked illegally. Downers are used to achieve subjective and physiological effects very similar to those of alcohol. In the 1950s scientists at the Addiction Research Center in Lexington, Kentucky, demonstrated that high doses of alcohol and barbiturates have almost identical effects, including a tendency to produce dependence and severe withdrawal symptoms.

In some respects severe barbiturate dependence is a more serious problem than heroin dependence. Abrupt withdrawal of the drug can produce a very unpleasant syndrome with anxiety, shakiness, insomnia, and sometimes delirium with tremors and convulsions. Another problem occurs when the excessive use of downers leads to an accidental overdose, especially when taken to get to sleep at night after consuming a fair amount of alcohol. Of drugs used to commit suicide, barbiturates are the most common.

The benzodiazepine family of drugs (*e.g.,* Librium, Valium, and Dalmane) are usually called "minor tranquilizers" and are very frequently prescribed for anxiety and insomnia. They have now displaced barbiturates in medical practice because they are safer, they produce less euphoria, and an overdose is less likely to be fatal. Nevertheless, these drugs can be habit-forming, and recent evidence of physical dependence has been reported. In years to come, the problem of dependence on minor tranquilizers, despite their relative safety, is likely to be more common.

Opium and heroin: God's own medicine?

During the major part of the 19th century, opiates in the form of patent medicines were as freely accessible as aspirin is today. In grocery and general stores these products were not called "smack" or "dope," as they are today, but were sold as Mrs. Winslow's Soothing Syrup, Godfrey's Cordial, and McMunn's Elixir of Opium. They were widely advertised as painkillers, cough mixtures, "women's friends," teething and soothing syrups for children, and cures for consumption. Laudanum, a mixture of alcohol and opium, was the choice of many of opium users, including Thomas De Quincey, the author of *Confessions of an English Opium Eater.* Morphine is the pure drug that gives opium its characteristic effects, and an early derivative of morphine was introduced into medicine as a cough suppressant toward the end of the 19th century. Its name was heroin.

Opium and its derivatives produce euphoria, drowsiness, and reverie. Heroin has, in addition, a powerful initial effect usually called a "rush." This is a feeling of ecstasy immediately following an injection. Withdrawal symptoms can be severe. Within the first 12 hours there will be muscle pain,

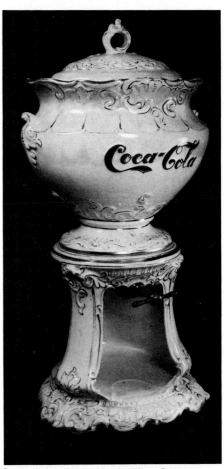

Cocaine, a stimulant and euphoria-producing extract of coca leaves, was an ingredient in Coca-Cola when the soft drink was first introduced in the United States around the turn of the century.

101

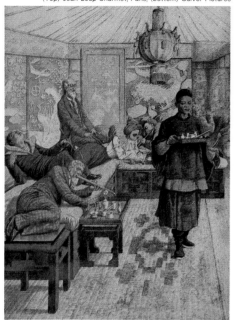

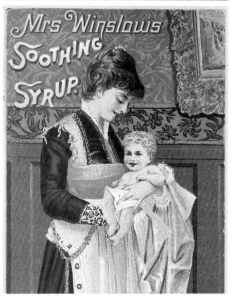

Opiates include a wide range of natural and synthetic substances that relieve pain and induce a state of indifference to threatening situations. During the 19th century the Chinese introduced opium smoking to many Western countries. The illustration above, entitled "Un Vice Nouveau," depicts a French opium den. Up until 1906 countless pharmaceutical preparations containing opium or morphine were widely marketed in the United States for such diverse ailments as diarrhea, dysentery, "women's trouble," consumption, and teething pain.

sneezing, sweating, crying, and yawning. Within about 36 hours the withdrawal symptoms will increase in intensity. Chills alternate with excessive flushing and sweating, and there will probably be an increase in heart rate and blood pressure as well as diarrhea and sleeplessness. These symptoms gradually subside over a five-to-ten-day period.

Today in most countries of the world, opioids are not available for recreational use. Those who want to achieve the opioid high must buy the drug (usually heroin) from an illicit source at a high price. Naturally, many people are deterred from using heroin under these conditions, and those who use it are more likely to come from a delinquent background or at least to be relatively unconcerned about social sanctions. That is not to say that every heroin addict is a delinquent.

Heroin use is a particularly tough habit to break, although many people do manage to escape. Follow-up studies of heroin addicts registered at London clinics found that about one-third were functioning well without the drug a few years after detoxification treatment. About half were still using other opioids prescribed by the clinics; the rest were in prisons or had died. Those who were able to stop using drugs usually attributed their success to a change in their social situation. Gaining the love and trust of a specific person, moving out of a drug subculture, obtaining a satisfying job, or some other change in life-style were the most frequently cited reasons.

Psychedelic drugs

The term psychedelic has been used to refer to the "expansion of consciousness" reported by users of hallucinogens including lysergic acid diethylamide (LSD), mescaline, and psilocybin. The last two substances are natural products, while LSD is a synthetic compound discovered by the Swiss chemist Albert Hofmann in 1943. Although these drugs can have harmful effects if used excessively, their addictive potential is very slight.

In 1896 mescaline was first extracted from the peyote cactus, which is found in Mexico and Central America. Peyote has been used for centuries in religious rites by some Mexican Indians. Psilocybin is the active ingredient of the sacred mushroom, *Psilocybe mexicana*. Both substances have effects similar to those of LSD, but they are not nearly as potent: only 0.0001 gram of LSD is needed to match the effect of 0.5 gram of mescaline; a three-pound bag of LSD would be enough to give a psychedelic experience to the combined populations of New York City and London.

The effects of LSD have been very closely studied in more than 2,000 research investigations. It produces dreamy, detached feelings and an unusually rapid flow of ideas but also was found to reduce intellectual proficiency on tests of memory, mathematical skills, and activities requiring focused attention. There is a distorted body image, heightened sensitivity to touch and smell, and a marked slowing in perception of time. Changes in moods and emotions are highly variable, ranging from ecstasy and "transcendental experiences" to great anxiety, depression, paranoia, and despair. As with other mind-altering drugs, the effects of LSD are dependent upon expectations and circumstances (set and setting). A "bad trip" can occur if the user is unprepared for the experience or psychologically disturbed.

102

(Top) Dan McCoy—Black Star; (bottom) Leonard Freed—Magnum

Marijuana

Of all the drugs likely to lead to habitual use, most scientists and users would argue that marijuana is the one that appears to cause the least harm and dependence. Nevertheless, there is still a great deal of controversy about legalization of the drug, mainly because the long-term effects of heavy use are still unknown. Three major studies carried out in Jamaica, Costa Rica, and Greece have carefully matched chronic users with nonusers of similar backgrounds and have found few important differences between the two groups. These investigations are often quoted to support the view that marijuana is totally safe; however, the total number of user versus nonuser pairs in all three studies was too small to detect the possible occurrence of less frequent consequences. It is unlikely, for example, that the well-established harmful effects of tobacco smoking would have been identified with similarly small samples.

In spite of this incidence of exposure to the drug, there are very few reports of severe dependence or compulsive use in Western societies. Furthermore, laboratory animals do not self-administer cannabis (whereas they will self-administer opioids, amphetamines, cocaine, alcohol, and barbiturates). In human users, withdrawal is not severely distressing. These facts must be assessed in conjunction with evidence that in Muslim and Hindu countries, where cannabis is more readily available than alcohol, the everyday heavy use of the substance does more frequently lead to dependence and difficulty in stopping. It may be that marijuana dependence would occur more often in Western cultures if "pot" were as easily obtained as cigarettes.

Volatile solvents

Since the peak of public interest in the use and abuse of inhalants in the 1960s, there has been a steady flow of information and research evidence on the problem. The glue for cementing model airplanes is the most widely used substance, but others include paint thinners, nail polish removers, lighter fluid, toluene, benzene, gasoline, and aerosol propellants.

Many of the sensations accompanying intoxication are similar to those produced by alcohol but, according to sniffers, the feelings of euphoria and omnipotence are much stronger. Most typically, sniffing occurs in groups, usually boys, and the aim is simply to get high. Unfortunately, many nasty side effects have been noted, ranging from immediate discomfort, nausea, muscle and joint pains, and double vision to brain damage and death.

There are a number of reasons for thinking that glue-sniffing will not go away and might be a greater problem in years to come. First, inhalants usually produce euphoria and produce it very rapidly. Second, glues and solvents are readily available; they can be found in most households in some form or other. Additionally, provided no permanent damage has been caused, the effects wear off quickly with little or no hangover.

Alcohol and alcoholism

For thousands of years in many cultures and historical periods, men, women, and even children have heeded Omar Khayyam's advice: "While you live, drink!—for, once dead, you never shall return." In moderation, alcohol is a

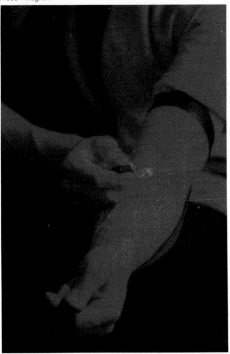

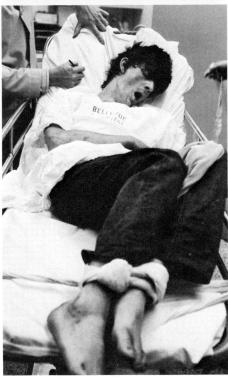

Heroin, a highly addicting morphine derivative, produces great euphoria in the form of a "rush" immediately following injection. Withdrawal symptoms can be severe and sometimes may amount to a medical emergency.

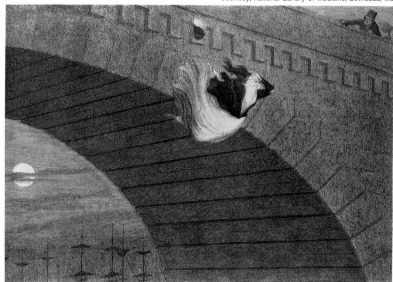

Courtesy, National Library of Medicine, Bethesda, Md.

Of all the dependence-producing drugs, alcohol is one of the most socially acceptable, yet it can also have disastrous social—in addition to physical—consequences, including the destruction of families. George Cruikshank's illustration is one of a series he called "The Drunkard's Children." Cruikshank was an enthusiastic promoter of temperance in the 1840s.

pleasure. However, there is now no doubt that alcohol can damage if taken in excess. Livers have been injured and families ruined; children have been harmed by their drinking parents; and alcoholics have destroyed their own self-esteem.

Although hundreds of books have been written on the subject and millions of people have asked, "Is my husband (or wife) an alcoholic?" the exact definition of alcoholism is still debated. The notion of an "alcohol dependence syndrome" is now beginning to replace the idea of a precisely defined disease that is either present or absent. The alcohol dependence syndrome begins to develop when there is an awareness of a compulsion to drink so that drinking takes priority over other activities. For lengthy periods drinking becomes more important than family, job, friends, and health. Tolerance to alcohol increases, and withdrawal symptoms such as shakiness, sweats, and depression tend to occur, especially on "the morning after the night before," when blood alcohol levels are reduced. Frequently, drink is consumed in order to escape and avoid withdrawal symptoms, with these symptoms typically disappearing very rapidly after a few drinks. The alcoholic begins to hide stocks of liquor at home or at work so that he or she is always prepared for the sudden onset of withdrawal symptoms. Finally, even if the severely dependent alcoholic is able to remain abstinent, he is still at risk. There is a strong possibility that if he starts drinking again, he will lapse into his old habits in a few days.

Of all the dependence-producing drugs, alcohol is the one that is the most widely available, the most socially acceptable, but at the same time the one that causes the most misery around the globe. Excessive drinking can cause damage to nearly every organ and tissue in the body, and it can harm families, careers, and the unborn fetus. Alcohol is frequently implicated in traffic, industrial, and domestic accidents. It has often been said that if alcohol had only recently been discovered, it would never pass the stringent safety tests required of marketable psychoactive substances today.

104

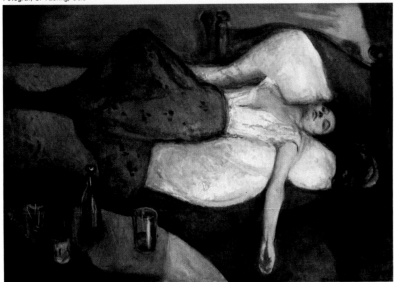

"The Morning After" is the title of this picture. After a night of indulgence in alcohol the drinker experiences headache and depression. Frequently the alcoholic will drink to avoid the loathsome withdrawal symptoms.

Tobacco dependence

Historically, attitudes toward the use of tobacco have varied widely. Sir Walter Raleigh enjoyed it and popularized pipe-smoking in England. King James I disliked tobacco's odor and prohibited its use. Unfortunately this edict had very little impact. The first Romanov czars instituted severe penalties such as whipping and exile to Siberia for tobacco smoking, and the 17th-century Chinese were even more violently opposed, with decapitation being the ultimate penalty. In spite of this sporadic opposition to tobacco, cigarette smoking is now one of the most prevalent forms of drug dependence to have afflicted both developed and less developed countries during the last 300 years.

One small change in tobacco curing in the mid-19th century has been partly responsible for the phenomenal spread of the habit. The production of so-called flue-cured tobacco enabled the cigarette smoker to inhale, thereby increasing addictive potential. Within just a few seconds of inhaling cigarette smoke, a strong concentration of nicotine travels from the lungs to the brain and strongly reinforces the smoking habit. Some researchers believe that nicotine releases the neurotransmitter substance noradrenaline from nerve cells in the brain that supply the heart. Brain-wave patterns after inhaling cigarette smoke show an increase in alertness similar to that produced by amphetamine. Certainly smokers often report an increase in energy and in their ability to concentrate.

The cigarette smoker experiences great difficulty in giving up the habit. In fact, many heroin addicts report that it is easier to give up heroin than cigarettes. Cases have been reported of smokers continuing to smoke after suffering awful consequences such as a peripheral vascular disease, amputations of limbs, and tracheostomy. After a tracheostomy, smokers have even been observed sticking the cigarette into the hole that has been made in their windpipe to allow them to breathe. If we were to draw up a list of drugs causing both dependence and harm throughout the world, tobacco would be

105

placed alongside alcohol right at the top. Yet both substances, with such enormous addictive potential, are legal, inexpensive, and easily obtained.

Predisposing factors: an addictive personality?

Many addicts, whether they be smokers, alcoholics, or hard drug users, attribute their problem to their "addictive personality." They assume that they were born with a predisposition to use drugs or that they developed such a personality at an early age. This is a popular view, and yet research workers have been searching high and low for such a personality and have found it to be as elusive as the Abominable Snowman. In fact, so many variables bear upon the excessive use of drugs and there are so many routes to addiction, that it does not make much sense to speak of the addictive personality, just as we cannot specify a single reason why cars break down. What then are the factors that allow us to say that a young person is at risk?

First, if we are trying to spot a potential addict, we would undoubtedly choose a person who is actually using a drug. An adolescent who is smoking regularly is more likely to become an adult addicted smoker than one of his peers who does not smoke. We would also choose a person who is using a drug with addictive potential, that is, cigarettes or heroin, rather than sarsaparilla or ginger beer or even LSD. Some drugs are more addictive than others, even for rats and monkeys. For example, cocaine tends to be preferred above all others by drug addicts, as well as by rats and monkeys.

The pharmacologic effect of the drug is important, but so is the psychological effect of being a part of a drug-taking subculture. Drugs have symbolic as well as chemical effects. This is clearly illustrated in the "mellow yellow" craze that swept California in the 1960s. Partly owing to a popular song by Donovan and an article in the *Village Voice*, it was widely rumored that banana skins contained a psychedelic substance. Consequently, thousands upon thousands of drug users contentedly smoked dried banana skins even though bananas are pharmacologically inert.

We would then look for a child whose parents were addicted. A child picks up many habits, good and bad, from his parents. Also, there has been some evidence of a slight genetic influence (but nothing yet conclusive). We would then ask whether the drug is cheap. For example, if we were betting that a child might become an alcoholic, we would choose a French child and not a Scandinavian, because in France wine is considerably less costly than it is in Sweden or Denmark. Not surprisingly, France ranks right at the top of world alcoholism and cirrhosis rates (*see* Figure 1).

Having chosen a young person who has started to use a highly addictive drug that is relatively cheap, in a drug-using subculture, and with a parent who uses the drug to excess, we would then consider occupations. Some occupations involve a high risk of addiction. A doctor is more likely to become a drug addict than is the schoolteacher. Business travelers, dock workers, sailors, actors, and musicians are more likely to become alcoholics. This is partly the result of social pressures and the stresses of the job, but it also has to do with availability. Availability is actually of paramount importance. For example, if a parent always left open cigarette packs strewn about the house, children would surely have easy access.

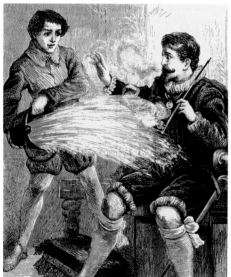

The etching depicts a boy dousing a man's pipe. Pipe smoking was popularized in England by Sir Walter Raleigh during the reign of Elizabeth I (1558–1603). Raleigh is credited with having brought two plants to England from America, the potato and the tobacco plant. It has been said: "How useful the one! How injurious to many the other!"

106

Finally, we would look for a boy rather than a girl. Women are indeed smoking, drinking, and taking drugs, but males still indulge in addictive habits more often than females.

There are also a number of factors that protect against drug addiction. The first would be a social environment that does not sanction excessive drug use. Some individuals suffer specific physical effects from certain drugs. The Chinese, for example, usually react poorly to alcohol. They tend to flush and feel sick after just a small dose. Experiencing such immediate unpleasant effects from a drug is likely to be a strong deterrent.

Of course, personality factors do have some influence. When a drug is illegal and not approved of socially, then regular users are more likely to have a delinquent background. In the United States more than 50% of heroin addicts had a history of delinquent behavior before they first used heroin. If a drug reduces anxiety then the anxious person is more likely to use it regularly. Some people enjoy being drunk and uninhibited, whereas others are more inclined to agree with Lady Nancy Astor, who said, "One reason I don't drink is that I want to know when I am having a good time."

How does dependence develop?

Many drug addicts, alcoholics, and smokers will argue that they are caught in the "iron grip" of physical dependence and are powerless to help themselves. Because of biological changes produced by the drug, continued use is necessary just to stay normal and avoid unbearable withdrawal symptoms. This explanation is now part of our folklore, but how credible is it? The answer: not very, for the following reasons. First, thousands of people every year receive strong opiates to kill the pain caused by fractures, burns, and surgical conditions. Often they experience withdrawal symptoms but no addiction. Second, drug addicts tend to use a larger dose of morphine than that required to prevent withdrawal symptoms. They are not simply using the drug to feel normal but are using a higher dose to produce a kick or euphoria.

In order to understand dependence, we must consider the way in which habits develop and are strengthened and the functional significance and rewards of the drugged state, as well as the psychological and social context in which the drug is used. The great thinker of Christian antiquity St. Augustine suffered for many years from a sexual compulsion. Of his compulsion he wrote: "When desire is given satisfaction, habit is forged and when habit passes unresisted a compulsive urge sets in. By these close links I was held." The pleasures of sex, food, money, and drugs can all strengthen a habit until it is difficult to resist. Psychologists call this positive reinforcement. In the field of addictions and compulsions, the avoidance of distress is also an important motivational force. The strengthening of a habit through the avoidance of pain, anxiety, frustration, and other unpleasant states is labeled negative reinforcement.

One of the assumptions made by many psychologists and neurophysiologists is that electrical activity in certain areas of the brain is associated with the experiences of pleasure and pain. In recent years our knowledge of the basic neurophysiology of motivation has been greatly increased by an experimental procedure known as electrical self-stimulation of the brain.

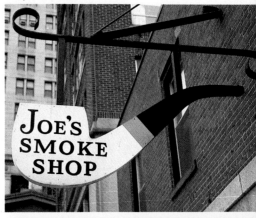

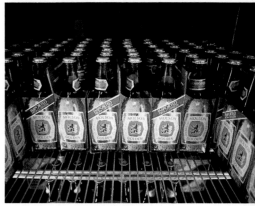

Among the drugs causing the most dependence and harm to millions of people across the globe are tobacco and alcohol. Yet in most parts of the world both substances are widely consumed— easily obtained, relatively inexpensive, and perfectly legal.

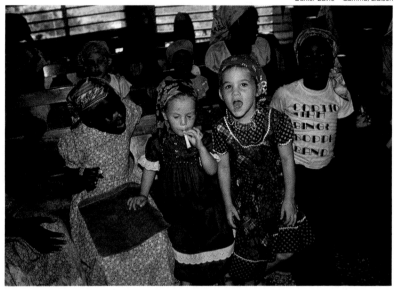

Having an addicted parent (or role model) and living in a drug-using subculture are certainly predisposing factors to addiction. These Rastafarian children are smoking marijuana—a common practice and part of the religious culture of this native Jamaican group.

James Olds, working at the University of Michigan in Ann Arbor, has been one of the pioneers of this approach. Olds and others have implanted electrodes in the brains of laboratory animals, usually rats. The rats are allowed to press a bar that either switches on a small electric current or switches one off. It has been found that with certain placements of the electrodes in the hypothalamus, the rat will press a bar for hours on end in order to keep up the electrical stimulation. With other placements the rat will press to stop the stimulation. It is not unreasonable to suppose that these areas of the brain (*see* Figure 2) directly influence the animal's pleasure and discomfort and that similar areas in human beings are activated by such things as drugs and distress and thus are involved in positive and negative reinforcement.

The pleasure, euphoria, or relief produced by some drugs is not only the result of an automatic arousal of certain brain centers, however, since the pleasure also depends upon a person's mental set and the setting. For example, in one experiment carried out at the Addiction Research Foundation in Toronto, it was shown that students who were given alcohol in a room by themselves tended to report tiredness and apathy, whereas students given the same dose in a social situation experienced an increase in sociability and found the experience to be very pleasurable. Such psychological and social factors are central to an understanding of human addiction. Nevertheless, the very fact that animals will quickly become addicted to various drugs suggests that the reinforcing effect of the drug can operate at a very basic level in the absence of the symbolism that is often invoked to explain addictions. We cannot argue for monkeys, as some have done for humans, that the misuse of drugs is the manifestation of dissatisfaction and loss of faith in the prevailing social system. Neither can we explain a monkey's addiction by suggesting it is the result of the search for different perceptions and ideas.

Indeed, most drugs have a pharmacologic effect that is either positively or negatively reinforcing, but whether or not an addiction develops depends largely upon the risk factors already outlined. The chain of events that leads

108

from initial experimentation to severe dependence is influenced at each stage by social pressures, modeling and imitation, price and availability, as well as the personality of the user and the social and cultural context in which the drug is used.

Inevitably the question arises: Why do people continue to use drugs—seemingly beyond all reason? On the face of it, compulsions and addictions have little to do with pleasure. They are self-destructive and actually reduce life expectancy, and yet the concepts of positive and negative reinforcement have been invoked to explain them. How can it be maintained that a drug habit is strengthened by increases in pleasure or reductions in distress when it is obvious that addictions often lead to catastrophic consequences? This is one of the paradoxes that psychologists have been addressing over the last 30 years or so, and they have produced a number of simple solutions.

First, the immediate pleasurable consequences of drug use have a more powerful influence on behavior than the delayed unpleasant effects. Second, a drug may produce a pleasurable effect on just a few occasions, but this intermittent reinforcement can have a powerful influence on the development of a habit. Also, pleasure is always relative, so that a drug that produces some negative effects will be rewarding if abstaining is even worse. It would appear that for these reasons the anticipation of illness, personal tragedies, and even death are not always sufficient to counteract the immediate, intermittent, or relative pleasurable effects. Drug use or abstinence then is associated with a pay-off matrix, or balance sheet, for a particular person, with the immediate rewards of the habit tending to predominate.

When some drugs start to be used excessively, the brain adapts to increased levels in the blood just as the body of an Arctic explorer will adapt to the cold. This process of neuroadaptation leads to tolerance and withdrawal symptoms. Tolerance refers to the tendency of the central nervous system to adapt to the intoxicating effects of the drug so that a larger dose is needed to produce the same effect. Withdrawal symptoms occur when the drug is stopped. Opiates, amphetamines, barbiturates, and alcohol all produce tolerance and very nasty withdrawal syndromes.

Most theories of neuroadaptation implicate a "compensatory adaptive process," which supposedly dampens the drug effect in order to maintain a stable state. These compensatory responses triggered in the brain then persist for hours or days after the drug has been stopped; bodily withdrawal symptoms are the result. According to this rather parsimonious view, tolerance and withdrawal symptoms are caused by a single process of adaptation.

The excessive use of a drug and the development of dependence, however, must be seen as a broader, more complicated process involving biological, psychological, and social factors. A person may be using a drug to reduce anxiety, feel more alert, be sociable, alleviate pain, or cope with a wide range of personal problems. After many repetitions, drug use can become a habit whatever the original reasons for using it and, probably, neuroadaptation leads to an increase in consumption in order to overcome tolerance and withdrawal. In attempting to understand, treat, and prevent addiction, this complex system of interactions has to be addressed.

Figure 1
Alcohol consumption and cirrhosis

	liver cirrhosis	consumption
France	57.2	16.4
Portugal	55.1	14.1
Italy	52.1	14.0
Austria	49.1	11.4
West Germany	39.6	11.3
Spain	38.8	11.7
U.S.	28.6	5.8
Czechoslovakia	28.1	8.0
Switzerland	24.6	10.0
Hungary	20.7	8.5
Belgium	20.5	8.3
Canada	19.6	6.5
Poland	17.2	5.5
Denmark	16.2	6.7
Sweden	15.6	5.7
Norway	7.6	3.4
Finland	7.5	4.1
Netherlands	7.4	4.8
South Ireland	7.0	4.5
United Kingdom	5.7	6.2

More people are likely to get hooked on a substance that is inexpensive, socially acceptable, available, and legal than on one that is considered illicit. Figure 1 shows cirrhosis mortality per 100,000 population among those 25 years of age and older and liters of pure alcohol consumed per capita in various Western countries. Not surprisingly, both rates are extremely high in France, where wine producing is among the major industries and wine drinking is so much a part of life.

Treatment strategies

Recent pharmacologic discoveries have ensured that the typical alcoholic or drug addict who is admitted to a hospital or detoxification unit will probably not experience very severe withdrawal symptoms. Within a couple of weeks his nervous system will be almost back to normal.

The main problem with all addictions is not in stopping but in remaining abstinent or developing permanent control. Mark Twain put his finger on this key dilemma: "Giving up smoking is easy. I've done it thousands of times." Therefore, treatment must be directed toward preventing relapse. There are three broad approaches to the treatment of drug dependence, with scattered evidence to suggest they are effective. Regrettably there is not the kind of cast-iron proof that would satisfy hard-nosed scientists.

Drug substitution. The use of methadone taken orally as a substitute for injected heroin is one example of drug substitution. Vincent P. Dole and Marie Nyswander of Rockefeller University in New York City, who pioneered the use of methadone as a treatment, believed that it counteracted the "drug hunger" that occurred during withdrawal and also that a sufficient dose of methadone produced a "heroin blockade." In sufficient doses, they argued, it would prevent the euphoric and sedative effects of heroin by blocking the sites in the brain that respond to opioid substances. Because methadone is taken by mouth rather than by injection, the effects wear off very slowly; consequently, it can be taken just once a day. Moreover, since methadone produces fewer sharp fluctuations in mood, the experience and behavior of an addict maintained on the substitute drug are relatively normal. There is still a great deal of debate about the usefulness of methadone, but the criticism voiced by some psychiatrists—that methadone maintenance is like "treating an addiction to Scotch with bourbon"—is probably an oversimplification.

Nicotine chewing gum is the other drug substitute for which there is emerging some promising evidence of effectiveness. Nicotine in chewing gum is slowly absorbed through the membranes of the mouth and throat, unlike the rapid absorption from a cigarette. Nevertheless, craving for a ciga-

Recent neurophysiologic experiments on animals which have demonstrated that certain areas of the brain are associated with pain and pleasure may enhance future understanding of the addictive process in humans. Figure 2 shows major portions of an animal brain. When electrodes are implanted in the medial forebrain bundle, the animal will self-stimulate; when electrodes are implanted in the periventricular system, the animal will work to terminate electrical stimulation that is applied by an experimenter.

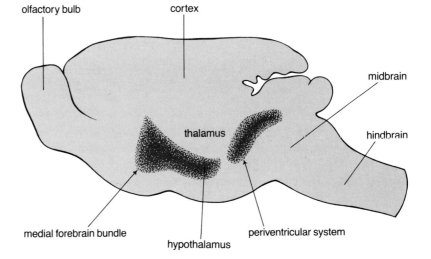

olfactory bulb

cortex

midbrain

hindbrain

thalamus

medial forebrain bundle

hypothalamus

periventricular system

rette appears to be counteracted by the gum, especially during the early stages of withdrawal. Further, it is then much easier to give up the gum than it is to give up cigarettes.

Many people, especially the less severely dependent, are able to give up their addictions without the use of a substitute drug; this, of course, is always preferable if it can be done. Oral methadone, nicotine chewing gum, and other drugs should be viewed as useful components of treatment. They are not as addictive or pleasurable as injected heroin or inhaled cigarette smoke and so they are ideal for the addict who worries about withdrawal symptoms and needs to give up in stages.

Coping with craving. People who are addicted to drugs, alcohol, and cigarettes are often resigned to the fact that they cannot cope with craving. When it starts to build up, for whatever reason, they feel helpless and powerless to resist. In recent years research has been directed toward methods of helping people to cope with temptation.

Alan Marlatt and his colleagues at the University of Washington in Seattle have been able to help alcoholics by having them identify high-risk situations and then repeatedly practice ways of dealing with these situations. High-risk events could involve social pressures, negative moods, stressful interactions with other people, or a small dose of alcohol. Coping strategies might be to avoid being "overwhelmed" by thinking about just one hour at a time; concentrating on the long-term benefits of abstinence; going for a walk or digging in the garden in order to ride out the craving; being assertive with other people, perhaps telling them not to put temptation in your way; or practicing relaxation or meditation. Any activity or thought that stands some chance of making the craving bearable is considered helpful. The aim of developing such coping skills is to "rehearse" these various strategies until they become second nature—as an airline pilot does when practicing emergency landings.

A slightly different approach to helping addicts cope with craving involves exposure to real-life temptations. At the Institute of Psychiatry in London researchers have shown that if craving is provoked and then resisted, two very beneficial consequences will follow. First, the urge will gradually go away, usually within an hour or two. Second, and of crucial importance, the

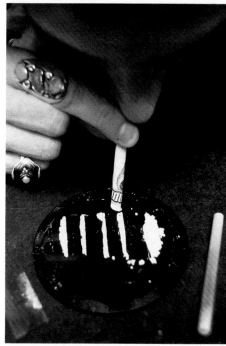

There is a mystique attached to cocaine use, largely owing to its very high price—per ounce, five times that of gold—and its limited supply. When snorted, this stimulant drug produces a quick and potent euphoric lift without hangover. Some of the drug's devotees have reported hallucinatory experiences involving the senses of touch, smell, hearing, and taste. The drawings (below) depict visual hallucinations described by recreational cocaine users in a study at the Neuropsychiatric Institute of the University of California, Los Angeles.

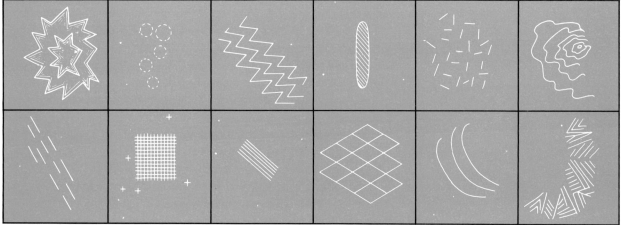

There are many approaches to treating drug dependence, with some evidence that many are successful. Unfortunately, controlled studies are lacking, as is absolute proof that any one method is 100% effective. "Aversion conditioning" is employed at the Schick Center for the Control of Smoking in Los Angeles. A technician gives a woman in a special booth a mild electrical impulse when she puffs on a cigarette. The impulses are irritating enough to create an aversion to smoking by building unpleasant associations with the habit. The overflowing ashtrays and cigarette advertisements on the wall are there to reinforce the ugly aspects of smoking.

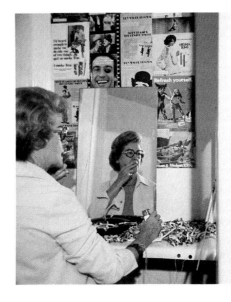
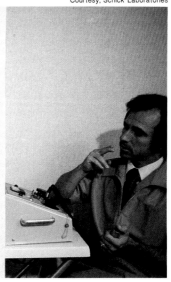

next exposure to a tempting situation will provoke a lower level of craving. This treatment approach is usually called "cue exposure" because it involves repeated exposures to the high-risk situations, or cues, that precipitate relapse. It is analogous to the methods that have been shown to be very effective in the treatment of phobias and obsessional compulsions. Although cue exposure is a relatively new scientific approach, it was anticipated by Shakespeare three centuries ago when his character Hamlet gave the following advice to his mother:

> Assume a virtue, if you have it not.
> . . . . Refrain tonight;
> And that shall lend a kind of easiness
> To the next abstinence: the next more easy;
> For use can change the stamp of nature
> And master ev'n the devil or throw him out
> With wondrous potency.

The excessive use of a drug and the development of dependence involve biological, psychological, and social factors; there remain many unanswered questions about the true nature of these complicated processes. Painting entitled "Drinker with Bottle" by Georg Baselitz (1981).

Although coping-skills training and cue-exposure techniques are being rigorously researched by drug addiction specialists, their "wondrous potency" has yet to be conclusively proved. Nevertheless, available evidence indicates that they are, at the very least, useful components of treatment.

The pleasures of sobriety. In the treatment of drug addiction and alcoholism, most clinicians take a broad approach, helping the addict to solve a wide range of psychological, social, vocational, and often marital problems. There is evidence to support the notion that these problems influence drug use. Solving some of the underlying problems gives the addict good reason to resist his or her self-destructive habit and to become committed to a sober life. Nathan Azrin, working at the Anna Mental Health and Development Center in Anna, Illinois, has had encouraging results in helping alcoholics with what he calls "community reinforcement."

Among other things, Azrin and his colleagues converted a tavern into a social club for abstinent alcoholics; they began a job-finding club; they persuaded foster families to develop links with isolated alcoholics to reduce the

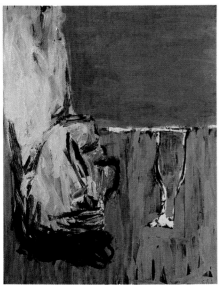

112

loneliness and alienation alcoholics feel within the community. The positive results reported are consistent with other research that indicates that those addicts who do well tend to be the ones who establish better interpersonal relationships or obtain satisfying jobs.

Self-help groups provide the addict with another way of making sobriety more rewarding; Alcoholics Anonymous (AA) is the most obvious and celebrated example. AA was first formed in Ohio in 1935, when "Bill W." and "Dr. Bob" got together to give each other mutual support. It is now a worldwide organization claiming over one million active members. The self-help process of AA involves not only providing mutual support but also "coping through involvement," so that sobriety is achieved and maintained by becoming actively involved in AA activities, attending regular AA meetings, helping others, holding office within AA, and so forth.

Many other methods have been proposed for the treatment of all kinds of addiction. These include aversion therapy, hypnosis, acupuncture, biofeedback, and sensory deprivation. Well-controlled investigations of these methods are either totally lacking or have not, as yet, shown them to be superior to any other. Nearly always, very good results are achieved in the first couple of weeks of any "therapeutic" program, but very poor results are reported when clients are reassessed one year later.

A final word

There are no easy solutions to the great many questions that have yet to be fully answered about the nature of addictions. What is the precise chain of events that leads from initial experimentation with a particular substance to dependency? Can this chain be broken? To what precise extent are addictions physical? Psychological? Biochemical? How can damage to individuals be minimized? How can young people be deterred from self-destructive habits? A particularly vexing question is: Why do only certain people get hooked when so many are exposed?

Man has always consumed substances that alter the mental state—that at first produce the most pleasurable sorts of euphoria. It is inevitable that some amount of abuse of and subsequent addiction to these substances occurs. It is most unfortunate that even today stereotypes persist of drug addicts and alcoholics as morally depraved, wayward, shameful, shiftless, and irredeemable creatures who "did it to themselves." The enduring stigma has probably stifled progress in conquering the problems of drug addiction and dependency. The reality is that these problems are both widespread and insidious and affect all classes of people.

It is an encouraging sign that the World Health Organization has recognized drug dependence as a problem worthy of attack and has included this as part of its overall commitment to dealing with mental health on a global scale. Although it seems a facile comment, perhaps the best approach to an enormous problem may be not looking the other way.

FOR ADDITIONAL READING:

Brecher, E. M. *Licit and Illicit Drugs.* Boston: Little, Brown, 1972.

Cohen, Sidney. *The Substance Abuse Problems.* New York: The Haworth Press, 1981.

De Quincey, Thomas. *Confessions of an English Opium Eater.*

Dupont, R. I., Goldstein, Avram, and O'Donnell, John (eds.). *Handbook on Drug Abuse.* Washington, D.C.: U.S. Government Printing Office, 1979.

Hodgson, R. J., and Miller, P. M. *Self Watching: Dealing with Addictions and Compulsion.* London: Multimedia Publications Ltd., 1982.

Jaffe, J., Petersen, R., and Hodgson, R. J. *Addictions: Issues and Answers.* London: Multimedia Publications Ltd., 1980.

Kalant, O. J. (ed.). *Alcohol and Drug Problems in Women.* New York: Plenum Press Inc., 1980.

Lipton, M. A., DiMascio, A., and Killam, K. (eds.). *Psychopharmacology: A Generation of Progress.* New York: Raven Press, 1978.

Marijuana and Health. Seventh Annual Report to the U.S. Congress from the Secretary of Health, Education, and Welfare. Washington, D.C.: U.S. Government Printing Office, 1979.

McLellan, T. A., *et al.* "Is Treatment for Substance Abuse Effective?" *Journal of the American Medical Association,* 12 March 1982.

Psychotherapies
by Leon Eisenberg, M.D.

No time rivals the present in the extent to which psychiatry and psychotherapy have penetrated popular consciousness, particularly the American consciousness—in books, in films, on television—sometimes in glamorous form, oftentimes in caricature. One wonders how many psychiatrists chose their profession in the hope of fulfilling the fantasy of being analyzed by as beautiful a psychoanalyst as the one Ingrid Bergman portrayed in *Spellbound.* D. M. Thomas's *The White Hotel,* a fictional portrait of a patient in treatment with Sigmund Freud, was a 1981 best-seller and, of course, a Hollywood motion picture will follow. *The Seven-Per-Cent Solution* (book and movie) imagined Dr. Freud and Sherlock Holmes working together to solve a crime. (In that case Freud came out one up on Holmes, whom he treated for cocaine addiction.) But no one in (or out) of his right mind would want to have his fate in the hands of the punitive and authoritarian staff of the hospital depicted in *One Flew over the Cuckoo's Nest* or to be treated by the zany psychiatrist (well-meaning but inept) in Mel Brooks's *High Anxiety.*

Jokes about psychiatrists parody the specialty in seemingly endless ways. As mind readers: the psychiatrist who greets a colleague with the comment, "You're fine; how am I?" As father figure: the repartee between two drunks in a bar; "My analyst can see right through your analyst!" As sexually obsessed: the patient beginning his 40th analytic session with the opening ploy, "What worries me is how I'm going to find a job and get my life in order, but if *you* want to talk about sex, it's O.K. with me." Then, of course, there is a light-bulb joke: "How many psychiatrists does it take to change a light bulb?" Answer: only one, but the light bulb has to want to change. Skeptics who are critical of psychotherapy have caricatured contemporary society as one in which half of the citizens are lying on a couch to be analyzed by the other half until the whistle blows, whereupon they change positions.

One does not have to be humorless to recognize that humor is serious business; it is a way of saying something important that might be offensive if it was said directly. The fact that the psychiatric profession is so commonly the butt of ridicule—humorous or otherwise—is a reflection of the fact that even in 1982 there remains a stigma to being a patient in treatment. Despite the fact that most violence in our society is perpetrated by individuals who are not psychiatric patients, the mentally ill are popularly believed to be dangerous. Employers often discriminate against individuals with a prior history of mental disorder despite the fact that most make good employees. We are

114

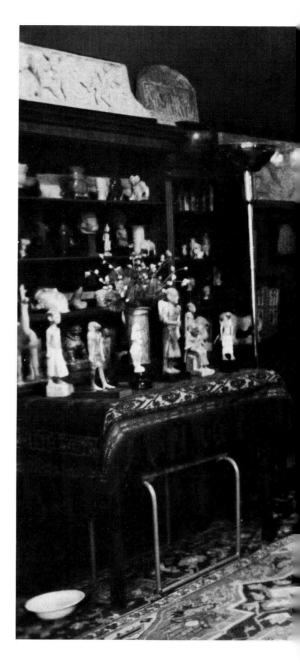

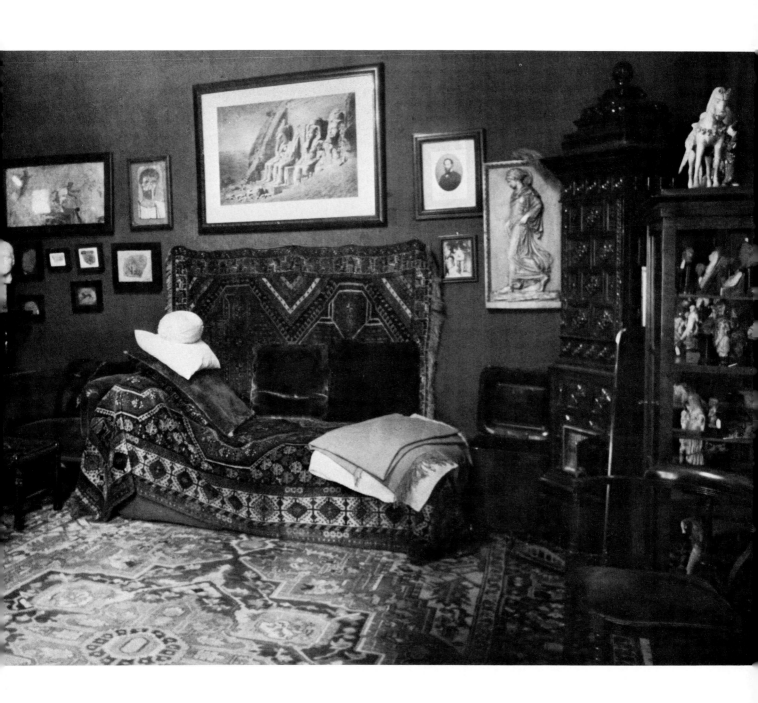

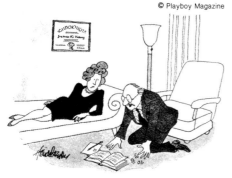

"The Electra complex is always a toughie, and on top of that, you were born under Aquarius. Let's see what the 'I Ching' says."

The consultation of psychoanalyst and client is a widely recognized comic situation, even for people who have never consulted a therapist. It is a circumstance that seems to exemplify the expression of human foibles.

Leon Eisenberg, M.D., *is Professor of Psychiatry, Maude and Lillian Presley Professor, and Chairman of the Department of Social Medicine and Health Policy at Harvard Medical School in Boston.*

(Overleaf) Sigmund Freud's office, Berggasse 19, Vienna.
© *Edmund Engelman*

not very far from the day when the mentally ill were thought to be possessed by demons and when mental illnesses were regarded as just punishment for sexual sins. Fortunately, the efforts of citizens' groups, such as the National Mental Health Association, have begun to reverse ignorance and suspicion.

What is curious is the extent to which popular culture has continued to lag behind changes in mental health practice. Psychiatrists (and psychoanalysts in particular) are now a minority of practicing psychotherapists, and most clients enter psychotherapy for mild and moderate rather than severe psychological disorders.

The scope of psychotherapy

Psychotherapy may be loosely defined as the treatment of discomfort, dysfunction, or disease by psychological methods. Several aspects of this definition merit emphasis. The treatment is defined by the *methods* it employs and not by the patients at whom it is directed. Psychotherapy is effective not only for the treatment of psychiatric disorders as such but also for the treatment of other medical problems, even those that have primary biological causes. Contrariwise, medication and other biological treatments have been shown to yield the best results for certain mental disorders. Some individuals seek psychotherapy in order to improve their ability to function on the job, to improve marital adjustment, or to achieve greater self-understanding; in such patients disease in the usual medical sense of the term is not present, but dysfunction or discomfort may be perceived by the patient.

The Report of the President's Commission on Mental Health, issued in 1978, estimated that about 15% of the U.S. population suffers at any given time from a diagnosable mental disorder. However, only two in five of those persons receive any form of care from mental health professionals. Three categories of illness account for four-fifths of the mental morbidity in Americans: depression, anxiety disorders, and alcoholism. The commission report recommended that the nation undertake a commitment to develop a network of accessible community mental health services, to plan for those services in a way that recognizes their close relationship to health and other human services, and to give priority to persons with chronic mental illnesses, the most neglected sector of the population. For many of these patients psychotherapy is only one component of the care they need, but it is an important component.

Although all methods of psychotherapy have in common the use of psychological methods, they differ widely in the theories on which they are based. They also differ in the techniques they employ as well as in the professional training required of the therapist.

Does psychotherapy work?

Although debate about the effectiveness of psychological treatment is far from new, it was drawn forcefully to public attention by hearings before the Health Subcommittee of the U.S. Senate Committee on Finance in 1980. The occasion for the hearings was provided by proposals to increase the coverage for outpatient psychotherapy under mandated benefit programs. Currently, policies sharply restrict the dollar amount provided for outpatient psychiatric care in contrast to broad coverage for the treatment of medical conditions. To the advocates for mental health—both lay and professional—this has long been regarded as unjust. However, even those senators sympathetic to this claim express concern about the ultimate cost to public funds if such care is made available without restriction. Cost control presents a particular problem owing to the difficulty of specifying precisely which conditions warrant psychotherapy. In addition, there are large numbers of "therapists" who differ in training and in methods of treatment but who contend they are legitimate providers of care. In consequence, staff members for the Senate committee put forth the proposition that proof of effectiveness should be required before a psychological treatment method is designated as eligible for reimbursement.

On its face the proposal is not unreasonable. Yet, the fact is that no such requirement is placed on what insurers term "usual and customary" (in contradistinction to "innovative") medical and surgical treatments. For example, tonsillectomy is regularly paid for even though most pediatric authorities contend that it is ineffective for all but a minority of the conditions it is used to "treat." Clearly, heart transplants are experimental (and this is why most insurance policies—except in California—will not cover them). However, many "standard" medical procedures have never been put to exacting test by a controlled clinical trial. Despite the lack of evidence for efficacy, such treatments have been exempt from fiscal challenge on the grounds that they are usual and customary in medical practice. The demand for proof in the case of mental health care then probably has far less to do with scientific issues than it does with cost containment.

What *are* the findings from studies of the outcome of psychotherapy? A vast literature can be summarized in one sentence: By far the majority of studies indicate that symptoms are substantially relieved and that social function is detectably improved at the end of treatment, even though all patients do not benefit. There are, of course, studies that show no improvement, but they stand in the minority. With some exceptions (which will be noted later) it has not been possible to demonstrate that any one method of psychotherapy is better than another. This does not prove that there is no difference; it may merely reflect the relative insensitivity of currently available methods for measuring outcome. A further reason for the difficulty in detecting potential differences in psychotherapeutic methods is that large-scale studies often employ beginning rather than experienced therapists because they are more available.

A significant variable in predicting outcome is the nature of the condition being treated by psychotherapy. By and large, the most favorable results have been obtained in the treatment of neuroses (anxiety states, phobias, conversion disorders, and adjustment disorders) and the least favorable in the treatment of psychoses (the schizophrenias and affective disorders). Even with psychoses, however, which in most cases respond best to psychoactive medication, psychotherapy has been shown to add to the benefit obtained from drugs.

Despite the confident claims of superiority made by psychotherapists of different persuasions, systematic comparisons of their results call to mind

In One Flew over the Cuckoo's Nest, *the movie adaptation of a novel by Ken Kesey, Jack Nicholson portrayed a recalcitrant mental patient who was endlessly locking horns with a punitive and authoritarian hospital staff.*

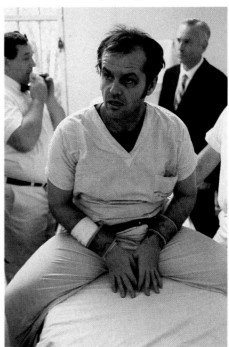

117

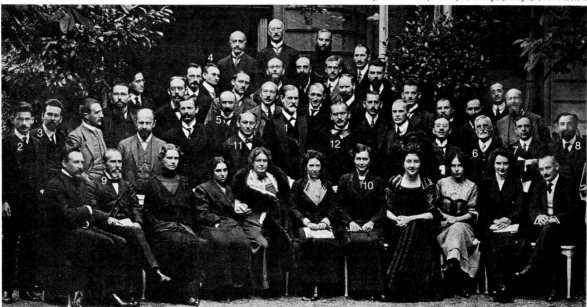

Many of the pioneers of psychoanalysis gathered for a group portrait in Weimar, Germany, in 1911. Included in the photo are (1) Sigmund Freud, (2) Otto Rank, (3) Ludwig Binswanger, (4) A. A. Brill, (5) Max Eitingon, (6) James J. Putnam, (7) Ernest Jones, (8) Wilhelm Stekel, (9) Eugen Bleuler, (10) Emma Jung, (11) Sandor Ferenczi, and (12) C. G. Jung.

the Dodo's comment in *Alice's Adventures in Wonderland:* "*Everybody has won and all must have prizes.*" In fact, the very success of various forms of psychotherapy raises a number of questions. When forms of psychotherapy based on theories as different as psychodynamic and behavioral, cognitive and nondirective, or individual and group produce similar results, it implies that there are some fundamental underlying components that are common to all therapies. What are these characteristics?

Psychiatrist Jerome Frank of Johns Hopkins University has suggested that the following aspects are common to all successful treatment approaches: (1) a therapeutic relationship that entails genuine acceptance of the sufferer; (2) a locale (an office, a hospital, or a clinic) designated by society as a place of healing; (3) a rationale that enables the patient to make sense of his symptoms; and (4) a set of tasks or procedures that provide the patient with new opportunities for learning. Frank believes that all therapies enhance the patient's hope of relief and provide opportunities for experiencing success: "When successful, all forms of psychotherapy relieve dysphoric feelings, rekindle the patient's hopes, increase his sense of mastery over himself and his environment, and in general restore his morale. As a result, he becomes able to tackle the problems he had been avoiding and to experiment with new, better ways of handling them."

Psychological treatment, far from being experimental, has been in use in healing the sick since the earliest of times. Indeed, until the fruits of the 19th-century revolution in the natural sciences began to be applied to medical problems in the early years of this century, most of the benefits doctors provided patients anywhere in the world were psychological.

Anthropologists who have studied preliterate societies around the globe confirm that there is no human group without healing practices intended to benefit the sick. Every human group has discovered at least a few medically effective herbal remedies by trial and error, and many tribes also had expert

118

bone setters and "specialists" in rudimentary surgery. But the great majority of procedures employed by traditional healers have had *symbolic* and *ritual* rather than pharmacologic actions. When the "medicine" worked, it was not because of the specific ingredients in the concoction; rather, the taking of the medicine was embedded in an elaborate transaction that had meaning for the patient and aroused expectations of cure.

Studies in outpatient medical clinics indicate that even today not less than half of patients who consult doctors have no discoverable biological cause for their problem. Of those with an ascertainable medical problem, a substantial fraction suffer from chronic diseases which are not fully reversible. Yet the majority of functionally impaired and chronically ill patients do obtain relief—relief based on the interpersonal transaction between "sufferer" and "healer." Even when potent drugs are the core of the treatment, psychological components remain an important ingredient. At the very least a prescribed drug has to be taken, which means a good doctor-patient relationship is essential to enlist the needed cooperation. But more importantly, along with the curative drug the ill patient needs to have his morale sustained by belief in his doctor.

The cynicism and widespread skepticism that abound about the effectiveness of psychotherapy defy the evidence for the power of psychological interventions that is visible in every sphere of life. Consider, for example, the "Hawthorne effect." In the 1920s researcher Elton Mayo, working at the Hawthorne Works plant of the Western Electric Co. in Cicero, Illinois, demonstrated that a change in working conditions could increase worker productivity. At first the increase was ascribed to the physical features of the change (increased illumination), but it was soon discovered that a change in the opposite direction (decreased illumination) could produce equal effects so long as the change was viewed by the workers as designed to make things better. Medical therapeutics is replete with similar examples of apparent benefit following a new treatment that, on further study, has been shown to have no intrinsic value other than that it aroused positive expectations.

Psychotherapy has been found to be an effective adjunct to medical therapy for diseases such as asthma that have a psychological component. At the National Jewish Hospital in Denver, Colorado, therapists help children who are severely sick with asthma deal with the problems of their illness. A psychiatrist uses a puppet (left) to help a child express his feelings.

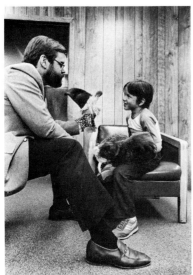

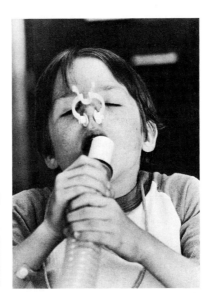

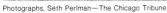
Photographs, Seth Perlman—The Chicago Tribune

So regular is this phenomenon, known as the placebo effect, that it must be taken into account in the scientific design of therapeutic trials. The outcome of a group of patients receiving a new treatment must be matched against that of a comparable patient group who receive either the standard treatment or, if there is no treatment thought to be effective, a placebo (an inert preparation made up in such fashion as to appear identical with the new agent being tried). Before physicians conclude that the new treatment is beneficial, they require statistical evidence that the rate of improvement it produces exceeds that which results from taking the placebo. The rate of placebo response varies with the nature of the condition being treated and the characteristics of the patients. It is usually not less than 20 to 30% and may be as high as 70 to 80%.

It is evident then that psychological effects are a major ingredient of every healing encounter. Systematic studies of psychotherapy have demonstrated its effectiveness in the treatment of a wide variety of medical as well as emotional disorders. The challenge for future research is to answer the still unanswered question: What type of treatment by what kind of therapist is best for which conditions and which patients?

Psychotherapists

The major categories of recognized psychotherapists have emerged from the fields of medicine, psychology, and social work. In recent years psychiatric nurses and mental health counselors also have been recognized as legitimate providers of psychological care. At the fringe of this group are many other self-proclaimed therapists whose qualifications may be limited to having undergone a course of an unorthodox "treatment" of the type they then propose to provide to others.

Unorthodox therapies extend from Erhardt seminar training (est) to religious cults that legitimize sexual acting out, from nude encounter groups to "marathons" (group therapy extending over several days without interruption), from Hubbard's dianetics (employed by the Church of Scientology) to spiritualism and voodoo rites. There is no question that each of these approaches can and does produce some temporary "cures" when the treatment mode happens to coincide with the psychological needs and cultural beliefs of particular communicants. For example, the disturbed person who believes himself "possessed" by an evil spirit may experience a loss of symptoms after an elaborate ritual of exorcism.

The risks involved in the practice of some of these unorthodox psychotherapies, on the other hand, are not trivial. Some individuals experience acute distress when they find themselves unable to adhere to the exhortations of a particular charismatic leader. The claims of these unorthodox therapies rest, for the most part, wholly on testimonials rather than any kind of systematic or scientific evaluation. Owing to the fact that there are more than 230 "brands" of psychotherapy and the number grows each year, the focus here is limited to the most common and best validated modes of psychological treatment.

Psychiatrists come from the medical tradition; in the United States they are physicians who have graduated from medical schools and have had three

120

years of post-M.D. residency training in psychiatry, in the course of which they have been supervised in diagnosing and treating a wide variety of patients with mental disorders. They are the only mental health professionals permitted to prescribe drugs and other biological treatments. In 1981 there were somewhat more than 25,000 members of the American Psychiatric Association (about two-thirds of them certified by the American Board of Psychiatry and Neurology).

Medically qualified psychoanalysts are psychiatrists who have completed additional training at psychoanalytic institutes. This training consists of seminars on theory and practice, a personal psychoanalysis, and the supervised completion of several "control" analyses of appropriate patients. The course of training requires five to seven years. (There are also psychoanalytic schools that provide similar, though not identical, training for individuals without medical qualifications—usually psychologists or social workers.)

Psychologists constitute another major category of psychotherapists. Most states in the U.S. have certification procedures for those legally entitled to practice as clinical psychologists. In addition to an undergraduate degree, they have completed a Ph.D. (doctor of philosophy) degree program plus an internship in clinical psychology. In some states an Ed.D. (doctor of education) degree or an M.A. (master of arts) degree plus three years of clinical experience may be substituted for the Ph.D. requirement in order to be admitted for certification. A much larger number of individuals with less training and without certification also provide psychological services. A survey conducted by the American Psychological Association indicates that about 32,000 of its 51,000 members provide clinical care.

A third recognized category of psychotherapist is that of social workers. It is unfortunate that this term is not limited to those with professional competence. For example, someone who works for a social welfare agency may be called a "social worker" despite a lack of any professional training. Membership in the National Association of Social Workers (which in 1981 exceeded 84,000) requires only a baccalaureate degree in social work, the minimum requirement in states that certify social workers. The Academy of Certified Social Workers (which accredits practitioners) requires at least an M.S.W. (master of social work) degree. Although the roots of social work lie in organized efforts to help groups of disadvantaged persons, recent years have seen an increasing emphasis on psychotherapy in case work. In the U.S. the number of social workers in full-time private practice has more than doubled in the past ten years (to an estimated 6,000 practitioners), and those in part-time private practice are estimated at about 15,000.

The last several decades have seen the emergence of new categories of mental health workers, although the patterns of training and the necessary qualifications have yet to be standardized. Special programs in psychiatric nursing, requiring specialization in addition to general nursing education, have long been in existence, but it is only in recent years that "psychiatric nurses" have begun to work in outpatient clinics and in private practice as psychotherapists. A number of organizations and institutions, such as the National Institute of Mental Health, have provided training programs for mental health counselors, individuals with a college degree who usually

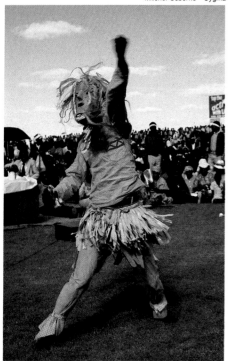

Until the advent of modern medical science, most of the benefits patients derived from treatments were purely psychological. A vast majority of methods used by traditional healers had symbolic or ritual rather than pharmacologic actions. The incantations of this modern-day witch doctor create a therapeutic atmosphere that may well have healing effects on believing participants in this Zimbabwe rally.

undergo two years of specialized training in outpatient mental health care. This category includes pastoral counselors.

Given these differences among psychotherapists, what criteria can an individual use to obtain competent mental health care when it is needed? The patient can verify whether the professional has the appropriate specialty certification and holds a staff appointment at a local hospital or university (which usually indicates peer approval of credentials). Neither certification nor a faculty appointment assures competence; gifted therapists may lack credentials and mediocre ones may have them. But generally it can be said that the odds for competence are better among the certified.

When should a psychiatrist be chosen and when another professional? Psychiatrists, because of their medical training, are best able to rule out organic disorders masquerading as psychological problems, to manage severe mental disorders for which medication as well as psychotherapy may be required, and to care for patients with coexisting medical problems. If the difficulty falls into the "problems of living" category, the psychologist (or experienced social worker or counselor) may be an equally competent psychotherapist and may charge lower fees (though not necessarily).

A smorgasbord of psychotherapies

Given the constraints of space, the following attempt to epitomize the essentials of theory and practice of some of the major schools of psychotherapy must necessarily be cursory and oversimplified. Nonetheless, it is useful to describe some of the elements of a number of them in order to emphasize the differences that exist among them.

Psychodynamic therapies. Psychodynamic psychotherapies are probably the most widely practiced form of psychiatric treatment in the United States. The psychodynamic approach is based on several overlapping theories about the organization and function of the human mind. Basically, the concept of psychodynamics has theoretical underpinnings in the notion that much of human emotion and behavior is rooted in the mind below the level of consciousness. There are, however, many conflicting factions among contemporary practitioners because the evolution of theory has left in question whether old concepts are to be discarded, modified, or kept intact.

Psychodynamic psychotherapies are relatively intensive talking treatments aimed at providing the patient with insight into his conscious and unconscious mental processes, enabling him ultimately to achieve a better understanding of himself. Psychodynamic psychotherapy attempts to enhance personality growth as well as to remove symptoms. It is usually conducted in face-to-face interviews at a frequency of one to two times a week in sessions that last 45 to 50 minutes. A course of treatment may take from six months to several years. A primary technique in many psychodynamic forms of treatment is "free association," which Freud characterized as the fundamental rule of psychoanalysis; in his words, the patient "is to tell us not only what he can say intentionally and willingly, what will give him relief like a confession, but everything else as well that his self-observation yields him, everything that comes into his head, even if it is disagreeable for him to say it, even if it seems to him unimportant or actually nonsensical."

122

"Empathy" on the part of the therapist allows the patient to express thoughts and feelings that permit the uncovering of underlying conflicts. The patient's maladaptive behaviors, feelings, and belief systems are also discerned from "the transference"—during which feelings and behaviors that originate in earlier significant relationships, particularly those with parents, are projected onto the therapist (who assumes a more or less passive role). A major therapeutic tool is interpretation. This technique helps the patient become aware of previously repressed aspects of conflict and the meaning of uncomfortable feelings evoked by the transference.

More supportive forms of psychodynamic psychotherapy are appropriate for patients in acute distress or turmoil or for those who cannot or do not wish to experience the anxiety of intensive treatment. Goals are generally more modest, and emphasis is on support more than interpretation. In supportive therapy useful defenses are strengthened (rather than challenged). The therapist is more active and is seen as a constant source of support. He may reassure, educate, inspire, and persuade. In the early phase of treatment the therapist and patient enter into an informal contract about the focus of treatment, its duration, and what each of the participants can expect of the other. The most important initial task is the attainment of a therapeutic alliance—i.e., a working relationship based on mutual trust and confidence. This alliance provides the context for focusing on specific problems that must be worked through.

As psychodynamic treatment proceeds, the therapist helps the patient recognize the historical determinants of his focal problem, the way that particular problem influences the patient's current life, and the way it manifests itself in relationship to the therapist. This tripartite effort was dubbed "the triangle of insight" by American psychiatrist Karl Menninger. The process of working through problems permits the patient to develop new and constructive styles of interpersonal relationships to replace the nonadaptive styles that led to the need for treatment in the first place.

Interpersonal psychotherapies. The importance of social factors and person-to-person interactions in the patient's maladaptive behavior are emphasized in the so-called interpersonal therapies. Adolph Meyer and Harry Stack Sullivan were principal pioneers of this therapeutic approach. In treatment patient and therapist meet once or twice a week and focus on current problems, conflicts, and wishes. Although early childhood experiences are recognized as important and may be acknowledged briefly in treatment, focus is on the here and now. The goals of treatment are symptom relief and improved social function. Treatment is time-limited and disclaims any attempt at fundamental personality change. The patient and therapist mutually agree on goals and time limits. Treatment is considered successful when the goals have been attained even if the patient is still afflicted with residual discomfort or dysfunction.

Psychoanalysis. Psychoanalysis is the most intensive form of psychotherapy, which, of course, originated with Freud. It is conducted with the patient lying on a couch for four to five visits a week, generally, for at least three years. In contrast to the once-or-twice-a-week psychodynamic therapy described above, the analyst is less active, fosters more regression, and aims

(Top) Dan McCoy—Rainbow; (bottom) Tony Korody—
Sygma

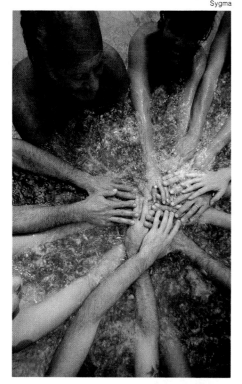

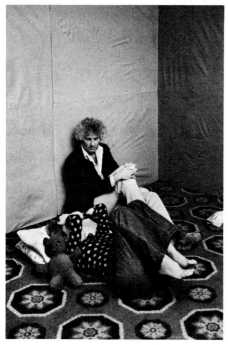

Nude encounter groups and primal scream therapy are two unorthodox methods of treatment that have arisen in the last couple of decades. Most claims for the effectiveness of these vogue therapies derive from testimonials of enthusiastic participants and not from science.

at greater structural changes in the personality.

In classical analysis the central focus is on the transference. To facilitate the development of the transference, the analyst endeavors to maintain a neutral stance toward the patient in order to serve as a "blank screen" onto which the patient can project his inner feelings, particularly those feelings that are of an irrational nature. This is, of course, an ideal but ultimately unattainable condition; the personality of the analyst, the patient's predispositions, and the actual relationship between analyst and analysand inevitably influence the process.

The key event in psychoanalysis is the resolution through interpretation of psychological events the patient has not hitherto understood. For this to occur, it is necessary for the therapist's personal (in addition to his professional) reactions to the patient to come into play (countertransference).

Psychoanalysis is the most demanding of the psychotherapies in terms of cost, time, and effort. Is there any evidence that the therapeutic yield from this very considerable investment is greater than that obtainable from other forms of psychotherapy? Unfortunately, despite 80 years of psychoanalytic practice, there is no such evidence. In part this stems from the lack of a scientific research tradition in psychoanalysis; in part it may reflect the difficulty of "measuring" changes in personality structure. Although psychoanalysis has had a profound influence on American psychiatry, which some view as quite astonishing in light of the absence of empirical evidence, that influence has waned significantly in the past decade. Fewer patients enter psychoanalysis, and many analysts now carry out short-term psychodynamic therapy. Freud himself wavered; he argued that psychoanalysis was a research tool at moments when he despaired of producing fundamental changes in the human psyche, and he contended that it was a method of treatment at times when its scientific inadequacies were criticized.

Two of Freud's onetime associates, Carl Jung and Alfred Adler, established their own approaches to psychoanalysis. Jungian analysis places far less emphasis upon free association, focusing instead on interpreting certain aspects of the patient's fantasies and dreams. The basic Jungian thesis is that there is a reservoir of shared unconscious wisdom—a so-called collective unconscious—which permeates each individual unconscious mind. Adlerian analysis concentrates on the patient's idealized concept of himself and is concerned with the relationship of the patient's personal aspirations and goals, both conscious and unconscious, to his social setting and total life situation.

During the last decade the importance of developmental deficits has been recognized as more important in some patients than intrapsychic conflicts—thus the proliferation of the various psychodynamic approaches and the waning of more traditional psychoanalyses. It is now recognized that empathic understanding is as important a therapeutic tool as insight. Moreover, such an approach tends to address more directly the needs of patients.

Human potential therapies. So-called client-centered (nondirective) psychotherapy was developed in the 1940s by Carl R. Rogers at the University of Chicago. It emphasizes the building of self-esteem in the patient, or client, by cultivating his internal resources for self-understanding and change. (Ge-

124

stalt therapy is a later human potential approach that promotes self-awareness by viewing the patient as a whole person—mind and body are considered inseparable.)

In Rogerian client-centered therapy the attitudes of the therapist rather than his technical training or skills are regarded as crucial to the success of the treatment. First and foremost the therapist must show empathy—genuine understanding of the experiences and the feelings of the client. The client's experience of being understood is considered to be a powerful impetus for growth. The therapist must also suspend judgment and evaluation in order to communicate caring for the client as a person with constructive potential. Additionally, the therapist must be open and honest in his relationship with the patient; of course, in following this precept, the therapist must be on guard against the risk of burdening the client with his own problems.

The available research on client-centered therapy provides evidence of positive outcome in the treatment of individuals with a wide variety of difficulties. This treatment method has been widely utilized in school counseling services and has been incorporated into training programs for teachers. Client-centered therapy is useful for individuals with psychological problems of mild and moderate intensity but not ideal for seriously disturbed persons.

Behavior therapies. The treatment methods of behavior therapy are based on the concepts of experimental psychology, particularly those of learning theory. Neurotic disorders are viewed as learned responses that have become maladaptive. Behavior therapy focuses on what can be observed (what is done and what is said) rather than on what must be inferred (motives, unconscious processes, and symbolic meanings). It begins by specifying desired changes in behavior.

A number of controlled clinical trials have shown that behavior therapy is the most effective form of psychotherapy for the treatment of phobias, for weight reduction, for training social skills in retarded children, and for diminishing psychosomatic symptoms such as tension headaches and chronic pain. However, the treatment plan must be acceptable to the patient; cooperation is essential to success. Since change is the goal, the patient must want to change.

Although behavior therapy is often discussed solely in terms of techniques, the relationship between the therapist and the patient is no less important in this form of treatment than it is in any other. The first task is to identify as precisely as possible the problems for which the patient wants help. By way of example, consider weight loss. Indeed, behavioral methods have been far more successful than other methods of treatment (including drugs alleged to suppress appetite) in achieving weight loss, with some success in maintaining the benefit. What distinguishes behavioral methods is the emphasis on modifying eating behavior rather than on calorie restriction per se, though decrease in calorie intake follows automatically from decreases in the frequency of eating and the amount eaten.

An overweight patient might be instructed first to keep a careful record (a diary) of each time he eats, what and how much is eaten, where and when it happens, and who else is present. This initial procedure may in itself be therapeutic by increasing the awareness—which many overweight patients

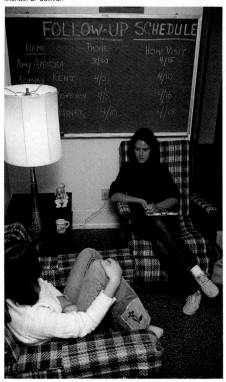

Today social workers form a major group of psychotherapists. In the U.S. there are more than 6,000 social workers in full-time private practice and an estimated 15,000 in part-time private practice.

125

lack—of his eating habits. Occasional successes have been reported from this step alone as an agent for change. It is, in any event, essential for the subsequent prescription of the changes to be made.

The second step is the control of the stimuli that precede and accompany eating; controlling events associated with eating helps the eating itself. Obvious steps include not keeping high-calorie foods in the home but having available instead supplies of low-calorie foods (celery, carrots, and so forth). The patient may be encouraged to eat in one place in the house (preferably the dining room), to use a distinctive table setting, and to eat at regular times. Behaviors such as eating in front of the television set are specifically discouraged. If paired with eating, watching television can itself become a conditional stimulus for eating whether or not it is mealtime or the patient is hungry.

The next step is to learn to control eating itself by focusing on every bite consumed and by decreasing the speed of eating. The patient may be instructed to count each mouthful, each chew, each swallow, and to put down his utensils at specified intervals. Increasing the delay between bites of food is a logical next step. Patients may have to learn to savor their food as they eat it and to make mealtimes enjoyable experiences.

Finally, each successive accomplishment (*i.e.,* keeping the diary, counting the mouthfuls, increasing the delay interval) earns "points," which are converted to tangible rewards. The rewards, of course, must be tailored to the patient's individual preferences (a new suit, a trip, a long-distance phone call, but not a box of fancy chocolates!).

In addition to this very rigorous and structured process, the patient needs ongoing psychologic support. Obesity is a source of great personal distress. The obese patient is the butt of humor, suffers social rejection, and may have difficulty at school or at work because of a general prejudice against fat people. This distress has long compounded the problem for the obese patient because it reinforces eating as a source of satisfaction when many normal opportunities for satisfaction are denied.

There is still a great deal to be learned about the enigma of obesity, of course. Behavior treatment, which attempts to alter permanently eating (and sometimes living) habits, has not been successful in all cases by any means. But it does seem to be the most effective method known of treating the widespread and refractory problem of overweight.

Relaxation techniques such as biofeedback, progressive muscle relaxation, autogenic training, transcendental meditation, and yoga are several behavioral methods that have in common the use of a quiet environment, the induction of a passive attitude (usually with eyes closed) in order to avoid distracting thoughts, and the use of some sort of mental device to draw attention away from external stimuli and onto internal stimuli. Whatever the method of induction, successful relaxation techniques decrease autonomic nervous system activity and can be very effective in the treatment of anxiety and a number of conditions that may have psychologic components, such as essential hypertension and headaches.

"Behavior modification" attempts to change behavior by shifting "reinforcements" from unwanted to wanted behaviors. Withdrawal of a reinforcement will, in principle, lead to the extinction of the behavior it has been main-

126

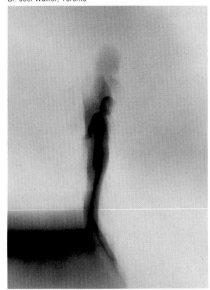 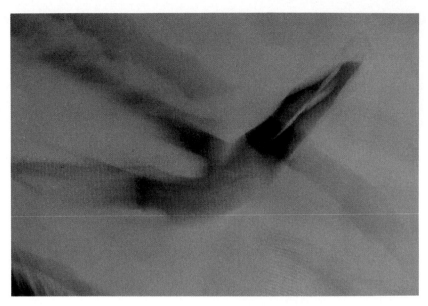

taining. For example, in children temper tantrums persist only so long as they gain results. If the parents are able to adhere to a program of deliberately ignoring the tantrums, then they will diminish. Behavior modification has proved to be a method of choice for teaching self-help skills and socially desirable behavior to mentally retarded children. It has also proved effective in reducing conduct problems in the classroom when employed by teachers with special training.

Cognitive therapy. Cognitive therapy, developed by A. T. Beck and his colleagues at the University of Pennsylvania, is an active, time-limited, and structured approach, particularly effective in the treatment of some depressions. Its techniques are designed to identify and to correct maladaptive concepts of the self in order to enable the patient to learn to master problems instead of giving up in the face of them. Cognitive therapy concentrates more on inner states (thoughts, feelings, wishes, and attitudes) than it does on overt behavior.

The depressed patient is helped to correct his extremely negative view of himself as defective, inadequate, and unworthy; to change his tendency to interpret the world as making exorbitant demands on him and presenting insuperable obstacles to his hopes; and to eliminate his persistently pessimistic view of the future, with expectations of frustration and failure.

A realistic view of the patient's situation (the one he comes to adopt if treatment is successful) leads to the recognition that difficulties can be overcome and that there are satisfactions to be had even in an imperfect world. Treatment must address the patient's "cognitive errors"—*e.g.*, drawing conclusions in the absence of supportive evidence, focusing on details taken out of context, drawing too wide a conclusion from a single incident (overgeneralization), and relating external events to the self when there is no such connection.

The efficacy of cognitive therapy for depression has been supported by more than a dozen controlled studies. This therapy was found to be more

A primary technique in psychodynamic psychotherapy is "free association," in which the patient is encouraged to reveal to his therapist as much of his inner life as he can, even those things that evoke feelings of anger, grief, shame, or confusion. Evocative images such as these photographs have been used by some psychiatrists as a device that can help the patient express his feelings through describing what he sees in them.

127

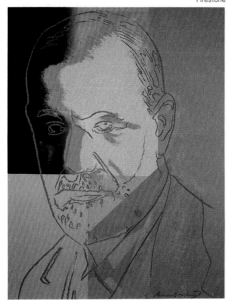

Psychoanalysis, which was originated by Sigmund Freud, is the most intensive form of psychotherapy. Its aim is to help the patient achieve alterations in his personality through a deep understanding of his past.

potent in relieving distress and changing behavior than alternative forms of psychotherapy. In addition, there is preliminary evidence that cognitive therapy may, in some cases, be superior to treatment with antidepressant drugs, but this observation requires further validation.

Family therapy. Family therapy, introduced in the United States in the 1950s, redefines psychological problems to include the entire family. It is thought to be the treatment of choice when the problems of an individual are best understood as manifestations of pathology within the family or when the family acknowledges its distress and seeks help in extricating itself from self-perpetuating destructive interactions. When the focus is on marital discord, treatment may be limited to the marital partners. More commonly, parents and children alike participate; sessions may include grandparents and other relatives if the extended family is in close contact.

There are a number of approaches to this form of treatment, which is one of the most rapidly expanding mental health specialties today. The task of the therapist is to attend to the continuing stream of family interactions, a task that requires considerable skill because individual members may demand disproportionate attention or withdraw from the action. When treatment is successful, communication within the family is increased, family members come to understand each other better, and the family develops more constructive ways of negotiating their differences and arriving at mutually acceptable solutions.

Of particular interest are recent reports of the successful use of family treatment methods in helping to maintain schizophrenic patients in the community after their discharge from the hospital. Studies have shown that emotional tension within the family is a stress poorly tolerated by schizophrenic patients. Helping patients and family to learn how to manage stress, therefore, has proved to be an effective adjunct to the use of medication in prolonging the schizophrenic's recovery.

Group therapies. Although there are a wide variety of theories and methods underlying different types of group psychotherapy, they share the essential feature of joining individuals in psychological distress into a group, guided by a therapist or "leader," on the premise that peer interactions enable such individuals to help one another in problem solving. Groups vary in size from 4 to more than 50 members but commonly consist of 8 to 10 patients plus a therapist and sometimes an "observer" or co-therapist.

A special kind of group is the peer self-help group, of which Alcoholics Anonymous (AA) is perhaps the best known example. AA is run entirely by and for alcoholics, and group meetings are devoted to confessions of the personal tragedies produced by drinking and inspirational testimonials by those who have overcome the problem. AA groups afford alcoholics the support of companionship with peers in a group whose norm is total abstinence from drinking alcohol. AA has been quite successful with alcoholics who are willing to join and to maintain membership. That excludes a considerable fraction of problem drinkers. Other successful self-help groups include Recovery Incorporated for patients recently discharged from mental hospitals and a wide variety of others organized for individuals who share a common problem: patients who have had surgery for breast cancer or abdominal cancers, abusive parents, paraplegics, diabetics, weight watchers, compulsive eaters, anorexia nervosa sufferers, and genital herpes victims. While some such groups have been organized by physicians or mental health professionals, others (like AA) abjure professional leadership and emphasize self-help.

In psychotherapy groups the function of the therapist is to facilitate interactions among group members. The goal is to create a climate in which participants shed their inhibitions. When members come to trust one another, they are able to provide feedback to each other—to respond to other group members in ways that may not be possible in ordinary social interactions owing to the constraints of social conventions. It is the task of the therapist to assure that matters do not get out of hand (*i.e.,* to intervene if, for example, one member is being mercilessly pilloried by the others). A successful group is marked by cohesiveness and increasing honesty in its interrelationships.

Group therapy usually takes place in sessions of an hour and a half to two hours on a weekly basis. Some groups are time limited (*e.g.,* to six weeks' duration). Others are ongoing, with participants leaving when they feel they have achieved maximum benefit. New members may occasionally join the group. There are many group approaches—supportive, analytically oriented, "transactional," those employing "psychodramatic" techniques—varying in intensity as well as in effectiveness. Some patients may participate in a group as an adjunct to individual treatment.

Treating Mrs. A

The proliferation of psychotherapeutic approaches used today reflects the fact that no single theory can explain all emotional problems. Nor can a single treatment method be applied. In fact, as Harvard University psychiatrist Aaron Lazare noted in 1973, a given emotional problem can be treated in quite different ways. Lazare outlined four "hidden" conceptual models and their distinct approaches. He showed that the individual psychotherapist

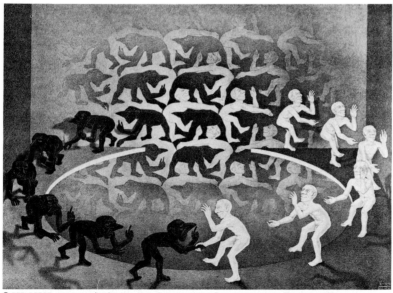

© BEELDRECT, Amsterdam/VAGA, New York. Collection Haags Gemmentemuseum—The Hague, 1981

One of Freud's major contributions to the field of psychotherapy was his elucidation of the process of transference. The patient undergoing therapy transfers to the therapist feelings that he has about his parents. It is the role of the therapist to recognize and interpret these feelings and to help the patient to acknowledge them.

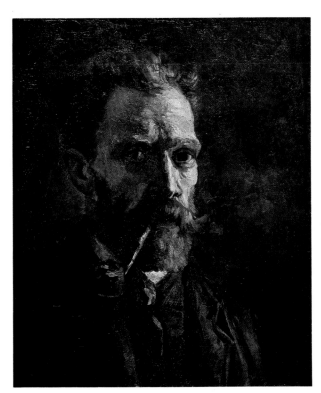
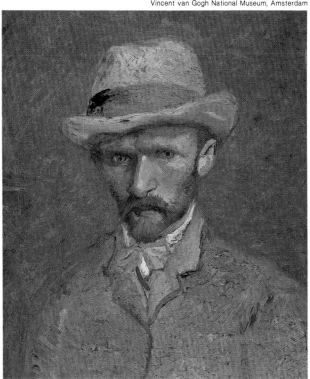

tends to interpret the symptoms presented by a patient in a way that fits his particular method.

Consider a common mental health problem: depression in a middle-aged woman, whom we shall call Mrs. A. A therapist who follows the "biological model" sees Mrs. A, a 50-year-old widow who has recently suffered a loss of appetite resulting in a 20-pound weight loss and a sleep disturbance characterized by early morning awakening. She reports her mood is "depressed" in the morning but improves as the day wears on. She exhibits slowed speech and complains of feeling hopeless and worthless. Her past medical history reveals a similar episode of depression 20 years earlier. Family history included a sister hospitalized for a depression that responded to electroconvulsive therapy (ECT).

The patient's age, symptoms, and history all correspond to the criteria for unipolar depression, a medical disorder that usually responds well to medication. Therefore, the therapist prescribes for this patient a trial of antidepressant medication, to which she responds. Should this course fail and her condition worsen, he might consider ECT treatments.

A therapist employing the "psychodynamic model" sees Mrs. A and notes first and foremost that she has been depressed for the several months since the death of her husband. Although her marriage had mostly been happy, there were also many stormy periods. Since the death of her husband, she has shown no visible signs of grief but has been depressed and has lost interest in her surroundings. She blames herself for traits that characterized her husband rather than herself. The therapist probes to learn she had a similar reaction after the death of her mother 20 years prior, when they had been

130

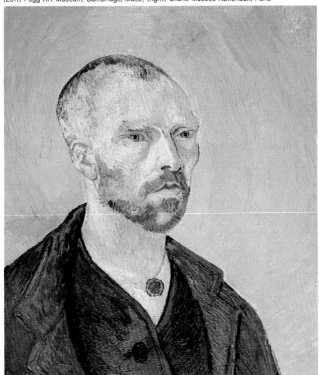 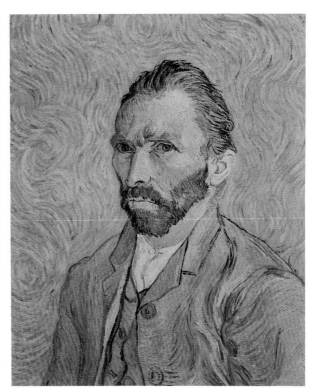

living together. The mother-daughter relationship was characterized by hostile dependency. It was six months after her mother's death that she married.

The therapist sees that the patient is intelligent, well motivated for treatment, and has considered psychotherapy in the past in order to understand herself better. The failure to mourn, followed by the onset of self-blaming depression, indicates to him that the symptoms are an expression of unconscious ambivalence. The relationship with her husband appears to have recapitulated many of the unresolved aspects of her relationship with her mother. He recommends that she come for dynamic psychotherapy sessions twice a week with special attention to the resolution of her delayed grief and her unconscious hostilities. In nine months she shows marked elevation of spirits and seems happy again.

A therapist following the "social model" sees Mrs. A and notes that she has been depressed since the death of her husband, who had been the major figure in her life. His loss has left her feeling utterly lonely and isolated. After his death she moved to a small apartment some distance from her old neighborhood. Although she was satisfied with her quarters, she found the community strange and unfriendly. Moreover, there was no access to public transportation, which might have enabled her to visit her friends and relatives. Since her husband's death, old strains between the patient and her children have gotten worse.

This therapist sees Mrs. A's depression as stemming from the loss of sustaining relationships, not only with her husband but also with her friends and children following her move from her accustomed neighborhood. His approach to treatment is aimed at helping the patient regain social ties. He

Among the goals of therapy are getting the patient to correct negative views of himself and helping him eliminate pessimism about the future. These four self-portraits by Vincent van Gogh reveal both the artist's evolution of style and his changing—and increasingly self-deprecating—perception of himself. The portrait at extreme right was painted shortly before deteriorating eyesight and recurrent bouts of depressive psychosis drove van Gogh to suicide.

131

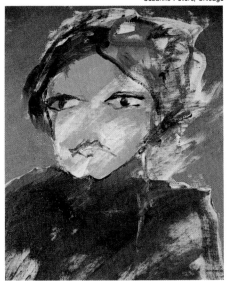

Various forms of psychotherapy differ greatly in their approaches to the patient's disorder. They all may agree on a single diagnosis, such as depression, but each may have a different opinion as to the cause of the disorder and the best way to approach its treatment.

encourages her to seek employment; in treatment he helps her develop social skills she had never acquired while her husband was alive.

Yet a fourth therapist, employing the "behavioral model," sees Mrs. A. He notes her symptoms: loss of appetite, sleep difficulty, feelings of hopelessness, and complaints of worthlessness. He views these as "depressive behaviors" that had begun shortly after the death of her husband, who had been a continuous source of positive reinforcement. This had been evident since the beginning of the marriage, at a time when the patient was still depressed from her mother's death. He learns that the husband had always ignored the patient's demands and pleas of being helpless, but he responded to the more positive aspects of her personality. After his death she began to complain to her children about her symptoms and her inadequacy. They responded to these complaints with frequent visits and telephone calls, but her depressive behavior only became worse.

In this therapist's assessment Mrs. A's symptoms are being maintained by the reinforcement provided by her children. He involves the children, encouraging them to reinforce her accomplishments rather than her complaints. He works with the patient to help her see how her ideas of worthlessness cause her symptoms; he helps her to acknowledge her many assets.

In the above case of Mrs. A, which therapist was "correct" in his approach? It can be argued that all were, because all were successful in helping Mrs. A overcome her depression. The reader may recall the great 1950 Japanese film *Rashomon,* in which the central story (the robbery and murder of a merchant and the rape of his wife) is told by each of the participants—the bandit, the merchant, and the wife—as well as an observer. Each presents a very different version of the same events. The viewer is left to ponder: Is each of the tales a separate aspect of the same truth? Is one right? In the hypothetical case of Mrs. A, one version of treatment is as "right" as the others. As Jerome Frank pointed out and a vast array of studies have demonstrated, success in psychotherapy is determined by many factors. Ultimately, what matters is that the patient is helped.

Group therapy can be effective in helping members solve their problems through their interactions. A special kind of group consists of members gathered because of a problem they have in common—overweight, alcoholism, or gambling, for example, or because they are peers in some other sense. These University of Wisconsin football players are participating in a group relaxation session led by a therapist. The aim is to help them work more effectively as a team.

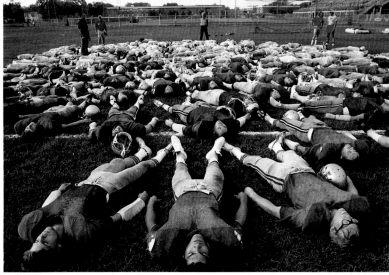

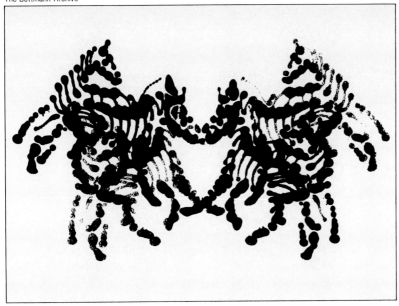

Hermann Rorschach's inkblots are a well-known diagnostic device for stimulating free association.

A final word

There is strong evidence that the psychotherapies *are* effective in relieving distress and in improving social function for most patients with emotional disorders. Yet we must await the results of systematic clinical research, which is presently under way, before we can confidently prescribe specific forms of psychotherapy for specific problems. Nonetheless, the important bottom line is that relief for sufferers *can* be provided by available treatments.

The fact that it *can* be provided, unfortunately, does not mean that it *is* being provided to most of those in need. The best available estimates of mental health needs in relation to services indicate that well under half of those who could benefit are receiving care. The major barrier to care is cost, because most insurance programs provide limited coverage or none. This denial of equity stems from an unwarranted fear of uncontrollable costs despite evidence that utilization is not excessive when coverage is provided. Some studies recently have shown that the addition of outpatient psychotherapy to insurance plan benefits results in some cases in cost savings by reducing repeated medical visits for psychosomatic complaints.

Among the most promising approach for making mental health services available is through health maintenance organizations (HMO's)—prepaid medical plans that provide comprehensive care to subscribers. Because HMO's distribute costs over a large population and can monitor the use of specialized as well as general medical services, they offer the best opportunity for cost containment.

A number of recent surveys have revealed that even patients who have mental health insurance coverage may not use it because they fear their emotional problems will be revealed to employers and will be held against them. For the same reason, others may forgo needed treatment. This is above all an indication that the greatest problem yet to be conquered may be the stigma so long associated with psychotherapy.

FOR ADDITIONAL READING:

Beck, A. T., *et al. Cognitive Therapy of Depression.* New York: Guilford Press, 1979.

Frank, J. D. *Persuasion and Healing.* Rev. ed. Baltimore: Johns Hopkins University Press, 1973.

Kleinman, Arthur. *Patients and Healers in the Context of Culture.* Berkeley: University of California Press, 1980.

Lazare, Aaron, ed. *Outpatient Psychiatry.* Baltimore: Williams & Wilkins, 1979.

Malcolm, Janet. *Psychoanalysis: The Impossible Profession.* New York: Knopf, 1981.

Parloff, M. B. "Can Psychotherapy Research Guide the Policymaker?" *American Psychologist,* 34 (1979):296–306.

Smith, M. L.; Glass, G. V.; and Miller, T. I. *The Benefits of Psychotherapy.* Baltimore: Johns Hopkins University Press, 1980.

Yalom, I. D. *The Theory and Practice of Group Psychotherapy.* New York: Basic Books, 1970.

Exercise and Mental Health
by Otto Appenzeller, M.D., Ph.D.

There is an energetic lobby today seeking to shift the primary focus of medical care from the relief of suffering to the prevention of disease and injury. These enthusiasts are urging that society adopt relatively cheap public health measures as a way of achieving expensive goals. The activists in health, mental or otherwise, have numerous recipes ready to assure a reduction in medical care costs by prevention of disease. One frequent advice is "aerobic" (endurance) training achieved through sports such as running, cross-country skiing, bicycling, and long-distance swimming. Recently, physical training has even been touted by some psychiatrists as a panacea for various forms of mental illness, those most vexing ailments.

Psychiatrists have described many single cases of the beneficial effects of exercise—as a means of reducing anxiety and tension, expressing aggression, working out sexual conflicts, repairing a "defective superego," and "curing" moderate depressions. Anecdotal, but not scientific, reports strongly support the notion that physical activity promotes a sense of well-being, which is, after all, what mental health is all about. Exercise *seems* to have a mystical quality that both renews and revitalizes the psyche. Of course, exercise cannot be "prescribed" based on these sheerly anecdotal observations. No one is sure whether this panacea works or is, in fact, worthwhile.

To many physicians, psychiatrists seem a species of theologian. They often evoke sarcastic remarks or perplexity from their colleagues. Other physicians, however, find psychiatric interests fascinating. Both psychiatrists and theologians are often faced with the problem of convincing others of the value of what they do. Running enthusiasts who claim psychological and spiritual benefits for the sport face much the same battle. In the limited studies that have been carried out to measure exercise's benefits for the relief of anxiety, depression, and so forth, mood generally is assessed by questionnaires, scores, scales, and inventories that depend largely on cooperative respondents. The answers before and after exercise or endurance training often provide eloquent and statistical evidence of improvement and benefit. But runners' responses are incomplete scientific measures, for they depend on language, which itself is not easily quantified.

Running enthusiasts are now gaining advantage in accumulating solid scientific evidence that gives weight for claims of the value of exercise, if not

Otto Appenzeller, M.D., Ph.D., *is Professor of Neurology and Medicine at the University of New Mexico School of Medicine in Albuquerque.*

(Opposite page) Runners in the 1981 New York Marathon cross the Verrazano-Narrows Bridge; photograph, Enrico Ferorelli—Wheeler Pictures

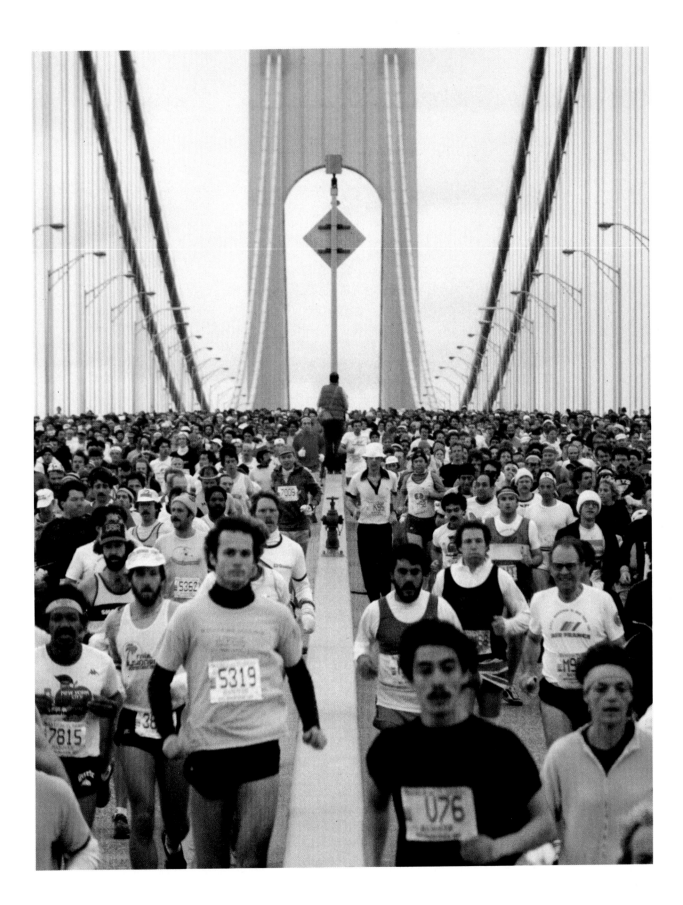

(Top) Richard Howard—Black Star; (center) The Bettmann Archive; (bottom) William McNamee—Woodfin Camp & Associates

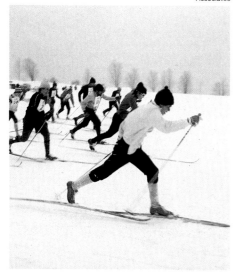

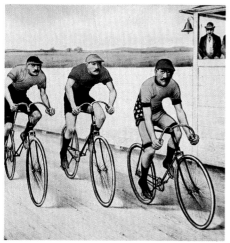

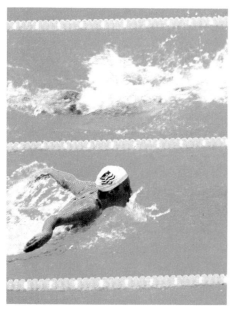

as a panacea, at least as a preventive measure of unprecedented effectiveness for many physical—and perhaps a number of mental—ills. Although they may not accept the quasi-religious trappings of today's exercise boom, many prudent physicians urge exercise on their patients with the same cautionary words used by some atheists: "There is no God, but it is wise to pray to Him from time to time."

Exercise and the nervous system: emerging evidence

Medical interest in exercise is not new. The Italian Bernardino Ramazzini in *Diseases of Workers,* published during the Renaissance, described a number of ailments in professional runners, whom he saw as excessively thin and compared with hunting dogs. He felt that their limited usefulness in service was due to their using up the "volatile elements of their blood" during their professional runs. Contrary to Ramazzini's views, it has now been clearly shown that runners are at no risk of exhausting their vital humors; surprisingly, they may even increase the levels of certain naturally occurring substances whose activity is similar to that of administered opium.

These naturally occurring opiumlike compounds, or peptides, among them beta-endorphin, have been found in the nervous system and many other tissues. They have been shown to influence pain sensation and, in abundance, produce a pain-free state, or analgesia (which has also been induced on occasion with acupuncture or with electrical stimulation of the brain). The effect of these substances, like the effect of opium itself, can be nullified by a drug called naloxone, which is a specific opium antagonist. These endogenous (originating within the body) opioids have many other effects. They influence hormonal secretion and the activity of hormones, temperature regulation and appetite, respiration and sleep, mood and sexual function, and they have tentatively been linked to drug addiction because they attach to the same sites in the brain where opium and its derivatives are effective.

When the changes in function produced by endogenous opioids are compared with measured alterations in internal balance of endurance-trained individuals, they closely parallel each other. It has been suggested that the exhilaration many runners feel several miles into their daily runs is due to an outpouring of these endogenous opioids. There is, however, no solid understanding of what has been euphemistically called the runner's "high" and its converse, the depression that often follows the inability to indulge in daily exercise and the exercise "withdrawal syndrome." It may, of course, be that any resemblance implied by these designations to the addictive properties of opium and perhaps its endogenous counterparts is purely coincidental.

Though endogenous opioids were first described in medical literature in 1975, a hint of the part they play in behavior and feelings during danger appears in David Livingstone's book *Livingstone's Africa: Perilous Adventures and Extensive Discoveries in the Interior of Africa,* published in 1872. The Scottish physician, missionary, and explorer described his feelings as a lion attacked and buffeted him: "The shake annihilated fear, and allowed no sense of horror in looking round at the beast. The peculiar state is probably produced in all animals killed by carnivora; and if so, is a merciful provision by our benevolent Creator for lessening the pain of death." Livingstone clearly recognized that somehow the "shake," or movement, was the trigger that extinguished fear and lessened his pain.

We now know that the so-called fight-or-flight response to danger—an alarm reaction that leads to adaptation or resistance—releases large quantities of catecholamines, substances that prepare the body for this response by increasing blood flow to muscles and the heart, which, in turn, also increases its pumping action. But simultaneously, with the release of catecholamines, there is also a secretion of endogenous opioids. During "fight" and "flight" reactions, prolonged muscular activity and movement is at first associated with pain and fear, but as the life-and-death struggle continues, the movement-induced secretion of endorphins may relieve the final agony.

A suspicion that the endorphin-release mechanism may have evolved as a means for dealing with inescapable pain led to investigations of the firewalkers who participate in religious ceremonies in the Balkans and other parts of the world. Lengthy preparation is required of celebrants, including dances that may parallel the violent movement that left Livingstone insensitive to pain and resigned to his end. These firewalkers, or pyrovats, complete their walks across the hot coals without the injury or burns that invariably harm the unprepared. But results of these investigations were inconclusive. After injections of naloxone, which nullifies the action of endogenous opioids and thus should have made the coal walks intolerable, the pyrovats were *unaffected,* except for an increase in the number and frequency of their footsteps on the hot coals.

In animals profound analgesia can be produced by inescapable electric shocks to the feet. This is antagonized by naloxone only if the shocks are intermittent, producing rhythmic movement, but not antagonized by naloxone when shocks are continuous, causing prolonged muscle spasm. Therefore, it appears that only particular sequences of intermittent movement bring about a release of endogenous opioids and opiod-related analgesia.

In humans a surge of endorphins has been demonstrated in the plasma after acute exercise. The capacity to release endorphins in response to physical stress also seems to increase with physical training and appears to be a normal and benign mechanism for coping with the stresses of long-distance running. In a 1980 experiment, however, high levels of endogenous opioids were maintained for only two hours after a 46-kilometer (28.6-mile) mountain race. It is not known whether these transient peripheral effects are associated with permanent alterations in endorphin-related brain function or behavior. But endorphins are known to be part of a feedback mechanism. After repeated stress their release may lead to maladaptive consequences. A persistent outpouring of endogenous opioids without appropriate feedback inhibition may cause stress-related pathologic states; suspicions that endogenous opioids are involved in depression, schizophrenia, and other mental illness are now being actively pursued. Moreover, in some fatal diseases of the brain, endorphin levels have been found to be very high. In highly trained endurance athletes, however, the plasma beta-endorphin levels decrease successively after repeated participation in the same 46-kilometer mountain race as though appropriate feedback inhibition of endorphin secretion preserves their sanity.

There is little doubt that physical exercise tends to raise the spirits. Some psychiatrists have even "prescribed" aerobic (endurance) activities such as running, cross-country skiing, swimming, and bicycling for patients suffering from anxieties and depression. There is, however, a paucity of "scientific" understanding of any specific psychological benefits that can be derived from regular participation in a given sport.

137

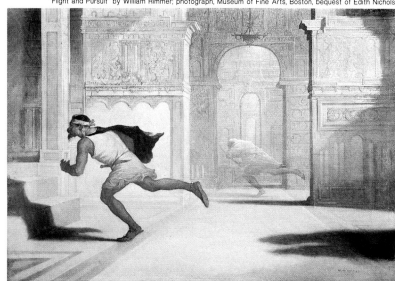

It is known that large quantities of substances secreted by the brain that produce a pain-free state are released into the bloodstream and go to the heart (increasing its pumping action) and to the muscles to prepare the body for a "fight-or-flight" response in times of danger. Recent research has suggested that the "high" runners feel several miles into their daily runs, as well as the withdrawal depression they report comes with inability to indulge in their sport, may also be related to an outpouring of naturally occurring opiumlike substances from the brain.

Psychiatric casualties of exercise

Neurotic breakdown of sudden onset in men devoted to sports has now been well-documented. In individuals with excessive, perhaps exclusive, preoccupation with fitness, the breakdown may occur about the age of 40—the age at which Ramazzini suggested retirement for professional runners.

Patients with "athlete's neurosis" are particularly difficult to treat. Most remain intractable chronic neurotics resistant to psychologic or physical therapies. They are constantly beset by gnawing hypochondriacal fears of illness, injury, and loss of function. These patients are known heroes of physical prowess and obtained satisfaction in life from a total devotion to sports. They have an enormous financial and spiritual investment in their bodies. They attach great importance to speed and strength—skills that deteriorate with age. The neurotic breakdowns in athletes are similar to those seen in some men devoted to work when they are forced to retire. It seems that the athlete's neurosis is a reaction to a loss of a part of the self, requiring readjustments that are not usually possible for such individuals. Such athletic crises are associated with an increased death rate, which is similar to the larger number of deaths found among creative geniuses when they are about to enter the same age group.

Sports heroes rarely retire voluntarily. They do so only after their fabulous earnings decline owing to progressive decrease in speed and skills. Few make a dignified exit from the professional arena to assume the relative sanity of the contemporary aging jogger who exercises for recreation.

A more recently observed, poorly understood phenomenon involves young women long-distance runners who take their sport to an extreme. In their pursuit of the "perfect runner's body"—lean, sparse, hard—these driven, highly competitive women and girls strive to achieve an inappropriate male ideal. Many not only run beyond exhaustion but also fall victim to anorexia nervosa, a complex psychiatric disorder characterized by self-inflicted starvation. The price of this fanaticism is sometimes death. An inordinate

For many aging men and women vigorous exercise seems to reduce the ravages of time on the physical decline of the body. It is probable that aerobic activity also preserves mental youthfulness. The graph on the opposite page shows a very slow and negligible decline between the ages of 30 and 70 in maximum performance of male marathon runners. One who in midlife runs a 3¹/₂-hour marathon ranks in the 99th percentile; not until he reaches the age of 73 would that time set an age-group record. Age appears to be a relatively unimportant variable. Similar observations have been made about intellectual capacity, memory, and social interactions in those who exercise.

138

desire for thinness may also account for the finding that female runners and swimmers who begin serious training before menarche frequently follow diets that are inadequately low in calories, protein, fats, and calcium.

Corporeal awareness is a perfectly natural phenomenon. Ordinarily it is unobtrusive, but it looms large in states of solitude. Even normal individuals often take an excessive interest in their appearance and subjective sensations. In women cosmetics, mirrors, and portraits may serve as outlets, and males indulge in elaborate adornments including whiskers, beards, and unconventional hairstyles. In primitive societies this body awareness that psychiatrists call narcissism may be expressed by deliberate deformation of the anatomy, and the recent vogue for tattooing among less primitive groups may be in this category.

Self-portraiture by artists might, of course, be motivated by vanity or the urge for self-perpetuation, but how can one explain the peculiar "dishonesty" of artist Beatrice Turner, who at the age of 58 painted a nude self-portrait portraying herself as a seductive voluptuous adolescent one year before she died of malnutrition? Perhaps this represents a narcissistic attempt to retain a youthful body well beyond its capacities to withstand the ravages of time and abuse.

The quest for "eternal summer"

To many nonparticipants even the relaxed runs of the recreational jogger lie outside the bounds of sanity. Many view the devotion to daily exercise as hedonistic and self-indulgent—an expression of narcissism—an attempt to stave off the effects of time and preserve an illusion of youth. Certainly the many physical complaints of today's jogger suggest narcissistic self-absorption. Joggers have myriads of ailments: aches and pains here and there mostly referred to legs, limbs, and backs. In almost all conditions of localized pain, the segment involved may intrude unduly onto the subject's awareness and inescapably direct attention to a leg, back, or bruised ligament and to the body as a whole.

Similar local enhancement of corporeal awareness can be seen with disease and also in ordinary circumstances of hunger, cold, heat, thirst, sexual arousal, or after exercise where it intensifies the relevant part of the body image. Perhaps, then, the daily exercise "fix" is a subtle form of narcissistic

Illustration by Kip Lott

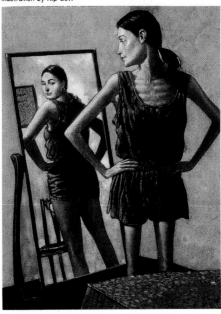

Exercise sometimes takes a negative psychological toll. Recently a phenomenon has been observed in some young women who devote themselves to long-distance running; they also fall prey to the complex psychiatric disorder anorexia nervosa. These perfectionistic women drive themselves to extremes and starve themselves to emaciation as well. Yet they are unable to see that their bodies are ever firm or lean enough.

World marathon records for men

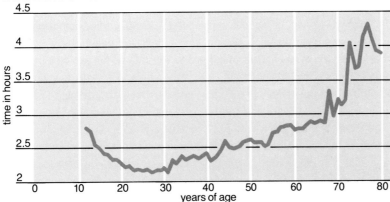

Adapted from "Aging, Natural Death, and the Compression of Morbidity," James F. Fries, *The New England Journal of Medicine*, July 17, 1980, pp. 130–135

(Top) Mark Kauffman, *Sports Illustrated;* (bottom) Neil Leifer, *Sports Illustrated*

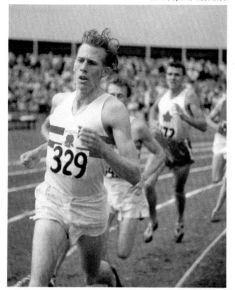

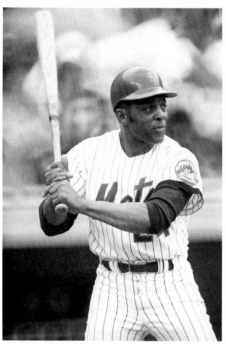

Roger Bannister (top), who broke the four-minute mile barrier in 1954 and is now a practicing physician, made a rare and graceful retirement from professional athletics. He has speculated that the casual sportsman may derive more healthy rewards from his sport than the champion who is forever obsessed with winning and has so much invested in his physical prowess. Indeed, facing retirement was not *easy but devastating for baseball superstar Willie Mays, whose exit from the major leagues came in 1973 at age 42.*

expression—now, of course, enshrined in linguistic approval as a "positive addiction" that serves to intensify "awareness of the body," a state now actively pursued by many members of our society.

Although legitimate questions are being raised about the mental health of millions of sporting adults in the United States, the sudden onset of athletes' neuroses are relatively unknown among those who jog, those who participate in aerobic dance classes, those who swim laps, and those who take daily long, brisk walks even though some do indeed become fitness fanatics. Of course, regular physical exercise to avert early disaster and perhaps postpone the inevitable end is in a totally different category from fanatic preparations for competitive excellence. Roger Bannister, who in 1954 was the first athlete to run a mile in under four minutes, has looked at the difference between the "champion" and the everyday "sportsman." (Bannister is also a physician who has investigated various aspects of the physiology of exercise.) The casual sportsman, Bannister has speculated, may derive more healthy rewards from his participation in a sport than the professional because his goals are moderate "and untarnished by the thought of success."

It might well be then that regular exercise rather than heroic competition prevents not only athletic neurosis but also the depression that commonly afflicts people when they happen to reach the middle-age juncture in their lives and careers. How aerobic exercise does this remains an enigma, and the role endorphins might play in the prevention of depression and various mental ills continues to be the subject of numerous studies on casual joggers and other exercisers.

Aging is of concern to all: to men, typically, as they approach the age of retirement, and to women, traditionally, much earlier, mostly related to matters of matrimony and childbearing. But athletic participation by age groups has led to eager anticipation of entry into the next older bracket in the hope that performance will not decline but will, even if static, be proportionately better than in the just-departed five-year segment. It is possible that man *is* as old as he feels and woman as old as she looks, and perhaps the changes brought about in bodily appearance and in feelings in women and men through exercise have some bearing on this.

As birthdays seem to come around with greater speed, we are apt to sigh, "How time flies"; it is good to remember, however, the wise words of Henry Austin Dobson: "Time goes, you say? Ah no! Alas, Time stays, *we* go." For many aging Americans the anticipation of competing in an older age group at the local weekend race seems to remove the common feelings of passing and sadness faced at each approaching birthday. Perhaps the completeness of life, which has usually manifested itself in three stages—the impetuosity and innocence of youth, the strength and steadfastness of middle age, and the crowning maturity of old age—could be changed, through exercise, to childhood, adulthood, and the terminal period of "you look wonderful."

No doubt this common flattery, "you look wonderful," in part motivates elderly women and men who now frequent our parks, parcours, and promenades. It may encourage the old to exercise regularly in their quest to prolong a useful independent existence, which has been epitomized by Oliver Wendell Holmes:

140

Call him not old whose visionary brain
Holds o'er the past its undivided reign.
For him in vain the envious seasons roll
Who bears eternal summer in his soul.

In the light of athletic performances by elderly men and women, it is obvious that training prevents or slows what have hitherto been considered the inevitable ravages of time on the human body. Visual evoked response times, which measure conduction velocities in the human brain's visual system and conduction velocities in nerves, suggest that measurable benefits can be obtained from endurance training. How these come about is not known. When, during the Renaissance, Ramazzini suggested that professional runners retire by the age of 40 as unfit for service, he correctly—if not consciously—anticipated the *emotional* breakdowns of athletic heroes as their physical prowess ebbs. In the case of nonprofessional runners, casual joggers, swimmers, cyclists, and aerobic dancers, however, it seems likely that exercise, particularly when used as an aid to change life-style, can preserve mental as well as physical youthfulness.

The mystique of aerobic exercise

Sense organs that are furnished messages via the nerves enable living things to survive, orient themselves in the outer world, and adapt to changes in it. This system has evolved through confrontation with an outer reality which we all experience. It is present in all of us before we meet the outer world, and it makes it possible to cope with the environment as we grow and develop.

Recent research in neurophysiology has allowed the discovery of some mechanisms that govern our ideation. For example, our perception of three-dimensional space is based on data supplied by the eyes about movement, size, and distance of objects and messages received from neck and inner-ear sensors that give information about the position of our body in space and also tell us about acceleration and deceleration, be it rotational or linear. These messages from the sense organs seem to be at the root of our concept of three-dimensional space, and yet we know that there are other dimensions we are incapable of sensing. Our capacity for self-generated movement evolved to help us cope with the environment; it is relevant to survival and perhaps provides us also with other as yet unrecognized "dimensions." These dimensions may well depend on movement-induced secretion of endorphins and their effect on mood and behavior.

Most of us use exercise as a common sense reaction to the public urging for change in life-styles in order to prevent disease. It is clear that the ideal for middle-aged American males and females has altered in recent years; it is now considered "bad" to be flabby and immobile. The new ideal of the exercising, dieting, nonsmoking American is really not new, however. In fact, it closely parallels the ideal prescribed by the Roman poet Juvenal (*c.* 55–130 AD) when he urged that man pray for a sound mind in a sound body. While there is yet no clear understanding of a cause-effect connection between healthy body and healthy mind, the few psychiatric casualties that might result from this quest are far outweighed by the benefits millions derive from exercise.

Detail of a Greek vase, 336 BC, The British Museum; photograph, Michael Holford

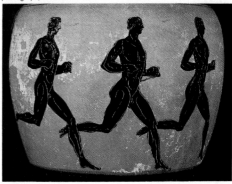

The current—and apparently spreading—obsession of so many men and women with physical fitness is really not new; the notion that man should strive for a sound mind residing within a sound body dates to ancient Roman times.

FOR ADDITIONAL READING:
Appenzeller, Otto. "What Makes Us Run?" *The New England Journal of Medicine,* 3 September 1981, pp. 578–579.

Appenzeller, Otto, and Atkinson, Ruth, eds. *Sports Medicine: Fitness, Training, Injuries.* Baltimore: Urban & Schwarzenberg, Inc., 1981.

Bannister, Roger. "The Meaning of Athletic Performance." In Talamini, J. T., and Page, C. H., eds. *Sport and Society.* Boston: Little, Brown, 1973.

Carr, D. B., Bullen, B. A., *et al.* "Physical Conditioning Facilitates the Exercise-Induced Secretion of Beta-Endorphin and Beta-Lipotropin in Women." *The New England Journal of Medicine,* 3 September 1981, pp. 560–563.

Critchley, Macdonald. *The Divine Banquet of the Brain and Other Essays.* New York: Raven Press, 1979.

Gallistel, C. R. "From Muscles to Motivation." *American Scientist* 68 (1980):398–409.

Henry, Sherrye, Jr. "The Price of Perfection." *The Runner,* March 1982, pp. 34–39.

Sacks, M. H., guest ed. "Psychiatric Aspects of Sports." *Psychiatric Annals,* March 1979.

———. *The Psychology of Running.* Champaign, Ill.: Human Kinetics Press, 1981.

Epidemiology: Challenges and Controversies

by Alvan R. Feinstein, M.D.

Epidemiology gets its name from human outbreaks of infectious disease. The outbreaks were called *epidemics* (from the Greek *epi* [ἐπι], meaning "upon," and *demos* [δεμος], meaning "people") to distinguish them from analogous events occurring in poultry (*epornitics*) or in animals (*epizootics*). Before bacteria and other microbial agents began to be identified in the late 19th century as causes of the outbreaks, the focus of epidemiologic studies had been air, water, and other features of the environment. The most famous of these studies was conducted in London in the 1850s by John Snow. From a map showing the pattern of water supply and the location of cases in a cholera epidemic, Snow concluded that a particular street pump was delivering contaminated water. He took the handle off the pump, and the epidemic ended.

The changing face of epidemiology

Snow's strategies and tactics set a new, enduring tradition for epidemiologic activities. Previously epidemiology had been concerned with descriptive data, often obtained from death certificates, about the occurrence of different diseases in groups defined by age, gender, occupation, geographic region, and other demographic distinctions. Snow's work helped epidemiology expand beyond these descriptive tabulations into two new domains: the analytic search for causes of disease and the use of active interventions to thwart them.

Snow had analyzed statistical information to make decisions about a disease's transmission, and he had taken direct action to prevent further outbreaks. Epidemiologists thereafter would continue to employ statistical analysis as a basic method of research into etiology, *i.e.,* the causes of disease, and would continue to emphasize prevention. In the late 19th century, the "sanitary movement" that followed Snow's work led to major improvements in sewage disposal, water purification, and other procedures that helped eliminate or reduce the spread of infectious disease.

One of the roles of modern-day epidemiologists—as etiologic detectives—has directly evolved from Snow's ancestral activities. Since the community epidemics that were common a century ago now occur only in countries where sanitation is still underdeveloped, the acute outbreaks that receive epidemiologic investigation today usually occur in relatively small groups of people. The detective work performed in checking the affected

Alvan R. Feinstein, M.D., *is Professor of Medicine and Epidemiology and Director of the Clinical Epidemiology Unit at Yale University School of Medicine, New Haven, Connecticut.*

(Opposite page) "The Doctor," oil on canvas, by Sir Samuel Luke Fildes (1891); photograph, the Tate Gallery, London

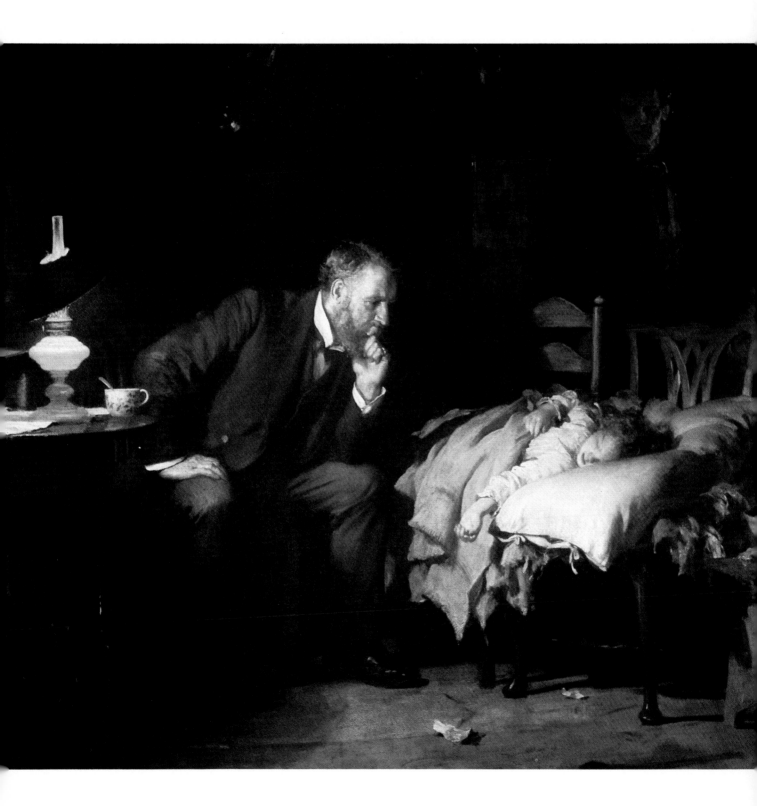

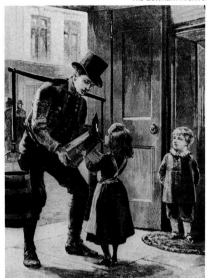 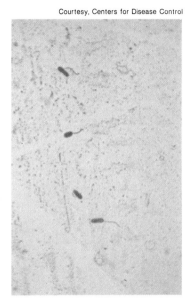

Cholera epidemics of the last century were probably unwittingly abetted by water carriers, who spread the disease through contaminated water and drinking vessels (left). Before the bacterium Vibrio cholerae *(right) was recognized as the cause of the outbreaks, epidemiologic research into their control focused on environmental sources of transmission. The sanitary movement that evolved from such studies led to improvements in the surveillance and purification of water supplies, in sewage disposal, and in food handling, all of which helped eliminate or reduce the spread of cholera and other infectious diseases.*

people and paths of exposure for these outbreaks has often revealed their sources in contaminated food, industrial toxins, or errors in the labeling or usage of chemical substances. Using modern techniques for identifying microbial agents, epidemiologic detectives have also found and christened the "bugs" responsible for such new ailments as Legionnaires' disease (in 1977) and in 1979 Lyme arthritis (a disease, transmitted by a tick, which can cause fever and inflammation of joints and of other parts of the body).

Another role of modern epidemiologists—as advocates and authorities for public health—is also derived from the heritage of Snow and his successors. The epidemiologists who work in modern-day sanitary activities may or may not be physicians, but the "patient" who receives the attention is the community. Their public health activities involve not only the traditional concerns about water and sewage but also the monitoring of cleanliness in food preparation and restaurants, the provision of suitable protection against occupational dusts and fumes, and arrangements for the proper disposal of industrial and nuclear wastes. In direct interventions with individual people, public health epidemiologists have helped in the vaccination campaigns that have sharply reduced the occurrence of poliomyelitis and measles and that led to the spectacular global eradication of smallpox.

These detective and public health activities are usually performed by epidemiologists working in municipal or state health departments, in such federal agencies (in the United States) as the Centers for Disease Control, the Environmental Protection Agency, and the Occupational Safety and Health Administration, and in such international groups as the World Health Organization. In recent years, as epidemiology has become established as an academic and investigative domain, appropriate departments have been created in medical schools, schools of hygiene or public health, national centers or bureaus concerned with vital statistics, and national research organizations, such as the National Institutes of Health in the U.S. and the Medical Research Councils of the U.K. and Canada.

144

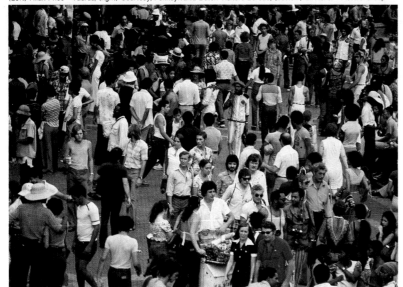

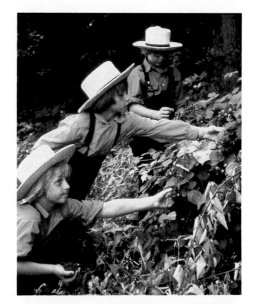

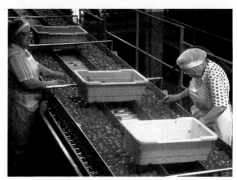

Some of the investigators working in these newer enclaves maintain the traditional epidemiologic focus on infectious disease, but others have expanded the scope of epidemiology to include research into the causes and prevention of the noninfectious or chronic diseases that constitute major "epidemics" in modern society. Among such diseases are cancer, hardening of the arteries (atherosclerosis), various forms of arthritis, and stones in various organs of the body.

The study of chronic disease has brought a new set of challenges and problems to epidemiology. Infectious-disease epidemiologists could (and still do) provide effective scientific proof of their etiologic suspicions by using experimental laboratory methods to induce the diseases in animals or sometimes in human volunteers and by applying sanitation or vaccination to prevent the diseases. For chronic diseases, however, the ailments have not been adequately replicated in laboratory animals, vaccines are not available, and the effects of preventive efforts have been difficult to demonstrate. The evidence to prove contentions about the causes and prevention of chronic diseases has thus depended mainly on statistical data, assembled in ordinary observational circumstances, without the scientific rigor of experiment.

If experimental evidence is demanded for scientific proof of a disease's cause, the necessary etiologic data can seldom, if ever, be obtained for the maladies of people living outside of laboratory environments. In the absence of definitive scientific proof, major controversies have arisen from philosophic differences about the requirements of acceptable evidence and from logistical difficulties in attaining the evidence. The main arguments refer to issues in determining what kinds of observational information, groups of people, and nonexperimental settings are satisfactory for scientific decisions and public-policy actions.

The legacy of John Snow has also created a precedent for current disputes about the accuracy of etiologic decisions and about the scope of effects to be considered when public health interventions are proposed.

Whereas most physicians deal with individuals, the epidemiologist's "patient" is frequently the community. Modern epidemiologists working in city or state health departments or federal agencies may act as detectives in mapping the spread of an outbreak of disease in the community or in certain population groups and in tracking it to its source. Their public health activities include monitoring sanitation in restaurants, stores, factories, and other places where food intended for distribution is handled.

145

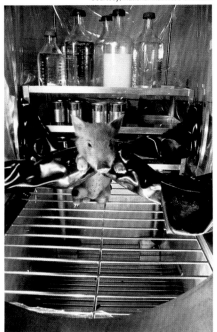

Epidemiologists often study animals in the laboratory to test their suspicions concerning the induction or transmission of infectious diseases and to find effective means of prevention or control. For many chronic diseases, however, adequate animal models do not exist, and investigators search for their needed evidence amid lists of statistics assembled from observations of people living outside the controlled laboratory environment.

Snow's reasoning was not entirely faultless. Although his action was credited with terminating the cholera epidemic, Snow had removed the pump handle at a time when new cases were occurring less frequently, so that the outbreak could have been expected soon to end spontaneously without specific intervention. As for the total scope of a public health intervention, there is no record of any arrangements having been made for the people deprived of the pump's supply to receive alternative sources of water.

Analogous problems in evaluating causes, effects, and interventions occur today in questions about whether statistical analyses can prove a cause-effect relationship, whether and when active interventions are warranted by these proofs, and what can be accepted as a suitable balance for the benefits and risks of the interventions. On one side of the controversies are proponents who urge prompt, vigorous action whenever the data are suggestive. On the other side are believers in strict scientific evidence, who are reluctant to act without convincing proof. In the nomenclature developed to characterize the opposing viewpoints, the activists, often accused of being too zealous, are called *evangelists*; and skeptics, often accused of excessive caution, are called *snails*.

In addition to these issues concerning causal analysis for the etiology and prevention of chronic disease, a new set of challenges has arisen in the past 15 years as epidemiology has expanded to include yet another new domain, called *clinical epidemiology,* which is concerned mainly with quantitative problems in evaluating the diagnosis, prognosis, and treatment of patients. The customary focus of clinical epidemiologists is on questions of patient care rather than public health, and the researchers have usually had substantial experience in clinical work. The development of this new domain has been prompted by the need to evaluate the advantages and disadvantages of the technological advances that have produced new radiologic devices, electronic equipment, pharmaceutical substances, surgical operations, and other procedures that can help identify and treat disease. Most of the cause-effect relationships in patient care must also be appraised from observational data, although certain agents can sometimes be studied with planned experiments called controlled clinical trials. With an additional new scope that includes etiology for chronic disease and evaluation for the clinical care of patients, the term epidemiology thus reverts from a specialized concern with contagious outbreaks to its more general etymologic meaning—the study of groups of people.

What do numbers tell us?

In research concerned with the etiology, prevention, and therapy of disease in human groups, both the older and newer forms of epidemiology are confronted with problems in cause-effect analysis. The epidemiologic approach to cause-effect reasoning for groups of people involves statistical comparisons of quantitative data. For example, surgery might be regarded as more effective than medical treatment for patients with coronary artery disease if the proportion of successful results were 50% for the surgical patients and 25% for patients treated medically.

This comparison of 50% versus 25% initially seems impressive as a

146

contrast of two percentages, since one of the treatments has been twice as successful as the other. On the other hand, the superiority of surgery might no longer seem impressive if we learned that only four patients were studied in each group, so that the 50% success rate for surgery represented the fraction of 2/4, and the 25% for medical therapy represented 1/4. In this circumstance, the number of treated people is so small that the observed results might easily arise by chance. A shift from success to failure of only one person would change the success rate of a treatment dramatically.

The cited statistical data would not be so "unstable" if the success rates of 50% for surgery versus 25% for medical therapy were obtained from such numbers as 200/400 versus 100/400. In this instance an addition or shift of several people in either direction would have no substantial impact on the overall results, and we would have no hesitancy in being impressed with the quantitative superiority of surgery.

The foregoing example indicates why tests of "statistical significance" have become basic to epidemiologic research. The role delegated to statistical tests of significance is to check the numerical data and to calculate the likelihood that the observed distinctions could arise by chance.

The statistical procedures begin with the temporary assumption that the agents under comparison are similar. With this assumption certain mathematical principles are used to calculate a probability (or P value), which indicates the likelihood that the agents and numbers of people under study would yield, by chance alone, a result as large as or larger than the distinction observed in the actual data. If this chance probability is sufficiently small, the observed distinction is deemed unlikely to have arisen from "the luck of the draw." When the P value is small enough, we reject the temporary assumption that the agents are similar, and we then proclaim the observed result to be statistically significant. The boundary that makes a P value small enough for this decision is usually set at or below 0.05; *i.e.,* a random chance of no greater than one in 20. For example, appropriate calculations would show a P value of 0.86 for the difference of 50% versus 25% success in the comparison of two treatments, if the results arise from the data of 2/4 versus 1/4. If the results arise from 200/400 versus 100/400, however, the corresponding P value is less than ($<$) 0.000001. Thus, if the two treatments are indeed similar, a difference of at least 50% versus 25% could occur by chance in about nine of ten studies containing 4 people in each group, whereas the same difference would be a chance occurrence in only one of one million studies containing 400 people in each group.

Although highly desirable in preventing credulous acceptance of data that are numerically inadequate, the epidemiologic quest for statistically significant results has had two important adverse scientific consequences. These consequences involve both intellectual issues in the interpretation of research and pragmatic issues in its performance. Intellectually, a focus on P values may produce misleading scientific interpretations and emphases, because the P value indicates the possible role of chance, not the importance of the observed distinction. Thus, for two treatments that produce the respective success rates of 40% and 41%—a difference that is quantitatively trivial—the results would be statistically significant at $P < 0.05$ if the "sam-

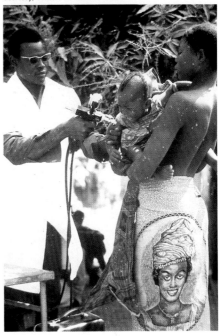

In vaccination campaigns epidemiologists deal directly with individual people. Their efforts have led to sharp reductions in polio and measles and have contributed to the worldwide eradication of smallpox.

147

ple size" were large enough to include 19,000 persons treated in each group. Conversely, for two treatments that produce the impressive quantitative distinctions of 0% versus 100% success, the P value may fail to achieve statistical significance if the sample sizes are too small, having such numbers as 0/3 versus 3/3. A focus on P values, rather than on the quantitative or clinical significance of the results, may therefore lead to an emphasis on trivia and a neglect of importance.

Pragmatically, the need for statistically significant results has brought about the enormous expense and complexity of clinical trials that require massive sample sizes and has also led to some of the peculiar research structures developed for studying causes of disease. To illustrate the sample-size problem, suppose that kidney stones occur spontaneously at a rate of 3 per 2,000 people. If we suspect that this occurrence rate is quadrupled in people who drink tea, about 4,000 people would have to be investigated for the observed difference in rates to be statistically significant. As will be noted later, the case-control and general association forms of epidemiologic research, despite their many scientific oddities and disadvantages, have the major attraction of avoiding the need to study such large numbers.

Studying cause and effect

The traditional scientific method of demonstrating that a particular agent causes a particular effect is to perform an experiment in which the events that occur after administration of the agent are compared with those that occur after administration of a "control," which can be an alternative agent, an inert placebo, or nothing. Such experiments can often be conducted for people receiving treatments intended to relieve a discomfort or to remedy some other manifestation of a disease. For other cause-effect relationships, however, alternative forms of research may be necessary.

Experimental trials are one method of researching cause and effect. In an experimental trial a planned design is used to assign the agents under comparison and to observe their effects. The structure of the research is

If it is suspected that kidney stones occur more frequently in people who drink tea (say, at a rate presumed to be up to four times that in the general population), and epidemiologists know that stones occur spontaneously at a rate of 3 per 2,000 people, they would have to investigate about 4,000 people for any observed differences in rates to be statistically significant. The need for statistically significant results has brought enormous expense and complexity to clinical trials that require massive sample sizes.

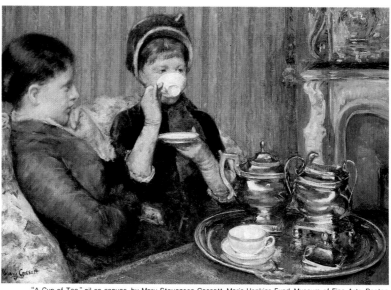

"A Cup of Tea," oil on canvas, by Mary Stevenson Cassatt, Maria Hopkins Fund, Museum of Fine Arts, Boston

shown in Figure 1. The people who enter the experiment are first checked for suitable eligibility. Their health must allow them to qualify for receiving either of the agents under comparison, and they must also be susceptible to developing the outcome event that represents the effect to be produced or prevented by the compared agents.

For example, the people admitted to an experimental trial conducted to test the suspicion that tea drinking causes kidney stones would be required initially to have evidence of stoneless kidneys and to be free of any specific reasons that might make them unwilling or unable to drink tea. The eligible volunteers would then be assigned, preferably at random, to receive either the active agent (tea drinking) or the control agent (avoiding tea). The members of both groups would thereafter be checked at regular intervals with clinical and radiologic examinations for kidney stones.

After a suitable period of observation, the occurrence of the outcome event (in this instance, kidney stones) would be counted in the members of each group. The rate of occurrence would be expressed as the risk of that event for the group. If the risk rate is higher in the actively exposed group than in the control group, if the difference is statistically significant, and if no other plausible explanation can be found for the difference, exposure to the active agent will be held responsible for the distinction.

Despite obvious scientific merits, the performance of such experiments is frequently thwarted by barriers in ethics or feasibility. In studies of etiologic agents that may cause disease, most investigators would be reluctant to ask people to become deliberately exposed to a possibly noxious substance; even if asked, very few persons will volunteer to receive a randomized assignment for exposure or nonexposure; and those who do volunteer cannot be coerced into faithfully maintaining the assigned regimen.

If the agent is intended, like the use of aspirin for pain, to remedy a manifestation of a disease, the trial is relatively easy to conduct, but if the agent is being tested for its prophylactic action in preventing or retarding a disease, the outcome event may have a low rate of occurrence, thereby requiring large numbers of patients to achieve statistical significance. Because the numbers may be too large to be attained at any single medical institution, the trial may acquire the added complexity, cumbersome logistics, and major costs of collaborating institutions.

Because the desired experimental trials can seldom be conducted, epidemiologists have often relied, instead, on observational studies of people who received the active agents through nonexperimental mechanisms of assignment. The observational studies can have several different structures.

Cohort studies are one such structure. The word cohort is commonly used for a group of people who are followed forward in time from the inception of a mutually common event until the occurrence of a subsequent outcome. In an experimental trial the cohorts are the groups receiving the assigned agents under comparison. In an observational cohort study, as shown in Figure 2, the groups are formed in the same way, but the agents are "chosen" (albeit sometimes unwittingly) by the personal decisions of the recipients. The agents may have been self-selected as personal habits, recommended as standard medical therapy, or imposed environmentally as at-

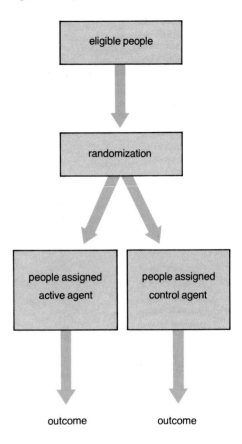

Figure 1: **Experimental trial**

eligible people

randomization

people assigned active agent

people assigned control agent

outcome

outcome

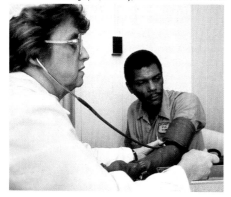

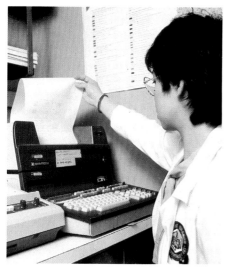

The people who take part in an experimental trial are examined to determine if they qualify for receiving any of the agents being compared and if they are susceptible to the outcome event being sought. They are then experimentally assigned to a group that is to be given one of the agents. At the end of a suitable period of follow-up observation, occurrences of the outcome event in the members of each group are tallied, and the rate of occurrence is expressed as the risk of that event for the group.

mospheric pollutants or occupational toxins. Except for the personal selection rather than experimental assignment of compared agents, an observational cohort study has the same basic arrangement and forward (or "prospective") direction as an experiment.

In a study of etiology the outcome event is the target disease whose rate of occurrence shows the risk for each group. The relative importance of the risks in the active and control groups is quantified by combining the two risk rates into a single index. The single index can be either a subtracted increment, which is called the attributable risk, or a quotient, which is called the risk ratio or relative risk. For example, if the customary risk of renal stones is 3 per 2,000, an investigator who suspects that tea drinking quadruples this risk might assemble a group of 2,000 tea drinkers and 2,000 non-tea drinkers. After arranging to follow the two groups for the next ten years, the investigator might find the results cited in Table 1. From these data, the rates of risk would be calculated as $12/2,000 = 0.0060$ for the tea drinkers and $3/2,000 = 0.0015$ for the non-tea drinkers. The distinction would be statistically significant at $P < 0.05$. The attributable risk would be $0.0060 - 0.0015 = 0.0045$, and the risk ratio would be $0.0060/0.0015 = 4$.

The elevation of the risk ratio above 1 would suggest that tea drinking may cause renal stones; the relatively small incremental value for the attributable risk would suggest that the hazard is not frightful; and the discovery of a small but distinct risk in the nonexposed group would indicate that tea drinking cannot be the only cause of renal stones.

Although the immediate problems of an experimentally randomized assignment of agents would be eliminated, this type of observational cohort study would still require that the investigator assemble 4,000 people and follow them for the next ten years. Very few investigators would be willing to make such a time commitment, and even if the investigators were willing, the people might not be easy to assemble and to maintain under protracted observation. Because these difficulties in logistics will occur whenever the outcome event has a low rate of attack and does not develop until long after exposure, cohort research will be difficult to conduct. To cope with this problem alternative research structures are often used to reduce either the duration of follow-up or the number of people under observation.

Cross-sectional surveys enable the investigator to take a "snapshot" of a large population. He is hoping to find the same relationships that might be revealed by the longer-term "moving picture" of a cohort study. As shown in Figure 3, a population is examined to note the concurrent presence or absence in each person of exposure to the agent and of the outcome event.

For example, if renal stones are not promptly fatal and if the stones are causally related to tea drinking, we might expect at any particular moment to find more stones present in tea drinkers than in non-tea drinkers. We might therefore survey a large number of people, asking about their tea-drinking habits and determining if they have renal stones. If the people are chosen from an older age group, so that they will have had a long exposure to tea drinking, we might expect to find that renal stones have occurred at rates shown in Table 1. The substantially greater frequency of stones in the tea drinkers would then help support the causal hypothesis.

150

In a cross-sectional survey, however, the investigator cannot deliberately use the option that is available in an experimental trial or observational cohort to select equal numbers of exposed and nonexposed people for follow-up. The relative proportions of exposed and nonexposed people found by the investigator would depend on their natural occurrence in the general community. In the proposed research, if about 80% of the population are tea drinkers, the investigator would encounter about four tea drinkers for every non-tea drinker. Thus, to find at least three cases of renal stones in non-tea drinkers, the investigator would need interviews with 2,000 non-tea drinkers and 8,000 tea drinkers. The total sample size would thus be increased to 10,000 people and would yield the results shown in Table 2.

The rates of risk, risk ratios, and incremental attributable risks calculated from Table 2 would be the same as those noted in Table 1, but they would represent the prevalence, rather than the observed new development (or incidence), of renal stones. Since the tea drinking and renal stones were noted concomitantly rather than serially, we could not be sure whether tea drinking had led to renal stones or whether people with early manifestations of renal stones had begun drinking tea as possible remedial therapy. Thus, although a cross-sectional survey will save the protracted time needed to conduct a cohort study, the required sample size will usually be larger than in cohort research, and the temporal relationship between cause and effect may be blurred.

Case-control studies offer an easy and relatively inexpensive substitute for the large sample sizes required in cohort or cross-sectional research. In this special epidemiologic structure, the investigator begins at the end of the causal pathway, by choosing a group of cases in which the outcome event has already occurred. A comparison group—usually called the control group but sometimes called the referent or compeer group—is then chosen from people in whom the outcome event has not been noted. The two groups are then "followed" in a backward direction with retrospective inquiries aimed at determining each member's antecedent exposure to the agent under investigation. The structure of the research is shown in Figure 4.

For example, in a case-control study of the relationship between tea drinking and renal stones, the investigator might use hospital records to identify and assemble 100 patients with renal stones. From patients with other diseases or from diverse community sources, the investigator might then choose 100 people without renal stones to serve as controls. If the prevalence of tea drinking in these two groups is similar to what was noted cross-sectionally in Table 2, the results of the case-control study would produce what is shown in Table 3.

The data of Table 3 would be calculated in a different way from those used in Tables 1 and 2. Because of the way the cases and controls were chosen, the risks of renal stones cannot be determined in the tea drinkers and non-tea drinkers. If the assembled numbers in Table 3 were arranged to express "occurrence rates" for renal stones, those rates would be 94/174 or 0.54 in the tea drinkers and 6/26 or 0.23 in the non-tea drinkers. Both rates are excessively high as estimates of the risk of developing renal stones, and their risk ratio of 2.35 (or 0.54/0.23) would be fallaciously low.

Figure 2: **Observational cohort**

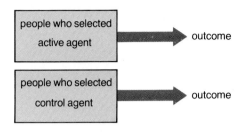

Table I:	**Hypothetical cohort study of tea drinking and renal stones**		
	number of people who developed		
	renal stones	no renal stones	total
tea drinkers	12	1,988	2,000
non-tea drinkers	3	1,997	2,000
total	15	3,985	4,000

risk for tea drinkers = 12/2,000 = 0.0060
risk for non-tea drinkers = 3/2,000 = 0.0015
risk ratio = 0.0060/0.0015 = 4.0

Figure 3: **Cross-sectional survey**

population under examination for exposure
to agent and presence of outcome event

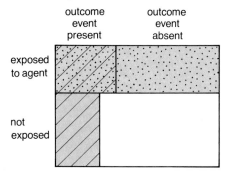

	outcome event present	outcome event absent
exposed to agent		
not exposed		

Table II: **Hypothetical cross-sectional survey of tea drinking and renal stones**

	number of people found to have		
	renal stones	no renal stones	total
tea drinkers	48	7,952	8,000
non-tea drinkers	3	1,997	2,000
total	51	9,949	10,000

risk for tea drinkers = 48/8,000 = 0.0060
risk for non-tea drinkers = 3/2,000 = 0.0015
risk ratio = 0.0060/0.0015 = 4.0

To avoid these errors epidemiologists examine the exposure ratios for tea drinking in the cases and controls. As shown at the bottom of Table 3, the "odds" for previous exposure to tea drinking would be 15.7 to 1 (or 94/6) in the case group and 4 to 1 (or 80/20) in the control group. A suitable algebraic derivation, not shown here, would demonstrate that the ratio of these two odds, which is called the odds ratio, approximates the risk ratio of a cohort study. In this instance, the risk ratio for the data in Table 1 is 4.0. The odds ratio for the data in Table 3 is 3.9 (or 15.7 ÷ 4).

Although the actual risks of exposure cannot be directly calculated, a case-control study can provide essentially the same risk ratio found in a cohort investigation but can do so with many fewer people and without the need for a protracted follow-up period. Because of these advantages, the case-control study has become probably the most frequently used mechanism in the epidemiologic investigation of etiologic relationships. In exchange for these advantages, however, the case-control structure creates a series of major scientific hazards which will be discussed later.

General populational associations are a quite different type of research structure. In all of the structures just discussed, the investigator assembles the pertinent data for each member of the groups under study. The data may be collected and arranged in diverse ways, but each person under investigation becomes marked as either positive or negative for presence of the "cause" and for presence of the "effect." In the general populational structure, no individual people are actually investigated. Instead, the investigator works with collections of data counted for different population groups. The numbers are then arranged into pertinent statistical associations.

For example, if data showed that the sales of tea in a particular geographic region had annual increases that paralleled a rising trend in the annual rate of renal stones for that region, an investigator might suspect a positive relationship between the two events. This type of statistical arrangement— based on changes with calendar time in a single geographic region—is called a secular association. In a variation of this theme, data for the sales of tea in a series of geographic regions might be correlated with data for the rate of renal stones in each of those same regions. The way such data might be arranged is shown in Figure 5. In this type of ecologic association, where the rates of two events are linked for different geographic (ecologic) regions, a concomitant rise in the rates for tea drinking and for renal stones would also denote a positive relationship between the two events.

This type of general populational study is so easy to do that it is sometimes referred to as "armchair research." All the investigator needs is an active imagination applied to the available tabulations of statistical data issued by suitable commercial organizations and by such official agencies as the census bureau and the bureau of vital statistics. One main hazard of the research is that statistical correlation does not imply causation, since correlations can be found for plausible but outlandish associations such as the birth rate in Copenhagen and the number of storks sighted flying over the city. Another hazard is the well-known ecologic fallacy, in which unrelated changes in exposure and in outcome take place in two different parts of the same general region but are then fallaciously linked together. Thus, the people who use increased amounts of tea may not be the ones who develop an increase in renal stones, although their data may be ecologically joined.

How valid is an association?

To make decisions about cause-effect relationships, epidemiologists have established a set of criteria that depends on fulfillment of five main principles. The first three principles refer to statistical features of the data, and the last two to biologic logic. Because the evidence is usually observational rather than experimental, the term association is regularly used for arrangements of data that describe the relationship between the alleged cause and its suspected effect. The five principles are: consistency, strength, specificity, temporal precedence, and coherence.

Consistency of the association requires that similar results be found when the association is studied in different localities and with different research structures. If contradictions occur, the results are not consistent and would not support the idea of a causal relationship. The occurrence of similar results in separate studies does not prove that a relationship is causal, however, since the same basic error may be made repeatedly. Different forms of distortion may produce consistent but erroneous results if investigators convinced of the causal hypothesis do not take adequate precautions to avoid biased observations or analyses. This type of problem occurred in recent years when three studies, published on the same day in the same medical journal, all supported the idea that breast cancer was associated with the drug reserpine, which is used in the treatment of high blood pressure. The association was later discredited when different sources of bias were demonstrated in the three studies and when subsequent research produced contradictory results.

Strength of the association involves two components. One is the magnitude of the risk ratio. Thus, a ratio of 7.5 is more impressive than 1.5. The second component is known as a "dose-response" curve, this concept referring to the assumption that an increased amount of exposure to the causal agent should lead to an increased risk of the effect. For example, the risk of lung cancer is higher in heavy smokers than in moderate smokers and higher in moderate smokers than in light smokers. (This principle can also be fulfilled erroneously, however, if the results are sufficiently distorted by bias; some of the sources of bias will be cited later.)

Specificity of the association refers to the idea of a distinctive relationship between the cause and the effect. If a single causal agent is held responsible for many other effects, or if many different causal agents are all regarded as contributors to a single effect, the individual cause and individual effect do not seem likely to be specifically related.

The principle is readily fulfilled in the relationships between microbial agents and their corresponding infectious diseases. The principle is more difficult to fulfill, however, for noninfectious diseases and their alleged causes. For example, because so many different cancers and other chronic diseases have been attributed to cigarette smoking, the principle of "specificity" has been violated. The etiologic role of cigarettes has been particularly disputed in atherosclerotic ailments where other causal agents—such as

Figure 4: **Case-control study**

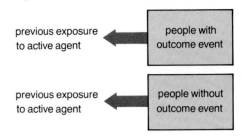

Table III:	**Hypothetical case-control study of tea drinking and renal stones**		
	cases with renal stones	controls without renal stones	total
tea drinkers	94	80	174
non-tea drinkers	6	20	26
total	100	100	200

odds for tea drinking in cases = 94/6 = 15.7
odds for tea drinking in controls = 80/20 = 4.0
odds ratio = 15.7/4.0 = 3.9

153

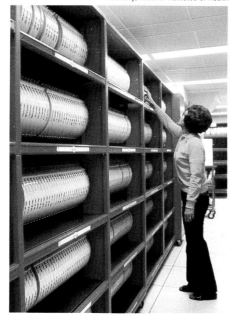

Hospital records offer one source of information for case-control research. In this kind of study the epidemiologist begins at the end of the causal chain of events, forming a group from cases in which the outcome event has already occurred. A control group of people in whom the outcome event has not been noted is also formed.

diet, metabolism of fatty substances, blood-clotting abnormalities, and personality factors—are also under suspicion.

Temporal precedence in the association means that there is evidence that exposure to the causal agent came before the development of the alleged effect. This demonstration is easily achieved in experimental or in observational cohort research where the admitted people are checked for their appropriate eligibility before exposure. The requirement is more difficult to attain in cross-sectional or case-control studies because of the possibility that early manifestations of the effect had led to a change in exposure to the causal agent. For example, after developing various gastrointestinal diseases, patients may reduce or stop their intake of coffee. If such patients later become the control group in a case-control study of pancreatic cancer, their relatively low intake of coffee may then make it spuriously seem to be a causal agent for the cancer.

Coherence of the association, the last principle, refers to the association's general plausibility and to its agreement with other forms of evidence in people or animals. For example, because cigarette smoke is inhaled directly into the lungs, it is more plausible as a cause of lung cancer than of bladder cancer. Because cancer of the uterus has been noted in rats receiving large doses of estrogens, the animal evidence helps support the proposed role of estrogen in causing uterine cancer in women.

Amid the emphasis on statistical and biologic issues, the five principles just cited do not include attention to the scientific quality of the data or to the scientific merits and hazards of the different methodologic structures with which groups are chosen, data collected, and results analyzed. Because no demands are made about scientific methods, the decisions about causation seem to require only a set of numbers that have appropriate statistical magnitudes and plausible biologic relationships. In the absence of more rigorous standards, epidemiologic research is vulnerable to a number of scientific problems.

Problems in epidemiology

Although the hallmarks of scientific research are high-quality data and unbiased comparison, neither is regularly achieved in contemporary epidemiologic research. The problem arises because of the difficulty of obtaining and arranging observational information about large groups of people.

How good are the data? In etiologic studies, when the investigator assembles data for each person's possible exposure and possible disease, neither type of information can be obtained with the type of quality control that is available for laboratory measurements. Information about exposure is often determined from medical records, which may have doubtful quality, or from interviews with the people under study. The accuracy of the information is often uncertain in case-control studies, particularly if the possible exposure took place long before the interview. Alternatively, the process of acquiring data about exposure may be biased if the interviewer or data excerpter knows the research hypothesis and knows whether each subject is a case or control. Epidemiologists have recently begun to recognize this problem and to improve the objectivity of the methods used for "ascertaining" exposure in

154

Courtesy, Centers for Disease Control

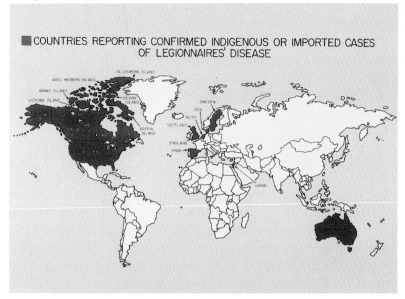

COUNTRIES REPORTING CONFIRMED INDIGENOUS OR IMPORTED CASES OF LEGIONNAIRES' DISEASE

The map depicts the geographical distribution by country of reported cases of Legionnaires' disease. In 1977 epidemiologic detectives painstakingly tracked down the Legionella pneumophila *bacterium, which was responsible for mysterious outbreaks of what appeared to be a new disease. Epidemiologists work with collections of data from different population groups, which frequently are delineated by geographic region. The numbers are then arranged into pertinent statistical associations.*

case-control studies—but many existing investigations were conducted without suitable precautions against biased ascertainment.

In general association studies, the information about rates of disease usually depends on the diagnoses that appear in tabulations of data from death certificates. Although most clinically oriented physicians are aware of the notorious inaccuracy of such tabulations, and although several epidemiologic studies have shown that the data are grossly unreliable, organizations such as the National Center for Health Statistics and National Institutes of Health, both in the U.S., continue to collect and analyze the data and to precisely arrange them for various regions and localities. The results may show rising or falling rates for heart disease, cancer, and other ailments in relation to county of residence, industrial development, water supply, and whatever other data have been amassed.

These analyses contain the statistical hazard, described later, that among the hundreds of thousands of associations under examination, many will yield statistically significant differences by chance alone. The massive computerized analyses also contain major scientific hazards because what is being analyzed is the rate of diagnosis, rather than the true rate of occurrence of disease.

With the availability of new technologic methods for diagnosing disease, the rates of identification of many ailments have changed substantially. The changes, however, may mean only that the disease is being identified differently, not that it has truly changed. For example, the rate of occurrence of systemic lupus erythematosus, a connective tissue disorder, has risen dramatically in the past four decades, but no one has proclaimed that an epidemic exists because the rising rate has been closely associated with new methods of diagnosis. A similar relationship is probably responsible for the rising rate of pancreatic cancer in the past decade, as exploratory surgery and new imaging methods have been increasingly used for diagnosing the disease. Nevertheless, epidemiologic research has seldom paid suitable

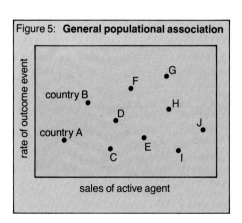

Figure 5: **General populational association**

155

attention to the role of changing diagnostic technology in changing the occurrence rates of disease.

The question of bias. The problem of unreliable data might be ignored if the errors occurred randomly enough to allow deviations in opposite directions to cancel one another. Unfortunately, major distortions in comparison can arise when data are collected and groups are formed without rigorous attention to scientific principles. Of the many different types of bias that can occur as "confounding factors" in epidemiologic data, three of the most common arise when groups of people are arbitrarily selected for comparison.

Susceptibility bias occurs if the effect of an agent is compared in two groups that initially are unequally susceptible to the effect. For example, to study the adverse results of employment in certain occupations, the longevity of people who worked in those jobs may be compared with the longevity of the rest of the population. When such data are collected, the investigators may be shocked to discover that the employed people, despite their "adverse" occupational exposure, had a longer life-span than the others. The bias that produces this situation has been noted often enough to receive a special name: the "healthy worker effect." It arises because of the screening examinations that people may receive before being offered work in certain occupations. As a result of the screening, the chosen workers are particularly healthy before they begin their employment—and they may then live longer (on average) than the rest of the population even if their occupational exposure has somewhat deleterious results.

The problems of susceptibility bias may have also impaired recent observational studies of the allegedly adverse effects of sex hormone therapy during pregnancy. For comparisons to be fair, the effects of giving sex hormone drugs must be noted in patients subclassified according to the reason (called the therapeutic "indication") the treatments were used. Since women who have had repeated miscarriages or other indications for hormone therapy may in addition be particularly likely to have children with birth defects, results will be distorted by susceptibility bias unless the groups have been suitably arranged to compare women who had similar clinical indications (or lack of indications) for the treatment under investigation. Such arrangements were not made in most of the studies that have showed "risks" for the use of sex hormones. In the few instances where such arrangements were made, no elevated risks were found.

The process of detecting an outcome effect involves (1) surveillance, (2) examination, and (3) interpretation. With surveillance the susceptible people are observed so that suitable events will be noted. With examination the events are tested, using procedures needed to identify the disease or other phenomenon that is regarded as the outcome effect. With interpretation the evidence acquired during the surveillance and examinations is appraised to decide whether the effect has actually occurred. When this three-part process is not similar in the groups under comparison, *detection bias* can occur. The similarity of the detection process for compared groups is particularly important in seeking a disease that often does not produce major symptoms, in applying criteria that identify a disease from the available evidence, or in deciding about "success" or "improvement" after treatment.

156

During clinical trials of therapy, this bias can be avoided or reduced if the medication can be given in a "double-blind" manner, with the identity of the particular treatment unknown to both the patient and the physician. In epidemiologic studies of causes of disease, detection bias is more difficult to avoid, because people exposed to certain agents may also be especially likely to receive the diagnostic tests that detect the diseases allegedly caused by those agents. Thus, the role of detection bias has not yet been convincingly eliminated in the statistical associations between oral contraceptive pills and thromboses (blood clots), between postmenopausal estrogens and uterine cancer, and between certain occupational exposures and chest cancer.

Constraint bias occurs when the people who are included in or excluded from one of the groups under study are chosen in a way that constrains the proportionate composition of the group with respect to either exposure to the cause or occurrence of the effect. Citations of success rates in patients discharged from the hospital after a specific type of surgical therapy might omit those who died during or immediately after the operation. Thus, of 100 patients receiving surgery (with 20 deaths occurring postoperatively), 60 patients could eventually be classified as successful, but the surgical success rate might be cited as the constrained value of 75% (or 60/80) instead of the correct value of 60% (or 60/100).

A different type of example is provided by a case-control study of the relationship between breast cancer and antecedent reserpine therapy for hypertension. Patients with cardiovascular disease were excluded from the control group. Since such patients would have been particularly likely to be users of reserpine, the constraint left the control group with a falsely low proportion of reserpine users, thereby producing an erroneous elevation of the odds ratio. In later studies, when this constraint was avoided, the odds ratio was found to be about 1.

"Fishing expeditions." In most forms of scientific research, data are assembled to test a specific hypothesis that a particular cause leads to a particular effect. During or after the research, an alert investigator may notice

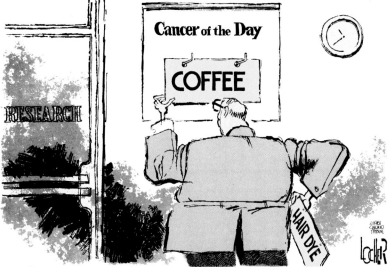

Locher © The Chicago Tribune

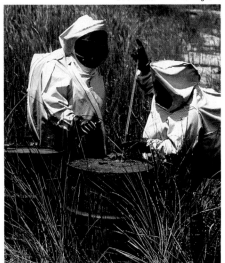

Certain workers who are exposed to major health hazards on the job may actually show longer-than-average lifespans. This phenomenon is known as the "healthy worker effect," and it can confound epidemiological investigations. Medical screening that prospective workers receive before being hired for positions known to present adverse occupational exposure often results in the chosen workers' forming a particularly healthy group.

things that lead to a change in the original hypothesis or that suggest a completely different hypothesis. If so, the new hypothesis is regarded as having been generated by the original evidence, but the new hypothesis is merely an untested idea. It must be checked with an entirely new set of data before it can be regarded as tested. This scientific principle—that a hypothesis cannot be tested with the same data used to generate it—is frequently violated in epidemiologic research.

The term fishing expedition is often applied to studies conducted without a specific hypothesis. A large set of data, usually available in computerized format, is examined in multiple ways as the investigator looks for "significant" associations. For example, if suitable information is available for the antecedent pharmaceutical therapy and the subsequent occurrence of new disease in a large number of people, the investigator can have a computer perform thousands of miniature case-control studies, searching for elevated odds ratios for the relationships between individual medications and their allegedly toxic effects in producing diseases.

Another version of a fishing expedition, sometimes called "data dredging," occurs when an investigator fails to confirm the original research hypothesis and then looks for supporting evidence in subgroups formed from the original data. For example, in a large case-control study of the relationship between saccharin and bladder cancer, the odds ratio was found to approximate 1, a value that would tend to exonerate saccharin. After exploring the results for many subgroups of people demarcated in various ways, however, the investigators found that the odds ratio was elevated in white male smokers. This elevation was then regarded as support for the original hypothesis that saccharin causes bladder cancer.

One main hazard of fishing expeditions or data-dredging explorations is the occurrence of "significant" results by chance alone. If a P value of 0.05 is used for making the decision that a difference is significant, the investigator can expect to find about one false positive result in every 20 explorations of associations in which no significant relationship exists. Thus, if 100 "negative" subgroups or associations are checked, about 5 can yield "positive" results by chance alone. Instead of recognizing the role of chance and instead of testing the hypothesis with new data, the investigator may accept the results as established and may then propose imaginative explanations to add biologic plausibility to the conclusions.

A different kind of scientific hazard in fishing expeditions is the decision that an "abnormal" event has occurred when two extremes of a normal range of events are compared. For example, if we tabulate the distribution of height for a large number of normal healthy people, we will find a group at one end who are about 58 inches tall and another group at the other end who are about 79 inches tall. The difference between the two groups is striking but would not itself be a cause for alarm or for declaring either group to be abnormal. Similarly, the rates of different diseases can be expected to vary in diverse localities, and the variations alone need not denote extraordinary etiologic influences—but the data are often used for indicting the etiologic role of such agents as water, air, nutrition, or industry when high rates of individual diseases are found in the different localities.

158

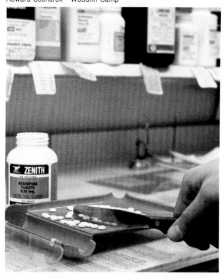

(Top) Courtesy, National Institutes of Health; (bottom) Howard Sochurek—Woodfin Camp

Triumphs, blunders, and controversies

Because human ailments are so difficult to study and because experimental evidence is so seldom available as a "gold standard" to confirm or refute the conclusions of observational research, perhaps the most remarkable aspect of epidemiologic investigation is not the occurrence of occasional blunders or frequent contradictions but the many triumphs that have been produced. In addition to the role of epidemiology in leading to the sanitation of sewage and water, epidemiologic methods were used to suggest the influence of different occupations on health, to identify dietary deficiency as the cause of pellagra, and to indict rubella (German measles) during pregnancy as a cause of congenital malformations. In the clinical epidemiology of the 19th century, the hospital studies of Pierre Louis helped put an end to centuries of therapeutic bloodletting, and Ignaz Semmelweis helped bring the sanitary movement indoors by showing that the unclean hands of physicians often transmitted puerperal sepsis (childbed fever).

Epidemiologic studies of blood from human populations helped set the stage for a vaccine against poliomyelitis by demonstrating that the etiologic virus, before attacking nervous tissue, had a bloodstream phase where it could be inactivated by antibodies. Epidemiologic studies helped demonstrate the now almost universally accepted role of cigarette smoking in causing lung cancer. In more recent years epidemiologic observations helped put an end to the deformed children produced by the use of thalidomide during early pregnancy.

Randomized clinical trials demonstrated that high concentrations of oxygen could blind premature babies; that rheumatic fever could be averted with appropriate antibacterial treatment; that vaccines against poliomyelitis, measles, and hepatitis were worthwhile; that treatment of hypertension could prevent long-term vascular complications; that beta-blocker drug therapy could reduce deaths after recovery from acute myocardial infarction; and that scores of new drugs do indeed perform as claimed.

Amid these and many other triumphs, epidemiologic methods have also produced some striking blunders. Despite Snow's demonstration of the influence of water in transmitting cholera, William Farr—the distinguished physician who is still revered as the founder of "vital statistics"—misinterpreted statistical data to conclude that high atmospheric pressure was a prime etiologic factor. Before Joseph Goldberger's heroic research in the early 20th century showed that dietary deficiency played a causal role in pellagra, a distinguished epidemiologic commission had concluded that pellagra was an infectious or possibly familial disease. In recent years, because of biased methods of research, peptic ulcer was erroneously associated with certain blood types, and reserpine, saccharin, and coffee have been improperly accused of being carcinogens.

The false conclusions drawn from observational data about clinical treatment led to such now rejected therapies as complete dental extractions for rheumatoid arthritis, gastric freezing for peptic ulcer, and radical surgery for many forms of cancer. Even the use of experimentally controlled clinical trials has not always resolved the therapeutic questions that the trials were presumably intended to answer. Thus, uncertainties still exist about the

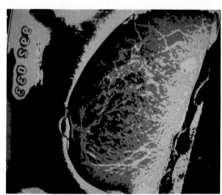

An example of a kind of bias known as constraint bias was provided by a study of the relationship between reserpine therapy for hypertension and subsequent breast cancer. Because patients with cardiovascular disease, who were likely users of reserpine, were excluded from the control group, this group was left with a disproportionately low number of reserpine users. The imbalance elevated the odds ratio. Later studies that avoided this error found no relationship between the drug and breast cancer.

159

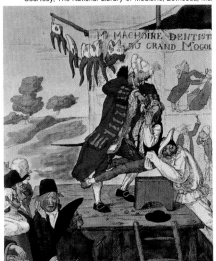

Complete dental extraction was once thought to be an effective treatment for rheumatoid arthritis. This epidemiologic blunder arose from false conclusions drawn from unscientific observations.

Computerized axial tomography (below) and nuclear magnetic resonance scanning (right) number among the many new diagnostic technologies that are changing the rate at which ailments are being identified. Epidemiologic studies must avoid confusing the changing rate of diagnosis of a disease with its true rate of occurrence.

value of such procedures as vaccination against tuberculosis, blood-lipid lowering (with the drug clofibrate) to prevent coronary artery disease, blood-sugar-lowering agents to avoid the vascular complications of diabetes mellitus, and anticoagulant or antithrombotic agents in preventing problems after myocardial infarction. Many of the uncertainties involve clinical and scientific disputes about the design of the trials, but other difficulties are inherent in the logistics of large-scale studies where the outcome event is a disease or complication that is to be prevented rather than remedied.

Somewhere between the accepted triumphs and the exposed blunders are the controversies produced when different studies of the same relationship yield conflicting data or when studies that show the same trend are later found to have been flawed by scientific problems. Consequently, many disagreements still exist about such proposed etiologic relationships as oral contraceptive pills and blood clotting, hormonal treatment during pregnancy and fetal abnormalities, estrogen replacement therapy and cancer of the uterus, and water fluoridation and cancer; about the role of smoking, diet, serum lipids, alcohol, and exercise in cardiovascular disease; and about the true etiologic impact of various industrial chemicals, food preservatives, low-level radiation, and air pollutants.

Some of the research (such as the initial claims that chromosomal damage had occurred in people living near chemical-waste dumps of the Love Canal area of Niagara Falls, N.Y.) has been of such poor quality that its fallacies are readily apparent to reviewers whose vision is unclouded by sociopolitical ideology. In many other instances, however, the research has been conducted with the customary practices of the craft and has sometimes come from well-known leaders in the field.

These difficulties have several sources. When no specific cause is known for a distressing event—such as the cancers, strokes, and other major chronic diseases whose etiologies are still uncertain—the human compulsion is to search for culprits. Among the culprits that might be considered are the "internal" roles of familial, genetic, psychic, and other constitutional

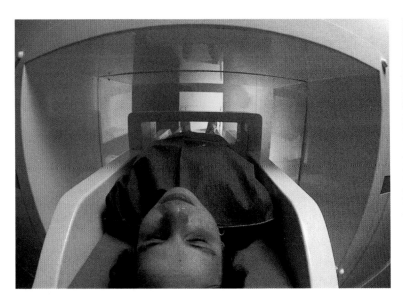

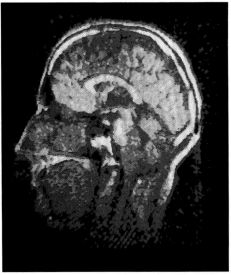

factors, but these factors are often difficult to discern and measure. Besides, epidemiology has traditionally been concerned with environmental and other substances that provide "external" exposure. Consequently, since chronic diseases have become prominent during an era of major "external" changes in industry, technology, nutrition, and life-style, these changes have become the main etiologic suspects. With increasing opportunities to acquire and analyze observational data addressed to these suspicions, and with the research stimuli provided by public and political pressures, many more studies can now be performed than ever before. The results of a particular study are often interpreted merely according to the prejudices of the beholder (not unlike beauty); the actual value of a study depends on a dispassionate appraisal of its scientific accuracy.

For such appraisals, however, rigorous scientific methods and standards have not yet been established in epidemiologic research. This deficiency is not surprising in a domain that is so relatively young in its modern evolution, that is confronted with so vast a set of challenges in studying free-living human beings, and that covers the full spectrum of human life from birth to death, from community to medical center, from health to disease, and from prevention to treatment. As modern epidemiology has become recognized as an essential activity in medical science, the investigators who do the research and the reviewers who appraise the results can better attend to the need for improving scientific quality.

The challenges are immense. They include the suitable identification of all the "internal" factors that have hitherto been neglected, the removal or reduction of all the biases that can occur in observational studies, and the solution of all the etiologic and therapeutic dilemmas that were previously cited for both infectious and noninfectious disease. Since epidemiologic research has become the main or the only procedure available for getting scientifically convincing answers to etiologic and therapeutic questions that cannot be suitably pursued with laboratory investigation, an increased attention to basic scientific principles and to the problems that require methodologic solutions will allow epidemiology to begin its maturation as a fundamental domain of modern science.

FOR ADDITIONAL READING:

Feinstein, A. R. *Clinical Biostatistics.* St. Louis: The C. V. Mosby Co., 1977.

————. "Clinical Epidemiology." *Annals of Internal Medicine* 69 (1968): 807, 1037, and 1287.

Fox, J. P.; Hall, C. E.; and Elveback, L. R. *Epidemiology: Man and Disease.* New York: The Macmillan Co., 1970.

Lilienfeld, A. M. *Foundations of Epidemiology.* New York: Oxford University Press, 1976.

Mausner, J. S., and Bahn, A. K. *Epidemiology: An Introductory Text.* Philadelphia: W. B. Saunders Co., 1974.

Roueché, Berton. *Annals of Epidemiology.* Boston: Little, Brown & Co., 1967.

————. *The Medical Detectives.* New York: Washington Square Press, 1982.

Sackett, D. L., and Holland, W. W. "Controversy in the Detection of Disease." *The Lancet* 2 (1975): 357.

Snow, John. *Snow on Cholera: Being a Reprint of Two Papers.* New York: The Commonwealth Fund, 1936.

Huntington's Chorea
by Harold L. Klawans, M.D.

In 1872 George Huntington, a Long Island general practitioner, described a form of adult-onset chorea in several families. Both his father and his grandfather had observed these same families for several generations, and because of their careful observations he was able to fully delineate this condition. He noted that it was "confined to certain and fortunately a few families and had been transmitted to them as an heirloom from generations back in the dim past." He described it as being "attended generally by all the symptoms of common chorea only in an aggravated degree, hardly ever manifesting itself until adult or middle life" and then progressing until the "hopeless sufferer is but a quivering wreck of his former self."

The tragic history of these families was played out in the early years against the famous witch-hunting mania that swept Europe and the American colonies in the 17th century. Unfortunate victims of the disease were persecuted and some even killed when their distressing and bizarre mental and physical symptoms were ascribed to contact with the devil. The gradual appearance of personality aberrations, garbled speech, and uncontrollable bodily movements in an otherwise healthy individual seemed to be obvious signs of demonic influence.

Huntington's description recognized the three marked peculiarities of this disease: its hereditary nature, the tendency for mental changes to occur in patients with chorea, and the tendency for the disease first to become manifest during adult life. Although these observations have been expanded and modified, they still represent the three major characteristics that distinguish Huntington's disease.

Huntington's disease (HD, or Huntington's chorea) is a hereditary, progressive disorder that usually begins to manifest itself during middle adult life. All of the signs and symptoms of HD are reflections of the changes that the disease causes within the brain. The most characteristic manifestation is spontaneous, involuntary movements known as chorea, which usually begin as brief, sudden, mild jerks of an arm or leg or part of the face. As the disease progresses, the movements become more frequent, more forceful, and more generalized. Since most adults with HD have these movements, the

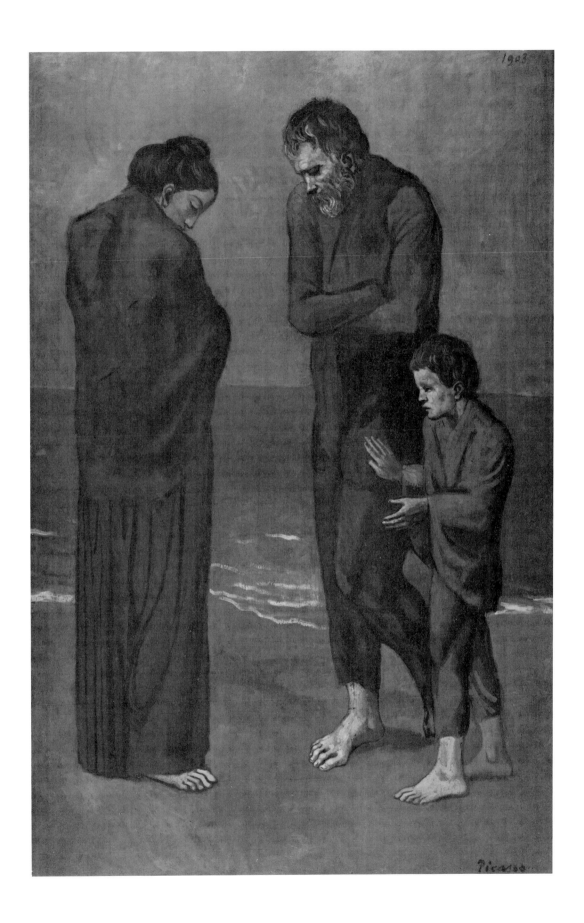

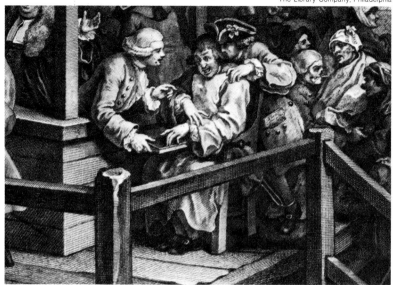

As Huntington's disease progresses, the patient develops chorea, a movement disorder in which the muscles of the face, limbs, and eventually the entire body are subject to uncontrollable jerky movements. There is also a deterioration of mental powers and personality. Before medical science had progressed to a degree that the cause of these movements could be understood, Huntington's patients were lumped together with other sufferers of brain disorders in a class of people who were regarded as both ridiculous and pitiable. "The Election," an engraving by William Hogarth (1697–1764), is part of a series satirizing corrupt electoral practices. It depicts a woman with a hereditary chorea being sworn in at a voting booth.

Harold L. Klawans, M.D., *is Associate Chairman and Professor in the Department of Neurological Sciences of Rush Medical College, Chicago.*

(Overleaf) "The Tragedy" by Pablo Picasso; photograph, courtesy, The National Gallery of Art, Washington, D.C.

disease is usually called Huntington's chorea. The second common set of manifestations consists of alterations in mental activity and personality. These include personality changes that vary from mild agitation and anxiety to frank psychosis and progressive intellectual deterioration.

There is no cure for Huntington's disease, nor is there a diagnostic test that can detect it before the symptoms appear. Of special poignancy is the fact that the disease is hereditary but does not appear until middle age, after childbearing is over. Therefore, an individual from a family that carries the HD gene cannot know if he or she has the disease and whether he is passing the disease on to his children. Each child of an affected person has a 50-50 chance of having Huntington's chorea. There are no "silent" carriers—if a person misses inheriting the disease, he will not transmit the gene.

"Leapings, strainings, and strange agitations"

Many U.S. families with HD can be traced back to 1630 and even earlier. This was a period of great turmoil in England. Charles I was continuing his father's avowed policy of driving nonconformists out of the land. The nonconformists, or Puritans, harassed by both the state and the Church of England, were leaving England as quickly as they could find ships to transport them. In 1630 a fleet led by John Winthrop left England for America with about 700 passengers. These immigrants included a number of residents from the small village of Bures in the county of Suffolk. Three men in this group seem to have brought chorea to America: William Knapp and two half brothers, Geoffrey and Nicholas Haste.

Geoffrey Haste was a member of the court of Ferrier of Bures. When his family objected to his chosen bride because her lineage could not be traced back to Norman times, Geoffrey took his wife-to-be and fled to America, settling in Stamford, Connecticut. Once there Geoffrey distinguished himself in various colonial criminal records by signing, with others, harsh verdicts against his fellow colonists. One of these was against a man who was held

164

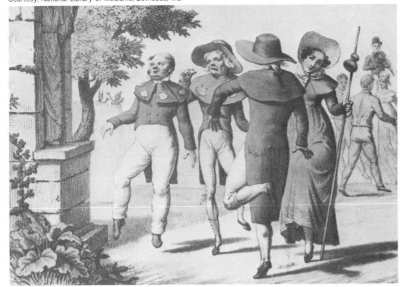

The word chorea is derived from the Greek word for "dance." The "dance" results when the random movements caused by the disease are superimposed over the ordinary purposeful movements of walking. "La danse de Saint Guy" is a caricature of a procession of epileptics and other neurological patients to the Eglise de Molenbeeck-St. Jean; from Charles Aubry's Album Comique de Pathologie Pittoresque, *edited by Ambroise Tardien, 1823.*

responsible for impregnating a young woman and was sentenced to stand upon the pillory to be publicly whipped, to have the letter R burned on his cheek, to pay the young woman's parents ten pounds, and, after all that, to marry the woman as soon as he recovered. Such extreme forms of punishment were common at that time. Geoffrey himself was fined in court for questioning testimony against him, and on another occasion was accused in court of retaining a stolen calf. His eldest son faced a death sentence on a charge of "bestialitie," but the magistrate decreased the sentence to two severe public whippings, a fine, and a halter to be fastened on his neck, which he was compelled to wear in public for two years. Following this punishment the son became quite religious and moved to another state. Many of his direct descendants were afflicted with Huntington's chorea.

At least one other of Geoffrey's sons gave birth to a long line of choreatic individuals. Yet another son, known in the neurologic literature by the name of Jefferson, deserves particular attention. He was one of the first settlers in Greenwich, Connecticut, a community that was not in sympathy with the spirit of the Puritans. On the border of the Dutch and Puritan settlements, Greenwich served as a retreat for treacherous and vicious men. In 1655 the deputies in neighboring Stamford complained to the General Court at New Haven about intolerable drunkenness among the English and the Indians in Greenwich, maintaining that the inhabitants were harboring runaway servants and that marriages in the community were often irregular. In the next year Jefferson and a few other settlers signed an agreement in court to yield themselves up to the lawful authorities. Jefferson later became a deputy for several years and retired from public life at the age of 44. It is known that he was ill for some time before his death at the age of 61. Jefferson had married the daughter of Nicholas, his father's half brother. From this union at least ten generations of patients with Huntington's chorea have descended.

Nicholas Haste himself was not without problems. He brought his wife, Ellin, with him from Bures on the Winthrop fleet. Ellin, the mother of Jeffer-

165

son's wife, was tried for witchcraft in 1653, found guilty, and hanged. One of their granddaughters, Mercy Disborough, was tried twice in the witch-mania epidemic of 1692 for that capital offense and then finally pardoned by the justices as the craze ran its course and the authorities, perhaps out of remorse, began reversing previous decisions. A son of Ellin and Nicholas gave rise to a family carrying the Huntington gene. It is usually believed that Nicholas and Ellin both had Huntington's chorea. It is less clear that Jefferson was affected.

The third affected family was that of William Knapp. William and his sons were notorious principals in some of the less savory aspects of colonial life. During his first ten years in the New World, the records of Massachusetts reveal several arrests for such offenses as public profanity, selling beer without a license, and making an offensive speech against the governor, John Winthrop.

William married Elizabeth Warne; one daughter of this marriage married a man named Mulfoot (later changed to Mulford), moved to East Hampton, Long Island, and formed the parent stem of what proved to be the historic Long Island group of Huntington's chorea—the sufferers who were studied by George Huntington and his forebears.

William Knapp and Elizabeth Warne had another daughter, called Elizabeth Knapp. In her early adult life this young woman achieved great fame as the celebrated Groton witch. In addition to William, Elizabeth Warne herself may have had the Huntington's gene. Following her husband's early death, Elizabeth Warne left her daughter, sailed back to England, and settled in Suffolk, where she was later accused of being possessed of the devil, was arrested, and even confessed to witchcraft. In the files of the British Museum records of the complaint brought against Elizabeth Warne by one John Buttery can still be found. Although there were hundreds of people accused of witchcraft in Suffolk in the 17th century, the county records have few details. Unfortunately there are very few accurate historical documents of

The unexplained personality alterations and bizarre physical symptoms of Huntington's chorea were, to the superstitious mind of the 17th century, an obvious sign of diabolical influence. Persons with the disease were accused of consorting with the devil, and some were tried and executed during the witch-hunting mania that swept through both Europe and North America.

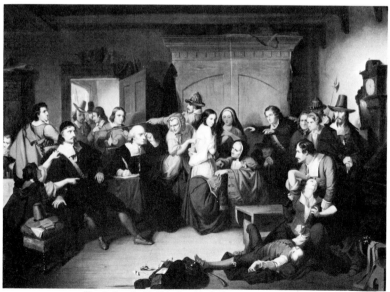

"Examination of a Witch" by Tompkins E. Matteson; photograph, Essex Institute, Salem, Mass.

witch trials held in England before 1690. It is of interest that Warne (Warren) descendants afflicted with Huntington's disease can still be found in the Boston area.

Like her mother in England, Elizabeth Knapp was accused of witchcraft. In 1671 the Rev. Samuel Willard, who was then minister of Groton, wrote a letter to Cotton Mather in which he described the younger Elizabeth's peculiar behavior.

This poore & miserable object, about a fortnight before shee was taken, wee observed to carry herselfe in a strange & unwonted manner, sometimes shee would give sudden shriekes, & if wee enquired a Reason, would always put it off with some excuse, & then would burst forth into imoderate & extravagant laughter, in such wise, as some times shee fell onto ye ground with it: I myselfe observed oftentimes a strange change in here countenance, but could not suspect ye true reason, but conceived shee might bee ill, and therefore divers times enquired how shee did it, & shee alwayes answered well; which made mee wonder. . . .

Several days later her abnormal behavior worsened:

. . . ye rest of ye family being in bed, shee was . . . suddenly throne downe into ye midst of ye floore with violence, & taken with a violent fit, whereupon ye whole family was raised, & with much adoe was she kept out of ye fire from destroying her selfe after which time she was followed with fits from thence till ye sabbath day; in which she was violent in bodily motions, leapings, strainings & strange agitations, scarce to be held in bounds by the strength of 3 or 4: violent alsoe in roarings & screamings, representing a dark resemblance of hellish form, and frequently using in these fits divers words, sometimes crying out money, money, sometimes, sin & misery with other words.

Willard, doing his duty as he saw it, questioned Elizabeth about her relationship with Satan. Under his questioning, she admitted that she had been receiving visits from Satan for three years but that he was continuing to torment her. Her consulting physician concluded that she had "Distemper" which was "Diabolicall" in origin. Whether Elizabeth actually had "Diabolicall Distemper," hysteria, or overt Huntington's disease remains unclear, but her father was choreatic and her mother also came from choreatic stock.

Certainly not all of the American "witches" had Huntington's chorea, but seven came from affected families and were at least subjects at risk. Of these, one certainly had abnormal movements that were apparent to her accusers. Of course, not all Huntington's families can be traced to these three families. Another group can be traced back to France, and their story has a familiar ring. In 1685 the Edict of Nantes was revoked, and religious tolerance in France came to an abrupt end. Many Huguenots fled France to avoid persecution. Some went to Nova Scotia and took Huntington's chorea with them. Other families with chorea have come from Germany, Ireland, and other countries of Europe.

Clinical features of Huntington's disease

The most characteristic motor manifestations of Huntington's chorea are the choreiform, "dance-like" movements. These movements are frequently the presenting complaint, the symptom that leads the patient to consult his physician. The word chorea is derived from the Greek word for "dance." The first dancelike disorder ever described was the dancing mania of the 15th

167

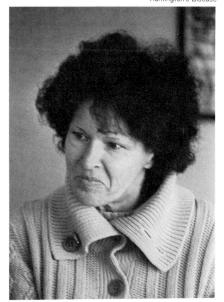

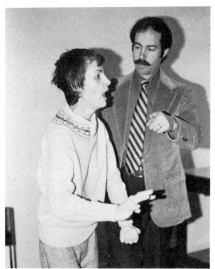

*The first manifestations of Huntington's
disease are subtle muscle malfunctions
caused by random spontaneous movements
of individual muscles. Movements of the
muscles of the face progress to episodes of
grimacing. In time, the movements in the
muscles of the limbs become more
pronounced, and gait is severely affected.
The patient's strength is unimpaired and
he is still able to initiate movement, but
his voluntary movement is combined with
sudden jerks of involuntary movement.*

century, in which sufferers of what is now felt to be some sort of mass hysteria grouped together and danced their way across western Europe. Since it was generally believed that only the intercession of St. Vitus could cure this affliction, it became known as St. Vitus' dance. In the 17th century the great English physician Thomas Sydenham described choreatic movements in children and adolescents. This disorder, now known as Sydenham's chorea or, incorrectly, St. Vitus' dance, is related to rheumatic fever and has in the last three decades become very uncommon.

The term chorea is now used to describe a type of abnormal spontaneous movement. Each is a single, isolated muscle action, a short, rapid, uncoordinated jerk. These jerks can be either proximal (involving the muscles close to the body) or distal (involving the parts of the limb furthest from the body) and are of enough magnitude to move the involved part. The simultaneous or successive occurrence of two or more such isolated movements can result in complex movement patterns, while the superimposition of these movements on normal movements can cause a dancelike gait.

Huntington's disease can appear any time from the first to the seventh decade of life but usually manifests itself when the victim is in his or her thirties or forties. The onset is almost always insidious. In cases beginning in middle adult years, the early motor symptoms are almost always related to chorea. Huntington's disease is not common. The incidence is said to be about one in every 20,000 births.

The first manifestations are often extremely subtle and may consist of a slight clumsiness or restlessness associated later with overt twitching of the fingers and grimacing of the face. Early in the course, the abnormal movements may be seen only during attempts to maintain a limb in a sustained posture. As the disease progresses, the chorea becomes more and more striking, and eventually all the patient's musculature is involved. At its most severe the chorea includes not only facial grimacing (involving lips, tongue, and cheeks) but also jerks of the head, weaving movements carried out by the patient to hide the otherwise obvious involuntary movements—an upward jerk of an arm may be fused into a voluntary scratching of the head. His gait is made up of jerky, lurching steps that are the result of a combination of voluntary and involuntary movements. Muscular strength is unimpaired, however, and the ability to initiate movement is intact, but the carrying out of a continuous movement is frequently impeded by superimposed muscle jerks that result in a severe and distressing form of incoordination.

While the choreiform movements can often be disabling, they are only rarely violent enough to result in harm to the patient. The great English neurologist Samuel Wilson described this quite vividly in two of his patients. The first was suddenly propelled through a shop window by a lurch of his body, while the second patient suffered a fatal broken neck when a sudden backward jerk of his trunk threw him down a hospital staircase. Fortunately, mass movements of the entire body are not common even in late stages of Huntington's chorea.

The voice is often affected by this disease. The abnormal movements can involve the muscles of both respiration and articulation, resulting in interruption of the normal sequence of breathing and speaking. The speech is often

168

markedly abnormal, erratic, and at times explosive. In severe instances it is virtually unintelligible.

Some patients with HD develop increased tone, or stiffness, in their muscles, which is called rigidity. This is often associated with a slowness in carrying out intentional movements and a paucity of movements. These two phenomena together are called akinesia (lack of movement). Some HD patients never develop chorea, their major motor difficulties being rigidity and akinesia. The akinetic form of Huntington's chorea is relatively more frequent among patients whose disease begins in the first or second decade. In patients with a very late onset of the disease, the first manifestation may be a to-and-fro tremor instead of the classic choreiform movements. This tremor consists of a rhythmic repetitive movement of the finger in which the same to-and-fro movement is repeated over and over again, contrasting sharply with the random, irregular jerks usually seen in HD.

Progressive intellectual deterioration is the second cardinal feature of Huntington's disease. The earliest mental symptoms may appear to be more emotional than intellectual. The patient becomes increasingly irritable and excitable, begins to lose his temper more easily, or develops other subtle changes in his personality. Alternatively, progressive indifference may culminate in severe apathy. The patient or his associates may note inattention or a decrease in the ability to concentrate. The usual complaints are vague and hard to attribute—inability to maintain interest in work or to get work completed, wandering of the mind, lackadaisical attitude, and so forth. These are often felt by the patient and his family and friends to be psychological in nature, due to stress or anxiety. However, as judgment, comprehension, and memory become affected, it becomes obvious that the patient is suffering from a progressive decline of the functions of the brain. The psychiatric manifestations are at times quite prominent, with instances of manic-depressive or schizophrenic reaction. While these are unusual, less marked alteration of personality, including paranoia and impulsive behavior, are more frequent.

It is quite common for the patient to accuse his or her spouse of infidelity or plotting to take away the patient's money or belongings. The accusations of infidelity are often both shallow and ludicrous—*e.g.,* meeting lovers in the bathroom of the home—but are nonetheless firmly believed by the patient. Sudden outbursts of anger and destructive behavior are less common but can occur. A tendency toward sexual promiscuity was noted by Huntington.

The course of HD is quite variable—either the mental changes or the choreiform movement may appear first. It is more common for the chorea to be noted prior to the onset of the mental changes or at least simultaneously with them, but this is not invariably true. In cases of juvenile Huntington's chorea in which rigidity predominates, the course usually is quite rapid. Children frequently have seizures, but they are not usually the first sign of the disease, so it is unlikely that the beginning of HD in childhood would be easily confused with other forms of epilepsy. Children in whom chorea is present usually have a slowly progressive course which mimics adult-onset Huntington's chorea. The average duration of life after the onset of the disease is said to be 13.7 years, but this can vary from 5 to 30 years.

Patients often experience several years of severe disability before death.

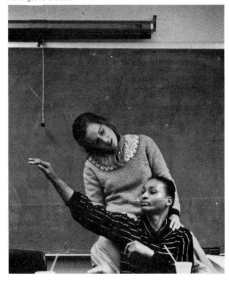

Huntington's patients can be helped by physical therapy that focuses on specific problem areas. Here a therapist helps a patient learn exercises to limber the neck and throat muscles. Some Huntington's patients develop rigidity of the muscles rather than chorea.

169

Photographs, courtesy, Dr. Edmond Chiu, Arthur Preston Centre, Melbourne

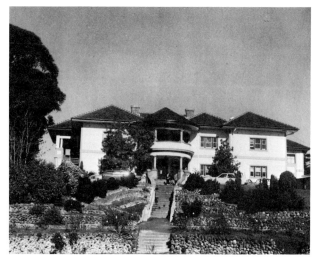
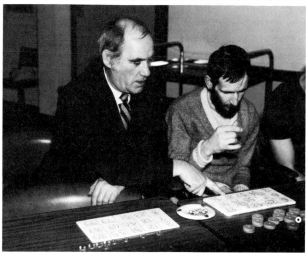
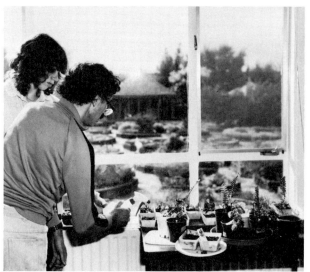
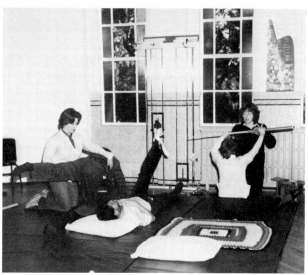

The Arthur Preston Centre in Melbourne, Australia, is the world's first facility exclusively for the care of patients with Huntington's disease. The center provides both day care and residential care. Patients are assisted in a variety of recreational and therapeutic activities as well as receiving specialized medical care.

Such patients usually have some degree of intellectual decline and impaired movement and often die as a result of pneumonia, pulmonary embolism, or cardiac failure. These are the problems common to patients who become bedridden because of chronic debilitating disease. Pneumonia occurs because of weakened resistance, weakened respiratory muscles, and because the patient has difficulty swallowing and coughing and may inhale food. Pulmonary embolism results from blood clots that form in the legs after a long period of immobility; the clots break off and travel to the lung, obstructing its blood flow. Cardiac failure results from poor muscle tone in the heart and inability to combat stress.

Establishing the diagnosis

There is no known test for HD. Diagnosis is based on recognizing the clinical manifestations and knowing the family history. A CAT scan revealing brain atrophy supports the other evidence but does not provide proof of the diagnosis, which is a clinical one. Huntington's disease is the only hereditary disease with personality change and chorea.

170

Pathology. It is important that an autopsy including study of the brain be obtained after death to confirm the diagnosis. It is the distinctive changes within the brain that characterize HD as a single specific disease (*see* page 172). The most significant feature is a primary loss of the nerve cells of the caudate nucleus and the putamen. These two structures are considered important in motor function, so their deterioration is thought to cause both the chorea and the rigidity-akinesia of HD. As the disease progresses, both the caudate and putamen, which together are known as the corpus striatum, become grossly shrunken and atrophic. At times the nerve cell loss is so marked as to give the corpus striatum a spongelike appearance. There are two normal neuronal cell populations in the striatum; the smaller appear to bear the brunt of the degenerative process, whereas the larger neurons are seriously affected only after the disease is well advanced.

Atrophy of the cerebral cortex is characteristic and is most marked in the frontal lobes. The ventricles of the brain, spaces between the lobes, are usually dilated. Microscopic examination reveals definite loss of neurons in all layers of the cerebral cortex, with certain layers being more affected than others. Since most mental functions are related to the activity of the cerebral cortex, it is the loss of cells in the cerebral cortex that causes the mental symptoms of HD.

Physiology. The mechanism by which the cellular changes in the caudate nucleus and putamen cause chorea is beginning to be better understood. It was once thought that chorea was due to loss of function of degenerated striatal cells, but it is now thought that chorea results from the abnormal function of living but diseased striatal cells.

The behavior of any nerve cell within the brain depends upon its ability to receive and respond to messages from other nerve cells. These messages are transmitted by specific chemical agents known as neurotransmitters. There appear to be at least three major neurotransmitters in the striatum: dopamine, acetylcholine, and GABA (gamma aminobutyric acid). The exact physiological abnormality in HD is not known, but a number of clinical observations have suggested that dopamine plays a role in the production of chorea in HD and other disorders. It is known that drugs that decrease brain dopamine improve chorea; drugs that block dopamine receptors and thereby prevent dopamine from acting improve chorea; and drugs that increase the activity of dopamine at striatal dopamine receptors worsen chorea.

Since brain dopamine levels are normal in HD, it is generally believed that the diseased striatal neurons respond in an abnormal, hypersensitive fashion to dopamine and it is this dopamine hypersensitivity which seems to cause the choreatic movements. The relationship of dopamine to chorea appears to hold true for other forms of chorea such as Sydenham's chorea and less common chorea of pregnancy (chorea gravidarium).

While much has been written recently about the possible role of dopamine in schizophrenia, it appears that most of the dopamine in the brain has as its major function the control of movement. Some 80 to 90% of the brain's dopamine is controlled by small cells in the midbrain of the *substantia nigra* ("black substance," so called because of the black pigment or melanin it contains). These cells release dopamine, which then acts on the dopamine

171

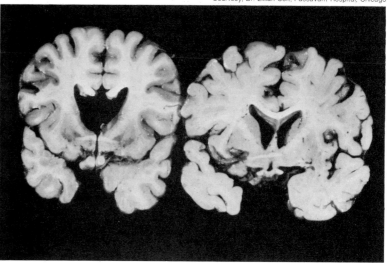

The most significant feature of the pathology of Huntington's disease is a loss of nerve cells in the brain. The brain (left) of the Huntington's chorea patient is markedly shrunken, compared with the normal brain. The ventricles, the spaces between the lobes of the brain, are dilated, and the caudate nucleus, the area bounding the lower sides of the triangle of the ventricles, is much deteriorated.

receptors of the corpus striatum. When the striatum responds in a hyperactive way because its cells are diseased, the result is chorea. Conversely, if not enough dopamine is released, the result is parkinsonism, a progressive neurologic dysfunction characterized by rigidity, tremor, and lack of movement. The lack of movement in parkinsonism is in many ways the opposite of the increased random body movements of HD.

It has recently been found that GABA is markedly decreased in specific regions of the brains (especially the corpus striatum) of patients dying with HD and that the enzymes necessary to produce this neurotransmitter are also decreased. The significance of reduced GABA concentrations in Huntington's chorea remains unknown. In parkinsonism there is a loss of dopamine, and replacement of dopamine activity by the drug levodopa, which increases brain dopamine, improves parkinsonism. By analogy, increased GABA activity might ameliorate chorea. Unfortunately, this has yet to be demonstrated, so it remains unclear whether GABA loss itself produces chorea. It is believed that the lack of GABA is the result of death of GABA-producing cells. The most significant question of all, why these cells or other brain cells die in HD, has not been answered.

The genetic gamble

Huntington's disease is inherited as an autosomal dominant trait: if a person has HD, each of his or her children has an independent 50-50 chance of developing the disease. If the child does develop the disease, then each of his or her children also has a 50-50 chance of developing the disease, but if he or she is free from the disease, then the offspring have no chance of having HD. In other words, there are no carriers for HD, only affected individuals who can transmit the gene or completely unaffected individuals. But since HD usually appears in the fourth or fifth decade, the patient has already completed his or her family, and the abnormal gene has been transmitted— or not. A person at risk for this disease must make decisions as to marriage and childbearing with this sword of Damocles hanging overhead. Because of this tragic problem there has been much interest in developing a test for HD

172

that can detect its presence before symptoms appear. If a person at risk knew at age 20 whether or not he or she was destined to develop HD, the decision to have children could be made much simpler, and a lifetime of anxiety could be eliminated for many people. There is at present no way to detect the presymptomatic patient and tell which children will pass on the abnormal gene to their children.

The British medical journal *The Lancet* recently reported the results of a model genetic counseling program for individuals in South Wales who were at high risk for developing HD. Since 1900 the incidence of HD in the area had remained nearly constant, about 7.5 persons per 100,000. In the studied area, 986 individuals were judged to be at high risk of having inherited the disease. Most cooperated with researchers. Genetic counselors visited persons who were at risk, informing them fully about the nature of the disease. Facts had been concealed by some older family members in some cases, and in others information came only after children had been born. The individuals or couples were not advised against having children, but alternatives to childbearing were discussed, with more specific information on contraception and sterilization available. Follow-up visits were to be made annually by nurses, aided by social workers.

By 1980, seven years after the start of the program, the births to individuals at risk showed a definite downward trend. For example, in 1973, the first year of the program, there were 26 births, and in 1980, 14 births. Researchers attributed the success of this unique program to the nonthreatening, noncoercive nature of the counseling and to systematic follow-ups and support. Of course, there is no present way of knowing how many of these parents or children will be affected by the disease—only time will tell.

Adding complexity to the problem of genetic counseling is the fact that HD can appear without any previous family history of the disease. This often raises the question of parentage, but it is thought that the gene can, on rare occasions, occur spontaneously as a mutation. It was at one time believed that the disease began to manifest itself at earlier ages in each successive generation, a phenomenon referred to as anticipation. It is now believed that this was an artifact of case-recording techniques and that such anticipation does not occur.

Hope for the future

There is presently no known way to prevent the progression of Huntington's chorea. Since the basic abnormality that causes the death of brain cells is not known, the process cannot be arrested or reversed.

However, help is available for some of the symptoms. The abnormal movements can often be improved with drugs such as haloperidol (Haldol) that block dopamine receptors. These drugs can improve the abnormal movement, but unfortunately the loss of mental function is not slowed, and the brain cells continue to die. The depression seen in many patients may improve with antidepressant drugs, and the psychosis and agitation often can be helped with antipsychotic agents.

Numerous investigations of the diagnosis, cause, and cure of HD are under way. The research includes studies of the chemistry of the brains of

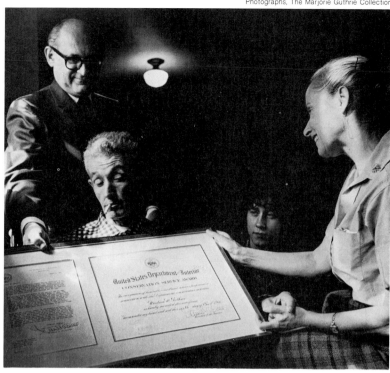

Woody Guthrie, folksinger, songwriter, chronicler of the hard times of the Depression, and author of the well-known song "This Land Is Your Land," died from Huntington's chorea in 1967. He is pictured in 1966 with his wife, Marjorie, and son Arlo, who is also a composer and folksinger, on the occasion of receiving the Conservation Service Award from the U.S. Department of the Interior. In 1967 Marjorie Guthrie formed the Committee to Combat Huntington's Disease to raise money for research, disseminate information, and provide counseling and support for Huntington's disease families.

Every child of a Huntington's disease patient has a 50-50 chance of developing the disease. There is no way of knowing if a child has inherited the disease before the symptoms begin to appear.

patients who have died with HD; studies of the chemistry of other tissues of living patients (since this is a genetic disease, all cells in the body carry the gene, and it is hoped that analysis of blood cells or skin cells will help to shed light on the basic biochemical or physiological defect); studies of brain metabolism in living patients using new noninvasive electronic devices which allow scientists to safely study metabolism of the brain as it functions; and studies of genetic linkage, which attempt to map out the exact gene that carries Huntington's disease in an attempt to predict which subjects at risk will develop the disease.

FOR ADDITIONAL READING:

Barbeau, A., Chase, T. N., and Paulson, G. W. *Huntington's Chorea.* Advances in Neurology, vol. 1. New York: Raven Press, 1873–1972.

Chase, T. N., Wexler, N. S., and Barbeau, A. *Huntington's Disease.* Advances in Neurology, vol. 23. New York: Raven Press, 1873–1972.

Harper, P. S., *et al.* "Huntington's Chorea: The Basis for Long-term Prevention." *The Lancet* 2: 346–349, 1979.

Harper, P. S., *et al.* "Decline in the Predicted Incidence of Huntington's Chorea Associated with Systematic Genetic Counselling and Family Support." *The Lancet* 2: 411–413, 1981.

Klawans, H. L. "The Curse of the Evanses." In *Torture in Vienna and Other Medical Entertainments.* New York: Raven Press, 1981.

Maltsberger, J. T. "Even unto the 12th Generation—Huntington's Chorea." *Journal of the History of Medicine and Allied Sciences:* 1–17, 1961.

174

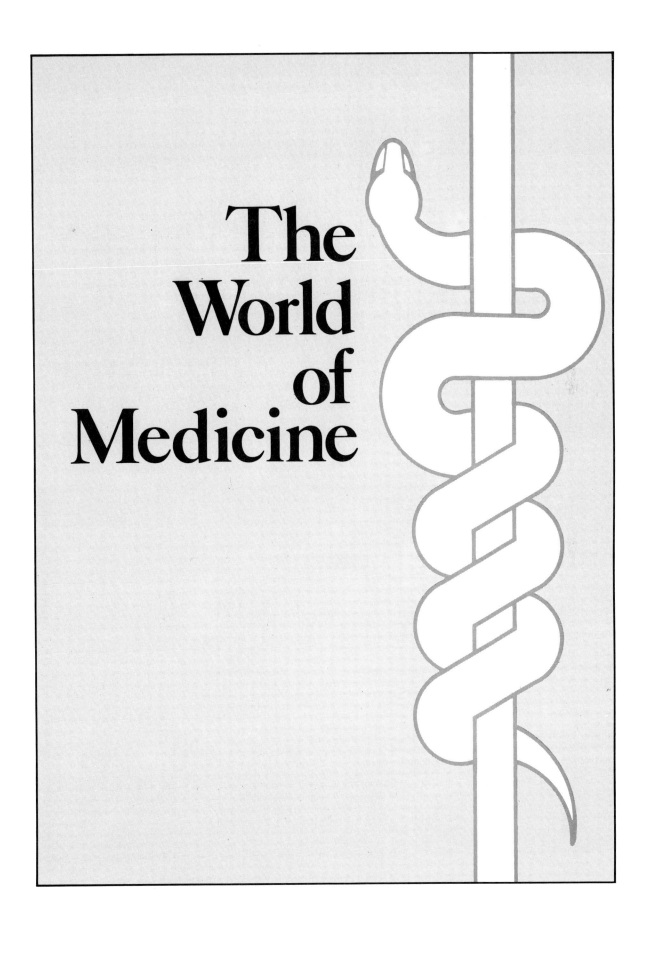

The World of Medicine

Contributors to The World of Medicine

Mark Abramowicz, M.D. *Drugs.* Editor, *The Medical Letter,* New Rochelle, N.Y.

George J. Annas, J.D., M.P.H. *Health Care Law.* Associate Professor of Law and Medicine, Boston University Schools of Medicine and Public Health.

L. Fred Ayvazian, M.D. *Diet and Nutrition Special Report: Do Ex-Smokers Gain Weight?; Lung Diseases.* Chief, Pulmonary Section, Veterans Administration Medical Center, East Orange, N.J.; Professor of Medicine, College of Medicine and Dentistry, New Jersey Medical School, Newark; Professor of Clinical Medicine, New York University School of Medicine, New York City.

Howard C. Baron, M.D. *Surgery.* Attending Vascular Surgeon, Cabrini Medical Center, New York City; Associate Professor of Surgery, New York University School of Medicine, New York City.

Lewis Bernstein, Ph.D. *World Medical News Special Report: Mental Health in China* (in part). Clinical Professor of Psychiatry, School of Medicine, and Adjunct Professor, Department of Psychology, University of California at San Diego; Professor Emeritus, Department of Psychiatry and Mental Health Sciences, The Medical College of Wisconsin, Milwaukee.

Rosalyn Bernstein. *World Medical News Special Report: Mental Health in China* (in part). Retired social worker, La Jolla, Calif.

Walter G. Bradley, D.M. *Neuromuscular Disorders.* Chairman, Department of Neurology, University of Vermont College of Medicine, Burlington.

Wilton H. Bunch, M.D., Ph.D. *Orthopedics.* Professor and Chairman, Department of Orthopedics and Rehabilitation, Loyola University Medical Center, Maywood, Ill.

Robert N. Butler, M.D. *Aging Special Report: The Teaching Nursing Home: A New Concept.* Director, National Institute on Aging, National Institutes of Health, Bethesda, Md.

Mitchell H. Charap, M.D. *Preventive Medicine.* Assistant Medical Director, Ambulatory Care, New York University Medical Center, and Instructor, Department of Medicine, New York University School of Medicine, New York City.

Robert R. Chilcote, M.D. *Blood and the Lymphatic System.* Assistant Professor, Department of Pediatrics, The University of Chicago, Pritzker School of Medicine.

Edward P. Cohen, M.D. *Allergy and Immunity.* Dean, School of Basic Medical Sciences, and Professor of Microbiology and Immunology, University of Illinois Medical Center, Chicago.

Elizabeth B. Connell, M.D. *Contraception; Gynecology and Obstetrics.* Professor, Department of Gynecology and Obstetrics, Emory University School of Medicine, Atlanta, Ga.

Peter Davies, Ph.D. *Aging.* Associate Professor of Pathology and Neuroscience, Albert Einstein College of Medicine of Yeshiva University, Bronx, N.Y.

Stephen E. Epstein, M.D. *Drugs Special Report: The Beta-Blocking Drugs; Heart and Blood Vessels* (in part). Chief of Cardiology, Cardiology Branch, National Heart, Lung, and Blood Institute, National Institutes of Health, Bethesda, Md.

Chris-Ellyn Johanson, Ph.D. *Drug Abuse* (in part). Research Associate and Associate Professor, Department of Psychiatry, The University of Chicago.

Warren A. Katz, M.D. *Arthritis and Connective Tissue Disorders.* Division Chief, Division of Rheumatology, Department of Medicine, Medical College of Pennsylvania and Hospital, Philadelphia.

John F. Keegan, Ph.D. *Diet and Nutrition Special Report: Life After Major Weight Loss* (in part). Director of Psychology, Clinical Nutrition Unit, Detroit, Mich.

Mary Jane Koren, M.D. *Emergency Medicine.* Director of Emergency Services, Wyckoff Heights Hospital, Brooklyn, N.Y.; Assistant Professor of Medicine, Albert Einstein College of Medicine of Yeshiva University, Bronx, N.Y.; Consultant Physician, New York City Poison Control Center.

Rose Kushner. *Cancer Special Report: Coping with Breast Cancer.* Executive Director, Breast Cancer Advisory Center, Rockville, Md.; Member, National Cancer Advisory Board.

Lynne Lamberg. *Preventive Medicine Special Report: Sleep: How Much Do We Need?; Skin Disorders* (in part). Free-lance medical journalist, Baltimore, Md.

Stanford I. Lamberg, M.D. *Skin Disorders* (in part). Associate Professor of Dermatology, The Johns Hopkins University School of Medicine; Chief, Department of Dermatology, Baltimore City Hospitals, Baltimore, Md.

Bernard Levin, M.D. *Gastrointestinal Disorders.* Associate Professor, Department of Medicine, Section of Gastroenterology, The University of Chicago, Pritzker School of Medicine.

Nathan W. Levin, M.D. *Kidney Diseases.* Head, Division of Nephrology, Henry Ford Hospital, Detroit; Clinical Professor of Medicine, University of Michigan Medical School, Ann Arbor.

Rachmiel Levine, M.D. *Glandular and Metabolic Disorders.* Director Emeritus of Research, City of Hope Medical Center, Duarte, Calif.

Charles P. Lucas, M.D. *Diet and Nutrition Special Report: Life After Major Weight Loss* (in part). Professor of Medicine, Wayne State University Medical School, Detroit, Mich.; Director and Chief, Division of Endocrinology and Metabolism, Clinical Nutrition Unit, Detroit.

James A. Merrill, M.D. *Gynecology and Obstetrics Special Report: Endometriosis.* Professor and Head, Department of Gynecology and Obstetrics, University of Oklahoma College of Medicine, Oklahoma City.

Drummond Rennie, M.D. *World Medical News.* Chairman of Medicine, West Suburban Hospital, Oak Park, Ill.; Associate Professor of Medicine, Rush Medical College, Chicago.

Joann Ellison Rodgers. *Drugs Special Report: Solved: The Riddle of Thalidomide; Surgery Special Report: Surgeries for Obesity.* National Science Correspondent, Hearst Feature Service, New York City.

Douglas R. Rosing, M.D. *Heart and Blood Vessels* (in part). Head, Cardiovascular Diagnosis, Cardiology Branch, National Heart, Lung, and Blood Institute, National Institutes of Health, Bethesda, Md.

Roger H. Scholle, D.D.S. *Dentistry.* Editor, American Dental Association, Chicago.

Charles R. Schuster, Ph.D. *Drug Abuse* (in part). Professor, Departments of Psychiatry and Pharmacological and Physiological Sciences, and Director, Drug Abuse Research Center, The University of Chicago, Pritzker School of Medicine.

Michael B. Shimkin, M.D. *Cancer.* Professor Emeritus of Community Medicine and Oncology, School of Medicine, University of California at San Diego.

Dallas W. Stevenson. *Diet and Nutrition Special Report: Life After Major Weight Loss* (in part). Psychologist, Clinical Nutrition Unit, Detroit, Mich.

Thomas B. Turner, M.D. *Preventive Medicine Special Report: Benefits of Moderate Drinking.* Dean Emeritus, and Professor Emeritus of Microbiology, The Johns Hopkins University School of Medicine, Baltimore, Md.

J. Ingram Walker, M.D. *Stress.* Associate Professor of Psychiatry and Staff Psychiatrist, Veterans Administration Medical Center, Durham, N.C.

Myron Winick, M.D. *Diet and Nutrition.* R. R. Williams Professor of Nutrition, Professor of Pediatrics, and Director, Institute of Human Nutrition, Columbia University College of Physicians and Surgeons, New York City.

Peter D. Wood, Ph.D., D.Sc. *Physical Fitness and Sports Medicine.* Adjunct Professor of Medicine and Deputy Director, Stanford Heart Disease Prevention Program, Stanford University School of Medicine, Stanford, Calif.

Aging

The currently accepted definition of dementia is a progressive deterioration in intellectual performance, always involving memory loss, that is severe enough to disrupt occupational or social skills or both. There is almost always loss of problem-solving ability and other aspects of abstract thinking, but a normal level of consciousness and awareness—including the awareness that something is seriously wrong—is maintained until late in the disease. By that time, memory even of familiar names and faces fades, as well as of how to perform day-to-day tasks. Ultimately dementia may cause death, often as a result of inactivity that leads to respiratory infections or heart disease. For most people familiar with this description, it corresponds to senile dementia, the irreversible mental deterioration often seen in the elderly.

Dementia and Alzheimer's disease

For many years the term Alzheimer's disease was used to denote what was thought to be a rare presenile dementia; that is, dementia in persons in their forties and fifties. Several lines of study that have been carried out during the past several years clearly indicate that this disease, in addition to being the major cause of presenile dementia, is almost certain to be the largest single cause of senile dementia. Estimates suggest that in the U.S. some 1.5 million to 2 million people suffer from Alzheimer's disease. This figure represents about 0.6 to 0.9% of the population, and as far as anyone knows, this proportion of the population of all developed nations is similarly afflicted.

Alzheimer's disease was originally described in 1906 by Alois Alzheimer, a German neuropathologist. His original patient was a woman of 55 years who died with severe dementia. At autopsy Alzheimer noted the presence in the brain of two abnormalities. The first was neuritic plaque, a structure that had been described previously in the brains of elderly people. It is now known that neuritic plaque is composed of degenerating nerve terminals, reactive glial cells (nonnervous cells present in nerve tissue), and fibrous material called amyloid. The second abnormality noted by Alzheimer was the neurofibrillary tangle, a fibrous structure within nerve cells, which showed up heavily with the use of a silver stain. The presence of the neurofibrillary tangle within nerve cells had not been described before, and it was really this abnormality that defined a new disease entity. It was perhaps unfortunate that the first patient in which this disease was discovered was so young, for this circumstance led physicians of the period to think of Alzheimer's disease as a presenile dementia. Because dementia in middle-aged people is quite rare, this attitude long held back research into the true nature of this disease; Alzheimer's was not perceived to be a major health problem. Happily this situation is now being remedied with ongoing investigative studies.

Reasons for concern

Two factors have reawakened interest in Alzheimer's disease in recent years. The first is a growing realization that, largely because of improvements in public health and living standards, an increasing proportion of the population of the developed nations is living to advanced age. In the U.S. in 1980 about 11% of the population were 65 years old or older. As health care improves, that percentage will also increase, making this age group the fastest growing section of the population. As the ranks of the aged swell, the economic and social problems associated with being old also increase in significance.

Perhaps principal among such problems are those associated with a decline in mental acuity; there are few handicaps as debilitating as a failing intellect. It has

Photomicrographs compare the concentration of neurons (dark bodies) in the nucleus basalis of Meynert taken from the brain of a person free of Alzheimer's disease (left) and from a disease victim (right). Degeneration of the nucleus may cause some of the memory loss and other symptoms seen in this disease.

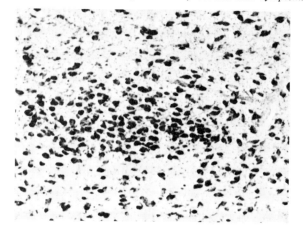
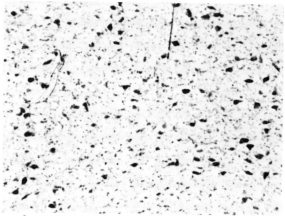

been estimated that about 15% of the U.S. population aged 65 or over suffer from senile dementia; in the early 1980s this represented more than 3½ million people. The proportion rises to over 20% for people over 80 years old. The economic cost of caring for these individuals is staggering. At least 50% of nursing-home residents suffer from dementia, and nursing-home costs in the U.S. in 1981 amounted to $26 billion. Probably the minority of dementia victims are in nursing homes, so that the hidden economic and social costs are truly enormous.

For the individual who suffers from senile dementia and for family and friends, the disease can have devastating emotional and financial effects. Fear, anger, embarrassment, and frustration pace its progress as everyone, the victim included, helplessly witnesses the erosion of intellect and personality that leads inexorably to a shutdown of the mind. Over a course of perhaps five to ten years or longer the family must cope with shortening attention span, sudden personality changes, bouts of paranoia, angry outbursts, disorientation and wandering, and, commonly in the later stages, incontinence and the inability of the sufferer to feed and dress himself. The economic burden on the victim and family for nursing-home or in-home care can quickly drain what under ordinary circumstances is a respectable life savings. And nursing care for senile dementia patients is usually not covered by health insurance programs, primarily because such care is interpreted as "custodial" rather than "medical" in nature.

The second factor that has rekindled interest is the realization that Alzheimer's disease is the single largest cause of dementia in persons aged 65 or over. Surveys by pathologists in the U.S., Europe, and Japan of deceased victims of dementia have found that 50 to 60% have the pathologic changes characteristic of Alzheimer's disease; that is, neuritic plaques and neurofibrillary tangles are the only abnormalities in the brain. A further 20% have plaques and tangles in addition to other pathologic abnormalities (usually as a result of one or more strokes). Therefore, Alzheimer's disease at least contributes to dementia in about 70% of dementia patients aged 65 years or more. The remainder are largely stroke victims, who make up about 20% of the total, or suffer from any one of about 50 conditions that can produce dementia, including brain tumors, hypothyroidism, pernicious anemia, head injuries, reactions to various drug treatments, and certain infections that affect the brain. Moreover, the apathy and lack of responsiveness often accompanying severe depression in the elderly are quite easy to mistake for symptoms of dementia.

A difficult diagnosis

There are two very important points to keep in mind: the majority of elderly suffering from dementia will turn

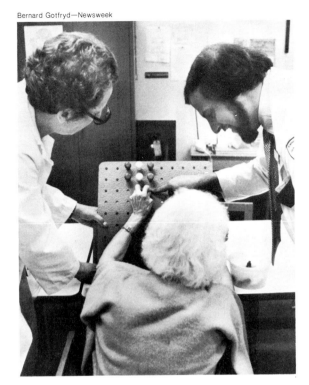
Bernard Gotfryd—Newsweek

Therapists train an Alzheimer's patient to maintain organized thought patterns. Hope for a definitive cure, however, lies in continued neurological research.

out to have Alzheimer's disease, but there exist other causes of dementia that are treatable. Perhaps the most important result of all the current interest in Alzheimer's disease is recognition of the importance of a good diagnosis. This is not a trivial matter, because at present there is no diagnostic test for Alzheimer's disease.

In practice, all other likely causes of dementia have to be ruled out. This means that a comprehensive neurologic examination is essential, blood samples must be analyzed for thyroid hormones and vitamin levels, and spinal fluid samples must be checked for the presence of abnormal cells or proteins. Computerized axial tomography (CAT scanning) can be used to search for evidence of strokes or tumors. The latest, highly sophisticated CAT scanners can detect the presence of even very small strokes and so are especially useful. When all other tests are negative, a diagnosis of Alzheimer's disease can be considered. This diagnosis can be confirmed, however, only by brain biopsy or at autopsy.

Alzheimer's disease and acetylcholine deficiency

Currently there is no established treatment for Alzheimer's disease, although research in this area has grown dramatically in the past few years. Stimulus for this growth has come from neurochemical investiga-

179

tions of brains removed at autopsy from patients with the disease. A breakthrough came in 1976 when three groups working in Great Britain uncovered evidence of a major deficiency in acetylcholine production in several regions of the brain. These regions included the cerebral cortex and hippocampus, both of which are probably involved in memory and other higher intellectual functions. This extremely important finding has since been confirmed and expanded in many laboratories around the world.

Acetylcholine is a chemical used by a small proportion of nerve cells in the brain to transmit signals to other nerve cells. Because there was abundant evidence from human and animal studies that interference with acetylcholine transmission impairs memory function, it was tempting from the start to speculate that at least some of the symptoms of Alzheimer's disease were due to a deficiency of acetylcholine. More recent work tends to support this speculation. Medical scientists now believe that the deficiency of acetylcholine results from the death of a small group of cells, called the nucleus basalis of Meynert, in an area deep in the brain. It is this small group of cells that is responsible for supplying a major portion of the acetylcholine in the cerebral cortex. This it does by sending long, branching projections (axons) up to the cortex, where acetylcholine is released from the axon terminals. Similarly, it is the death of cells in the septal region, near the midline of the brain, that results in the deficiency of acetylcholine in the hippocampus.

One of the most vexing questions at this time concerns the specificity of the deficit in acetylcholine production. At least 20 compounds in the brain are now thought to be used as transmitters of information between cells, and more and more such transmitters are being identified every year. Is the production of all transmitters affected by Alzheimer's disease, or is it just acetylcholine? This question is important because if there is only one deficit, the chances of finding a successful treatment are much greater than if there are multiple problems.

Unfortunately, this question has not yet been completely answered. In light of the 11 other transmitters so far investigated, the best that can be said is that acetylcholine deficiency seems to be the most consistent and dramatic. Some problems have been reported to occur in nerve cells that use noradrenaline as their transmitter, but currently available information indicates that these are present in only a relatively small proportion of Alzheimer's patients. The same may be true of nerve cells that use serotonin, somatostatin, or gamma-aminobutyric acid as their transmitter. Nerve cells that use vasopressin, vasoactive intestinal peptide, cholecystokinin octapeptide, thyrotropin releasing factor, substance P, dopamine, or LHRH as transmitters seem to be largely unaffected by Alzheimer's disease, except perhaps in the very late stages. The emerging picture portrays a dramatic loss of acetylcholine-producing cells in all Alzheimer's patients, with a lesser and quite variable involvement of other nerve cells, especially in very severely affected, late-stage cases. This picture makes it quite reasonable to assume that if a treatment could make good the deficiency of acetylcholine, it would alleviate the symptoms of the disease considerably, especially in patients in the early stages. The question now is: How can this be accomplished?

Attempts at treatment

The first rational attempts to treat Alzheimer's patients involved giving them large doses of choline chloride. The rationale was simple: choline is converted to acetylcholine in the brain; more choline means more acetylcholine. There was also a striking precedent for this approach. The brains of patients with Parkinson's disease, a degenerative disorder of the central nervous system, are deficient in the transmitter dopamine, and the administration of L-dopa, a precursor of dopamine, not only increases amounts of dopamine in the brain but also lessens symptoms considerably for most patients. There was a further stimulus: choline is a natural product found in many foods and thus was not likely to have any unpleasant side effects. The unfortunate thing is that choline, even in large doses, does not seem to help patients with Alzheimer's disease. Attempts to treat patients with lecithin have also met with failure. Lecithin is a natural product that contains choline in a bound form, and large doses of lecithin raise blood choline levels even higher than does choline.

The reason choline and lecithin do not help seems to be that increasing amounts of choline *in* the brain simply does not increase the amount of acetylcholine *made* by the brain. Precisely what does govern the rate of acetylcholine production is not known despite a great deal of work over the past decade, and there is no clear idea how one might increase the rate of synthesis of this compound in the brains of patients with Alzheimer's disease. This is an area ripe for future research.

Another approach to rational treatment for Alzheimer's disease that has begun in a few research centers is to reduce the rate at which acetylcholine is broken down in the brain. One drug that has this action is physostigmine, an alkaloid found in betel nuts. This drug inhibits the activity of acetylcholinesterase, the enzyme responsible for halting acetylcholine's action when it is released to transmit nerve impulses. Very preliminary reports of the effects of physostigmine on patients with Alzheimer's disease are encouraging; the drug does seem to improve performance on tasks involving memory. This is not to say that the drug restores all of the afflicted patients' former intellectual capacity, but it does appear to produce measurable improvements. Similar preliminary results with another inhibitor of acetylcholinesterase, tetrahydroaminoacridine (THA), seem to indicate that research to find a treatment for acetylcholine deficiency is on the right track at last.

Because acetylcholine transmits signals from nerves to muscles in many parts of the body including the heart, the diaphragm, and the gut, problems are likely to arise in trying to use acetylcholinesterase inhibitors to treat Alzheimer's patients. If the breakdown of acetylcholine were inhibited too much, nerve-muscle communication would be disrupted because of an excess of acetylcholine—with fatal results if adequate medical attention were not immediately available. Consequently drugs like physostigmine and THA are potentially very toxic; indeed, many of the nerve gases developed for chemical warfare are irreversible inhibitors of acetylcholinesterase. Research directed toward finding much safer ways of treating acetylcholine deficiency is urgently needed, especially since work with physostigmine and THA implies that clinical improvements can be obtained even with some drugs that are considered less than perfect.

Search for the underlying cause

A successful treatment for the acetylcholine deficiency that seems to cause the symptoms of Alzheimer's disease is not the whole solution, however. Medical scientists need to understand why the acetylcholine-producing cells die. What is it that has the ability to seemingly select these particular cells for destruction? Several theories have been advanced, but at this time the available evidence is so limited that a clear favorite is hard to pick.

The most popular hypothesis is that a viral infection causes the cell death. This idea has gained support because of work on a rare form of dementia called Creutzfeldt-Jakob disease, which has been shown to be transmissible from people to a variety of animals, including monkeys. Transmission is usually accomplished by the injection of brain tissue from patients who died with Creutzfeldt-Jacob disease into the brains of animals. The presence of a transmitting agent that can multiply in the animal brain is beyond doubt, but so far the nature of the agent is not clear. If it is a virus, then it is a rather unusual beast: it takes a very long period to cause disease (one to five years in monkeys), and it cannot be found with conventional virus-detection methods. The relevance of this work to Alzheimer's disease is not yet clear. The pathologies of the two diseases are very different, and numerous attempts to transmit Alzheimer's disease to animals have met with no success. Again, conventional virus-detection methods have failed to reveal any evidence for the presence of a virus. Therefore, if virus does cause Alzheimer's disease, this virus must be even more unusual than the causative viral agent of Creutzfeldt-Jacob disease.

Possibility of inheritance

A major concern to the relatives of patients with Alzheimer's disease is the possibility that it is inherited. This seems to be true in only a very small percentage of cases. In a few families there is evidence that the disease results from a genetic error passed down from generation to generation, with an average of 50% of the offspring inheriting the error. For the vast majority of cases, however, the disease appears to occur as a random event. The most detailed surveys conducted in the U.S. have been unable to find an abnormally high incidence of dementia among the close relatives of patients age 65 or over. Although there are several other possible causes of Alzheimer's disease, including environmental factors and abnormalities in the immune defense system, there is so little evidence that medical scientists can only guess at their possible significance.

Awaiting a cure

For the many people concerned with Alzheimer's disease, there are several reasons for optimism. When all the figures are compiled, it is clear that most people will avoid this condition, whatever the age group. Even among those over 80, four out of five will live out their lives without any signs of dementia.

On the other hand, these statistics bring little comfort to the large number of present and future victims and their families. For them perhaps the most important immediate consequence of the upsurge of interest in Alzheimer's disease is the knowledge that they do not have to carry the burden alone. In the past few years support groups have sprung up throughout the U.S., and research centers have instituted workshops to help family members cope with the problems of dementia. In 1979 several support groups formed the Alzheimer's Disease and Related Disorders Association, which currently has its headquarters in Chicago and more than 50 chapters around the nation. The organization works not only to exchange information but also to make the public, the medical profession, and the country's lawmakers more aware of the plight of the afflicted and to encourage research. Alzheimer's disease and other disorders of aging will be conquered only if there is substantial support of research scientists and facilities.

The very dramatic progress research has made toward understanding Alzheimer's disease offers real hope that in the next few years medical science will develop a successful treatment for the symptoms of this condition. It is becoming clear that Alzheimer's disease is a specific neurological disorder and not an inevitable result of growing old. It seems almost obligatory that a treatment be found, for it would indeed be a hollow victory were we to prolong life without ensuring that the additional time could be enjoyed.

—Peter Davies, Ph.D.

Special Report:
The Teaching Nursing Home: A New Concept
by Robert N. Butler, M.D.

At its worst the principal institution of long-term care, the nursing home, is bereft of skilled nursing and unqualified to be a home. It is feared and scorned as a warehouse for the dying. Instances of abuse of patients and profiteering have been documented repeatedly. Happily, some nursing homes are caring residences where chronically ill or disabled persons receive high-quality medical and social support services. Relatively rare are nursing homes that participate in research, professional training, patient and family education, and innovation in long-term-care services. At any given moment there are more patients (1.3 million) in the 18,000 or so nursing homes in the U.S. than are in its 5,830 community hospitals. Yet compared with the country's intellectual and professional investment in hospitals, the investment in nursing homes is minuscule.

In the 19th century, hospitals were in transition. The quarantine houses of the 18th century had given way to the warehouses of the chronically disabled poor in the 19th. Symbolic of the formal integration of education, science, and patient care was the building of a teaching

In some nursing homes elderly residents receive high-quality care. But employees are not always trained to meet all the needs of the chronically ill and disabled.

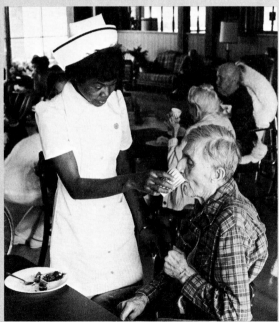

Peter Menzel—Stock, Boston

hospital adjacent to a medical school by Johns Hopkins University in Baltimore, Md., inaugurating the modern university medical center. Only graduates of four-year colleges were accepted as medical students. They were introduced to the bedside as well as to the laboratory. In the 20th century, hospitals in general became scientifically oriented as a consequence of innovations emanating from teaching hospitals. Not only did significant improvements in the quality of medical education occur but patients also began to receive better and better care.

There were 1,005 hospitals affiliated with medical schools in 1979. But few medical centers, hospitals, or medical schools were affiliated with nursing homes. Long-term care, including nursing-home care, remains the largest segment of the health-care system in the United States to remain remote from research and training.

The distance between nursing homes and academic centers has had unfavorable consequences for developing and applying knowledge about the medical care of older people (geriatrics). The needs of the elderly for social support services (individual and family counseling, social casework, arrangements for housing, and other help) are not filled systematically. Professional specialists and assistants are not well trained to meet the social and medical needs of the patient who is receiving or likely to require long-term care. New procedures are not properly conveyed to the nursing home and assimilated into its ordinary practice.

This is dismaying in itself and all the more discouraging as the nation becomes "grayer." Some 25 million Americans, one in nine, are aged 65 and older. This population is expected to double by the year 2025. The proportion of elders may reach one in five or six if birthrates remain low in the next half century. Therefore, the same sort of transition that occurred at the turn of the century with the advent of the scientifically oriented teaching hospital—as students entered the wards of hospitals to learn medicine firsthand—not only is long overdue but also will soon be crucial to the well-being of a huge segment of the population.

The costs of a "graying" America
With age the chances of having a chronic disease rise. Over 80% of older U.S. citizens have at least one chronic condition. Many have two or more. The most frequently reported are arthritis, hypertension, hearing

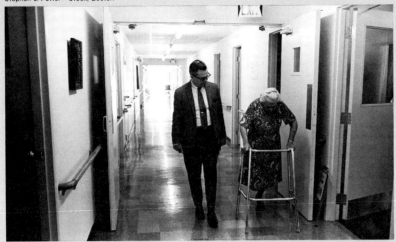

The distance between nursing homes and academic centers is unfortunate. A long overdue concept is the "teaching nursing home," which would bring more physicians, medical students, and allied health professionals to these often neglected facilities, where they would learn from and contribute to the improved care of the elderly.

impairment, heart problems, visual impairment, and diabetes. However, only one elderly citizen in six reports being severely restricted, and only one in five has any limitation in normal activity.

The aged population, as these data might suggest, relies more heavily on health-care services than the younger adult population. Constituting 11% of the U.S. population, the elderly account for 30% of all personal health-care spending. Of $250 billion spent in the U.S. annually for health care, about $75 billion is for services to the elderly, chiefly those over age 75. About one-third—$25 billion—is for nursing-home care, half of which is paid by government and half by private sources, including the elderly and their families. The cost of this care has been rising at rates greater than for inflation generally. Nursing-home costs are projected to reach nearly $77 billion a year by 1990.

The population needing long-term care is difficult to determine exactly. An estimated 30 million Americans of all ages have activity limitations, including 6 million so disabled as to require assistance in personal care, locomotion, or basic living activities (such as grooming, bathing, and meal preparation). The majority of these 6 million are elderly (4 million).

About 1.8 million of the disabled live in institutions like the nursing home, mental hospital, and rest home. The remaining 4.2 million, although living in the community, are most at risk of needing institutionalization. A change in family-support arrangements, a disabling accident, a worsening of circulatory problems or mental capacity, or other change in ability to manage on one's own may be the precipitating cause of institutionalization.

The main provider of care to the aged—the family—is changing: fewer children, children later in life, higher divorce rates, adult children living far away, and middle-aged women in the paid workforce. These patterns tend to make family members less available to provide elements of long-term care at home.

A new approach: long overdue

"Long-term care" refers to the range of health and social support services required by people with a variety of functional limitations due to chronic illness or impairment. The range includes the services of persons such as physician, nurse, social worker, minister, family counselor, legal adviser, physical therapist, speech therapist, occupational therapist, home-health aide, mental health worker, nurse's aide, homemaker, chore or repair person, friendly visitor, chauffeur, and companion or attendant.

Effective strategies and techniques of long-term care are needed. The teaching nursing home concept offers ways to meet these and other challenges by bringing the long-term-care field into close contact with new knowledge, professional training, and service development.

Steps already are being taken to meet the challenges. These steps are meant to reverse the neglect in care for the aged. This is being accomplished with the creation of teaching nursing homes as a means of dealing with the sociomedical problems of later life. The National Institute on Aging (NIA), part of the federal National Institutes of Health, recently invited universities and nursing homes to cooperate. The NIA has set aside funds to help create several teaching nursing homes and to help support biomedical and health-related psychosocial research in them. The Robert Wood Johnson Foundation, one of the nation's major philanthropic organizations devoted to improving the nation's health care, has begun a grant program to help support the association of ten nursing homes and university schools of nursing.

The U.S. Administration on Aging has initiated a program of support for long-term-care gerontology centers based at universities. Major national representatives of nursing homes, such as the American Association of Homes for the Aging (AAHA) and the American Health Care Association (AHCA), have found the teaching nursing-home concept attractive. (The AAHA chiefly represents voluntary nonprofit institutions; the AHCA, for-profit institutions.)

Based on a university affiliation, the teaching nursing home would have the following objectives: (1) to foster systematic clinical research on disease processes of the aged and to develop diagnostic techniques and methods of treatment adapted specifically for the elderly; (2) to train both young and established physicians in principles of geriatrics and their application; (3) to train nurses, allied health workers, social workers, and a variety of other professionals in the care of geriatric patients; (4) to study ways to improve care of the elderly in nursing homes and other settings, such as the home and the physician's office; (5) to study the community living patterns of the elderly and to design community-based services and strategies of care and health maintenance aimed at postponing or, whenever possible, preventing institutionalization; and (6) to devise and demonstrate methods of improving services and minimizing costs.

Into such model facilities would come regular faculty members and students of medical, nursing, social work, and allied health schools. Observation and instruction at the bedside or in the clinic would supplement classroom activities and readings. The rapport of patients and well elderly persons with care givers would be demonstrated, as well as effective working relationships of practitioners as members of a team. Young practitioners would be accustomed to the synergistic effects of research, training, and service in a sophisticated institution.

None of this would occur, nor could it have occurred, in an environment laden with negative attitudes toward aging and the elderly. In the past, medical school students were introduced to elderly patients as having intractable problems rarely worth extensive diagnostic and therapeutic investment because of the relatively few years of expected life remaining. Frustration among care givers was often masked by trivialization of the elderly patient and his or her chronic needs.

The frustration also stemmed from the low quality and quantity of geriatrics. Little new, usable information was becoming available to replace procedures that seemed to be useless rituals. The intellectual challenges that attract capable people into a field of activity were virtually absent. Geriatrics was regarded as a second-rate specialty. The few physicians who held themselves out to be geriatricians often lacked adequate experience and orientation. As recently as 1977 a survey indicated that hardly 700 of the 320,000 U.S. doctors claimed geriatrics as a specialty, and few of these had superior professional backgrounds.

The teaching nursing home would attract scientists to study processes of aging and diseases associated with old age. These model institutions, like the teaching hospital, would bring together patients whose illnesses

or problems are under study, the supporting professional and other personnel necessary for clinical and laboratory research, and the supplies and equipment essential to the conduct of the studies. The teaching nursing home would be useful to patients by maintaining a roster of clinicians interested in research and care of specific diseases and problems. Patients could be referred to special treatment centers.

Ongoing neglect

Relatively uninvestigated are the major causes of admission to nursing homes. These include the following:

Senile dementia. The various forms of senile dementia, a progressive condition marked by deterioration of memory and personality, afflict three million to four million Americans. One million have such severe memory loss that they cannot manage their own lives. It has been estimated that at least half a million nursing-home patients have senile dementia as the major or contributing cause of admission to the homes. Even if those patients who also have another disabling disease could be cured of the latter, the dementia would bar their return to community living. Patients with senile dementia are concentrated in nursing homes for custodial care because the disease has been considered to be an untreatable or incurable result of normal aging. Placement in institutions without academic ties has put them beyond reach of research.

Incontinence. Inability to control urination and defecation requires constant nursing attention. The individual soiled with urine or feces is prone to skin ulcers. Families that otherwise may be able to provide care for the disabled person may be unable to cope with the problems of incontinence. While there are passive control measures such as adult diapers, possibilities exist for training individuals to control bladder and anal sphincters for a half minute or so in order to reach a bathroom.

Immobility. The third major biomedical cause of nursing-home residence, immobility, involves loss of movement due to arthritis, stroke, and other diseases of the muscle and nervous systems as well as impaired vision and fragile bones. Research is greatly needed to improve prostheses (such as artificial hip joints), equipment to facilitate movement (electric wheelchairs and hoists), drugs to ease pain and reduce joint inflammation, vision and hearing aids, environmental designs for safety and easy motion, and physical rehabilitation to assist the individual in regaining control of limbs.

Social handicaps. In addition to medical reasons for admission, there are many important social causes. Many nursing-home patients are older widows who have no children at all, no children at home to provide care during the day, or no children living nearby. The placement of a patient in a nursing home may reflect the unwillingness or inability of family members to give care. It may also reflect absence of community-based

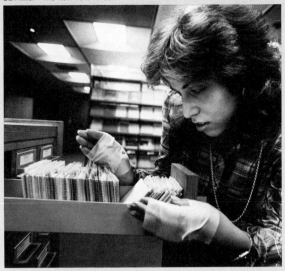

This medical student's hands are taped to simulate arthritis as part of an innovative course in geriatrics at the Medical College of Pennsylvania.

services—such as home-health services, family counseling and education, and services to make a household safe and usable for the handicapped—which could otherwise help the family to help the patient. Lack of money to buy drugs, equipment, and services, unfortunately, may prompt the family of a poor elder to request state-supported institutionalization.

The study of nursing-home patients has value to individuals at earlier stages or at risk of needing institutional care later. One benefit is the development of information helpful in preventing aggravation of the disease or in fashioning the social supports necessary for care at home. Studying why some people with the same sociomedical problems require institutional care while others do not can be valuable in developing community and family supports. Patients can be advised on how to avoid risks to well-being. Or they can be assisted in planning ahead for probable needs, such as switching to congregate housing (*e.g.,* an apartment house with meal and other services) or adapting their own house. Such studies are relevant to planners and to those who finance health and social services.

Methods of defining an elderly patient's sociomedical condition and needs for support are essential to effective plans of care. Unfortunately, assessment approaches and procedures adapted specifically for the elderly are relatively undeveloped and untested. Ideally, a plan should include objective measurements of progress, so that unproductive strategies are quickly identified and replaced.

The teaching nursing home would permit studies of the adaptation of patients to life in institutions. Since one-third of patients remain in nursing homes for at least three years, environmental design and staff practice should be studied and tested to promote patient satisfaction.

The facility would be a base for studies of patient-family interactions, visiting patterns, staff morale and attitudes toward patients, and the reasons for the decision to institutionalize or for selecting nursing-home over community-based care. The impact of death on surviving family members and nursing-home patients and staff could be studied to help identify those needing counseling and methods of support before or after the death. Hospice service—dignified care for the dying patient at home as well as in the institution—could be planned and evaluated.

The model facility would be a base for research conducted beyond its walls (such as studies of the frail elderly living at home). It could extend its health services to private homes, housing projects, senior centers, and other institutions. It could provide, or assist in developing, screening for disease and education on healthy living. It could furnish consultation to other nursing homes, physicians, and hospitals.

Realistic hopes

Assuming that lay and professional communities want to establish such an institution, which would so greatly benefit both the elderly and the rest of the population, what steps need to be taken? The primary step is the affiliation of a nursing home and a university medical center through its teaching hospital and medical, nursing, and other professional schools. The affiliation must respect the "home" components of the nursing home and the social needs of the long-term-care patient.

The facility must have space for its teaching and research activities, a place for consultation with patients and families, and, if possible, an area for the continuing education of established physicians, nurses, and other professionals. Arrangements should be made to share laboratory services in the teaching hospital and to transport patients there for special studies. Offices should be available for outpatient medical and social services. Curricula in the university medical center should be adjusted to incorporate long-term-care subjects and practices. Medical, nursing, and other students should be required to spend some clinical practice time in the teaching nursing home. Regular faculty members would hold teaching rounds in the facility.

If such relatively simple plans are followed, the professional graduates of the university center, now augmented by a teaching nursing home, would be prepared to deal with the realities of an aging population. Their services would be more effective because of new knowledge and better means of applying it. Modern research, training, and service would, at long last, have reversed the neglect and serious gaps in care and embraced the problems and opportunities of later life.

Allergy and Immunity

Before the era of antibiotics doctors sometimes treated patients who had pneumonia with injections of serum from a horse that had been immunized previously with killed pneumococcal organisms, the bacteria responsible for the disease. The treatment was carefully controlled. The horse serum contained antibodies generated in response to the precise type of bacteria that was causing the illness. Pneumonia, then as now, was a serious and often fatal illness.

In many instances such antiserum therapy was quite helpful. The antibodies in the injected serum circulated throughout the patient's body, seeking out and helping to destroy the infectious organisms. At times, however, one serum injection was insufficient to cure the patient, and after a week or two a second had to be given.

The second injection, in contrast to the first, often led to a severe allergic reaction. Within moments some patients would begin wheezing, perhaps experience a drop in blood pressure, and even die. They had experienced a generalized reaction called anaphylaxis. Those surviving would develop hives, a red itchy rash over most of their body, and perhaps blood in the urine. After several days or weeks the reaction would gradually subside.

Allergic reactions

The term anaphylaxis is used to describe the severe reaction following the second or subsequent injections of animal serum or other foreign substance. The first injection gave protection (prophylaxis); the second was without protection (anaphylaxis). The unusual feature of the reaction was that it could be caused even by portions of the same vial of serum that had been used previously without harm. Because it occurs so suddenly, an anaphylactic reaction is also called an immediate hypersensitivity reaction. It may be local, i.e., confined to one portion of the body, or generalized, depending upon the severity of the reaction. The term allergy, or altered reactivity, is more commonly used to describe a localized, immediate hypersensitivity reaction.

For example, persons who have hay fever (allergic rhinitis) have an immediate hypersensitivity reaction in the nose shortly after breathing substances, such as ragweed pollen, to which they are sensitive. In the U.S. alone approximately 30 million individuals have asthma, an allergic reaction occurring in the lungs. Patients with this illness experience wheezing because of the narrowing of air passages after they breathe substances to which they are sensitive. Ragweed pollen is a notorious cause of asthma as well as of hay fever, both of which often coexist in the same individual. People with ragweed-induced asthma have symptoms in the fall of the year, when pollen is abundant. The air flowing around mucus in the narrowed air passages in the lungs causes the characteristic high-pitched respi-

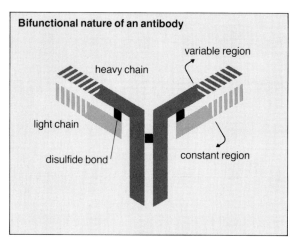

Structurally most antibodies are composed of four protein chains—two light chains and two heavy chains—linked together by sulfur-sulfur bonds. The variable (V) region, which is different for each antibody, is responsible for combining with the antigen. The unvarying, or constant (C), region triggers a host of immunologic functions.

ratory wheeze. Patients allergic to one substance, such as ragweed pollen, often are sensitive to other substances as well; for example, other types of pollen, house dust, or mold spores.

What causes anaphylaxis and other allergic symptoms? Why does the body sometimes react so violently, damaging itself when it is exposed to harmless substances? Clearly, not everyone responds to ragweed or other substances in an allergic fashion. Why some do and others do not is unknown. The tendency to develop allergies is inherited; children of people with allergies are more likely to develop allergies than other children. The precise allergen, or environmental substance causing symptoms, depends on exposure. Patients leaving one part of the country to escape their allergic symptoms often develop symptoms several months after arriving in another region; they develop allergies to the "new" allergens that are present there.

Role of IgE antibodies

Although little is still known about the underlying cause of allergy, much has been learned recently about its mechanism in the body. In their studies of the mechanism of allergic reactions, medical scientists have found that a normal individual can be rendered allergic if transfused with serum from an allergic donor. This is the case even if a small amount of serum from an allergic donor is injected into the skin of a nonallergic recipient. An immediate hypersensitivity reaction is provoked at the site if a small amount of test allergen is injected there. This passively transferred "allergy" gradually disappears as the donor's serum is metabolized and degraded. (Unlike injections of horse serum, serum transfer from one human to another does not lead to anaphylaxis because major antigenic differences between donor and recipient are not present within members of the same species.) The substance in the serum that is responsible is called reagin; it is now known to be a special class of antibodies known as immunoglobulin E, or IgE.

Antibodies are proteins—long chains of amino acids—formed by the body in response to an antigenic challenge. For example, when children receive polio vaccine, their bodies form antibodies that react specifically with polio virus, protecting them against the disease. Most antibodies including IgE contain four protein chains: two identical light chains, each having a molecular weight of approximately 20,000 daltons, and two identical heavy chains, each of approximately 55,000 daltons.

One portion of the molecule, the variable (V) region, is responsible for combining with the antigen; the other, the constant (C) region, triggers a host of biological functions, including the allergic reaction. The variable region, in which the sequence of amino acids is different in each antibody, determines the specificity of the antibody-antigen reaction; *i.e.,* which antigen "fits" the combining site of the antibody. For most antibodies the "fit" with the antigen is precise.

The C region of IgE antibodies is made up of amino-acid sequences that do not vary with antibodies of different specificities; *i.e.,* reacting with differing antigenic substances. This region combines with specific receptors for it on the surface membranes of mast cells, or basophils, so called because they contain large round granules that stain with colored dyes possessing a net basic charge. These granules contain chemical mediators of the allergic reaction, including histamines, which are released after IgE-coated mast cells interact with the antigen that fits the exposed variable region. Thus, IgE-coated mast cells in the lung of a patient with asthma release their contents after the patient inhales substances to which he is sensitive. Among other phenomena the mediators stimulate the flow of mucus in the breathing passages and cause the contraction of smooth muscle, the type of muscle that surrounds the breathing passages and regulates their size and shape.

Newly discovered substances

In 1938 Charles Killaway, an Australian, first discovered a material called slow reacting substance of anaphylaxis (SRS-A). Like histamine it was found to be a mediator of the allergic reaction. Freshly isolated smooth muscle from a guinea pig, suspended in a special solution to keep it viable, contracts if it is exposed to SRS-A. (A device of this sort is a common means of studying the mechanism of the allergic response.) The rate of muscle contraction under these conditions is slow and sustained. In contrast, histamine causes rapid contractions of brief duration.

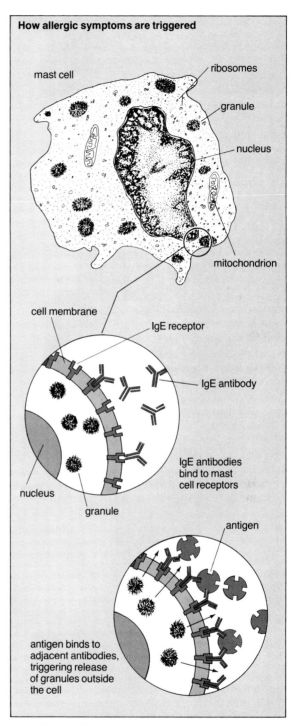

How allergic symptoms are triggered

mast cell
ribosomes
granule
nucleus
mitochondrion

cell membrane
IgE receptor
IgE antibody
nucleus
granule

IgE antibodies bind to mast cell receptors

antigen

antigen binds to adjacent antibodies, triggering release of granules outside the cell

Typical mast cell (top) contains granules filled with mediators of the allergic reaction. On its cell surface are receptors that bind to the C region of IgE molecules (center) and thus allow the cell to become coated with antibodies. When the proper antigen bridges the V regions of two or more adjacent bound antibodies, mast cell granules migrate to the cell surface and are released to the surrounding medium (bottom).

In 1979 SRS-A was found to be a combination of previously unknown substances. These were called leukotrienes because they were found in leukocytes and because their structures contain three double bonds in a certain arrangement. Leukotrienes are derived from arachidonic acid, a common precursor of several biologically active substances, including prostaglandins and thromboxanes, which are involved in such inflammatory diseases as rheumatoid arthritis. It had taken about 40 years from its initial description for scientists to identify and characterize the active substances in SRS-A. In part the difficulty arose because the effect of leukotrienes on the smooth muscle of the breathing passages is so strong and so pronounced that only minute quantities are required for an effect. In some instances they are a thousand times more potent than histamine in causing smooth muscle contraction.

Asthma is a disease primarily of small airways in the lungs called terminal bronchioles. They are immediately adjacent to the minute air sacs, the alveoli, where oxygen in air and carbon dioxide in blood are exchanged. In asthma, mast cells in terminal bronchioles release mediators of the allergic reaction after they come in contact with an airborne substance to which the patient is sensitive. Doctors now believe that leukotrienes are involved in asthma because these substances strongly stimulate the smooth muscle surrounding terminal bronchioles to contract, effectively narrowing the breathing passages.

What triggers allergic symptoms?

How does an antigenic substance stimulate the release of leukotrienes and other mediators of the allergic response, leading to the symptoms of asthma, hay fever, and other allergic diseases? The surface of each mast cell contains as many as 500,000 receptors for the C region of IgE. These receptors bind IgE produced elsewhere in the body and thus allow the mast cell to become coated with antibodies. The antigen-combining-portion of each bound IgE molecule is oriented toward the exterior of the cell, where it can combine with antigen. An antigen that bridges two or more IgE molecules bound to the surface of a mast cell stimulates mediator-containing granules to migrate to the cell's surface, where they are released into the surrounding region in a process called degranulation.

The receptors for IgE have been partially characterized. They are carbohydrate-containing proteins with a molecular weight of about 50,000 daltons. Not all of the IgE receptors on mast cells are occupied by IgE antibodies. In most people less than half of the receptors present are bound at any one time. In allergic individuals, however, such as those with asthma and hay fever, the quantity of IgE formed and its concentration in the blood are so high that virtually all receptors on mast cells for IgE are occupied.

The combination of antigen with IgE on the surface of mast cells leads to degranulation and mediator release through a complex series of biochemical events. An increased level of adenosine monophosphate (cyclic AMP) inside the cell inhibits mediator release; some drugs used successfully to treat allergic illnesses—theophylline is an example—inhibit the breakdown of cyclic AMP. Mast cells are not killed in the process of degranulation and mediator release; the granules reform, and the same cells can be involved in a later reaction.

New strategies for treatment

There are many approaches to the treatment of patients with allergies. For many, removing the antigen from the environment is a simple, effective measure. Thus, a cat owner who is sensitive to cat dander and wheezes after inhaling it may have no symptoms whatsoever if the animal finds another home. For someone allergic to plant pollens an air conditioner, which would allow the person to keep the windows closed during summer months when pollens are abundant, may relieve many symptoms. Under a doctor's care some patients take such medicines as adrenalin to dilate breathing passages and theophylline to inhibit mediator release. In more severe cases corticosteroids such as cortisone are required. Although corticosteroids are quite effective, they are used only in severe cases because of their potentially serious side effects.

In the future allergies may yield to new and innovative strategies. One approach under current study is to prepare substances that partially mimic IgE. When introduced into the body they would occupy receptor sites on mast cells but would not be able to combine with antigen. In this way antigen-sensitive IgE produced by the body would not find "open" receptors, and mediators could not be released.

Another new approach involves the synthesis of substances that effectively act as antagonists to leukotrienes. The use of antagonists in the treatment of allergy is well established. Antihistamines are commonly administered to patients with hay fever and other allergies to counteract the histamine released by mast cells. (Antihistamines usually are not recommended for asthma sufferers because they have a drying effect upon mucus in the lung, making it difficult to clear.) A substance that counteracts the action of leukotrienes in contracting the smooth muscle of the bronchiolar airways could prove to be of immense benefit to patients with asthma and other allergic diseases.

—*Edward P. Cohen, M.D.*

Arthritis and Connective Tissue Disorders

Should I exercise? But I don't like to exercise! What kind of exercises can I do? Will jogging hurt my joints? These are some of the questions and comments fre-

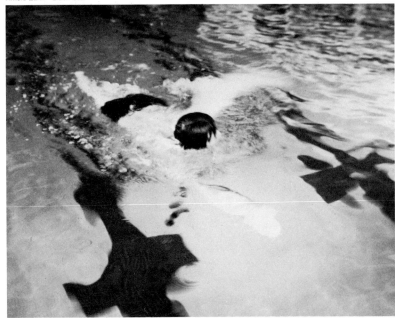

Swimming is an especially valuable form of exercise for many arthritics. The surrounding water buoys the body, thus reducing pressure on the joints, and allows great freedom of movement.

quently posed by patients to their physicians. For the many people immersed in a body-conscious, exercise-oriented society, the issue of exercise is more germane now than ever before. Jogging and running have become a way of life; there are now thousands of long-distance races held for amateurs each year. Exercise clubs are commonplace; even many senior citizens groups place major emphasis on exercise programs. Many hospitals conduct physical fitness programs for both the sick and healthy of their communities. Health spas as vacation spots have sprung up all over the world. They are big business, some of the more elite ones charging several hundred dollars a day.

The visual and printed media have picked up on the popularity of exercise. Keeping fit is a favorite topic of radio and television talk shows, and some daily programs are dedicated to exercise technique. Several monthly magazines exist that deal with a variety of forms of exercise. Many newspapers run a regular column, and "exercising to live a longer life" is a current topic of newspaper tabloids. Most bookstores now have entire sections reserved for physical fitness.

Deciding to exercise and choosing the type of activity pose an even greater problem for victims of arthritis than for their healthy counterparts. Although arthritics too have become caught up in the enthusiastic wave of health fitness, in considering an exercise program they must cope with pain, stiffness, fatigue, and limitation of joint motion. For each patient with arthritis the problems related to exercise are different. In some rheumatic conditions only a single joint may be affected, such as in bursitis of the shoulder. Diseases like rheumatoid arthritis, however, tend to affect all of the joints in the body. Systemic lupus erythematosus is a disease

of connective tissue that causes such symptoms as fatigue and shortness of breath even more often than joint pain. In the past patients and physicians were not so concerned about exercise because drugs were the mainstay of therapy. Today, even though there is a renaissance of drug therapy for arthritis, medication has become but one modality in a comprehensive management program in which exercise plays a key role. Proper exercise appears to enhance the value of drug therapy.

Benefits of exercise for arthritics

Concepts of exercising vary from patient to patient. For some it means a few minutes of haphazard limited-range calisthenics or a casual game of golf once or twice a week. For others exercise entails vigorous weight lifting, running several miles, or a taxing singles tennis match daily. Arthritic patients readily become aware of their physical limitations regarding exercise. Pain deters participation in many sports. Yet properly designed physical activities may actually raise the pain threshold and thus diminish pain.

The muscles of most arthritic patients are expected to be weak and somewhat atrophied because of the inactivity that pain and limited mobility have caused. Physical stress has a greater punishing effect on arthritic joints than normal ones because the shock-absorbing function and synchronous motion are lost. Large effusions (fluid-filled swellings) in a joint may in fact prevent full range of motion, increase pain, hasten muscle atrophy, and cause the joint to be unstable. In recommending an exercise program the physician or therapist has a specific purpose in mind; it may be pain relief, muscle strengthening or maintenance of existing strength, facilitation of endurance, correction of deformity, prevention of deformity, or overall conditioning.

Most normal people feel stiffness in their joints and muscles from time to time in the morning upon arising. The natural reaction is to stretch and put the stiff joints through a brief range of motion. For the arthritic patient, however, morning stiffness is profound and may last for several hours. The tendency not to use the joints for fear of pain causes contractures, a permanently contracted state of muscle. Yet, despite such caution a sudden reflex movement of that joint may still induce considerable pain. A daily exercise program that emphasizes gradual increases in the range of motion will eliminate these contractures and render the joints and muscles more supple. Hence, exercises actually may be analgesic. Furthermore, there is some evidence that regular exercise raises the pain threshold because of the increased production of endorphin, one of the body's natural opiates.

Exercises that strengthen the muscles that put a joint through its motions serve to stabilize the joint and to protect it against sudden undesirable movement. This state can be best achieved by isometric exercise, which maximally increases muscle contraction against resistance without putting the joint itself through a range of motion. An example is sitting on a chair and holding the leg outstretched with a weight on the ankle. The opposite approach is isotonic exercise, in which the joint is repeatedly placed through a full range of motion. Isotonic exercises provide more endurance and strength, but isometric exercises are recommended initially for the arthritic patient because muscle strength is preferred over endurance and because isometric exercises are much less painful to perform.

Range of motion and stretching exercises, whether or not they are performed to the extent of increasing endurance, are sometimes extremely helpful in correcting deformity. But they serve their most valuable role when performed to prevent contractures. Faulty posture and joint positioning promote contractures of the flexor (joint-closing) muscles, especially of the hands, wrists, knees, and hips. Prolonged sitting in a chair while watching television results in permanent deformity of the hips and knees. Such problems are preventable with just minutes of daily exercise. Herein lies the key to a successful program. Exercise makes the arthritic patient feel well psychologically. The tonic effect of fitness and activity cannot be overemphasized. Bed rest, necessary for a short time in the treatment of active rheumatoid arthritis, has its virtues, but the deconditioning effects of prolonged bed rest and inactivity are well known. The aphorism "use it or lose it" applies quite well here.

Precautions and recommendations

Although exercise and fitness should be considered critical to successful rehabilitation of the arthritic pa-

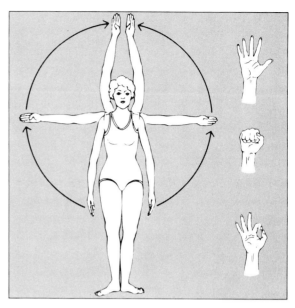

At-home exercise programs developed for arthritis victims emphasize the conditioning of muscles and joints that are most vital for daily functioning. One exercise shown improves the range of motion of the shoulders; the other works the joints and muscles of the hands.

tient, common sense must dictate the type, frequency, and extent of activity. All professional athletes warm up thoroughly before they undertake any demanding exercise. The arthritic patient should be even more compulsive about preliminary graduated exercises. Local application of heat to involved joints will assist the warm-up process. Physiologically, vigorous daily exercising is not required for the athlete, but daily range-of-motion exercises are necessary for the arthritic patient to keep the joints flexible.

Too much exercise may be as bad as no exercise at all and can lead to severe problems. For example, injudiciously increasing the number of repetitions of an exercise or the weight on a joint may increase pain and perhaps induce inflammation. Effusions become worse when an arthritic joint is excessively exercised. The inflammatory process may lead to permanent destructive changes in the joint cartilage and soft tissues. Both the patient and the therapist must be cautious not to overstretch and perhaps rupture already weakened ligaments and tendons. Many patients with rheumatoid arthritis and certain other rheumatic conditions also have osteoporosis, a demineralization of the bones. Excessive stress on the thinned-out bones may result in fracture.

Physical exertion is inappropriate if the patient must take to bed regularly for a day or two after a sporting activity. Exercise-induced pain is to be expected, but it should subside within two hours. For the minimally afflicted arthritic most sporting activities within reason

190

are permissible; in the patient with severe joint disease activity will have to be restrained. In general, sports involving prolonged twisting and weight bearing, such as tennis, should be avoided in favor of bicycling and swimming.

Opinions vary as to the effects of running and jogging on normal joints. There is some inconclusive evidence that, because of accumulated impact-loading in the joints, healthy joggers may be more susceptible to arthritis in later years than nonjoggers. The effect of running on joints already affected by arthritis is clearer. Pain and swelling of the joints are predictable consequences, and running should be avoided if such symptoms develop. Severe stress will worsen arthritis.

Proper exercise is in keeping with attempts to make the lives of arthritic patients as normal and as satisfying as possible. This goal can be achieved only if the patient has the will both to cooperate and to overcome his or her illness.

—Warren A. Katz, M.D.

Blood and the Lymphatic System

Sickle-cell disease, or sickle-cell anemia, is a serious hereditary disease that most often affects Africans and people of African descent. In the U.S. some 50,000 blacks, or about one in 500, are estimated to have the disorder, and worldwide the number is in the millions. To date sickle-cell disease is still incurable, but the outlook for sufferers is not nearly as grim as was once believed. Clinical experience in the U.S. indicates that only a few percent of afflicted individuals will die by the age of 20. Early diagnosis and appropriate supportive medical care has played a critical role in reducing death rates and serious complications. Continued advances, particularly on the genetic and molecular levels, into the nature of the disease and its control are improving prospects for sickle-cell victims.

Sickle-cell trait and malaria

Sickle-cell disease is now known to be an indirect result of man's genetic adaptation to the parasite responsible for one of the great scourges of mankind, malaria. With their bite, mosquitoes inject the malaria organism, a protozoan, into the bloodstream. There it meets the body's immune defenses, which attempt to limit its multiplication and eradicate its offspring. The host-parasite relationship in malaria, however, is precariously balanced through a series of immunologic measures and countermeasures. The parasite has evolved a mechanism to elude the host's defenses by drilling into red blood cells, the cells that carry oxygen, where it hides from the immune defenses circulating in the blood. So protected, it divides and increases its numbers before erupting back into the bloodstream, where it may invade more red cells.

In Africa and other parts of the world where malaria has long been endemic, the human host has responded by taking advantage of certain chance genetic mutations that allow the immune system to recognize cells containing the parasite and to destroy them. Among the more important of these mutations are glucose-6-phosphate dehydrogenase (G6PD) deficiency, thalassemia trait, and sickle-cell trait. For populations of humans that are under constant siege from malaria-carrying mosquitoes, these mutations represent an advantage for surviving and multiplying in areas where people without such a mutation cannot thrive. Such selection pressure accounts for the presence of these mutations in people—primarily blacks and a few groups of Mediterranean and South Asian origin—whose racial stock has had a history of involvement with the malarial parasite.

Sickle-cell trait is a disorder of hemoglobin, the protein pigment within the membrane of red blood cells that allows them to carry oxygen to and carbon dioxide from the tissues of the body. The type of hemoglobin

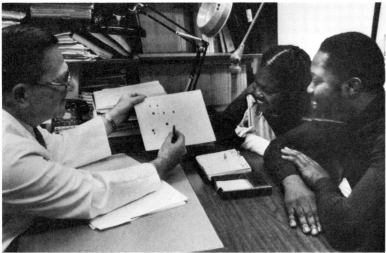

Bernard Gotfryd—Newsweek

Recent advances in the prenatal diagnosis of sickle-cell disease now allow most couples who carry the trait to know with certainty whether their child will have the disease. This knowledge can help them make better informed decisions about continuing or terminating the pregnancy.

that a person possesses depends on the pair of hemoglobin genes that he or she inherits. Normally two adult hemoglobin (HbA) genes are inherited, one from each parent. The term adult distinguishes this variety from fetal hemoglobin (HbF), which is produced by the developing infant in the womb. Ordinarily by the age of four months the body ceases manufacturing HbF, replacing it with the adult form. In sickle-cell trait one of the two genes for adult hemoglobin is altered and produces sickle hemoglobin (HbS). Molecules of HbS still carry oxygen satisfactorily but tend to crystallize readily, particularly in situations of decreased oxygen concentration. About one out of five black Africans possesses one gene for HbS; i.e., 20% have sickle-cell trait. In the U.S. the number of blacks so affected is nearly one out of ten.

Within the red blood cell, hemoglobin is maintained at an extremely high concentration in order to carry large amounts of oxygen. In cells with sickle trait the normal gene and the sickle gene each fill the red cell with roughly 60% HbA and 40% HbS. At this concentration of HbS there are few, if any, clinical problems. To the advantage of the carrier of sickle-cell trait, if conditions within the red blood cell are changed by a rapidly proliferating malarial parasite, the HbS molecules crystallize. Crystallization of HbS stiffens the cell, damages the membrane, and marks the cell for destruction within the spleen, the principal filter of the bloodstream. There the parasites are killed, preventing invasion of the brain and other organs.

Sickle-cell disease

Unfortunately, persons with sickle-cell trait can pay a high price for their survival advantage. When a father and mother both carry the sickle trait, i.e., each possesses one HbA and one HbS gene, there is a one-in-four chance that each child born to them will receive an HbS gene from each parent. Such children, who have two genes for HbS, develop sickle-cell disease. After four months of age these infants produce red cells that contain nearly 100% HbS. When deoxygenated, HbS molecules at this concentration spontaneously (without the presence of parasites) aggregate into crystal-like strands, which align to form fibers. These long fibers damage the membrane of the red blood cell, deforming the cell from its normal concave-disk shape into a characteristic sickle shape.

Each time the red cell of a patient with sickle-cell disease circulates through the arterial and venous circulation the cell sickles and unsickles often, losing bits and pieces of the extended tips of the sickle in the turbulence. Finally the cell becomes more spherical and less flattened, losing much of its flexibility, and can no longer deform to slip through the smallest passageways in the circulation. It lodges in a tiny blood vessel and, caught there, it loses more oxygen and vital metabolites. Its damaged membrane leaks potassium and wa-

ter, dehydrating the cell and concentrating the hemoglobin within. The hemoglobin becomes so viscous that the cell retains the sickled shape even when reoxygenated. This so-called irreversibly sickled cell is soon ruptured. White blood cells degrade hemoglobin to its amino-acid building blocks and with the help of the liver produce the yellow pigment bilirubin. In a few patients red cells are destroyed so rapidly that bilirubin accumulates in quantities sufficient to stain the whites of the eyes yellow, a condition termed icterus or jaundice. Iron from the red cells is reused; thus, despite low blood counts, iron supplements are not needed.

Effects of cell sickling

Although irreversibly sickled cells are rapidly destroyed, the anemia that results from sickle-cell disease is perhaps one of the less severe problems with which afflicted individuals must cope. For reasons not yet understood, the blood of these people often suddenly and preferentially clogs small blood vessels that supply bone, depriving this tissue of oxygen. Despite the blocked blood flow the demands of the bone for oxygen continue, and carbon dioxide and other products of tissue metabolism accumulate. Nerve endings in the bone detect the lack of oxygen and the accumulating toxins and cause intense pain in the back, chest, or extremities. The attack may last from a few hours to several days depending on the extent of blood deprivation. Such painful crises are the most frequent complication of sickle-cell disease.

On the average, minor attacks occur every few weeks in about half of patients; major attacks requiring hospitalization occur as often as once or twice yearly in about 25% of patients. Many patients never have severe pain, and nearly one-half go several years between major crises.

The factors that predispose some victims to have more frequent painful crises than others have recently been the subject of study by a group of collaborating university hospitals. In the minority of instances serious infections, extreme exercise, exposure to cold, or loss of body fluids through diarrhea or vomiting play a role. In the majority of instances, however, no clear-cut predisposing factor can be found. Often the individual will wake from sleep with the pain. Pain may start in one bone and move to others. The striking appearance of irreversibly sickled cells has intrigued researchers, but as yet no one has connected its presence to the development of crises. Surprisingly little is known about this very important problem, but progress is expected in the next several years.

Individuals with sickle-cell disease are prone to certain infections, which fortunately are rare and of only a few specific types. In the first few years of life the spleen loses its function because of repeated episodes of blood deprivation and becomes reduced to a useless nubbin of scar tissue. In the absence of the

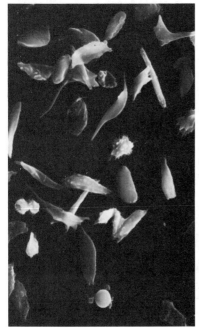 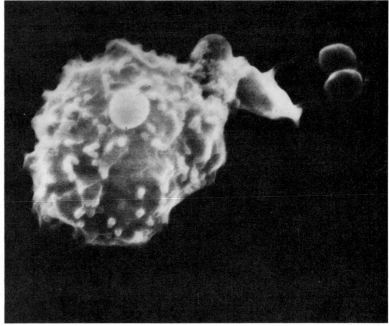

Under magnification, sickle cells (left) show their characteristic shape, a result of the spontaneous crystallization of hemoglobin. (Right) White blood cell, part of the body's immune mechanism, consumes a bacterium. This normal defense function is impaired in victims of sickle-cell disease.

spleen's filtering activity, bloodstream infections of the bacterium *Streptococcus pneumoniae* can proliferate rapidly and spread to the coverings of the brain (meninges), causing pneumococcal meningitis. If not treated promptly, the blood infection and meningitis may overwhelm the body's defenses and cause death. Paradoxically, individuals with sickle-cell disease are also more susceptible to cerebral malaria than either normal or sickle-trait individuals. The absence of splenic function allows the infected cells to disseminate even though they may have sickled.

Another bacterial species, *Salmonella,* infects bones of patients with sickle-cell disease, causing salmonella osteomyelitis. Instances of this infection may be difficult to differentiate from a painful crisis. Salmonella osteomyelitis, however, is far less frequent, developing in only a small percentage of patients. Absence of the splenic filter, which allows these organisms to spread to bone, and low concentrations of oxygen within bone may impair defenses against this organism. Victims of sickle disease suffer from common childhood viral infections no more frequently than normal individuals.

Repeated blood deprivation in bone can lead to long-term complications like hip disease and degenerative arthritis. Sickling may also block blood vessels to other tissues and organs and thus cause stroke, kidney disease, painful erections in males, vision disturbances, respiratory problems, and skin ulcers. Bilirubin may accumulate in the gallbladder, solidify into stones,

and obstruct the flow of bile, producing abdominal pain and intense yellow skin discoloration. Surgery may be necessary to remove the stones.

The bone marrow of sickle-cell disease victims must labor at at least five times its normal capacity to make up for the sickled red cells lost through destruction. As an adjustment to the demand, the bone marrow actually enlarges at the expense of yellow fat within the bone. Whereas in normal individuals common viral infections may slow red cell production very little, in sickle-cell patients, because red cells may survive only a week or two in the circulation instead of the normal four months, the red cell count may fall precipitously to levels that require transfusion. In a young child whose spleen has not yet been completely destroyed by sickling, clogged blood vessels within the spleen may suddenly cause it to trap, or sequester, ever increasing numbers of circulating red cells. The spleen enlarges, and the resulting lowered blood volume and sudden decrease in oxygen-carrying capacity may cause shock and death. Splenic sequestration is rare, but in the age range of four months to a few years it may be the most common cause of death of children with sickle-cell disease.

Diagnosis and treatment

Diagnosis of sickle disease in children relies on tests that detect the presence of HbS in samples of red blood cells and further blood tests to differentiate the disease from certain closely related disorders of hemo-

193

Cancer

globin. It is now possible to diagnose the disease prenatally by amniocentesis. In this procedure the obstetrician samples cells from the fluids bathing the fetus by
means of a needle inserted into the abdomen and uterus under the guidance of sound-wave images. DNA is
extracted from the cells and the mutation in the hereditary material identified directly. This comparatively recent breakthrough in prenatal diagnosis allows a family
to choose whether to continue the pregnancy or, in
view of the complications of the disease, plan an
abortion.

Current treatment for most of the complications of
sickle-cell disease is unsatisfactory. Physicians administer strong pain relievers during painful crises and treat
associated infections with antibiotics. If dehydration is
present intravenous fluids may be necessary. Oxygen
is of no help because it cannot reach the tissues beyond the blocked channels. Transfusions are used for
severe exacerbations of anemia. In individuals who
have suffered stroke, long-term transfusion therapy
may be necessary to prevent recurrent strokes. A high
level of normal transfused blood suppresses the patient's own marrow from making sickle cells. If continued for several years, however, such "hypertransfu-
sion" therapy may provoke liver and heart failure or an
immune response to the transfused blood.

Lacking satisfactory treatment, medical centers that
deal with this problem encourage children with sickle-
cell disease to attend regular classes, participate in
physical education classes, including swimming, and
avoid missing any more school than is absolutely necessary. In short they are encouraged to lead a normal
life. Early statistics derived from African populations
had shown that most victims of the disease did not survive for more than a few years. Unfortunately, many
physicians uncritically extrapolated these figures to
American children, predicting a dire prognosis and unnecessarily alarming parents. In retrospect, the high
death rate for sickle-cell victims in Africa may have
been caused by cerebral malaria. In the U.S. most children with sickle-cell disease need not miss much
school and in general cope well with their problem; very
few are lost to infections, stroke, or splenic sequestration when they receive appropriate medical care. The
minority of children who do have severe limitations
need appropriate supportive care in a center experienced with these problems.

New therapies

Many researchers are now seeking agents to relieve
the severity of the disease. Several approaches have
been proposed, but none tested thus far has proved
very satisfactory. Among the more promising are drugs
that pass through the red blood cell membrane and retard or prevent the crystallization of deoxygenated
HbS. These include chemical derivatives of tryptophan
and phenylalanine, which are two of the natural amino-

acid building blocks of proteins, as well as certain short
amino-acid chains called peptides that contain phenylalanine. Another agent, dimethyladipimidate, has been
shown in tests outside the living body to completely
prevent crystallization of fully deoxygenated HbS. Other therapies under study reduce the concentration of
deoxygenated HbS in the red blood cell membrane and
so delay its crystallization. A drug that makes it harder
for HbS to release its bound oxygen would have this
effect, as would some safe technique for physically
increasing the size of the red blood cell. Yet other
therapeutic agents being investigated act on the red
blood cell membrane, rather than on HbS, to inhibit
sickling or to prevent damage to the membrane. One
drug, Cetiedil, which is used in Europe as a local anesthetic, has been shown to insert itself in the red blood
cell membrane and somehow alleviate sickle-cell crisis. To date all of these approaches have been highly
experimental. The ideal compound that can be given
by mouth, crosses the red cell membrane, affects only
the HbS molecule, and has few side effects of its own
is not yet known. It is important that the therapy is not
worse than the disease.

Continuing advances in genetics also offer exciting
possibilities for controlling abnormal HbS production. It
is conceivable that future approaches may delay or
prevent the switch from fetal hemoglobin to adult sickle
hemoglobin in early infancy, or even restart HbF production in the adult. Because red cells containing HbF
transport oxygen nearly as efficiently as normal red
cells and lack the sickling problem, the approach has
many advantages. It may also be possible to insert
genes coding for normal HbA directly into the bone
marrow cells of sickle-cell victims. However, a good
deal more research is necessary if sickle-cell disease
is to be conquered in the near future.

— *Robert R. Chilcote, M.D.*

Cancer

Definite advances toward the eventual control of cancer continue to be made. Improvements in treating
some forms of cancer, identification of carcinogenic
environments, and a better understanding of the mechanisms by which normal cells become cancerous have
highlighted recent progress in cancer research.

Clinical aspects

Total incidence and death rates from cancer have continued to increase in the United States. It was estimated that during 1982 there would be 835,000 new cases
and 430,000 deaths from cancer in a population of 230
million.

Much of the rise in the cancer death rate is due to
lung cancer caused by tobacco smoking. A sharp rise
in lung cancer among American women began in the
early 1960s, and lung cancer soon will replace breast

194

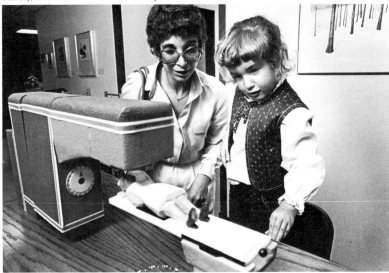

Young leukemia patient at the University of Rochester (New York) Cancer Center works a toy replica of the center's accelerator before confronting the real machine. Such play reduces children's fears of treatment by giving them some control over the situation.

cancer as the most common form in women, as it long has been among men. Cancer of the stomach and of the uterus continue to decline, but their lower incidences do not compensate for the self-induced pandemic of lung cancer.

Since the 1950s the death rate from cancer has decreased among people under the age of 45 and especially among children. This decrease has been attributed to advances in treatment, but a drop in the number of new cases also may have contributed to the decline. Only 10% of cancers, primarily those of the blood-forming and lymphatic systems (leukemias and lymphomas), occur before the age of 45. The decrease among the younger population is offset by the increase among the older population, in which the more frequent cancers, such as those of the lung, colon, or breast, arise from cells of the epithelial lining.

The five-year survival of cancer patients living during the late 1970s (except those with skin cancer, which is almost always curable) was estimated to be about 45%. This is an improvement from about 40% recorded a decade earlier, although the baselines for the two sets of data are not entirely comparable. Moreover, the rates are "relative," being adjusted for deaths of cancer victims from causes other than cancer. Better diagnosis and treatment of cancer has been stimulated by the availability of trained oncologists (cancer specialists) and the network of cancer centers deployed throughout the U.S. under the second National Cancer Act, passed in 1971. Better education of the public in matters of health, including cancer, also has made an important contribution.

Surgery and radiation remain the most important forms of curative treatment for cancer. Some traditional radical operations, however, are being replaced by simpler, less extensive ones. For example, radical mastectomy, which entails removal of the breast, un-

derlying chest muscles, and the fat and lymph nodes under the arm of the corresponding side, is being supplanted by less disfiguring surgery and cosmetic reconstruction of the breast. Radical surgery for cancer of the pancreas practically has been abandoned as ineffective. More and more, clinical trials are being performed to determine the most effective forms and extent of surgery and radiation therapy.

Better diagnostic procedures have contributed to improved results. Such techniques as computerized axial tomography (CAT) and ultrasonic imaging are allowing tumors to be detected at an earlier, smaller stage of development. Timely detection is motivated by the availability of promising therapy. As an example, bone cancers diagnosed in 1980 were less extensive on the average than they were 20 years earlier and thus more amenable to therapy.

Most impressive results were recorded in the treatment of advanced Hodgkin's disease, a type of lymphatic cancer, by Vincent DeVita, Jr., and others of the National Cancer Institute (NCI) in the U.S. Intensive courses of four anticancer drugs known acronymically as MOPP yielded a ten-year disease-free status in 70% of patients with a previously fatal form of the disease. Complications of the rigorous treatment included an increase in secondary cancers and leukemia induced by the treatment. Nevertheless, advanced Hodgkin's disease now joins choriocarcinoma of women (a rare cancer that develops from the placenta during pregnancy) and acute lymphatic leukemia of children as types of cancer that can be cured with systemic chemotherapeutic agents.

Chemotherapy in combination with surgery and radiation continues to increase the chances for survival of children with Wilms' tumor, a rare kidney cancer; rhabdomyosarcoma, a cancer of muscle; osteogenic sarcoma, the most common form of bone cancer; Ewing's

195

tumor of the bone marrow; and some lymphatic cancers. Cure or prolongation of life is achieved in a high proportion of patients with testicular cancer and with small-cell cancer of the lung. For many other patients with advanced, disseminated cancer, chemotherapy can alleviate symptoms and prolong life.

New agents continue to be added to the list of some two to three dozen drugs that have been found to be useful against cancer. Among the more significant ones are the broad-spectrum anthracycline antibiotics derived from the microorganism *Streptomyces peucetius* and introduced from the Farmitalia Research Laboratories of Milan, Italy. Doxorubicin (Adriamycin) and daunorubicin are two examples, to which Bisanthrene is being added. The platinum complexes (*e.g.,* cisplatin) discovered by Barnett Rosenberg of Michigan State University have found useful clinical application for cancer of the testes and ovaries. To the list of anticancer alkaloids derived from the periwinkle (*Vinca rosea*) has been added yet another agent, vindesine, which is active against adenocarcinoma of the lung. A new estrogen inhibitor, tamoxifen, is useful in the management of advanced cancers of the breast that depend for their growth on the availability of estrogen hormones.

Interferon, the antiviral protein that is a natural product of mammalian cells, and the interferon stimulator Poly I:C thus far have yielded disappointingly mediocre results as anticancer agents. Difficulties in extracting enough interferon from human cells for therapeutic use are being overcome with genetic engineering techniques that allow its production in bacteria, an achievement that should permit broader investigations with larger doses.

Public pressure led to the clinical testing of amygdalin (laetrile), a reputed anticancer agent derived from apricot pits, at several cancer centers and under NCI sponsorship. Charles Moertel of the Mayo Clinic and others reported that no substantive improvements were produced in more than 150 patients who received oral and intravenous laetrile plus "metabolic therapy" of diet, enzymes, and vitamins as espoused by the proponents of laetrile. High levels in the blood of cyanide, which laetrile releases, was the main toxic effect. Although there were no matched controls, the total absence of beneficial effects should close the issue.

More specific use of chemotherapeutic agents would be possible if there were reliable methods by which the clinical response could be predicted. Such procedures would spare patients who would not respond from the rigors of chemotherapy.

Ways are being devised to test agents outside the body for chemotherapeutic activity against human cancer, similar to tests that use cultures of bacteria to predict their sensitivity to antibiotics. Sydney Salmon and Anne Hamburger of the University of Arizona have used tumors excised from the body and kept alive in culture for this purpose. Transplants of human tumors into mice that lack the normal immune response to reject them also have been investigated at the University of California at San Diego and other centers. In each case further work is needed to establish how closely the response of these tumors to various agents predicts the response within the body. One limitation is that such tumors are composed of different subpopulations of cells that may change their character. This variability may eventually yield tumor specimens that are not representative of the original tumor in structure or behavior. On the other hand, tumors with widely variable cell populations may provide a means for understanding and assessing the effectiveness of combinations of chemotherapeutic agents.

Psychological, social, and economic problems that confront cancer patients and their families are becoming better recognized. Cancer clinics are being expanded for the rehabilitation of successfully treated pa-

St. Christopher's Hospice, which opened in England in 1967, realized the need for humane care for terminal cancer patients. These small, specialized facilities, several of which have now been established in the U.S., emphasize pain relief and provide psychological support and cheerful surroundings so that the dying patient can enjoy strength, spirit, and dignity.

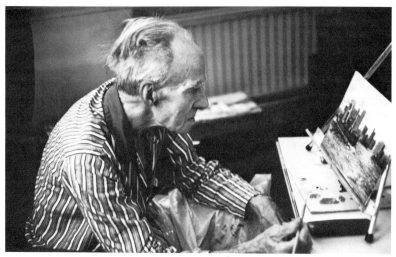

Grace Goldin

tients, and provisions are being made to encourage their reemployment. The care of patients with terminal cancer, who still represent the majority of all cancer patients, is receiving long-neglected attention. Special facilities for the dying, called hospices, were introduced in the 1960s by Cicely Saunders in Great Britain and have since spread to the U.S. and other countries. Psychological support and freely administered opiate analgesics are important features of this useful humanitarian concept.

Chemical causation

To date, cancer prevention has been limited to identifying cancer-causing situations and recommending avoidance. During the 1970s public concerns in the U.S. about pollution of the environment with genetically harmful chemicals and ionizing radiation peaked, and a national program was organized to test chemicals for carcinogenic activity. The method selected, a form of bioassay, was to feed mice and rats maximum tolerated amounts of these chemicals during their lifetimes and compare the occurrence of tumors in the treated groups with untreated controls.

About half of some 200 tested chemicals were defined on this basis as being carcinogens in laboratory animals and thus of possible hazard to human beings. This interpretation was challenged on several pharmacologic grounds, especially when test animals received exposures and dosages that seemed far removed from those likely to be encountered during ordinary human lifetimes. Industry particularly challenged the applicability of the findings to governmental regulations. The controversy over saccharin provides an example of the problems that are involved. A similar problem may have arisen concerning formaldehyde, specifically over the hazards of its presence in urea-formaldehyde foam insulation installed in homes and schools during the past decade. Persistent complaints about the release of irritating and toxic formaldehyde gas from the foam insulation, coupled with a recent report that formaldehyde vapors cause nasal tumors in rats, led to a government ban on the insulation in early 1982. Among factors clouding the issue were the results of an epidemiologic study of cancer mortality among chemical plant workers, which revealed no elevation of risk of cancer, compared with controls, among workers occupationally exposed to formaldehyde.

More rapid, less expensive substitutes for bioassays in animals have been suggested, but their relevance for humans also remains to be shown. Most chemicals that induce cancer in humans or in animals also induce genetic mutations. This relationship has been exploited in tests that use bacteria to assess the mutagenic potential of suspected carcinogens, especially substances that have first been treated with enzymes to simulate their metabolic conversion in the body. The results of these tests, however, are as difficult to ex-

trapolate to humans as the results of bioassays in rats and mice. Agreement between the two kinds of tests thus is of little help. Tests on the cancerous transformation of mammalian cells maintained in the laboratory are a promising field for research, but these also remain to be demonstrated as convincing predictors of hazard to humans.

Carcinogens can be endogenous—*i.e.,* be manufactured by the body—as well as be of environmental origin. Estrogens, female sex hormones that are metabolic products of cholesterol, induce a variety of cancers in man and other animals. Nitrosamines, shown to be powerful carcinogens in many animal species, are produced in the body from nitrites and amines. Yet the role of nitrosamines in causing cancer in humans remains to be demonstrated.

Industrial exposures are particularly informative sources of information regarding possible carcinogenic hazards. It has been urged that rosters of workers in chemical plants and other suspected industries be maintained for surveillance. The synergistic effects of exposure to different agents was emphasized by the work of Irving Selikoff of the Mount Sinai School of Medicine in New York City and others. They found that workers who inhale asbestos, a known carcinogen, and smoke develop more than 20 times more lung cancers than asbestos workers who do not smoke. A similar synergism was discovered among workers who smoke and who handle uranium ores, as documented by Victor Archer of the National Institute for Occupational Safety and Health and others.

Viral causation

The causative role of viruses in some forms of animal cancer is now firmly established. The leukemia-lymphoma complex in chickens, cats, and cattle is caused by viruses called retroviruses, whose genetic instructions are carried by RNA rather than DNA. In chickens and in cats it behaves as a classical infectious disease with animal-to-animal transmission, in which actual tumors are the "tip-of-the-iceberg" manifestations of a complexity of underlying effects. Protective vaccines have been or are being developed for some forms of these diseases.

A causative role for viruses in some human cancers also no longer can be doubted. The Epstein-Barr (EB) virus, which is associated with Burkitt's lymphoma (a childhood cancer of the lymphatic system), is perhaps the clearest example. The hepatitis B virus, which has been strongly linked with primary liver cancer, is another likely possibility.

The search for a human leukemia virus, which has had several false starts in the past, is productively active again. In 1981 Robert Gallo and his associates at the NCI reported isolating a retrovirus from cancerous cells cultured from a patient with a rare lymphatic cancer. Antibodies to the virus were found in the serum of

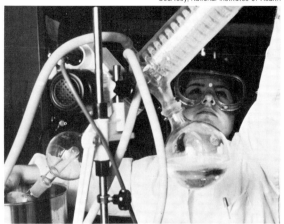

Cancer will be conquered only if research is supported. Research depends on substantial financial backing of well-qualified scientists.

patients with a form of adult lymphatic leukemia. Work by Yorio Hinuma and colleagues of Kyoto University in Japan with a similar, if not identical, virus supported and extended Gallo's findings. This virus may be the first human RNA tumor virus to be eventually linked to human cancer.

An outbreak in the U.S. of Kaposi's sarcoma, an uncommon type of cancer that usually appears in the form of skin tumors of the lower extremities, came under investigation in 1981 by the Centers for Disease Control in Atlanta, Ga., after it had received numerous reports of occurrence among homosexual men. Continued surveillance eventually uncovered more than several hundred cases among homosexual and bisexual men, the great majority in their late 20s to early 40s, in New York City, California, and England. These details were unusual since the affliction, although indigenous in Africa, is rare in the U.S. and Europe. The epidemiologic pattern of the outbreak related it to a form of pneumonia caused by the parasitic microorganism *Pneumocyctis carinii* and associated with a deficient immune defense mechanism. The evidence implicates some transmissible agent, perhaps a virus, which has not yet been identified.

Binding between virus and cell appears to be more intimate in the induction of tumors in humans than in cats and fowl. Also, tumor induction seems to require enviromental stimuli. Thus, the EB virus alone causes infectious mononucleosis, a nonmalignant, self-limiting disease, but it requires additional stimuli (repeated malarial attacks have been suggested) for the induction of lymphoma. Viral carcinogenesis in humans may constitute a process of induction by viruses followed by promotion by environmental and other factors. At the present time, environmental carcinogenesis and viral carcinogenesis appear to be separate research endeavors, primarily because different scientific talents

are addressing the problems. This distinction should fade out in the future.

Host factors

Studies have intensified on the familial and genetic factors in human cancer. Families with a history of cancer have a greater chance of having additional occurrences than families in which cancer has been rare. This tendency of course may be due to sharing the same environment or life-style as well as to genetic characteristics. Regardless of its nature, it has obvious implications for public health.

The influence of genetic factors was recently demonstrated by Michael Swift of the University of North Carolina. His work showed that relatives of individuals with certain rare recessive diseases associated with cancer also have an increased risk for cancer.

Biochemical definition of genetic traits that are related to disease, including cancer, is an important research field. For example, such findings may resolve the question of why lung cancer occurs in fewer than half of heavy smokers; perhaps susceptible persons will be found to have a genetic deficiency that prevents the activation of detoxifying enzymes and will be identified on that basis. Technology already available for the separation and identification of all proteins present in the blood may also define groups of people who have a particular susceptibility, or resistance, to cancer.

Research on cancer and the role of diet, an important environmental risk factor in carcinogenesis, has been expanded in recent years. Statistics of cancer in various populations, as well as laboratory studies on animals, suggest that consumption of unnecessary calories and excessive use of animal fats and meat are related to a higher occurrence of cancer. Religious groups who eschew tobacco and alcohol and subsist on modest diets that are high in plant products and low in animal protein and fat have a 30% lower incidence of cancer than the general population of the U.S. Of course, membership in such groups involves selective factors other than nutrition.

Although identifying foods and the substances within them that cause cancer is an important concern of cancer research, attention is also being given to dietary substances that restrict or inhibit cancer. Certain food substances and food additives, for example, have been shown to retard the appearance of spontaneous and induced cancers in laboratory animals. Lee Wattenberg and co workers at the University of Minnesota reported such effects from supplementing the animals' diets with antioxidants like butylated hydroxyanisole (BHA), a common preservative added to cereals and other foods for human consumption.

Michael Sporn of the NCI has found that retinoids, synthetic isomers of vitamin A, inhibit the appearance of experimental epithelial cancers. Gerhard Schrauzer of the University of California at San Diego and others

198

have reported that selenium, a dietary trace element that is present in many foods, inhibits carcinogenesis in laboratory animals. The concept of chemoprophylaxis, or cancer prevention by means of chemicals, that is emerging from such studies is now to be tested in humans in field trials under the auspices of the NCI.

Cellular aspects

Research in molecular biology remains the cutting edge against cancer. It is now clear that in many cases the transformation of normal cells to cancerous ones involves a change in the DNA of the cell genome, the cell's total complement of genetic instructions. The change can result from viral infection of the cell and the subsequent incorporation of a viral genome into the cell genome. The discovery in retroviruses of reverse transcriptase, an enzyme that transcribes RNA into DNA, clarified the mechanism by which RNA viruses as well as DNA viruses accomplished this incorporation. The transformation to cancer cells also can be the result of mutations of short segments of DNA through the action of carcinogenic chemicals or radiation. In either case, the changes to DNA thus produced lead to the loss of inhibitions of cellular behavior that are inherent in the biological contract among individual cells existing as multicellular organisms. The DNA changes are replicated and passed to subsequent generations of altered, cancerous cells.

All cancer, however, may not arise from a single underlying process. That cancer cells can be reversed to normal behavior, as reported by Barry Pierce of the University of Colorado, suggests that some cancers may be the result of mechanisms that spare the DNA genome and instead act at some other point along the pathway from gene to final product.

With the discovery that some genes can move between chromosomes, the distinction between viruses and genes becomes increasingly hazy. As Wallace Rowe of the National Institutes of Health points out, cancer may be the result of a genetic infection or of an infectious gene.

Recent work by Robert Weinberg and others at the Massachusetts Institute of Technology demonstrated that certain segments of DNA extracted from cells of several kinds of human cancer can transform noncancerous mouse cells into cancerous cells and become incorporated into the mouse cell genome. The active DNA segments from three different human tumors were distinct from each other. If replicated and extended by others, this work represents the isolation and identification of human cancer genes, or oncogenes. Moreover, there is evidence that at least some of these genes are identical to those found in cancer-causing retroviruses.

The following scenario for future research can now be suggested. Oncogenes from human tumors would be reproduced in quantity by means of recombinant

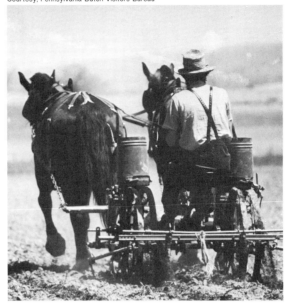

Such groups as the Amish, whose religious practices include certain life-style and dietary restrictions, have a lower incidence of cancer than the general U.S. population.

DNA technology. Such oncogene antigens could lead to vaccines against some forms of cancer. Using monoclonal antibody technology, medical researchers would induce cultures of special hybrid cells to generate large amounts of antibodies that are highly specific for oncogenes. These antibodies then would be applied to diagnostic and therapeutic investigations. The basic technology required for this scenario is already available, and experiments along these lines could actually be performed by the end of the century.

Research support

Cancer will be conquered by scientific research. Research requires support: finances, facilities, and ever freshened manpower. The generous governmental subsidy of U.S. biomedical research that followed World War II is being reduced. As biological products become profitable, new patterns of industrial-academic arrangements are emerging. In Japan and Italy, as well as in the U.S., chemotherapeutic agents against cancer already have become profitable commodities. Judicial rulings that biological systems and products of recombinant DNA are patentable have stimulated industrial-academic relationships. There is resistance to such relationships, just as there was a half-century earlier against the intrusion of government into biomedical research. The government-academic partnership was a glorious era, during which discoveries flourished. There is little reason for premature fears that adding industry to the partnership will be any less fruitful or more restrictive.

—Michael B. Shimkin, M.D.

199

Special Report:
Coping with Breast Cancer
by Rose Kushner

All potentially fatal illnesses—especially cancer—cause disability, economic hardship, changes in lifestyle, and, often, disfigurement. All are accompanied by some psychological trauma. Over and above this, to women of all past and current cultures, the female breast is the foremost visible symbol of femininity, sexuality, and maternity. Its loss or even its threatened loss causes immeasurable anguish; the emotional pain of breast cancer is therefore unique. One in every 11 women will develop breast cancer in 1982; this means that there will be about 112,000 new cases and more than 37,000 deaths in this year alone.

History of breast cancer treatment

Breast cancer has plagued the world since the dawn of written medical history, and its treatment is detailed in an Egyptian papyrus dating back to 3000–2500 BC. In his chronicles of ancient Greece written centuries later, Herodotus described how Atossa, daughter of the Persian king Cyrus the Great, hid her cancerous breast from her husband, Darius I. Only after the breast ulcerated did she call the court physician, Democedes, for help. Even in those long-ago days, women delayed seeing a doctor.

Until the mid-1800s breast cancer was treated by cutting off the afflicted breast as swiftly as possible, after which the wound was seared by fire-cautery. Without anesthesia, mastectomy was agonizing torture, and many women survived amputation only to die afterward of hemorrhage or infection. After William Morton introduced ether in 1846, surgeons had time to worry more about the appearance of the scars left by surgery. Having patients unconscious also allowed surgeons to probe and follow the spread of the cancer to the adjacent chest musculature and axilla (underarm area).

In 1889 William Stewart Halsted, a pioneer of modern surgery, perfected his radical mastectomy technique. In this procedure the breast, its underlying tissue, all of the axillary lymph nodes, and both pectoral (chest) muscles are removed. Women who had Halsted radical mastectomies were left with extensive scars and hollowed areas where the muscles had been removed. But for the first time a diagnosis of breast cancer was no longer an automatic death sentence.

The psychological effects of the amputation and mutilation, however, were devastating. In the January 1975 issue of the *American Journal of Psychiatry* a report entitled "Psychoemotional Aspects of Mastectomy" declared that "while mastectomy performs a gratifying service by saving a woman's life, her appreciation is muted by the price she must pay for that service—the loss of a breast and permanent disfigurement. Within the value system of American society, that price is a considerable one." The article urged public and private agencies and individual psychiatrists and psychologists to make provisions for postmastectomy counseling.

In April 1975 the National Cancer Institute (NCI) published statistics of hospital admissions which revealed that there were at that time about 677,000 women in the United States who had known histories of breast

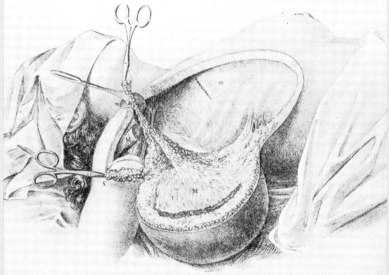

Until recently the standard operation for breast cancer was the Halsted radical mastectomy, developed in 1889 by William Stewart Halsted, a pioneer of modern surgery. The operation removed the entire breast, underlying chest muscles, and all of the lymph nodes in the underarm. Although the operation was often life-saving, it left the woman with deep, difficult-to-conceal scars. Today, less extensive surgery, often coupled with drug or radiation therapy, spares the woman with breast cancer a great deal of the psychological and physical trauma of extensive disfigurement.

From "History of Radical Mastectomy," William A. Cooper, *Annals of Medical History* (1941), vol. 3, no. 1, p. 47

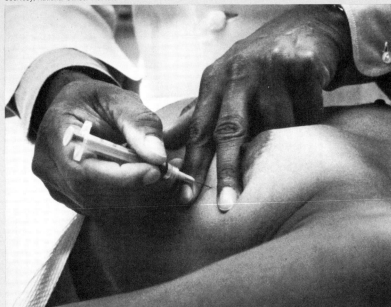

A needle biopsy determines whether a breast lump is a solid tumor or a fluid-filled cyst. If it is a cyst, it can be drained by this procedure. Although the great majority of lumps that women find prove to be noncancerous cysts or harmless growths, all women live with some degree of fear of developing breast cancer. In the U.S. one woman in every 11 will develop breast cancer.

cancer. Yet only 300,000 to 350,000 of them were mentioned in psychiatrists' and social workers' records or in membership lists of supportive organizations such as the Reach to Recovery program of the American Cancer Society (ACS). This meant that many thousands of women had never tried to get help in their recovery from mastectomy.

Since 1975 there have been numerous studies of women's emotional suffering after losing one or both breasts, but no researchers dealt with women's emotional suffering *before* breast cancer struck. The problem was not even recognized until the late 1960s, when research proved that breast self-examination (BSE) could detect tumors at early, curable stages. Health professionals were surprised to discover that women's refusal to think about breast cancer was an obstacle to their looking for symptoms in their breasts. Society's obsession with two firm, beautiful breasts seemed to outweigh women's fears of dying of cancer. Their response was "denial"—an inability to even think about the disease.

Coping: the extremes

Diane Scott is a vivacious, dark-eyed beauty who was first runner-up in her state's Miss America contest. She moved to New York to follow a modeling career immediately after her graduation from high school, and at 23 Diane's junoesque figure is in great demand for lingerie and bathing-suit advertisements. But Diane lives with a secret terror. Her mother had a mastectomy for cancer in one breast when she was 28, and her second breast was lost two years later. Diane knows she has at least a 60% risk of developing the disease two to five years earlier than her mother did. But in spite of her anxiety,

Diane refuses to examine her breasts or even to permit her gynecologist to do so.

Her doctor has urged her to see a plastic surgeon about having prophylactic (preventive) mastectomies, a procedure in which the skin and nipples are lifted up, the breast tissue is removed, and silicone implants are inserted. But Diane cannot bear the thought of willingly losing her own precious breasts. Instead, she works hard and plays hard, consciously determined to ignore her high-risk status.

Women's refusal to look for a symptom of early breast cancer triggered a 1973 Gallup Poll to study "How Women Think About Breast Cancer." In an attempt to identify their attitudes before breast cancer struck, the ACS asked 1,007 women older than 18 what they considered their most serious potential medical problem to be. Almost half (43%) specified cancer, and of these, 13% specified breast cancer. Even so, only 18% of the women interviewed had practiced BSE during the preceding year.

At the end of 1974 the well-publicized mastectomies of Betty Ford and Happy Rockefeller triggered a breast-cancer panic; women lined up outside doctors' offices and screening centers for examinations. Six years later, to see if the panic had effected a permanent change in attitude, the NCI commissioned another poll, "Breast Cancer: A Measure of Progress in Public Understanding." Asked what their most serious potential health problem was, the majority (58%) of 1,580 healthy adult women said, "breast cancer." Yet, paradoxically, about 60% of those surveyed had never examined their breasts.

When the nonpracticing women in the survey were asked why they did not do BSE, many replied that they

201

"didn't think of it." Since breast cancer was cited as the most serious medical problem facing women, many health professionals decided the problem was really a lack of confidence in the technique. The solution would be more publicity, better teaching materials, training classes, and perhaps personal instruction by a doctor or nurse. A growing number of health professionals, however, now believe that women do not examine themselves because they do not want to find what they are looking for—a symptom of breast cancer.

Women who practice BSE usually feel anxious and apprehensive before and during every examination, but they check themselves in spite of these feelings. They endure the same feelings every time they have a regular gynecologic checkup. When it is over, they breathe a sigh of relief—until the next time.

More often, however, women do not do BSE or see a doctor. They (or their partners) may discover a symptom accidentally while making love, dressing, or when a bump or bruise causes them to rub the injured spot. Only about 10% of breast cancers are discovered by physicians. Diane, for example, discovered a dimple near her nipple during a photography session. Remembering her mother, she became rigid with terror but did nothing more about it.

Such denial behavior has two possible outcomes. The symptom, even if it is invasive cancer, may remain static in the breast, never disappearing and never growing to become life-threatening. While no one believes a woman should take this risk, there are documented cases of malignancies that remained encapsulated and dormant for decades. It is possible, though not probable, that Diane could live her normal life-span with a cancer in her breast. A more likely outcome is that the small lump would get larger and spread, invading her lungs, liver, or brain. Cancer in a breast does not kill; it is metastasis—spread to vital organs—that causes death.

The ACS-NCI data showing that millions of women in the United States are afraid of breast cancer prove that anxiety about the disease—"coping with breast cancer"—begins long before a scalpel touches a woman's breast. Regrettably, the most common coping mechanism is the one Diane is using: denial. Denial prevents women from learning anything about the disease; it stops them from seeing their doctors immediately if they should find a symptom; it blocks their accepting a diagnosis if cancer is found. Some women have such a strong tendency to denial that they stop seeing or feeling a symptom entirely.

Wilma Lewis had never had a breast problem, nor does she have a family history of the disease. After her 50th birthday in 1981, when her doctor ordered a mammogram (breast X-ray) to which future tests would be compared, a lump was found deep inside her left breast. A surgical biopsy revealed that the mass seen on the mammogram was harmless, but a 4-mm cluster

of abnormal cells lay next to it. Not visible on the film, this was diagnosed as "lobular carcinoma in situ," or LCIS. Wilma was informed that breast cancer is a multicentric disease; one spot means there may well be others. This is common with in situ carcinomas.

Wilma had taken the Pill for 15 years and was 34 years old when her first child was born—both established high-risk factors. Her doctor, like Diane's, suggested prophylactic mastectomies. Wilma, unlike Diane, accepted his recommendation. She began looking for a second job to pay for her surgery. In the meantime, she cannot keep her hands from feeling her breasts, even when she is fully clothed.

Diane and Wilma are both "coping with breast cancer" although neither has the disease. Diane denies a problem exists, while Wilma permits it to dominate her life. Both women are extreme examples of how high-risk women cope with the knowledge that they will probably develop breast cancer. All women, however, live with a certain amount of dread of the disease. There are about 50 million women in the U.S. over the age of 35; the sheer magnitude of numbers makes it impossible to study their fears and, unfortunately, very little can be done to assuage the concerns of so many millions of symptom-free women.

Helping women cope

A great deal can be done for the hundreds of thousands of women who examine themselves and find breast problems of some kind. It should be emphasized that only one of every ten of the symptoms will prove to be mammary carcinomas; most lumps and thickenings are either normal changes that accompany hormonal fluctuations of the menstrual cycle or are harmless, nonmalignant (benign) growths. Few women escape finding a symptom at some time in their lives, but their emotional pain is no different from the suffering of those who will be found to have cancer.

More than a million women will endure weeks or months of "preclinical anxiety," even though the vast majority of symptomatic women will not have breast cancer at all. These women can be helped by information, referrals, and support during the time they must wait for a diagnosis.

Most women with symptoms wait for days, weeks, or months before calling their doctors (usually their gynecologists) in the hope "it" will go away. If it does, they resume their routine of watching, waiting, and worrying. If they do find something suspicious, it is common not to want to seem panicky or paranoid, and they decide to wait until the next menstrual period has passed before calling a gynecologist. These women confide in no one, not even husbands, family, or friends; there is no point in worrying loved ones, they rationalize. Although they try to avoid touching the bump, like a cavity in a tooth it magnetizes their attention—they cannot leave it alone.

Photographs, courtesy, National Cancer Institute

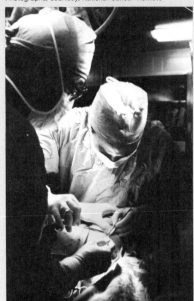
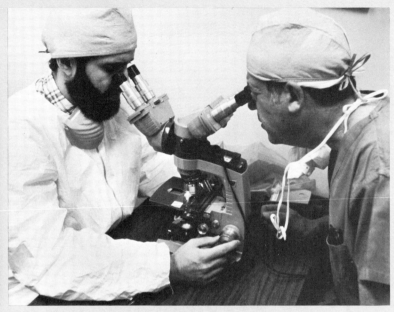

If the needle biopsy shows the lump to be a solid tumor, a surgical biopsy is done to remove the lump so that it can be studied under a microscope to check for the presence of cancerous cells. Both the surgeon and the pathologist examine the tissue.

Choosing a doctor

Waiting will have one of two outcomes: the lump will disappear or it will stay. If a symptom remains, most women finally call their gynecologists for an appointment. In the United States 90% of women who use any doctor at all see their obstetrician-gynecologists (OB/GYN's) for every health problem. Not all OB/GYN's, however, are qualified to deal with breast diseases, and they may immediately refer patients to surgeons who do "breast work."

How can a woman evaluate a doctor who treats breast disease? The best way is by judging his or her breast examination. A thorough exam should include not only the breasts but also an exploration of both axillas. The patient should be asked to lift and extend her arms to be sure both breasts respond identically to the movements. There should be no dimpling or puckering. The nipple should be squeezed gently to see if there is any discharge. If a doctor does not follow these general guidelines, women should request referrals to another physician.

Some women choose to go directly to a surgeon for evaluation of their symptoms; they do not see a gynecologist, internist, or family practitioner first. By doing so, they eliminate much of the expense, as well as the anxiety, of interim appointments.

In the examining room, the woman undresses from the waist up and waits anxious minutes for her doctor to come in. She is too nervous to chat; she wants to show the suspect spot immediately. The doctor palpates (feels) the mass to see if it seems to be attached to other tissues. If it moves freely and is perfectly

round, the woman may be assured that it is a cyst and that the contents can be aspirated by a surgeon.

Aspiration biopsy

The surgeon repeats the gynecologist's examination and agrees that the lump appears to be a cyst filled with fluid that can probably be biopsied by aspiration. This is done with an ordinary hypodermic needle and requires no anesthesia, even though it looks menacing. Once the cyst has been aspirated, the contents will be evaluated by a cytologist (cell specialist).

If the mass had been solid, nothing would have flowed into the syringe. Some surgeons use a special needle that can actually carve a small bit of tissue out of a lump. Wide-bore needle biopsies are popular in many countries but not in the United States. The main reason is that most tumors are "heterogeneous"— they are composed of both malignant and harmless cells. In such a "blind biopsy," finding malignant cells is a conclusive diagnosis of cancer, but removing benign cells may mean only that the needle penetrated a harmless area.

Often nothing can be withdrawn by either type of needle aspiration. The doctor's next step depends on the patient's age and personal-risk profile. Some physicians recommend that women under 30 who have no family history of breast cancer return for another examination after one or two menstrual cycles. If a close relative did have the disease, even younger women may be referred to other specialists for additional diagnostic studies. Certainly all women older than 40 regardless of family history will have more examinations.

203

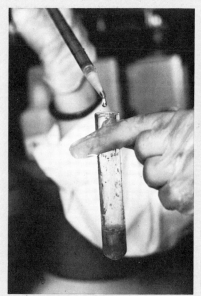
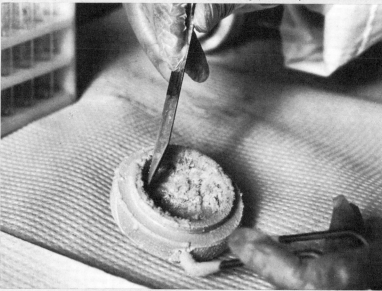

*Today it is very important that an estrogen-receptor assay (left) be done to determine if the cancerous tissue needs
the female hormone estrogen to grow. Tissue used in the test must be frozen (right) immediately after its removal.
The test helps determine which treatment is most likely to be effective.*

Mammography

Mammography, X-raying the breasts, is the most reliable diagnostic tool for breast cancer available today, although it is only about 85% accurate. Women undress from the waist up, and their breasts rest alternately on a specially treated plate. To get as accurate a picture as possible, the breasts are gently squeezed by a special device that flattens them.

Two views of each breast are usually taken, from different angles. For one, the beam comes from above; the second is taken from the side toward the center. In 1977 the NCI recommended that women under 50 not be X-rayed routinely for screening to look for lumps, because mammography uses ionizing radiation that itself can cause cancer.

Some doctors believe X-rays should be taken if a persistent mass is in a breast regardless of a woman's age. Others believe all lumps should be biopsied and, therefore, see no reason to expose women to potentially harmful irradiation when surgery will be done no matter what the mammogram shows. However, women under 30 who have chronically cystic breasts may be sent first for evaluations by other methods.

Other tests

Thermography. The temperature of diseased tissue is often higher than that of healthy tissue. A thermograph visualizes these temperature differences on a televisionlike screen, and experts can interpret the images to detect abnormalities. While this technique is not yet reliable enough to make a firm diagnosis of cancer, it is useful for monitoring younger women who should not be mammographed but who are at high risk or have lumpy breasts.

Ultrasonography. While thermography measures the varying heat patterns of tissues, diagnostic ultrasound is based on the fact that different tissues also have varying densities that emit distinctive sound waves. These are "heard" as echos by a painless acoustic beam that penetrates the breasts. Like heat radiation, the echos are converted into waves of light by a computer that projects the image onto a screen. For a breast examination women lie, face down, on a special table with a small water tank at its upper end. Their breasts are submerged in the water while the beam does its work, and the patient feels no sensation from the ultrasound.

Ultrasonography has been used for years for diagnosing problems in hollow organs and for monitoring pregnancy. In Japan "echograms" are used routinely and successfully for diagnosing breast cancer, but for reasons that are not understood, the technique is not as reliable as mammography for Occidental women. Like thermography, ultrasound is used primarily as a screening and monitoring tool for younger women.

Diaphanography. Diaphanography, or DPG, is a sophisticated form of transillumination, shining a strong light through the tissues to assess their state. With the circling motions of BSE, an instrument containing an ordinary light bulb is pressed against the breasts and into the axillas. Again a computer is used, this time to pick up light waves the human eye cannot see and to project an image of the inside of the breast onto a screen. There is no pain. Best of all, the patient knows the results immediately; there is no anxious period of waiting. Although DPG is widely used in Sweden, its reliability for detecting breast cancer has not yet been tested in the United States; like thermography and ultrasound, it is used as a monitoring tool.

Surgical biopsy

All women with persistent breast symptoms—who began by visiting OB/GYN's, internists, or family practitioners after months of BSE, watching, waiting, and worrying (and perhaps spending hundreds of dollars)—must eventually face a surgical biopsy. More than a half million women will wait anxiously for a space on an operating-room schedule. Most will be asked to sign a form giving the surgeon permission to perform an immediate mastectomy if cancer is found. While the majority of symptoms will be benign, all of these women endure the anguish of not knowing if they will wake up with one breast or with both.

There are two kinds of surgical biopsies, incisional and excisional. The first is a procedure in which only a part of the mass is removed. This is not commonly done in the United States for the same reason widebore needle biopsies are rare: the danger of removing a benign segment of a heterogeneous tumor and having a "false negative" diagnosis. In an excisional biopsy the entire mass is removed for examination under a microscope by a pathologist.

Surgical biopsies are usually done in hospitals, and for decades it has been routine to perform them under general anesthesia. While the woman is asleep, the tissue is sent for a "frozen section" analysis; if cancer is found, the surgeon proceeds to remove the breast immediately.

It was once believed that a mastectomy had to be done immediately after a biopsy or the disease would "spread like wildfire." Now, however, it is known that separating the two procedures by a few weeks does not affect survival. In 1979 the NCI recommended that a diagnostic biopsy be separated from further treatment in a two-stage procedure. As a result, the practice of routinely doing both operations at the same time is slowly ending. Many surgeons are now doing biopsies under local anesthesia in ambulatory "walk in–walk out" clinics.

Of course, many women prefer to be asleep when any surgery is done. For breast cancer diagnosis, many do not want to be awakened and be forced to cope once again with preoperative anxiety and stress. But the 1979 NCI recommendation was welcomed by most women because it gives them time to get second opinions on the diagnosis and an opportunity to investigate treatment alternatives other than mastectomy. Furthermore, it is estimated that about 15–20% of all early breast cancers can be eradicated simply by excising the tumor, so it is possible that some women could be cured by only the "lumpectomy" done for a biopsy.

A woman who chooses to have her biopsy done separately must endure an additional waiting period of anxiety during the two or three days it takes for the pathologist's diagnosis by "permanent section." Instead of being quick-frozen for study under a microscope, the tissue is stained and embedded in wax. Although frozen sections are rarely inaccurate, there are certain benign cells that may look like cancer unless a paraffin study is done.

Estrogen-receptor assay

All women must be sure their surgeons order that an estrogen-receptor assay (ERA) be done on the tumor if it is found to be malignant. The ERA is a test that can measure whether or not a cancer needs the female hormone estrogen to grow. If it does, the tumor is estrogen-dependent, or ER+; if not, it is estrogen-independent, or ER−.

If the mass is benign, of course, the assay is unnecessary. If a patient has no malignant axillary lymph nodes and the disease never returns, the results of the ERA are never needed. However, it must be done whenever cancer is diagnosed, whether a woman has a one- or two-stage procedure. At this time the assay gives oncologists (cancer specialists) the only clue for choosing appropriate anticancer treatment if there are future problems.

The test requires at least one gram of fresh tissue. The specimen is usually sent to a commercial laboratory for analysis. To obtain reliable data the tissue must be frozen to −73° C within 15 minutes of its removal. Large medical centers prepare specimens for the ERA routinely, but this is not always the case in smaller hospitals. Women should ask their surgeons to make the necessary arrangements in advance of a biopsy.

Staging

"Staging" is for many the most stressful part of preclinical anxiety. The term applies to certain examinations that must be done to see if the disease has already spread to other organs. While most women believe cancer usually spreads from one breast to the second, this is not so. If breast cancer does metastasize, the disease usually spreads to the bones, liver, lungs, and, less commonly, the brain. The only reason for removing a breast is to try to stop the cancer while it is localized, so if there are signs that it has already spread, the mastectomy is unnecessary.

A bone scan can frequently find occult (hidden) metastases too small to be seen on conventional diagnostic X-rays. Special blood analyses (liver-function studies) or scans may detect spread to the liver; chest X-rays are done to examine the lungs for metastases. Unfortunately, however, the technologies available today are still not sensitive enough to find all microscopic spots of cancer that may be present in other organs. As a result, many breasts are removed even though the women have metastatic disease because there is still no reliable way to find it. But about 25% of distant metastases can be identified with the tools available today, and for those whose disease has spread, mastectomy is not indicated.

If the patient and her surgeon decide on a two-stage procedure, the waiting period gives ample time to have these vital tests done. Women who choose to have a one-stage procedure should have the tests done before the biopsy.

Choosing the treatment

Most surgeons in the United States believe amputation is the only safe treatment for breast cancer, but it is important to remember that there are different kinds of mastectomies. In addition, many breast-cancer specialists are now treating the disease by procedures in which the tumor and axillary lymph nodes are removed but the breast is left intact. Radiotherapy (high doses of therapeutic X-rays) is used to eliminate any spots of cancer that may be left behind. Women anticipating a one-stage procedure should discuss these options with their surgeons in advance of the diagnostic biopsy.

Mastectomy. The Halsted radical mastectomy, as was previously mentioned, was routinely done for all cases of breast cancer until the 1970s, but it is rarely done now. The "modified radical" mastectomy has replaced the Halsted as the most common breast-cancer operation in the United States. Also known as a "total mastectomy with axillary dissection," this procedure involves removing the breast and underarm lymph nodes. The pectoral muscles are left in place so the woman does not have the chest and axillary defects caused by their removal. This operation also makes reconstructive plastic surgery easier.

In a simple, or total, mastectomy only the breast is removed. This procedure is not commonly done, because at least some of the axillary lymph nodes must be removed and examined to see if cancer cells are present. However, there are cases of elderly or infirm women who would not be given drugs even if they had malignant nodes. For them an axillary dissection or even a sampling is unnecessary surgery.

Segmental resection. A growing number of surgeons now treat small breast cancers by lumpectomy, removal of only the tumor, along with a complete axillary dissection. Others excise the lump plus a rim ("margin") of healthy tissue; some feel an entire wedge of the breast must be removed in a "quadrantectomy." Because of such variances, all less-than-mastectomy procedures are often grouped under the general term segmental resection. In all such cases, at least a sampling of axillary nodes is also taken to see if the woman will need some kind of adjuvant therapy.

Most doctors who do lesser procedures insist that women also receive high-dose X-ray treatments to destroy any other foci of cancer that may be in the breast.

Since 1976 the NCI has been conducting comparative clinical trials to find out if such radiotherapy is needed, but even preliminary results have not yet been announced. Until final data are reported, such radiation therapy is recommended.

Postsurgical radiotherapy involves visiting a hospital daily for four or five weeks. At the end of the external treatments an extra "booster" of radiation is given to the area where the tumor was located. This is done either by temporarily putting tubes of radioactive material in the site or by using special high-dose "particle beam" radiation therapy, which is delivered to the breast by a special apparatus.

The presence of cancer in the lymph nodes is the only way to know which women are at high risk of developing metastases in other organs. If any nodes are malignant (positive), adjuvant therapy using drugs, hormones, or antiestrogens must be given as soon after nodal surgery as possible. This is the time when the results of the ERA are important; women whose tumors were ER+ receive different anticancer agents from those with ER− breast cancers.

If the pathologist reports that none of the nodes contained cancer cells (node-negative), women who had mastectomies can breathe a sigh of relief and make plans for reconstructive mammoplasty. Those who chose segmental surgery followed by radiotherapy can begin their X-ray treatments as soon as the incision is healed. If cancer is found in even one node, plans for reconstruction to replace the lost breast must wait six months or a year until adjuvant therapy is completed. Node-positive women who have segmental resections and radiotherapy are usually given adjuvant treatments during the five weeks of radiation.

Living with fear

Statistics indicate that about 25% of node-negative women will develop metastatic disease in spite of the absence of cancer in their axillas; those who had positive nodes and received adjuvant therapy have, of course, a higher risk of recurrence. So all women treated for breast cancer face added years of watching, waiting, and worrying about unusual bone pain, hoarseness, coughing, and digestive problems. Moreover, women who have had cancer in one breast have a higher risk of developing it in the remaining breast. Periodic follow-up examinations, with all their accompanying anxieties, become new patterns of their lives.

The lucky hundreds of thousands whose biopsied lumps were benign also face years of anguish and anxiety because they are now in the high-risk category. Some will respond like Diane and deny; some, like Wilma, will opt for prophylactic mastectomies. All women, after suffering through weeks or months of waiting, multiple examinations, and, finally, diagnostic surgery, will again face the harrowing ordeal of coping with the fear of breast cancer.

Contraception

Ever since people first began to try to devise ways to prevent unwanted pregnancies, they have pursued an elusive ideal—the perfect contraceptive. The ideal contraceptive would be 100% effective, 100% safe, esthetically acceptable, reversible when pregnancy was desired, low in cost, easy to use, and would be unaffected for long periods of time under variable storage conditions in a wide variety of climates. Furthermore, it would not require interrupting the sex act or be otherwise dependent upon being used at a precise time before or after each act. Since a perfect contraceptive does not (and possibly never will) exist, all forms of fertility regulation are measured against this hypothetical ideal. Today's birth control methods fall into three main categories: hormonal methods, intrauterine devices, and barrier methods.

Hormonal methods—systemic regulation

More than 150 million women have used or are now using oral contraceptives (OC's). These drugs are the most thoroughly studied drugs in medical history. Originally felt to be an "ideal" method, the oral contraceptives are now recognized both to have a number of minor side effects and to present serious health risks to a small percentage of users. Both adverse and beneficial side effects of the Pill have been documented. The former, of course, have received far greater publicity than the latter.

Combined pills. The Pill has undergone considerable change since it was first introduced more than a quarter of a century ago. The original Pill was a combination of two hormones, a synthetic estrogen and a progestin; it acted by stopping ovulation. Somewhat later, the mini-Pill was developed, containing only a progestin; it stopped ovulation in only some of the women taking it. Other hormonal effects on the reproductive tract produced temporary infertility. Most recently developed is the biphasic combined Pill, in which the progestin dose is higher in the second half of the cycle, simulating a woman's normal hormonal pattern.

The dosage of estrogen in the combination OC has been steadily decreased. It has now dropped to a minimum level, below which pregnancies begin to occur and irregular bleeding becomes a problem. As the amount of estrogen has been reduced, the frequency of serious vascular complications such as pulmonary embolus (blood clot carried from the legs to the lung), heart attack, and stroke has also declined. In addition, it has been demonstrated that the risk of developing these conditions does not apply equally to all women. A recent study has shown that if women over the age of 35, particularly those who smoke, stopped using the Pill, 75% of the serious complications could be averted. The risk of major complications to young, healthy, nonsmoking women is almost negligible.

A number of metabolic changes have been noted with the use of the combined OC's. In most instances, their occurrence and magnitude vary directly with the type and dosage of the hormones employed. However, it is still unclear what long-term significance there is, if any, to these observations.

In addition to the serious vascular side effects, some women experience certain minor but annoying side effects, especially during the first few months of use. These include breakthrough bleeding, skipping of menstrual periods, areas of increased pigmentation of the face, and weight gain. These problems often cause women to discontinue taking the Pill.

On the other hand, a number of beneficial effects have been documented with use of the OC's. Many women report the same feelings of well-being that they experienced during their pregnancies. It has also been found that Pill users are partially protected against venereal diseases and their complications, the rate being half that of noncontraceptors. In addition, because of the reduction in the quantity of menstrual flow produced by the OC's, there is a decrease in the incidence of anemia.

It is particularly interesting to find, given the frequently expressed concern about the possible induction of malignancies of the female reproductive tract by the oral contraceptives, that they produce exactly the opposite effect. Pill users have fewer benign breast tumors, fewer benign and malignant ovarian tumors, and probably also fewer endometrial carcinomas.

Progestin-only pills. During the development of oral contraceptives, it was felt that the risks arose primarily from the estrogen component. Therefore, studies were started to see if giving a progestin alone in a continuous fashion would be effective. It was found that the progestin-only mini-Pills produced fewer metabolic changes than did the combined medications. However, it has more recently been discovered that the progestins too may pose certain risks. It appears that their use may be associated with an increased incidence of high blood pressure, superficial venous thrombosis, and, possibly, some forms of arterial disease.

It has also been found that mini-Pill users have a somewhat higher pregnancy rate and less regular cycles and that bleeding problems such as spotting and irregular menses are more common than with the combination Pill. Thus the progestin-only medications are used primarily in certain selected situations—for women with estrogen-related side effects, those who wish to begin oral contraceptives while lactating, those who have increased cardiovascular risks.

Virtually complete protection against pregnancy can be obtained with combined OC's—if they are taken exactly as directed. However, their actual effectiveness rates are often much lower. This is usually due to the failure to follow instructions properly as well as to the early discontinuation of Pill use because of side ef-

Unexpected benefits of the Pill
cancer of the womb* hospitalizations expected: 4,000 ///////////// averted: 2,000
cancer of the ovary* hospitalizations expected: 3,400 ///////////// averted: 1,700
benign breast disorders† operations expected: 40,000 ///////////// averted: 20,000
pelvic inflammatory disease† hospitalizations expected: 27,000 ///////////// averted: 13,000
iron deficiency anemia† cases expected: 68,000 ///////////// averted: 27,000
*based on total of 40 million American women who have ever used the Pill †based on total of 9 million Americans currently using the Pill

Studies among women who use oral contraceptives show that the Pill apparently has prevented thousands of cases of uterine and ovarian cancer and other disorders.

fects. As a result, the demographic impact of the oral contraceptives has been less than was originally anticipated. They remain, however, a highly effective form of birth control and one that is safe for the vast majority of women who take them.

Morning-after pills. For many years a synthetic estrogen, diethylstilbestrol (DES), has been employed as a postcoital contraceptive, administered after unprotected midcycle intercourse at the time of presumed ovulation. However, use of the morning-after pill began to decline after a rare cervicovaginal malignant tumor was found in a small percentage of the daughters born to women who took this agent during pregnancy. At the present time DES is recommended primarily for emergency situations; for example, to prevent pregnancy from rape or incest. Moreover, it is suggested that if the DES fails to work, termination of pregnancy should be seriously considered.

Because of the potential risks of DES, other estrogens are now being evaluated as morning-after pills. In addition, both estrogens and progestins are being looked at as agents to use either just before or just after each act of intercourse. This method would be particularly suitable for a woman who has intercourse infrequently. However, because of the complexities of studies of this sort, involving both the woman and a po-

tential fetus, it is unlikely that these products will become available in the near future.

Proposed pills for both men and women. A number of approaches are being taken which may make the oral contraceptives of the future equally effective but safer and easier to use. For women new hormonal agents, both progestins and estrogens, are being evaluated. Certain of the progestins such as norgestimate appear to have fewer side effects than those currently being prescribed. Natural estrogens such as estradiol are being studied to see if their use would reduce the incidence of estrogen-related side effects. A new agent, RU-486, has just been reported to induce early abortion when taken monthly just prior to the time of anticipated menses. These new approaches are all still in the research phase.

Researchers are also looking at new and better ways in which to administer hormones. These include preparations that are given only once a week or once a month; the triphasic Pill, in which the hormones are given in three different doses during the cycle; and the miniestrogen Pill, in which a progestin is given daily but an estrogen is administered only every second or third day. Again, it is too early to know whether or not these preparations will offer significant advantages over the present OC's.

Although there is a widely perceived need for an oral hormonal contraceptive for men, there is no such Pill available at the present time, despite a considerable amount of research. The steroids used in the female preparations have been extensively evaluated in men. Although certain of them will stop the production of sperm, their side effects make them completely unacceptable; men taking these agents undergo breast development, lose all interest in sex, are unable to have erections, and cannot ejaculate. Research efforts are currently under way, however, to see if the additional use of male hormones, given by injection, can make this combination a practical approach to male contraception.

Injectable hormones. It has been recognized for many years that there are numerous clinical advantages to having an injectable method of contraception available for women. These include ease of administration, high levels of safety and effectiveness, and the generally favorable acceptance of this type of contraception by women. In fact, a number of surveys have shown that injectables rank highest among all currently available techniques for these reasons.

The preparation that has been most carefully studied and widely used to date is a progestin, medroxyprogesterone acetate (Depo-Provera, DMPA). This agent has been registered and is now being used in more than 80 countries, the most recent approval being obtained in Sweden. Depo-Provera is currently approved in the United States for the treatment of endometrial and metastatic renal cancers. However, it has still not been approved by the U.S. Food and Drug Administration (FDA) for use as a contraceptive, despite the fact that the FDA's own advisory committee has twice recommended that this be done. The reasons given by the FDA have included: lack of need in the U.S., increased risk of cervical cancer, induction of breast tumors in test dogs, bleeding problems (excessive blood loss and temporary cessation of menses), delay in the return of fertility, and, most recently, endometrial malignancy in a few rhesus monkeys given several times the human dose of this drug.

Depo-Provera has, over the years, been violently attacked by a number of women's groups and has been the subject of several congressional hearings. At the same time, there has been and continues to be great debate about the scientific validity of the expressed concerns of the FDA. Many scientists now believe that most of the fears expressed about Depo-Provera have not been confirmed by careful evaluation of the existing data. These publications point out that Depo-Provera has been well received by many U.S. women, and that its use as a contraceptive continues despite the lack of FDA approval. No association has been found between treatment with Depo-Provera and cancer of the cervix. While abnormal bleeding patterns do occur and there is, on occasion, a delay in establishing a pregnancy once use is discontinued, these have not proved to be major clinical problems.

Beagle dogs, used for laboratory testing, are known to have a high incidence of spontaneous breast tumors and are no longer used in some areas as a test animal for this reason. It also now appears that the tumors found in the monkey uteri have arisen from a type of tissue not present in the human uterus. Moreover, these same tumors have now been identified in monkeys that have never been exposed to Depo-Provera. Therefore, the question remains as to what, if anything, these animal findings mean as regards the use of DMPA in women. Finally, Depo-Provera has been administered to thousands of women all over the world for many years; to date there have been no serious side effects reported in those receiving this drug.

Of key importance in international family-planning programs is the effect that this long continued controversy is having on the use of Depo-Provera in those less developed countries that do not have their own drug regulatory agencies. Despite its high level of acceptance by women, the long delay in securing FDA approval is producing adverse effects on both the initiation and continuation of the use of DMPA, as doubts about its safety become more widespread. A hearing before the FDA was requested several years ago and as of 1982 was still pending. However, the FDA has now set up a public board of inquiry which will evaluate the entire situation and presumably come up with appropriate recommendations.

Because of the generally perceived need for inject-

able methods, work is now under way to synthesize, screen, and evaluate a number of new long-acting agents and techniques. Hormones such as levonorgestrel, progesterone, and norethisterone are being manufactured as injectables, incorporated into polymers such as polylactide and polyglycolide. One interesting new approach is the development of microcapsules that have a potential for sustained release, lasting from one month up to several years following injection. While they are still in the research phase, the early clinical studies show considerable promise.

In men a number of male and female hormones have been injected alone or in combination to suppress the production of sperm. Estrogens cannot be used alone because of their feminizing side effects. Progestins used alone will depress sperm development but will also decrease the secretion of male hormones (androgens), leading to impotence. Androgens used alone must be given in very large doses that could produce adverse side effects. Lower doses of male hormones have been found to produce incomplete suppression of sperm, and thus they have unacceptably high rates of failure.

The most promising current approach is to combine testosterone (given by injection or implant under the skin), which will maintain potency, with a progestin, which will suppress sperm production. However, no combination tested to date has produced total and continuous suppression of sperm without significant side effects.

Hormonal implants. Considerable effort continues to be expended in attempts to find ways to administer hormones in ways that are as effective as the OC's but that are easier to use and have fewer adverse side effects. Several new approaches have been taken, two of which will probably become available sometime in the mid-1980s.

The first of these is the implant. A number of hormones have been incorporated into capsules or rods made of Silastic, a synthetic rubberlike substance. The current implants are of two general types, biodegradable and nonbiodegradable. The former variety has an average duration of action of one year and the latter of four or more years. While the biodegradable products have the disadvantage of being very difficult (if not impossible) to remove if adverse side effects develop, they avoid one disadvantage of the nonbiodegradable variety. This second type of implant is usually injected beneath the skin of the forearm and can easily be felt and may actually be visible. This feature makes them unattractive to some women and, consequently, implants are now being tested in other areas of the body.

To date, hormonal implants have produced no major adverse side effects. Their minor effects are quite similar to those of the oral and injectable hormonal contraceptives, the most frequent problems being related to abnormal bleeding and cycle irregularity. Numerous studies have shown that the implant technique is highly effective and has been well accepted by women in many areas of the world. In fact, they are viewed by many as being equivalent to temporary sterilization.

Implants have been found to have a number of advantages. They are generally inexpensive and relatively easy to manufacture. They require only one visit to a health-care facility to obtain long-term contraception, and they can be inserted by paramedical personnel. When reinsertions are carried out at appropriate intervals of time, they offer the potential for many years of fertility regulation.

Studies are also being conducted in men, using testosterone-releasing implants along with orally administered progestins, attempting to produce long-term suppression of sperm production. Although some effect is observed for several months to a year, in many cases a small but significant number of sperm continued to be released. Another problem has been the development of the "escape phenomenon"; men will inexplicably, after a period of use, once again begin to produce sperm. Since this escape cannot be detected clinically, until this problem is resolved the male implant will probably not be approved for general use.

Vaginal rings. Another relatively new approach to the cyclic use of hormonal contraception is the development of vaginal rings. These are usually made out of Silastic and contain a progestin which is slowly released at a rate that will prevent pregnancy. The original rings were formulated using medroxyprogesterone acetate; more recently norethisterone and norgestrel have been tested. A vaginal ring is inserted by a woman high into her vagina after her menses; three weeks later she removes it, has a menstrual period, and then replaces the ring. The major advantage of this method is that only one "use" gives a month's protection, unlike the Pill, which must be taken daily. In addition, some researchers believe that it has an advantage over the implants in that use of the device is controlled by the woman herself. A somewhat different approach has explored the possibility of using continuous hormonal medication from vaginal rings, comparable to the use of the mini-Pill. In this instance, the rings are left in place for several years.

The major problems encountered during the development of the rings were related to abnormal bleeding patterns. A second but less frequent complication, one related specifically to this vehicle, was vaginal irritation and erosions in a small percentage of women using the vaginal rings. Considerable variation has been found in the acceptability of this approach, some women finding it a major improvement and others feeling that it offers no major advantage over existing methods.

Intrauterine devices

Intrauterine contraceptive devices (IUD's) were used in the late 1920s but were generally abandoned in the

early 1950s because of concerns about infection. There was a resurgence of interest in the late 1950s, and since then numerous devices have been studied, mostly in two major categories. The first are nonmedicated devices made of plastic or metal. Plastic IUD's such as the Lippes Loop and the Saf-T-Coil became a reality following the development of new plastics that had the property of memory, assuming their original form after insertion. Stainless steel IUD's such as the Hall-Stone ring, the Majzlin spring, and the "M" device were also tested, but they proved to cause unacceptably high rates of abnormal bleeding and embedment in the uterine wall.

As research continued on the early IUD's, two general observations were noted. First, the larger the device, the lower the pregnancy and expulsion rates but the higher the pain and bleeding rates. Second, and conversely, the smaller the device, the higher the pregnancy and expulsion rates but the lower the pain and bleeding rates.

The next step, the so-called second-generation medicated devices, stemmed from these observations. It was found in 1966 that a small T-shaped plastic platform had minimal side effects but low effectiveness. However, when coupled with a metal such as copper or a hormone such as progesterone, these devices were as effective as the nonmedicated devices but with fewer side effects. With the development of the Copper 7 and the Tatum-T, copper became the first medication to be delivered to the uterine cavity by an IUD. Other metals have been looked at as possible additives, but at the present time none has achieved the level of effectiveness, reliability, durability, and safety of copper.

One of the problems with the earlier copper devices was the gradual fragmentation of the copper wire, which limited their duration of use. Presently used devices are now being approved for three years. However, the addition of a small silver core in the center of the wire seems to have resolved this difficulty. In addition, the use of solid copper sleeves may extend the period of use up to as much as 10 to 15 years.

Another medicated device, the Progestasert, was developed by adding progesterone to a T-shaped base. The principal advantage of this IUD is a reduction of total menstrual blood loss. In contrast to the larger, nonmedicated IUD's, blood losses are less than those occurring during a normal menstrual period. In the present device, the progesterone is depleted after one year *in utero,* requiring removal and replacement with a new device. However, 18-month and three-year models are currently being tested.

New steroid-bearing IUD's are undergoing intensive clinical evaluation. One of these is the norgestrel Nova-T. It appears to be very effective, reduces blood loss, protects against infections, and has the potential of providing significantly longer contraception than the

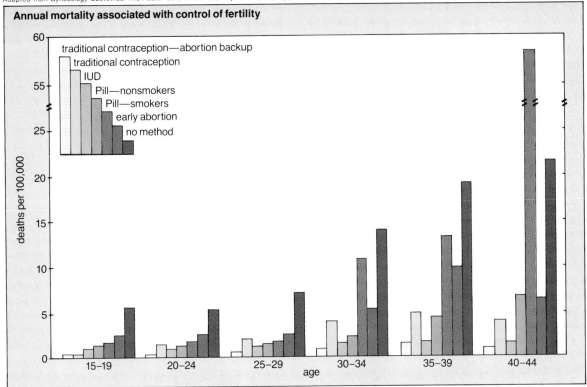

Annual mortalities associated with various methods of birth control and no contraceptives are compared for women in six age groups. Risk of death varies considerably with the method and with age.

progesterone-bearing IUD's. Of considerable interest is the fact that there are preliminary data that suggest that the incidence of pelvic inflammatory disease (PID) with progesterone-releasing IUD's may be less than that observed with the nonmedicated IUD's.

All IUD's have been found to have adverse side effects, the actual rates varying from one device to another. The major reasons for the removal of IUD's are perforation of the uterus, partial expulsion, cramping, bleeding, pregnancy, and infection; these adverse effects have been observed with all IUD's. It was previously believed that the removal of the IUD in a pregnant women would tend to produce an abortion. However, continued research has shown exactly the opposite; the chances of carrying a pregnancy to term are doubled if the IUD is removed.

Pelvic infections that occurred in IUD wearers were originally felt to be mainly gonorrheal in origin and thus were unrelated to the presence of the IUD. More recently, however, it has become clear that there is a slightly increased risk of PID associated with the wearing of an IUD, and that these infections are caused by a variety of organisms. This observation has particularly affected the use of this method by teenagers, although it was originally believed that the second-generation IUD's were ideal for this age group. However, studies have shown that there is a direct relationship between

the rates of PID and the number of sexual partners, and thus IUD use remains a possibility when a young woman has only one sex partner.

IUD's are very useful following induced abortions. Motivation is usually very high at this time, and the insertion of an IUD immediately following the termination of the procedure is a safe and effective (but often neglected) option. Studies are also now being carried out attempting to find devices suitable for insertion after giving birth. It is very important in many areas of the world to be able to offer contraception to women following delivery while they are still under medical care and highly motivated to prevent another pregnancy. IUD's are now being evaluated that progressively biodegrade as the uterus involutes back toward its normal nonpregnant size.

Although certain of the older devices did not have a tail that protruded through the cervix, most of the currently used devices have tails. They are used for identification purposes and for removal. There has always been concern about the role of the tail of an IUD in the induction of PID. Consideration is now being given to the development of tailless IUD's, but there are two practical problems that must be solved. First, an accurate, safe, and inexpensive way must be found to locate the IUD once it is inserted. Second, safe and easy methods of removal must be developed. Research ad-

Contraception

dressing both of these issues is now under way.

The work done to date suggests that the IUD's of the future will probably be medicated. For example, antifibrinolytic agents are being evaluated in attempts to cut down on abnormal bleeding. Agents that inhibit contractions are being looked at to see if their addition to an IUD would decrease uterine cramping.

None of the currently available IUD's is as effective as the combination Pill when it is taken properly, but since this is frequently not the case, continuation rates remain higher for the IUD. In general, IUD's have been shown to have higher morbidity (incidence of disease) but lower mortality rates than the OC's.

The IUD continues to be widely used because it has a number of very specific advantages. Intrauterine contraception requires only a single act of motivation. IUD's act locally and thus do not have a major impact on a number of body systems as do the oral contraceptives. Finally, in areas with limited health care, the devices can be inserted by paraprofessionals and require, in most instances, minimal follow-up.

Barrier contraceptives

A barrier contraceptive is one that prevents the sperm from reaching the egg by setting up either a chemical or a physical block or both. Barrier methods were the only effective techniques generally available prior to the introduction of the Pill and the IUD. Once the use of newer, noncoitally related methods became widespread, the use of barriers declined sharply. In recent years, however, with the growing concern about the adverse side effects of Pills and IUD's, there has been a gradual return to the use of barrier methods by both men and women.

Barriers for use by women. The contraceptive diaphragm is a shallow rubber cup with a rubber-covered steel spring in the rim. The diaphragm covers the cervix and the upper portion of the vagina. A diaphragm must be properly fitted and used with a spermicide if it is to be an effective barrier to the ejaculated sperm. Since the vaginal walls have been shown to contract and relax spasmodically during the excitation phase of sexual intercourse and to expand during orgasm, a diaphragm should be of the largest size that can be worn without discomfort.

Cervical caps were used a number of years ago and are now the subject of new research efforts. They are small cup-shaped devices that are filled with a spermicide and placed over the cervix, being held in place by suction. The caps must be custom fitted if they are to be well retained. Many women have considerable difficulty putting the caps on properly and subsequently removing them.

Cervical caps appear, at the present time, to offer few advantages over the conventional vaginal diaphragm, their chief advantage being their small size. While it has been suggested that the caps may be left

on for several days, the discovery of the toxic shock syndrome associated with the use of vaginal tampons strongly suggests that prolonged obstruction to the normal outflow of uterine secretions may be potentially dangerous. One design, however, has a one-way valve that allows mucus from the cervix and uterus as well as menstrual blood to flow out.

Spermicides play an important role in fertility control. These include jellies, creams, foams, and suppositories for vaginal use, some alone and others in conjunction with a diaphragm. In addition to being quite effective when used properly and consistently, chemical barriers provide considerable protection against sexually transmitted diseases (STD's).

Concern about spermicides has been generated by a recent report that indicated a possible increase in the risk of certain congenital disorders to babies born to women who had used vaginal spermicides. The report, however, did not establish whether or not the women were using spermicides at the time of conception. Moreover, it did not establish the presence of a well-defined set of anomalies that could be causally linked to the spermicides, as would have been anticipated. In fact, the incidence of certain of the abnormalities was actually lower than in the general population. Other similar studies currently under way have failed to confirm this earlier observation.

Soft drinks, laundry detergents, and innumerable other solutions have been used for douching. However, the contraceptive effectiveness of douches is very poor. The reason is obvious; studies have shown that sperm are already in the fallopian tubes 90 seconds after ejaculation. Consequently, it would be unrealistic to expect cleansing to have any major effect on conception rates.

There is increasing interest in vaginal sponges as a form of fertility control. Research is currently under way on sponges made of materials such as polyethylene foam. Their effectiveness is usually enhanced by the addition of spermicides such as nonoxynol 9.

It has been reported by Chinese scientists that gossypol, a pigment from the cotton plant, depresses sperm production when administered orally to men. This substance has been widely tested in China and has been shown to be effective, but there are serious problems with side effects and with reversibility. It has been shown more recently that gossypol has a direct spermicidal effect. Thus, this material might be more useful as a vaginal barrier contraceptive.

Barriers used by men. Condoms are currently one of the most widely used forms of contraception. They are quite effective; when used properly and consistently, the effectiveness of the condom is better than 97%. Moreover, if the condom is employed in conjunction with a vaginal barrier, a success rate close to 99% can be attained. They also play an important role in protecting against STD's.

212

The only complications directly related to condom use are rare instances of allergic reactions to the lubricant. The popularity of the condom has been jeopardized in the past because of the stigma of their association with illicit sex, prostitution, and venereal disease. However, the condom is now gaining popularity because of its safety and because of the growing need men feel for assuming their share of the responsibility for birth control.

Attempts have been made to dispel the previously negative image of the condom. Many of these devices are now brightly colored, lubricated, thinner, and some contain a spermicide for added effectiveness, especially in the event of breakage. Research has recently been undertaken on water-soluble condoms made of polyethylene oxide which contain a spermicidal agent. They are being fashioned into a cap that fits over the end of the penis.

Potential future methods

A number of potential contraceptive methods are currently under investigation. Hormonal contraceptives under research include several substances that are analogues of hormones such as LHRH (luteinizing hormone releasing hormone) which are made in the brain. These neurohormones play a major role in the reproductive cycles of both the male and the female. For all of the reasons noted above, in the male the analogues would have to be given with androgens. In the female two modes of action are possible, depending upon the dosage used and at what point the drug is given in the menstrual cycle. First, ovulation may be inhibited if higher doses are administered. With lower doses they will act approximately like the mini-Pill. A second use could be to induce hormonal changes that would cause the very early interruption of a pregnancy.

A variety of routes of administration are being considered. A nasal spray has already been tried successfully. Other possible routes include oral, vaginal, and the various prolonged-release systems. To date, the animal and human studies have not shown any serious adverse effects, but much more work will have to be done to establish the long-term safety and effectiveness of these agents.

It now appears that a long-sought substance, follicular inhibin, which controls the process of follicular development and ovulation, has been identified in animals. Thus, it is possible that this type of agent could be developed to block ovulation in the human female.

Preliminary work has also been done to try to find drugs that would block the transport of the ovum to the tube and would block the orderly development of the sperm and their transport through the vas. Thus far, unfortunately, many of the agents found to be effective in animals have proved to be toxic to humans.

Given our present state of knowledge, it seems reasonable to assume that it should be possible to vacci-

nate someone against a part of that individual's reproductive tract, against a part of the reproductive tract of the opposite sex, or against some part of the developing embryo or its supporting placenta. Considerable work has been done on developing a vaccine against human chorionic gonadotropin (HCG), a hormone elaborated during pregnancy. However, it is essential, before administering such a vaccine to large numbers of women, that the problem of potential autoimmune diseases and the possibility of damage to a developing fetus (in the event of contraceptive failure) be thoroughly investigated.

—Elizabeth B. Connell, M.D.

Dentistry

Until as recently as five years ago one could assume that a dentist practicing in the United States practiced alone, drew patients from the public at large, and expected those patients to pay a fee for whatever services were provided. This "traditional" dentist could be expected to have ultimate responsibility for all professional and business aspects of his, or less frequently her, practice. Also, by tradition, the patient could assume to have freedom of choice of the dentist and the dentist, freedom of choice of patients. Today, increasingly, these assumptions are no longer as valid.

Changing concepts in dental care delivery

Although for the foreseeable future the traditional, independent, fee-for-service form of dental practice will continue to remain the major source of dental health care in the United States, alternative modes and settings for providing dental care are emerging more frequently than ever before. The reasons for the development of these alternatives are varied and complex; several of the more decisive factors bear mentioning.

Of primary importance has been the success of the dental profession in encouraging the use of fluorides in community water supplies, in dental care products for home use, and in topical applications in the dentist's office. It is currently possible to measure a decrease in the prevalence of dental caries (decay) of up to 50% in some U.S. communities. This factor, in turn, has had a profound effect on the character of dental practice. For example, of total services rendered by dentists, extractions have decreased from 14% in 1950 to 4% in 1979. In 1979 diagnostic services accounted for 34% of dental services performed, preventive services 21%, and restorative care 17%. Clearly, the emphasis on preventive care has resulted in a decreased need for fillings and dentures.

Consumers, too, have demonstrated an increased awareness of the value of preventive care. Their demand for dental insurance reflects, in part, the desire of the public to enter programs of regular dental care. Presently, about one of every three Americans is as-

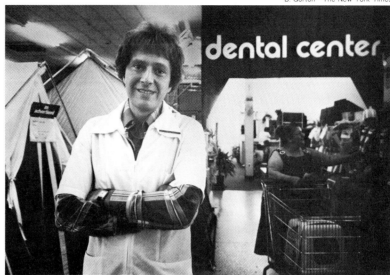

D. Gorton—The New York Times

A new trend in dental care is the dental clinic located within a retail store or shopping mall, which charges fees substantially below local rates for private practice.

sisted by some form of dental insurance, and it has been estimated that by the end of this decade half the population in the United States will be covered by such insurance.

Two factors that have had a significant effect on dental practice relate to activities of the federal government. The use of financial incentives to increase dental school enrollments permitted the government to directly influence the number of practicing dentists in the nation. During the 1970s the supply of dentists rapidly expanded by 25%. And in 1977, after a decision by the U.S. Supreme Court, the Federal Trade Commission directed that the advertising restrictions observed by health care professionals should be lifted. Both the abundant supply of dentists and greater freedom to develop innovative advertising and marketing concepts have resulted in a predictable increase in competition within the profession.

Still other factors that have influenced the delivery of dental care include scientific advances that have improved the productivity of the dental work force, a more efficient use of dental auxiliaries such as dental assistants and hygienists, and the entry of nonprofessionals such as denturists into the dental delivery system. (Denturists are individuals who do not have a dental science degree but who maintain practices providing dentures. These practices are illegal in most U.S. states. In Canada they are more common.) An economy beleaguered by inflation has also had a major impact on the provision of dental care. In fact, virtually every aspect of the dental profession has been challenged to modify its traditional concepts and values. The question to be answered now is how dentistry can better serve the diverse dental health needs of today's society. The following are alternative forms of dental practice that currently seem most significant in their bid for public and professional acceptance.

214

Retail store dentistry

In a new kind of dental practice, services today are offered to the public within a retail store setting. Typically, space is leased in a department store, shopping mall, or drugstore by a separate administrative group that subleases the space to a dentist or to a dental group. The first retail store dental facility opened in 1977 in California. Since that time approximately 90 such facilities have opened in at least 17 states and the District of Columbia.

These facilities generally operate during the same hours as the retail store in which they are located, and in many, if not most, of these practices, prearranged appointments are not required. Proponents of retail store dentistry emphasize the high visibility and convenience of the facilities. Detractors claim that the traditional long-term doctor-patient relationship is being disrupted and question whether the quality of care is at an acceptable level. These various assertions about retail store dentistry remain unverified by scientific studies.

Franchise dentistry

When the marketing of dental practices is accomplished under a system providing a uniform trade name for each practice, it is termed "franchise dentistry." The dentists who participate in these facilities often receive such benefits as media advertising, patient referrals, and financial management services.

The firms or individuals offering franchise agreements frequently assume essentially all marketing and management responsibilities for the practice, such as site selection, maintaining patient record systems, and advertising of the availability of dental services. The dentist entering a franchise practice generally pays a substantial initial fee and a yearly or monthly fee thereafter that remains a significant economic factor in this kind of practice.

Individual practice associations

For some dentists the individual practice association (IPA) offers the opportunity to more directly compete with nontraditional forms of dental practice while still retaining most of the traditional characteristics of a private practice. An IPA is defined as a partnership, corporation, association, or other legal entity organized and operated on behalf of health care professionals.

This form of practice permits a group of dentists to contract for their services collectively and to enroll special patient populations, such as the employees of a large corporation. In an IPA the participating dentist can retain his or her own office and continue care for patients not covered by contract as well as those who are. According to the terms of the contract, the dentists are reimbursed for care provided either on a fee-for-service basis, a table of allowance, or by a fixed monthly premium.

The concept of the IPA is one that originated in medical practice. The viability of the IPA as a model for dental practice, particularly in regard to patient acceptance, is largely untested. In both the medical and dental IPA's the patient's choice of health practitioner is limited to those physicians and dentists participating in the associations.

Health maintenance organizations

The health maintenance organization (HMO) is a system in which a group of health care professionals agree to provide a comprehensive set of services for a voluntarily enrolled number of patients. A prenegotiated and fixed periodic payment is made on behalf of each individual or family unit enrolled. There are currently more than 11 million members utilizing such HMO services in the U.S.

Only approximately 25% of the HMO facilities, however, offer comprehensive dental benefits to plan members, usually on an optional basis. This rather low percentage is not surprising in that the HMO system can reduce health care costs more efficiently for medical rather than dental services. The cost savings of an HMO result primarily from a reduction in the incidence of surgical and hospital care requirements of the enrolled patients. The savings have largely been attributed to the preventive medicine thrust of the HMO. By contrast, surgical and hospital care costs are not major factors in the economics of dental care, and dentists have emphasized preventive measures in private practices for many years.

Although federal funding in the form of grants and loans to HMO's has been sizable in the past, such financial support is expected to be greatly reduced in the near future. This threat to the potential growth of HMO's may prove more apparent than real, however, as there is evidence that major private insurance carriers and other national health corporations will increase their financial commitment to HMO systems of health care in the near future.

Capitation dentistry

In a dental capitation program subscribers receive predetermined services as appropriate and necessary, while the dentist is compensated monthly at a fixed rate per subscriber. It has been estimated that approximately 5% of practicing dentists have some patients in capitation programs along with their regular, fee-for-service patients. Those persons enrolled in a specific capitation program must receive their care from a dentist who has contracted with that program.

Dentists involved with capitation programs assume some financial risk since the dentist is compensated by virtue of the number of enrolled patients, rather than by the number of patients who actually receive services. Utilization of services can vary from 25 to 75%. Some

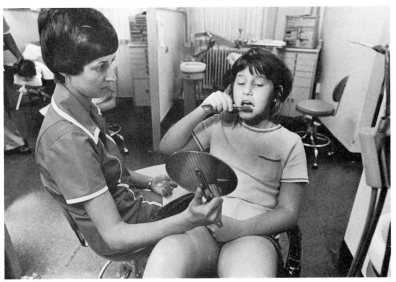

In recent years there has been a significant decrease in dental disease in the United States, which has resulted in part from an important emphasis on preventive care and a more efficient use of well-trained auxiliary personnel.

Photographs, National Foundation of Dentistry for the Handicapped

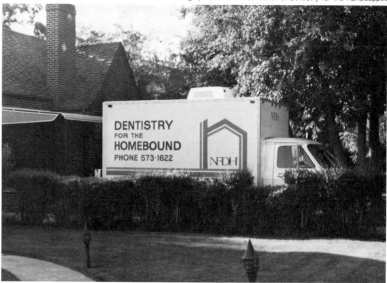

Home dental care for housebound people and nursing home residents in Denver, Colorado, is provided by dentists using a customized van. Modularized equipment carried in the van can be set up within a residence to form a complete dental office, including chair, drills, and X-ray machine.

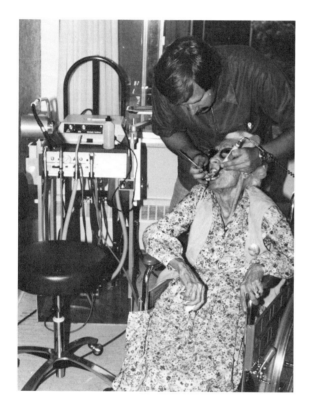

would argue that patients are also at risk as the profits of the dentist increase and as the treatment provided decreases. Whether capitation actually encourages undertreatment remains uncertain.

Corporate dentistry

A small number of major corporations have found it advantageous to own and operate dental facilities to serve the needs of their employees. In most instances

dependents of employees are also eligible to receive dental services in these company-sponsored facilities. In several of these corporate plans the dental clinic is simply a part of a medical clinic. Often employees are permitted to seek treatment during working hours without a loss of pay.

The largest of the corporate facilities is that of R. J. Reynolds Industries of Winston-Salem, N.C. The clinic is housed in a 47,000-sq-ft building and is operated by a staff of about 200 persons. There are approximately 30 dentists and dental specialists working within this corporate facility.

Other alternative dental delivery systems

Although not a new system of dental health care, more and more dentistry in the U.S. today is being performed in the nation's hospitals. Essentially half of the U.S. hospitals have at least one dentist on the medical staff, and about one-third of all practicing dentists have hospital privileges. For these dentists the hospital serves as an extension of the private dental office. The hospital environment can be essential for certain patients with medical problems that complicate dental treatment. In addition, the hospital can provide an element of safety for patients requiring extensive dental therapy that may temporarily compromise their general well-boing. A number of hospitals employ dentists on a full- or part-time basis in conjunction with dental education programs and in the provision of care to special population groups, such as the handicapped, the elderly, and the poor.

Convalescent centers and nursing homes, which are the primary settings for the long-term care of the impaired elderly and disabled patients in the U.S., often also serve dental needs. The oral health problems of these patients are considered to be more serious, in

216

many instances, than those of the general population. Neglect of appropriate oral hygiene care is prevalent among long-term-care patients. There currently is no reliable estimate of the number of nursing homes providing dental services. Clearly, however, in years to come there will be a growing demand by the elderly population for dental care as the size of the older population increases and as fewer of the elderly lose their natural teeth.

The alternatives to the solo, fee-for-service practice of dentistry mentioned here represent only the more prominent examples of the new methods of dental care delivery. Still, other alternatives will be developed in an attempt to bring dental health within the reach of all. Improvements in the methods of delivery can be instrumental in closing the gap between the need and the demand for dental care. There is still a long way to go. Surveys indicate that although 90% of the U.S. population is afflicted with dental disease, only 50% of the population seeks dental care in any given year.

Dentistry is constantly changing in response to the social, political, and economic influences of the times. The dental profession therefore must be committed to providing high quality care accessible to all at a reasonable cost through practitioners who demonstrate genuine concern for individual patients. And only those forms of dental practice that serve all these patient needs will succeed.

— Roger H. Scholle, D.D.S.

Diet and Nutrition

One of the great mysteries of science is how the body is able to regulate its weight over long periods of time. There is no doubt that a system of communication exists between those factors that regulate energy intake and those that regulate energy output. As activity increases, so does appetite. The athlete may consume twice as much food as the sedentary individual. Conversely, if the amount of food is restricted, a marked reduction in physical activity will take place. One of the first responses of the body to starvation is a drastic curtailment of all nonessential physical activity. It is as though the body is trying to maintain some hypothetical weight level by constantly adjusting its energy input and output.

The nature of this system of communication is almost entirely unknown. Messages must be constantly passing between centers in the brain that regulate food intake and centers that regulate energy expenditures. Some of these centers have actually been located, and their destruction in experimental animals has resulted in drastic imbalances in the system. For example, the hypothalamus regulates appetite; destruction of one part of this center will result in uncontrolled eating, while destruction of another part results in total loss of appetite. Scientists assume that similar centers for modulating activity must also exist, but these have not yet been located. Moreover, how the centers that regulate food intake and activity communicate with each other is still a great mystery. Why some people maintain an almost constant weight no matter how much they eat or how active they are whereas others are constantly struggling to keep from gaining or losing a few pounds is still not understood. And it is an understanding of the nature of these differences that is crucial to unraveling the mystery of how the body controls its own weight. Recently we have begun to identify some of these differences.

Recent revelations about body weight

A person's ultimate weight depends not only on the amount of food energy consumed but also on how efficiently that food energy is converted into heat for maintaining body temperature, and into work energy, which will fuel both voluntary and involuntary activity. By way of example, two individuals consume 2,500 cal per day in their diets. The body of one is much more efficient, however, than that of the other. The efficient individual needs only 2,000 cal to maintain body temperature and perform all its necessary voluntary and involuntary work. The less efficient individual uses all 2,500 cal to fuel these processes. Thus the more efficient individual has 500 cal left over after expending the *same amount* of energy on maintaining the *same amount* of activity. These 500 cal are stored, as body fat, presumably for use if food becomes scarce. From the standpoint of the chronic food shortages that plagued mankind for millions of years, the more efficient individual would have the greater chance of survival. Therefore we would expect this group to have been selected for and to make up a large percentage of the population of the world.

But when (in certain populations) food becomes extremely abundant, the *more* efficient individual begins to gain weight and deposit body fat at a *lower* caloric intake than the *less* efficient individual. Now a price is being paid for efficiency in converting food calories into useful energy. The price is obesity, which if carried to extremes will shorten life expectancy and presumably in the next million years will increase the number of inefficient converters.

In this sense, many obese individuals suffer from having a particular type of metabolism, which under other circumstances would serve them well. In societies of abundance, however, it places them at a disadvantage. For them obesity is not a disease in the usual sense but rather a price they pay for being able to convert food calories to work calories more efficiently. They must keep their food intake lower than another individual of similar build.

Recent studies in both Great Britain and the United States have begun to shed new light on this problem. Obese persons who have reduced to their ideal weights have been placed in a special environment where all activities can be carefully monitored and the energy required for those activities can be calculated. Food intake is carefully controlled. The previously obese individual begins to gain weight at a calorie intake that is lower than the intake of a person who has been thin all his life, even though both begin at the same weight and the energy expenditure is the same in both. Thus two individuals of the same build at 150 lb get the same food, perform the same activities, and expend the same energy. The one who was always 150 lb remains at that weight; the one who has previously reduced begins to gain weight even though 150 lb is his "ideal weight." This ability to gain weight on fewer calories may be the most important reason for obesity in many people. For these people to lose weight they must eat less than their thinner counterparts or exercise more, or both. Only by paying special attention to what they eat and carefully controlling their calories can they hope to lose weight and to maintain their weight loss over a long period of time.

This problem of constant calorie control to maintain ideal weight is much more prevalent in women than in men—in part because women often set their goals at weights lower than are ideal for them and their systems are constantly struggling to restore what they perceive to be their proper weight, and in part because there is some evidence that women are more efficient calorie converters than men. During periods of food scarcity women survive longer than men and are able to utilize the limited calories available more efficiently. During periods of abundance, however, this increased efficiency allows them to reach a surplus in calories sooner than men and consequently to deposit fat on a relatively smaller calorie intake.

For women, then, weight control is a double problem. Many are obese—more women have this problem than men. On the other hand, even greater numbers are too thin, perhaps not too thin for their own body image, perhaps not thin enough to threaten their health or longevity, but thin enough to be at constant war with their own metabolism and thin enough so that the only way to maintain their weight is to constantly be on a diet. It is estimated that at any given time more than half the women in our society are dieting—many because they are truly too fat, many more because they wish to become or remain too thin, and a large number, perhaps the majority, who suffer from a combination of these two problems.

What is true obesity?

Obesity, by definition, is an excess of body fat. Although this definition might sound simple, it really is not. Only if precise data are available that define the "normal" amount of fat in the human body at any stage of its development can we define excess. The standards currently in use are at best approximations. Ap-

propriate standards are difficult to set because what we are interested in is not really normal or average weight but rather ideal weight—the weight at which an individual has the best chance to live longest and maintain optimal health.

Defining this ideal weight still remains a major problem. Added to this is the problem of actually measuring body fat. Precise measurement requires complicated procedures and therefore cannot be done on large populations. The most common method used for estimating body fat is looking at an individual's weight at a given height. This method has certain obvious drawbacks; for example, the 250-lb lineman on a professional football team may be heavy, but he certainly is not obese because most of his increased weight is muscle. However, for most people excess weight and excess fat tissue are strongly associated. If we accept this, then the task is to determine a range for ideal weight for height for men and women and to decide how much above that constitutes obesity.

Traditionally this ideal weight has been determined by the life insurance companies by establishing at what range of weight for height people live longest. This method, upon which most of our public health knowl-

Skin-fold thickness offers one measure of the amount of fat in the human body. Setting standards for the "ideal" weight that will optimize health is a difficult goal.

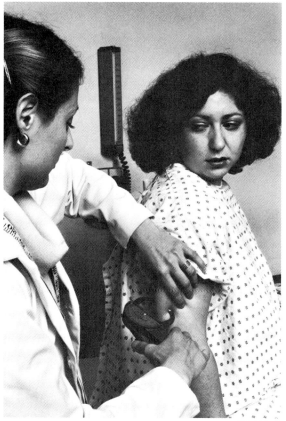

Bob Adelman

edge of obesity depends, has some serious flaws. First, the population used for determining the ideal weight is highly selected, since only people who seek insurance are included. Second, small subsamples of the overweight population may be contributing much more to the risk than others. For example, if the risk of dying early is increased considerably in obese people with a particular kind of family history, these people will bias the overall sample; statistics then might falsely suggest that a person of similar weight without such a family history also had the same risk. Third, the only criterion for ideal weight using this method is longevity. Nothing relating to other aspects of health is considered. And finally, the standards in present use are more than 20 years old, and today's weights may be quite different. In fact we know that today an individual 5 to 10% heavier than the ideal weight on the 1959 life insurance charts is closer to the weight at which maximum longevity can be predicted. The life insurance tables are currently being modified to reflect this increase.

It is important to understand that the concept of ideal weight implies that people above or below this weight are at increased risk. Although it is true that the risk increases much more rapidly for people who are significantly above their ideal weight than it does for those who are significantly below it, this latter group is also somewhat at risk. Being too thin can present its own health problems.

Notwithstanding all of the difficulties outlined above, we have learned a great deal about the health risks of obesity in the last few decades. While arguments may be presented as to what should constitute ideal weight and how much above it constitutes a significant health risk, certain facts are clear.

People who are 20% or more above their ideal weight have an increased risk for certain serious diseases, many of which can be life threatening. The risk for developing any of these health problems increases in direct proportion to the degree of obesity. Conditions in which obesity is a primary causal factor include diabetes, menstrual abnormalities, reproductive problems, heart failure, arthritis, gout, and high blood pressure (hypertension). Obesity is also a contributing factor in cancer of the uterus. There is a strong association between obesity and atherosclerosis, gallbladder disease, and premature death.

For certain of the above conditions the risks are greater in men (*i.e.,* gout); for others the risks may be exclusively in women (*i.e.,* menstrual abnormalities or cancer of the uterus). For most, however, the increased risk is present in both sexes. Since more women than men are obese, obesity presents a greater health risk in women than it does in men. However, since the incidence of the disease with the highest mortality rate on this list (atherosclerosis and its complications) is considerably higher in men than in women

at *any weight,* obesity as a contributing factor to early death may be more serious in men than in women.

There are two ways of looking at the importance of obesity as a health risk. On the one hand, obesity significantly increases the risk of a person's developing one or more of the diseases listed above. On the other hand, most obese individuals do not develop these diseases prematurely. Suppose a person of a particular sex and age and family background has a 20% chance of developing high blood pressure when he is at his ideal weight and a 40% chance if he were 25% above his ideal weight. Obesity thus would double the chances for high blood pressure. However, more than half (60%) of obese people with this background will *not* have high blood pressure. Should that 60% lose weight? This question presents a dilemma that medical science has been trying to grapple with: which obese person is at risk and which one is not? If we could accurately classify obese people into various categories, separating those at increased risk for one or more of these serious health problems from those at no health risk at all, we would be able to counsel a person with some assurance that our counsel, if followed, would benefit him.

At present we can do that only to a limited extent and often only after the fact. For example, if one is obese and has a tendency to high blood sugar (hyperglycemia), we can predict with some certainty that the chances of developing diabetes are very high and can be considerably reduced by losing weight. From a practical standpoint this ability to predict health risks only after certain warning signals are present means that obese people should pay particular attention to these signals and should be seen by a physician more often than their nonobese counterparts. In addition, they should have their blood pressure checked frequently and their blood sugar and cholesterol levels determined at least once a year, particularly if they are over 40. Of course, many experts will argue that since there are no known benefits of being obese and since we cannot predict which obese person will develop the problems on the list, all obese people should lose weight. While, for the most part, weight loss is considered advantageous, there are two problems that must be recognized with this approach. First, there is some evidence that obese people who do not develop any of the complications listed above live slightly longer than their nonobese counterparts. Thus for many obese people, losing weight may actually *shorten* life expectancy. Second, most obese people are unable to attain and sustain their ideal weight. Thus a significant portion of the population is obese and will remain obese until medical science learns how to manage the problem much better. Given this reality it is essential that obese people understand that *some* of them are going to develop the complications outlined above.

Clearly, anyone who is significantly obese should try

weight (lb)	X	10-light activity
		15-moderate activity
		20-heavy activity
age 25–34	-	subtract 0
35–44	-	subtract 100
45–54	-	subtract 200
55–64	-	subtract 300
65+	-	subtract 400

Many overweight persons have used the above method to estimate the caloric requirement needed to reach their target weight; the target weight is multiplied by an activity factor and then reduced by an age factor.

to lose weight, since sustained weight reduction may significantly reduce one's risk of developing serious health problems. To deny this would be like saying that heavy cigarette smokers need not stop, since not all of them will get lung cancer, emphysema, or heart disease, or that heavy drinkers should not stop because not all of them will get cirrhosis or other serious complications of alcoholism. To continue any of these practices is a form of Russian roulette. Though the odds may differ the game is the same. With obesity, however, we are beginning to have ways of predicting the odds for at least some of its complications before overt disease is present. Therefore, since many people will not or cannot lose weight, it is important that the obese person take advantage of what little prediction is possible to help him understand more precisely the actual risks of obesity to his personal health.

Losing weight: changing concepts

From the preceding discussion it should be clear that weight reduction is neither healthy nor desirable for everyone. Even a person who is truly obese may not derive any health benefit by losing weight. However, the more weight an individual carries beyond his or her "ideal weight," the greater the chances are that undesirable health consequences will follow. Therefore, there is little question that anyone who is significantly obese should attempt weight reduction. However, we have also seen that weight reduction may be particularly difficult for the obese person, not because of any lack of motivation, but because of physiologic mechanisms within the body that favor the deposition of fat. From a practical standpoint this means that many obese people will have to reduce their caloric intake more than a lean person in order to lose the same amount of weight.

The first principle of weight reduction in obesity is reducing caloric intake. The amount of reduction will vary from person to person, but in extreme cases 1,000 cal per day or less may be necessary. This degree of caloric reduction leads directly to a potentially serious prob-

lem. It is difficult on any diet that allows 1,500 cal or less to meet the requirements for all the known vitamins and minerals and undoubtedly for other essential nutrients for which we have not yet determined the requirements. This means that the foods used should be of high nutritional density. That is, they should contain the largest quantity of essential nutrients *per* calorie that is practical. To meet these requirements, the diet should be as varied as possible, including foods from as many of the various food groups as it can.

The second principle of a weight reduction diet then is variety, to heighten the probability of getting all of the essential nutrients. In fact, if it takes a diet of fewer than 1,200 cal per day to achieve weight loss, a vitamin and mineral supplement is indicated.

The third principle of weight reduction is patience. Although it is exciting to see the pounds come off rapidly, and the motivation to continue the diet is better if weight loss is rapid, this way may not be practical for many obese people. As long as *any* weight loss is occurring, the diet is working. Finally, it is important to increase energy expenditure while keeping calories limited. This will increase the negative energy balance and therefore the rate of weight loss. However, exercise alone without calorie control usually will not work, particularly in obese people.

Maintaining reduced weight

Weight maintenance after successful weight loss is much more difficult than losing the weight initially. Part of the difficulty stems from setting unreasonable goals in the first place. From what we have seen, a previously obese individual, owing to efficient conversion of food energy to metabolic energy, may have a much harder time maintaining his or her ideal weight than a nonobese individual. At the same caloric intake many obese individuals gain weight whereas their lean counterparts do not. To maintain ideal weight many obese individuals must limit their calories to a degree that is very difficult to achieve and that in some cases is unattainable and even unhealthy. To do this would mean a life of constant dieting.

From a health standpoint it is important to remember that the more a person is above ideal weight, the greater the risks. Thus if a person who was 30% above ideal weight can hold his weight to only 10% above, he has still reduced his chances of developing health complications significantly. The key then may be compromise—setting a long-term goal that may not be ideal but is achievable. This may still mean eating less food or at least consuming fewer calories than previously, but at least the level sought is attainable. Success will require a change in life-style or at least in the overall eating pattern, and it is for this reason that behavior modification techniques in weight reduction have worked better than most methods.

There is no reason for rigidity either in a reducing diet

220

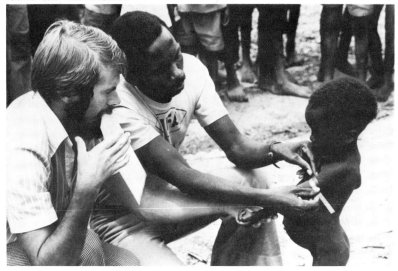

Protein-calorie malnutrition bordering on outright starvation is the most serious disease afflicting third world countries. Children who survive this condition often suffer permanent physical and mental retardation.

or in a weight maintenance plan. The number of calories need not be lowered to the same extent each day. It is illogical to assume that any animal, including man, takes in the same number of calories each day. In fact, the reverse is true, particularly when food is scarce. One day may be feast and the next famine, or one week there may be very limited food and the next relative abundance. The body has ways of adjusting to these variations over an extended time without major shifts in weight. A successful weight maintenance program for a person who was obese means keeping at a desirable weight (significantly below the previous weight) but not necessarily the ideal weight and changing the overall pattern of consumption to reduce calories over a long period without necessarily setting caloric goals on a daily basis.

Starvation

It is ironic that while obesity is probably the most serious nutritional disease in the United States, starvation or at least semistarvation is the most serious disease in the countries of the third world. This "disease," which takes several forms, is referred to as protein-calorie malnutrition, or PCM. It is most serious in young children because it can result in permanent damage. PCM often strikes infants who are not breast-fed and who cannot be properly bottle-fed. Growth stops, fat tissue disappears, muscles waste, and the infant becomes emaciated. Often the child will hardly cry and will be so weak that there is very little movement. Even if these infants "recover" from this severe form of semistarvation, they will carry the stigma for the rest of their lives. These include permanent stunting of growth and retarded mental development unless special care is taken to enrich their environment.

A second critical period during which PCM often strikes is around the time of weaning. Often the child is

weaned to a diet that is low in calories and in protein. Growth begins to slow down while at the same time the body begins to swell as it retains water (edema). The hair turns a lighter, almost reddish color, and the skin often shows a severe rash. The liver enlarges as fat is trapped within it, and the concentration of certain essential blood proteins drops to dangerously low levels. This picture is so specific and so dramatic that the name given it in Africa, kwashiorkor (the disease of the displaced child), has been adopted all over the world. Again, even if the disease is cured, permanent growth stunting and retarded development are likely to occur. It has been conservatively estimated that 300 million people in the world today are survivors of severe PCM as children. The cost of this "disease" in human lives, in human misery, and in the loss of productive capacity is staggering.

Semistarvation has periodically afflicted large adult populations and continues to do so today. One of the best medical descriptions of semistarvation was left to us by the Jewish physicians in the Warsaw ghetto in Poland in the 1940s, who, even while suffering Nazi-imposed starvation themselves, studied what they termed hunger disease. They divided the disease into three stages: utilization of reserves, adaptation, and deterioration.

During the first stage the body uses up its fat and carbohydrate (glycogen) reserves for energy. In addition, muscle tissue is also broken down to supply needed fuel. This stage can last from a few days to many weeks, depending on how much fat tissue the person has to begin with.

The stage of adaptation will last from two to three months in complete starvation to many years if the degree of semistarvation is minimal. It involves a series of changes in the overall metabolism of the body which are all aimed at utilizing available energy in the most

221

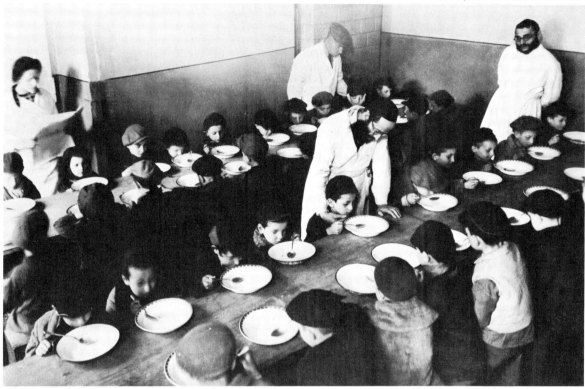

When the Warsaw ghetto was isolated in the 1940s Jewish physicians observed and left precise descriptions of the progressive effects of semistarvation, or hunger disease.

efficient manner possible. Thus the basal metabolic rate or the energy expended at rest drops. The amount of activity declines, heart rate slows, blood pressure drops, and the blood is pumped around the body more slowly. Body temperature falls, often by several degrees, as a way of cutting down the energy required for heat production. The changes, although not identical, are very similar to those that occur in hibernating mammals.

There are prices to be paid for this abnormally severe level of energy conservation. Fluid shifts from inside to outside the cells, and the volume of blood increases. The body feels cold, and the tips of the fingers and toes may turn blue as the circulation slows. Energy is diverted from tissue repair, and the cells normally lost from the lining of the gastrointestinal tract are not replaced. This inevitably leads to digestive problems, severe diarrhea, and a vicious cycle as the malnutrition is increased. Thus as the adaptation becomes more severe, the person becomes sick and health begins to deteriorate. If this unhealthy situation prevails for too long, the process becomes irreversible and death will occur. Often the heart will fail because it has been weakened by the long periods of starvation and is not able to handle the extra load imposed by the changes that have taken place in the rest of the circulatory system.

Although this degree of starvation is rarely seen in the United States, we are beginning to see lesser degrees of caloric restriction much more frequently. Perhaps this is the result of the dieting obsession that pervades our society. Whatever the cause, a disease called anorexia nervosa is becoming much more prevalent. This disease, seen mostly in adolescent girls and in young women but occasionally in males, is a psychologic aversion to food that results in a self-imposed form of starvation. In its most severe form, all of the changes described above may occur and even death may ensue. In its less severe forms various degrees of the adaptive response may occur. These patients often are extremely thin, having totally expended their reserves. In addition, there may be a wide variety of medical complications—*e.g.,* their temperature may be low and their circulation sluggish.

There is a great deal medical science does not understand about the body processes that generally work to enable a person to maintain a relatively stable weight. However, whatever the nature of these processes, they are being rendered inoperable in huge numbers of the world's population, in some cases by too many calories and in others by too few. In both instances serious and often life-threatening consequences may be the result.

—Myron Winick, M.D.

222

Diet and Nutrition

Special Report:

Life After Major Weight Loss
by John F. Keegan, Ph.D., Charles P. Lucas, M.D., and Dallas W. Stevenson

The obese person has frequently been stereotyped as jolly, generous, considerate, and undemanding. The actual psychological profile, however, is quite different. It is more likely that the obese person is self-conscious, rejected, nonassertive, and unhappy with his or her lifestyle. This reexamination of the obese personality has resulted from observations of individuals who have lost a great deal of weight through recently developed weight-loss methods (modified fasting, behavior modification, and intestinal bypass or gastric surgery). Studies of personality have shown that the obese individual changes dramatically after losing weight, showing greater assertiveness and more self-confidence. A striking example is a patient who, prior to weight loss, was willing to cook a meal for her husband at any time of day. After weight loss she responded to his untimely requests for dinner by tactfully suggesting that he prepare his own.

Origin of obesity and its problems
During adolescence most children become sensitive to their growth and weight, especially in comparison with their peers or what they think to be the ideal. During this time a third of all boys and half of all girls become sufficiently concerned about some aspect of their growth to consult a physician.

When researchers questioned adolescents about how they would like to change their body size, girls responded that they would prefer to be smaller in all aspects, while boys wished that they had a greater proportion of bone and muscle. According to Boston nutritionists Johanna T. Dwyer and Jean Mayer, adolescent girls whom they studied believed they developed obesity because they somehow lacked determination, ambition, and willpower. The young women thought that they were overeating when, in fact, their food intake was found to be within normal limits. Psychological tests revealed that adolescents who perceive themselves to be obese often feel isolated and rejected by their peers.

At the University of Pennsylvania obesity researcher Albert J. Stunkard discovered that negative body image was most evident in adults who developed obesity in childhood or adolescence. He also found that people with early-onset obesity frequently viewed their bodies as loathsome. Many of these individuals refused to have photographs taken of themselves, avoided looking in mirrors, and shunned crowds to escape inspection. By contrast, Stunkard found that those who be-

came overweight or obese as adults did not report similar feelings.

Many obese youngsters find it hard to compete in the same athletic activities enjoyed by their leaner peers. While physical differences are likely to be minor or unnoticed at a very young age, the disparity in physical agility between the lean and the obese begins to increase with puberty and adulthood. When middle age is reached, the more grossly obese shy away from sports and even are reluctant to join in leisurely activities, such as walking, dancing, and family games. This attitude may stem from the negative experiences they encountered during their early failures in attempts at athletics or other physical activities.

The morbidly obese (whose excessive weight is a hazard to their health) may find it physically demanding to appear in public places, to shop, to attend concerts or sporting events, and to perform simple maneuvers like getting in and out of an automobile. The obese person is more likely to develop diabetes, high blood pressure, or chest pains (angina pectoris) and to seek help for these conditions. His doctor is usually able to treat his symptoms but often fails to offer a comprehensive treatment of the obesity and its associated problems. The net effect for the patient is increased physical and social isolation. The psychological consequences that result from this isolation include lack of assertiveness, loss of self-esteem, feelings of rejection, limitations on the variety of coping mechanisms for stress, and the pain of isolation.

At some point in this sequence of events, most obese individuals try to lose weight. Frequently their attempts are met with some degree of success, but often the lost weight is gained back. This cycle is often repeated dozens of times; many individuals eventually give up the battle forever. It is encouraging to note that today an increasing number of patients have succeeded in attaining the goal of normal weight through the use of weight-loss methods that help dieters both lose weight and adjust their habits so that their weight stabilizes. These advances have made it possible for scientists to examine changes in the lives of individuals who have achieved a massive weight loss.

Massive weight loss
A recent study of the social consequences of massive weight loss was conducted at the Clinical Nutrition Unit of Wayne State University in Detroit. The persons studied had been involved in a program consisting of a

223

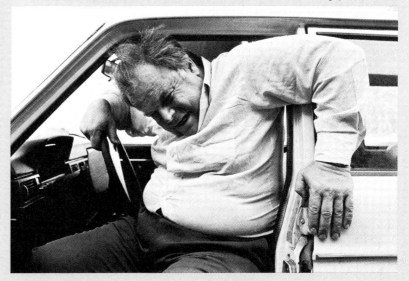

Extreme obesity can present practical problems, such as trying to fit behind the wheel of a car. The man at right finds it a tight fit at 305 pounds. A year later, after participating in a program of diet and "life rearrangement" at the Weight Control Unit of St. Luke's-Roosevelt Hospital Center in New York City, he had lost 115 pounds (opposite page).

modified fast with nutritional supplements and a program of behavior therapy. Seventeen patients who had achieved weight loss ranging from 40 to 135 lb (averaging 77.5 lb) were asked to complete a questionnaire. The questionnaire consisted of items with a five-point scale on which subjects could indicate agreement or disagreement with 24 statements. The items covered four primary areas of interest, asking questions regarding the patient's satisfaction with family relations, intimacy in relationships, friendships, and work.

The patients felt that there had been improvement in every area. More than half the patients reported an improvement in family relations, 13 out of 17 an improvement in intimacy in relations, 11 out of 17 an increase in the development of friendships, and 9 out of 17 a more satisfying work life. It is of interest that a degree of deterioration in each of these areas was reported by a small number of patients. However, overall there was a great deal of improvement in these 17 individuals. Extremes of those who enjoyed improvement and those who suffered deterioration are illustrated by the following two cases.

Case one: Martha, a 55-year-old married woman and mother of four children, was overweight as a child. In contrast to many obese youngsters, she was very athletic and full of energy. As an adult she maintained a very busy schedule of civic activities, hobbies, sports, and volunteer work. Over the years her weight increased to 250 lb. As a result, her physical activities decreased both in and outside the home. She developed high blood pressure that required hospitalization at the age of 40. Five years later she had the first of two heart attacks, which left her unable to do even light housework without getting short of breath. Her relationship with her husband and family seemed to change during this time. While she had once been assertive and socially active, she now became increasingly de-

pendent in her relationship with her husband. Consequently, he became less attentive and more demanding at home and less attentive to her at social gatherings. Then, through a carefully supervised weight-loss program, she lost 110 lb in six months and was able to maintain her new weight for a full year. As she approached her ideal weight there was marked improvement in her physical stamina. She returned to tennis and golf and once again became active in her home and social life. In addition, her assertiveness returned, and she became less dependent in her relationship with her husband. Her husband responded by being more attentive and less demanding. The result was improvement in family relations and heightened intimacy with her husband. Outside her home, her friendships improved in quantity and quality; she began to do volunteer work again.

Case two: Helen, a 26-year-old lawyer, also had been overweight since childhood. She became interested in losing weight to improve her appearance. At the onset of her weight-loss program she weighed 180 lb and hoped to attain her ideal weight of 115 lb. As she lost weight she became more physically and socially active. She began to play tennis and joined a local tennis club. At work several of her male associates began to treat her differently. Many men who had paid her little notice in the past now began to ask her to go out. She accepted many of these invitations, but when asked a second time she usually refused. Helen stated that this change in attitude was due to the development of anxiety over the sexual advances of her male companions. She responded by dropping out of the weight-loss program and regaining the weight she had lost.

In another study in 1977 psychiatrist Charles Solow at Dartmouth College Medical School studied 29 patients who lost a considerable amount of weight through bypass surgery, which shortens the length of

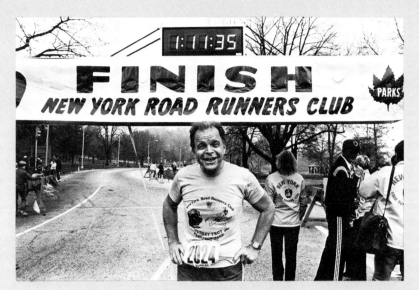

the intestine so that less food and fewer calories are absorbed. The response of these individuals to weight loss included an increased level of activity and an improvement in mood, self-esteem, interpersonal relationships, and effectiveness at work. Solow noted that individuals who lost weight felt that they had more control over their lives. Twenty-three of the patients showed an increase in physical and social activity. Over a three-year period half of all the patients either became employed or improved their job positions. Eighteen patients reported that they were more assertive. One consequence of the reduction in weight loss was a decrease in the use of denial. For example, marriages that had been erroneously portrayed as quite satisfactory before weight loss were more realistically evaluated later on. In general, there was a turnabout from the chronic sense of helplessness and failure that characterized these individuals before their weight loss to feelings that they could effectively make changes in their lives.

At St. George's Hospital Medical School in London, 22 people were studied who had lost an average of 80 lb through bypass surgery. With weight loss many of these patients showed an improved self-image. Doctors noted improvement in assertiveness and autonomy, as well as a similar degree of improvement in mobility and physical activity. Job performance and employment improved in 75% of the patients. Psychological test data indicated that weight loss was associated with less anxiety, fewer physical complaints, and a reduction in depression. Two women were of particular interest. After they lost a considerable amount of weight, they gradually began eating large amounts of food in an attempt to avoid further loss, despite the fact that they were still considerably overweight. Interviews with these patients revealed that they feared further weight loss would lead to a negative alteration of their personalities. One woman expressed the concern that she would return to the promiscuity in which she engaged prior to marriage if she lost more weight.

Consequences of obesity versus benefits of reducing

Efforts at public health education have made the public well aware of the negative consequences of obesity; the obese individual has a higher likelihood of developing high blood pressure, diabetes, stroke, and heart problems. The well-known Framingham Heart Study, begun in 1948, has been continuously gathering information on the health and habits of the adult inhabitants of Framingham, Mass. Data from the Framingham project have shown that obesity is one of the more important health problems in the United States today. It is estimated that successful treatment of obesity would result in a 25% reduction in the incidence of death from heart attack and stroke. Actuarial data from U.S. insurance companies show that individuals who lose weight live longer than those who remain overweight.

It cannot be overemphasized that the psychological impact of obesity is as significant as the physical diseases it may be a factor in causing. This is especially clear when one considers the years of social stigma, feelings of failure, and the resultant social isolation often experienced by overweight people. The obese person is often handicapped by lack of self-esteem, by rejection, and by unassertiveness. Successful weight reduction has yielded many psychological and social improvements. Although in rare instances there have been negative consequences from weight loss, the beneficial psychological, physical, and social effects have been clearly demonstrated. These findings imply that there are great gains to be made for millions of people by developing effective weight-loss and weight-maintenance programs.

Special Report:
Do Ex-Smokers Gain Weight?
by L. Fred Ayvazian, M.D.

It is often said that persons who quit smoking may expect to gain weight and that the exact cause of this weight gain is unknown. An excuse smokers commonly use for refusing to abandon their habit is fear of gaining weight, and ex-smokers sometimes resume smoking in efforts to shed unwanted pounds. Articles in both scientific journals and popular magazines often open with the assumption or implication—unattributed, unreferenced, and unchallenged—that smokers can enjoy greater freedom in dietary indulgence without adding weight. Are these attitudes defensible? Is there in fact scientific evidence of an inverse association between smoking and body weight?

Data gathered about smoking and weight

Few studies of important statistical magnitude have specifically looked into the "weigh less, eat more" phenomenon claimed for smokers. Much of the hard data linking smoking and weight is gleaned from long-term screening and intervention programs. The primary concerns of such studies—the Framingham Heart Study and the Oslo Study are two outstanding examples—may be assessment of risk factors for coronary disease, hypertension, maternal or neonatal health, or cancer and other diseases with high mortality. The Framingham Heart Study screening for coronary risk factors began in 1948 with an initial cohort of 5,209 men and women between the ages of 29 and 62 years in the Massachusetts town from which the study takes its name. It has since continued short-term and long-term observations (habits, physical characteristics), measurements (blood chemistries, standard cardiac and respiratory tests), and documentation of diseases among this population. The Oslo Study, initiated in 1972, also investigated coronary risk factors. It followed a group of 16,525 "healthy" individuals, all men, at the outset aged from 20 to 49 years. A more recent study, the Ontario Perinatal Mortality Study, reported in 1978, examined the effects of maternal smoking on pregnancy and the fetus.

The findings from such studies confirm that differences in body weight between smoking classification groups do indeed occur in both men and women. The following premises are now considered beyond dispute:

1. In large population groups habitual smokers weigh less than nonsmokers of comparable age.

2. These differences are least noticeable in persons 20 to 39 years old and quite marked in the 40- to 59-year-old group.

3. Ex-smokers tend to be heavier than those who never smoked, while smokers of 15 to 29 cigarettes per day consume at least as many calories daily as persons who have never smoked, yet have lower body weights.

4. Smokers who succeed in overcoming their habit experience an initial gain in weight within weeks or months, rarely extending beyond the first year.

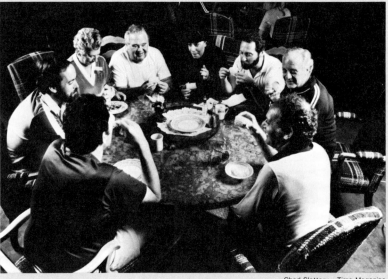

Ex-smokers need not trade the cigarette habit for extra pounds. Support groups such as this one in Santa Monica, California, help members learn new eating habits to maintain a healthful life-style.

Chad Slattery—Time Magazine

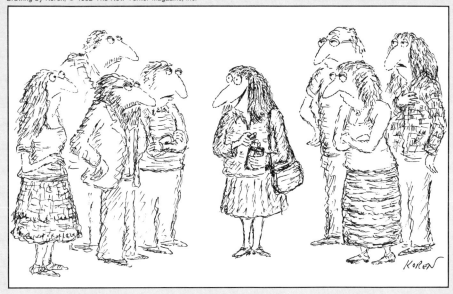

"Does anyone mind if I smoke?"

5. Those smoking the most cigarettes before quitting gain more weight than those smoking a lesser amount.

6. The weight gain is temporary unless alterations in dietary habits become permanent (a phenomenon that might be attributed to "substitute consumatory behavior").

7. Few individuals who quit smoking gain weight if they are being supervised by a dietitian or if they have the support of self-management programs that build strong scruples against overeating.

8. Overweight smokers in weight-reduction classes who succeed in reaching their goal weights under strategies stressing positive life-style values do not increase their rate of smoking.

9. The hazards of smoking dwarf those of obesity.

Among possible explanations for the negative effect of smoking on weight are: increased metabolic utilization (or waste) of calories; increased bowel motility, with a resulting calorie loss; decreased food absorption from the intestine; appetite suppression; changes in food preferences; psychological patterns; and combinations of these factors. The tendency of smoking to increase gastrointestinal activity, to speed food transit time, and to diminish calorie absorption is established and unquestioned but is thought to contribute only trivially to the control of body weight.

Some public health workers point out that a goal of total physical fitness often becomes an obsessive pursuit and that for the normal individual who does not have diabetes, high blood pressure, or heart disease, moderate overweight need not imply a hazard to health. It has been repeatedly demonstrated that nonsmokers as a group have substantially lower overall mortality than smokers, but the benefits of physical fitness have not been fully documented in the same way. It may be surprising, but statistically the lean athlete who smokes carries a greater risk of coronary disease and cancer than the overweight nonsmoker.

In a British report of sudden deaths in active sportsmen, of 19 deaths (including three with unknown smoking habits) 13 occurred among smokers, 11 of whom had smoked more than 20 cigarettes a day; this is a finding of some interest because smoking is rare among keen sportsmen. Current tallies show that the principal causes of mortality in older age groups—heart disease, stroke, diseases of the respiratory system—correlate poorly with weight alone but are all known to be increased by smoking.

The Framingham Heart Study, continuously analyzing a large general population since 1948, provides an opportunity to document changes that occur after substantial alterations in smoking habits. The study found, for example, that smokers used more alcohol than nonsmokers and that the more a person smoked, the more he tended to drink. The leanest subgroup in the Framingham group included those smoking 10 to 19 cigarettes per day, while men and women smoking 40 or more cigarettes daily weighed nearly as much as nonsmokers. Thus, while this study found weight closely related to smoking, it did not find that people who smoked the most weighed the least.

The Framingham study merely documented facts about the studied population's habits; it made no special efforts to change them. However, an unforeseen bonus was that during the first 18 years of the study a substantial number of men (39%) and a smaller group of women (22%) discontinued cigarette smoking. The study found that weight remained stable (within one-half pound) among those with fixed smoking habits, but the group who quit smoking showed short-term gains of 3.8 lb within a few weeks, 5.1 lb within six months, and then held constant for up to two years. A prompt loss of over one pound regularly followed the resumption of smoking.

Physiological factors affected by smoking

The Oslo Study of over 16,000 "healthy" men found that increasing daily exposure to cigarette smoke (in the order: never-smoker, ex-smoker, noninhaling smoker, inhaling smoker, and present nonfilter smoker) was paralleled by rising blood cholesterol values, and that among ex-smokers both body weight and blood cholesterol tended to increase according to the number of cigarettes smoked before quitting. As in other studies, weight gain that occurred after smoking ceased was found to be temporary, applying mainly to the first year. During the rise in body weight in the early weeks following cessation of smoking, documented metabolic differences included falls in cellular oxygen needs, heart rate, and thyroid activity and improvement in physiologic activity of the lungs.

In controlled laboratory studies simulated cigarette smoking in dogs significantly elevated both total oxygen consumption and arterial concentrations of free fatty acids, and in rabbits similar cholesterol changes were induced with the inhalation of carbon monoxide, a gaseous constituent of tobacco smoke. The Tobacco Institute objects, perhaps with some justification, to the extrapolation to humans of data from animals.

In the human, carbon monoxide from cigarette smoking during pregnancy is thought to interfere with the blood and oxygen supply to the unborn child. A number of well-designed obstetrical studies have established that maternal smoking during pregnancy diminished weight gain, as well as fetal weight, length, and head circumference; maternal smoking also led to more frequent placental abnormalities and accidents. Moreover, when pregnant smokers increased their food intake, although they gained more weight, this gain failed to protect the fetus and the newborn against the deleterious effects of the mother's cigarette smoking. The maternal use of tobacco reduces neonatal birth weight in a dose-related manner; that is, the more the mother smoked, the smaller the baby tended to be. While a reduced total pregnancy weight gain among light smokers may be entirely accounted for by the smaller size of the newborn infant (and placenta), the lessened weight gains of heavy smokers are only one-third due to the lower-weight newborn. Low-birth-weight infants are subject to increased tendencies toward a host of difficulties, being in general weaker and less robust.

Smoking and eating patterns

In another report a careful evaluation of seven volunteers who successfully overcame the smoking habit again confirmed a prompt gain in weight, fall in heart rate, and other physiologic changes. An additional finding was an alteration in glucose metabolism, with a fall in blood sugar 30 minutes after eating, possibly leading to increased appetite. The one in seven who did not gain weight showed an impressive rise in activity levels.

Looking into the eating patterns of 42 Columbia University students ranging in age from 18 to 36, investigators found that when given free choice, the smokers ate fewer sweet foods and more salty foods and the nonsmokers consumed the most sweet foods. This study suggests that smoking acts specifically to decrease desire for sweet-tasting (and often high-calorie) foods. National studies matching cigarette consumption with total food sales in large populations found that sugar sales increased significantly during 1968 to 1972 (the same years cigarette sales dropped dramatically following a highly publicized antismoking campaign by the federal government), a relationship that did not hold up with other foods.

Of related interest are often-quoted experiments indicating that nicotine causes rats to increase their consumption of sugar-water and thus increase their body weights, and that carbon monoxide increases heart activity in rabbits. These studies, however, again reflect nonhuman metabolism, and they arbitrarily single out individual water-soluble (nicotine) or gaseous (carbon monoxide) elements of tobacco smoke while ignoring the vast complex of other solutes, nonsoluble substances, tars, gases, and particulates, which may have biologic activity alone or in combination.

Advice for the soon-to-be ex-smoker

What, then, can the person who plans to quit smoking anticipate? Many successfully break their habits and remain stable in weight; others, even with unchanged calorie intake, become heavier. The likelihood of obesity, however, has been exaggerated. The magnitude of the ex-smoker's weight gain generally is small and transient and is reversible with sufficient motivation. Precautions against unwanted weight should be taken from the outset of a program to quit smoking. They should include minor (and often virtually imperceptible) dietary adjustments or small but daily increases in physical activity, or both. Such vigilance may amount more to healthy correction of life-style habits than to punitive hardships.

Support and skilled counsel are available from such national organizations as Weight Watchers and TOPS Club (Take Off Pounds Sensibly) and from health clubs that promote safe exercises for all age groups. Literature is available through local medical and nursing societies, dietetic and fitness groups, and state lung associations. For the long-term maintenance of goal weight it is wise to follow a nutritionally sound diet. Unfortunately, there is an overabundance of well-promoted, gimmicky fad-diet plans on the market. Some people are wise, in the end, to tolerate a few extra pounds above "ideal" weight in return for the status of ex-smoker, with all the health benefits that state brings.

Drug Abuse

In the 1960s and 1970s drug abuse became a pervasive feature of life in the United States. The psychedelic 1960s introduced millions of college students and young adults to marijuana, LSD, mescaline, and other mind-altering substances, opening the gates to a flood of experimentation with herbal, pharmaceutical, and illictly manufactured substances. From cities and campuses the trend spread until, in the 1980s, drugs could be bought in virtually every hamlet, and users were as young as grade-school age. In 1982 it was estimated that marijuana was the number one cash crop of California. It has been said that if all the international cocaine dealers were to form a corporation, it would be the seventh largest in the U.S., passing Standard Oil (Indiana) Corp., which had $29.9 billion in revenues. Street sales of cocaine netted $30 billion in the U.S. in 1981; of marijuana, $24 billion.

Such huge sales totals indicated that these drugs were being consumed on a regular basis by millions of people from all socioeconomic levels and age groups. Furthermore, many people viewed regular drug use by adults as merely a life-style choice and favored only mild (or no) legal penalties. This change of attitude marked one of the major social changes in the U.S. in the second half of the 20th century.

Despite massive efforts at education, dangerous personality-altering, physically damaging drugs continued to be consumed throughout the U.S. In 1981 drug-enforcement officials cited trends that seemed to indicate that drug abuse was on the rise after declining through the 1970s. Of special concern was the "garbage" habit, taking a variety of drugs simultaneously.

Heroin

When the average person in the United States thinks of a drug addict, he is most likely to conjure up an image of a heroin user. Heroin addiction is a major public health and social problem; in 1981 there were at least 450,000 addicts in the U.S. It is estimated by the National Institute on Drug Abuse that this figure represents a fourfold increase since 1960. A 1982 report to the governor of New York estimated that there were 163,000 to 177,500 heroin addicts in New York City alone—one out of every 40 to 43 residents. A Rand Corp. study of California prison inmates revealed that heroin addicts each committed an average of 167 crimes a year—robberies, burglaries, and thefts—to support their habits. This represented a massive economic toll exacted from the victims of these crimes and from the public at large, since the costs ultimately filter down to the taxpayers.

Heroin is a derivative of morphine that was developed in 1898 by the Bayer Co. of Germany. It was initially thought to be less addicting than morphine and was briefly used as a treatment for morphine dependence. It was quickly recognized, however, that heroin was simply a more potent form of morphine. Despite its effectiveness as an analgesic, heroin is not approved for this use in the U.S. Although recent efforts to legalize the medical use of heroin for terminal patients have stimulated research comparing heroin with morphine, studies have failed to show any significant differences in the efficacy of the two drugs.

Although it was once primarily encountered only in ghetto areas of big cities, heroin and its attendant problems have spread through large areas of the U.S. Its use is no longer confined to people on the fringes of

Drug abuse has become so pervasive that theaters and other facilities that stage rock concerts now routinely have medical teams standing by to treat fans who are overcome while attending the performances.

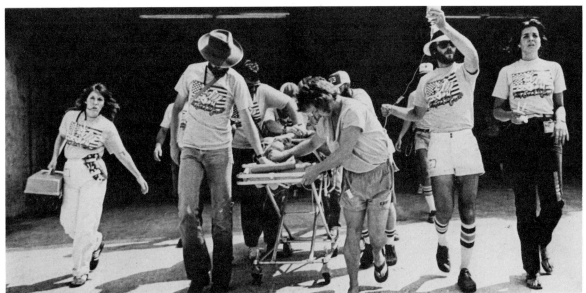

Terrence McCarthy—The New York Times

society. Street heroin varies widely in its quality but generally averages about 2–3% pure heroin. In 1981 and 1982 authorities in several large Eastern and Mid-western cities noted a resurgence of white heroin from the Middle East, which had declined in use in the 1970s, when brown heroin from Mexico was more common. The Middle Eastern heroin was much more potent—up to 16% pure. It is adulterated with milk sugar (for its bulk), mannite (for its fluffiness), and qui-nine (to give it a bitter taste similar to heroin). Although it is sometimes inhaled or injected subcutaneously (called "skin-popping"), heroin is usually injected intra-venously, since this route produces the most rapid on-set of effects with the smallest amount of drug. Unfor-tunately, this route is also responsible for the majority of the heroin addicts' medical problems because of contamination and infections from the use of unsteril-ized equipment.

Statistics indicate that the typical heroin addict in the U.S. is a male between the ages of 18 and 30 who is a minority group member (usually black or Puerto Rican) and lives in a large urban ghetto area. However, both male and female business and professional people—even health professionals—many of whom manage to hold regular jobs, also are heroin addicts. Some were experimenters with "recreational drugs" who dabbled in heroin, believing they could use it only occasionally or in moderation. In general, though, heroin addicts are poorly educated, have minimal skills for legal jobs, and have engaged in criminal activities prior to becoming addicted. Once addicted, most commonly the addict turns to crime to support his habit, which can cost hundreds of dollars per day; he may need to inject heroin three or more times a day to avoid the discom-fort of withdrawal. For most heroin addicts procuring the drug is a full-time occupation filled with risks and frustration. It is probably the arduousness of the heroin addict's life that leads to the cessation of drug use in older addicts. The price of heroin, its poor quality, and the uncertainty of maintaining a supply have, in addi-tion, led many addicts to seek substitutes for heroin.

"T's and Blues" — a heroin substitute

Pentazocine (marketed as Talwin by Sterling-Win-throp) is an analgesic drug useful in the treatment of moderate to severe pain. In the first years after its introduction in 1967, abuse of Talwin was rare and generally limited to health professionals who believed they would not get hooked. In the late 1970s, however, pentazocine, particularly in combination with tripelen-namine, became an attractive substitute for heroin. This combination, known as T's and Blues (from the color of some tripelennamine tablets), was particularly popular in cities where the heroin supply was low and the price was high. Although pentazocine is active when taken orally, it was most commonly injected intra-venously by abusers. The U.S. government's Drug

Abuse Warning Network (DAWN) reported that pentaz-ocine-related deaths and emergency room visits in-creased significantly in the early 1980s, particularly in the cities of Chicago and Philadelphia.

The typical pentazocine abuser is an ex-heroin user, although there are individuals addicted to T's and Blues who were not previously addicted to heroin. Most pentazocine abusers report that they use the drug as a substitute for heroin because it is cheaper and of more uniform quality. If given the choice, there is little ques-tion that most would prefer good-quality heroin.

Pentazocine has both morphinelike actions and weak morphine-blocking activity (antagonism). In con-trast to morphine and other opiates, pentazocine does not prevent or attenuate the heroin withdrawal syn-drome. Because of its antagonistic actions the drug actually precipitates withdrawal in individuals physical-ly dependent on heroin. After an addict has been with-drawn from heroin for several days, however, pentazo-cine (particularly in combination with tripelennamine) is reported to produce heroinlike physical and subjective effects (those resulting in mood alteration). If repeated-ly administered over a period of several weeks, pentaz-ocine will produce physical dependence of the opiate type, just like heroin.

The toxic effects of high doses of pentazocine are both psychological and physical. Overdosing may bring on manifestations similar to those of psychosis, includ-ing hallucinations (usually visual) and even psychotic behavior, delusions, and feelings of depersonalization. One of the most common physical complications of pentazocine abuse is ulceration and sclerosis (harden-ing) of the skin, subcutaneous tissues, and muscles resulting from repeated injections of the drug at the same site. In addition, the combination of pentazocine and tripelennamine has been found to produce convul-sions that can lead to death. Further, overdosage deaths from pentazocine can also result from respira-tory depression.

At the present time the pharmacology of the combi-nation of T's and Blues has not been investigated. Animal studies have shown that tripelennamine poten-tiates the analgesic effects of certain opiates, but whether this is true with pentazocine is unknown. Fur-ther, it is not entirely clear whether the addict is taking T's and Blues for the pentazocine or the tripelenna-mine effect. Many antihistamines have been abused by heroin addicts both alone as well as in combination with opiates. Although further research is necessary, it is clear that T's and Blues appeal to the same portion of the population that become addicted to heroin if it is available at a competitive quality and cost. Prevention of drug abuse in this population involves a combination of efforts including not only reduction of drug supplies through law enforcement but social change as well, which will provide meaningful alternatives to excessive and dangerous drug use.

Methaqualone — Quāāludes

Methaqualone is the generic name for a nonbarbiturate, sedative-hypnotic drug introduced into medical practice in 1950 by M. L. Gujral of India. Subsequently, alone or in combination with diphenhydramine (an antihistamine with sedative properties), it was marketed in Europe as a sleeping aid and daytime sedative. Methaqualone became available in the United States in 1965 under the brand name of Quāālude by W. H. Rorer, Inc. It was subsequently marketed by a number of other companies as well.

Because methaqualone is chemically unrelated to the barbiturate sedative-hypnotic drugs, it was initially believed that it did not share their dependence and abuse potential. However, within a few years after its introduction cases of street abuse, overdose, and both physical and psychological dependence were reported in the U.S., United Kingdom, and Australia. It is now generally acknowledged that despite its chemical differences methaqualone is pharmacologically equivalent to the barbiturate sedative-hypnotics. By the early 1970s it was widely abused in the U.S. It was particularly popular on college campuses, where it was also known as the "love drug" because of its purported aphrodisiac properties. Although it is the opinion of most experts that methaqualone does not directly stimulate sexual activity and pleasure, the drug, like barbiturates and alcohol, does reduce inhibitions and thus could indirectly lead to an increase in sexual activities in some individuals.

As a consequence of its widespread abuse in the United States, in 1973 methaqualone was placed under the strictest regulatory control possible for prescription drugs (*i.e.,* Schedule II of the Controlled Substances Act, which includes such widely abused drugs as opiates, amphetamines, and barbiturates). Although the methaqualone problem in the U.S. declined during the mid-1970s, in 1978 the prevalence of its abuse showed a sudden increase which continued into the 1980s. In addition to its older street names ("sopors," "ludes"), it is now also called "pillows," "disco biscuits," and "vitamin Q." Officials of the Drug Enforcement Administration (DEA) have recently stated that methaqualone was the second leading drug of abuse in the U.S., after marijuana.

Methaqualone at low to intermediate doses produces an intoxication very similar to that of alcohol. In 1981 reckless driving resulting from motor incoordination, slowing of reflexes, and loss of judgment and inhibitions produced by methaqualone was estimated to be a contributing factor in 20% of the fatal car accidents in some areas of the U.S., notably in Florida. Loss of inhibitions and judgment may also result in antisocial behavior. Overdosage with methaqualone presents special medical problems because of the complex effects that high dosages of this drug produce. In 1980, 5,300 emergency room "mentions" of

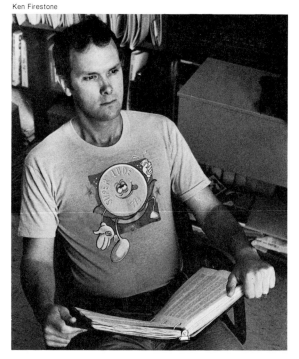

Ken Firestone

Quāāludes are a sedative-hypnotic drug used largely by students and middle- and upper-income groups. They are among the top-ranking drugs of abuse in the U.S. today.

methaqualone were recorded by the DAWN system, an increase of 137% in three years. When the drug is taken repeatedly over several days, tolerance to it develops, leading the user to take higher doses. Repeated use of methaqualone on a daily basis can lead to the development of physical dependence with a withdrawal syndrome similar in both its symptoms and severity to that of the barbiturates. In 1980, however, most individuals used methaqualone on a spree basis rather than in the continuous manner necessary to produce physical dependence.

In the early 1970s methaqualone was obtained largely from forged prescriptions, and the drug was therefore of standard quality and purity. In the 1980s, however, the vast majority of methaqualone sold on the illicit market is smuggled into the U.S. (much of it from Colombia) and is variable in its quality and purity. In 1980 it was estimated that over 100 tons of methaqualone were smuggled into the U.S., whereas fewer than 4 tons of the drug were manufactured and distributed legally. In addition to smuggled methaqualone, it is alleged that a number of Quāālude "look-alike" tablets (which contain other drugs such as aspirin, phencyclidine, or phenobarbital) are being sold by unethical pharmaceutical firms. In addition to these illegal sources of methaqualone or methaqualone substitutes, there have recently developed so-called stress clinics, where licensed physicians prescribe vitamins and methaqualone. Such stress clinics, which charge

231

$100–$150 per visit, give only peremptory physicals to their patients before providing a prescription for methaqualone. Since the price of methaqualone obtained in this manner is approximately half of the $5–$10-per-tablet street price, these clinics are very popular.

In 1982 a bill was introduced in Congress proposing to reclassify methaqualone as a Schedule I drug, confining its legal use to research only (as heroin is classified). Such laws had already been passed in Florida and Georgia in an attempt to close down the stress clinics. Medical supporters of the bill said that replacements for the drug were widely available.

In the latter part of 1980 and early 1981, data from DAWN indicated a slight decline in the abuse of methaqualone. Whether this reflects a significant trend in the abuse of methaqualone or only a temporary change remains to be seen. Only increased public awareness of the dangers associated with methaqualone abuse will have a major impact on this public health problem.

Cocaine

Cocaine, like morphine, nicotine, and caffeine, is a plant product that possesses psychoactive properties. Cocaine is found in significant quantities in only 2 of the over 200 species of the coca plant. *Erythroxylum coca* grows in the Andes in Ecuador, Peru, and Bolivia. *Erythroxylum novagranatense* is found in drier mountainous regions of Colombia as well as on the Caribbean coast of South America. This latter species is cultivated in Peru for export to the U.S., where after the cocaine is extracted the remainder is used as a flavoring in cola drinks. Coca-Cola once contained cocaine (hence its name) but eliminated the drug in 1906.

Archaeological evidence indicates that coca-leaf chewing has been practiced in Ecuador for over 5,000 years. In the Incan empire coca was considered a plant of divine origin, and its use was generally restricted to the ruling class. The appropriate occasions for coca-leaf chewing were highly ritualized, and casual use was considered a sacrilege. Following their conquest of the New World, the Spanish rapidly discovered that coca-leaf chewing produced a striking increase in the endurance of Indian workers, enabling them to work long hours at cold, high altitudes with little food. The coca leaf became a form of payment for Indian workers by their Spanish employers. Exportation of coca leaves to Europe occurred, but the practice of chewing the leaves never became popular, presumably because they lost their potency during the long sea voyage from South America.

The modern history of coca began when cocaine was extracted from the coca leaf and discovered to have local anesthetic properties in addition to its stimulant effects. Cocaine's stimulant properties were vividly described by Sigmund Freud. Freud experimented on himself with cocaine and found that it alleviated boredom and depression and increased his endurance for work. He felt that cocaine might be useful in the treatment of depression and other mood disorders. In addition, he attempted to use cocaine to treat a physician colleague addicted to opium, a treatment practiced in the U.S. at that time. This attempt, however, ended in disaster since the patient became dependent upon cocaine and used it in sufficient quantities to produce a toxic psychosis. Although Freud continued his personal use of cocaine, his interest in it as a psychotherapeutic drug waned. Cocaine's potential for creating serious problems was recognized by the German psychiatrist Albrecht Erhlenmeyer, who accused Freud of having unleashed "the third scourge of humanity" (the other two being alcohol and opiates). On the other hand, cocaine's use as a local anesthetic, which was pioneered by Freud's colleague Carl Koller, led to major advances in painless surgery. Although as a local anesthetic cocaine has been largely supplanted by other less toxic drugs (*e.g.*, procaine), it is still used in certain types of surgery of the nose and throat.

It was not long after its introduction that cocaine's powerful euphoria-inducing properties led many to consume the drug at frequencies and in quantities that produced toxic consequences. Both the seductiveness of cocaine and its toxic consequences were amplified when the drug was injected intravenously or snorted intranasally. The public's gradual recognition of cocaine's dangers led to its being removed from Coca-Cola as well as from a variety of other popular beverages containing cocaine (*e.g.*, Mariani wine). Its inclusion in the Harrison Narcotic Act in 1914 removed it from legal access to the general public except through medical prescription.

Cocaine has remained available through illegal sources, which are currently profiting to an incredible extent from the popularity of the drug. The National Narcotics Intelligence Consumers Committee has estimated that the retail value of cocaine imports is almost $30 billion per year. The profits involved are staggering because a gram of cocaine, which can be produced for a few cents, currently sells for $100 to $140 even after being cut with other substances by 50% or more. This quantity could easily be used by a single cocaine user in an evening. The mystique and reputation of cocaine today are at least in part influenced by its high price; it has been associated with sports figures and entertainers and in general with "life on the fast track." Although the price of cocaine would seem to limit its access to the affluent, it was estimated that over ten million Americans took cocaine in 1979, compared with an estimated 10,000 people in 1959. Among high school seniors interviewed in 1981, 16.5% reported they had tried cocaine, while 5.8% stated that they had used it in the past month. Prevalence figures for cocaine use are even higher at the college level but decline when people reach age 30.

The effects of cocaine depend both upon dose and

route of administration. By far the most common method of use is "snorting" the drug intranasally. Less frequently the drug is injected intravenously or chemically converted to a "free base," which is smoked with tobacco or marijuana. Cocaine produces effects virtually identical to those of other stimulant drugs such as the amphetamines. In recent experiments conducted at the University of Chicago, experienced cocaine users could not distinguish the *immediate* effects of intravenous cocaine from those of amphetamine. These effects include euphoria, feelings of self-confidence, energy, talkativeness, increased sociability, and in some individuals an increase in sexual interests. Cocaine also diminishes fatigue as well as appetite for food. The duration of cocaine's effects is much shorter than the amphetamine's, leading most users to multiple drug administrations. For some individuals the seductive effects of cocaine are sufficiently powerful that they continue to take cocaine every 30–60 minutes until the drug supply is exhausted. Since cocaine diminishes fatigue, individuals who have large drug supplies may consume cocaine for several days without stopping to rest. When totally physically exhausted or when drug supplies are finally used up, these compulsive users collapse and sleep for long periods of time ("crashing"). When they awake they often experience a period of depression (the so-called cocaine blues), which may lead them to seek out cocaine to get high again. This pattern of drug "runs" and "crashing" is typical for all stimulant drugs, but it is important to emphasize that this type of compulsive drug use occurs only in certain individuals.

The toxic consequences of cocaine are both physical and psychological. In addition to clinical reports of amphetamine-induced psychosis, it has been experimentally demonstrated that if amphetamines are taken repeatedly at high doses over only a few days, a toxic psychosis closely resembling paranoid schizophrenia will be produced in normal volunteer subjects. Symptoms of this toxic psychosis disappear as the drug is eliminated. Although it has not been experimentally demonstrated that cocaine can produce a similar psychosis, clinical reports of its occurrence are well documented. Of particular concern is that the paranoia that is prominent in this toxic psychosis can lead to violent and aggressive actions. Further, many clinicians feel that for certain individuals who may be predisposed to schizophrenia, the drug-induced toxic psychosis may exacerbate the underlying propensity.

Physical toxicity produced by cocaine is both direct and indirect. At high doses cocaine can produce convulsions, hyperthermia, cardiovascular collapse, and death. The repeated administration of sublethal doses often indirectly leads to physical problems because of cocaine's antifatigue and antiappetite properties, since exhausted, malnourished individuals may be less resistant to disease.

National Institute on Drug Abuse

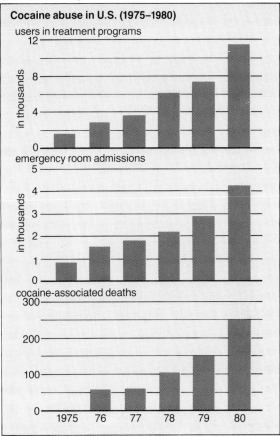

There is currently no uniformly successful therapy for individuals who compulsively abuse cocaine. Psychotherapeutic techniques as well as behavioral modification are currently being explored to determine their usefulness in treatment. At this time the single most important preventive factor limiting the public health consequences of its abuse is cocaine's high price. Continued efforts to diminish the quantities of cocaine smuggled into the U.S. are aimed not only at reducing supplies but at keeping the price of cocaine at a prohibitively high level.

Difficulties in drug-abuse monitoring

Despite the existence of large-scale systems set up by the federal government (*e.g.,* DAWN) to monitor drug abuse, estimates of the prevalence of abuse and the problems resulting from such abuse must be interpreted carefully. For example, a decline in the number of emergency room visits associated with a particular drug may reflect a decrease in its abuse, a more cautious use of it, or the development by a counterculture of the means for coping with drug-induced emergencies. Further, national statistics may not reflect the prevalence of drug abuse in a particular community. Finally, accurate self-reports by drug users are difficult to

233

obtain because of fears of exposure. Thus, statistics concerning the abuse of drugs must be viewed only as crude estimates.

It is also difficult to give an accurate description of the effects produced by a given drug. Credibility gaps often develop when people who have experimented with a drug read a description of its effects written by a supposed drug expert. The effects of a drug depend on the dose, route of administration, the individual's age, sex, previous drug use history, as well as expectations and the setting in which the drug is taken. Although it is common for many individuals to report the same drug experience, some find it horrible whereas others wish to repeat it as soon as possible.

It has often been assumed that those who find the drug experience pleasurable have an underlying psychopathology. Although it is true that many drug abusers do show some form of psychiatric disorder, it has not been established that the pathology has led to the abuse or vice versa. It is hoped that longitudinal studies currently being conducted will better enable us to determine the characteristics of individuals who are more prone to abuse drugs.

— Charles R. Schuster, Ph.D.,
and Chris-Ellyn Johanson, Ph.D.

Drugs

Aspirin is a drug that calls for superlatives. It is the most widely used of all medications; thousands of tons are consumed annually in the United States. It is one of the oldest and least expensive of all drugs and probably the most underestimated by the people who use it. If aspirin were first introduced in 1983, it would be heralded as a wonder drug because of its effectiveness for so many different maladies, it would probably be available only by prescription because of the dangers associated with its use, and it would certainly be expensive.

Before the Christian era physicians knew that ingesting the bark of a willow tree could relieve pain and fever. In the 19th century European scientists isolated and purified the active ingredient in willow bark and identified it as salicin, which was also present in many other trees and plants. From salicin these scientists prepared salicylic acid and tried it in patients. Salicylic acid proved to be effective in relieving pain, fever, and the symptoms of rheumatoid arthritis, but it was too irritating to the stomach to be acceptable for general use. A scientist working at the Bayer Co. in Germany synthesized a derivative of salicylic acid that proved equally effective and much less irritating; this was acetylsalicylic acid, which Bayer renamed aspirin just before the turn of the century.

Aspirin for pain relief

The effectiveness of aspirin in relieving pain is widely underrated. A single dose of two aspirin tablets is about

as powerful a weapon against pain as modern medicine possesses. For pain due to cancer, for example, aspirin has been found superior to oral narcotics such as propoxyphene (Darvon) and codeine. For pain after childbirth aspirin is as effective as such expensive prescription drugs as ibuprofen (Motrin) or naproxen (Naprosyn). For postoperative pain aspirin probably provides as much relief as any painkiller that can be taken orally. Only injected narcotics such as morphine have a clear-cut advantage over aspirin for relief of pain.

How aspirin works

Aspirin has three types of action that have been known throughout this century; in addition to its analgesic effect (relief of pain), it is antipyretic (lowers fever) and anti-inflammatory (reduces inflammation). However, as with so many other drugs, the mechanism of action by which aspirin achieved these effects was unknown over decades of extensive worldwide use.

In the early 1970s scientists discovered that pain, fever, and inflammation are all caused at least partly by chemicals called prostaglandins (which are manufactured by cells in the body in response to injury) and that aspirin inhibits the synthesis of these substances. Aspirin relieves pain by preventing the formation of prostaglandins that sensitize nerve endings at the site of the pain. It lowers fever by preventing the release of prostaglandins from those parts of the brain that regulate body temperature. Aspirin reduces inflammation by di-

"Personally, I never take anything but aspirin."

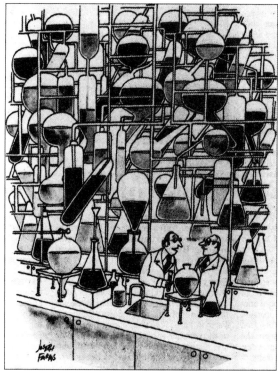

Drawing by Joseph Farris; © 1978 The New Yorker Magazine, Inc.

minishing the liberation of prostaglandins from cells that have been injured.

This inhibition of prostaglandin synthesis leads to a fourth therapeutic (or sometimes toxic) effect of aspirin that was, surprisingly, not recognized until long after aspirin became the world's most popular drug. Aspirin interferes with the function of platelets, cells in the blood that play a vital role in blood clotting. Just two aspirin tablets can double the time it takes blood to clot (the bleeding time), and this effect can persist for a week. This anticoagulant effect of aspirin can be useful therapeutically in preventing strokes caused by clots in the arteries of the brain or heart attacks caused by coronary artery thrombosis. But aspirin can also cause an undesirable tendency to bleed that can have serious consequences in hemophiliacs, in patients who have stomach ulcers, in people undergoing an operation, and in a number of other circumstances.

Effect on the stomach

For most people who take aspirin the effect of the drug on the stomach is the most important factor limiting their ability to use it. This is especially true of patients who regularly take large amounts of aspirin to relieve the symptoms of rheumatoid arthritis. Aspirin particles irritate the lining of the stomach and can cause bleeding; the anticlotting effect of aspirin can then make the bleeding worse.

Most people who take aspirin are unaware of the bleeding, which usually is very slight, but many do notice symptoms of dyspepsia (indigestion), heartburn, and nausea. The incidence of bleeding is highest with aspirin preparations that dissolve slowly and are deposited as large particles on the lining of the stomach.

Plain aspirin

In order to reach the bloodstream, aspirin tablets must first disintegrate and then dissolve. In some cases improperly manufactured tablets may be packed so tightly that they will not disintegrate, or they may crumble in the bottle and break down into salicylic acid and acetic acid, which smells like vinegar when the bottle is opened. Salicylic acid is probably as effective as undegraded aspirin but is considerably more irritating to the stomach. Many claims have been made, on the one hand, for the superiority of one brand of plain aspirin over another and, on the other hand, for the equality of all brands regardless of price. But so far no scientifically acceptable test has shown either that any brand of plain aspirin is more effective in relieving pain than any other or that expensive or inexpensive brands are equally effective.

Buffered aspirin

Particles of buffered aspirin tablets dissolve more quickly than particles of plain aspirin, so there is some basis for believing that buffered products might begin

Adapted from Thomas G. Kantor *et al*, "Oral Analgesic Studies: Pentazocine Hydrochloride, Codeine, Aspirin, and Placebo and Their Influence on Response to Placebo," *Clinical Pharmacological Therapeutics*, July–August 1966, vol. 7, no. 4, p. 449, © The C. V. Mosby Company

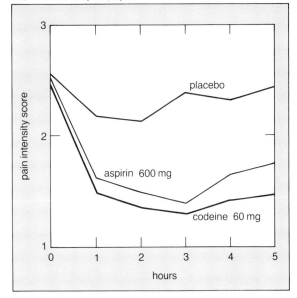

Analgesic time-effect comparison of single oral doses of aspirin, codeine, and a placebo in 49 surgical patients, each as measured by pain intensity scores and percent of patients with 50% relief.

to act more quickly than aspirin. However, this theoretical advantage in the rapidity of pain relief with buffered aspirin tablets has not been demonstrated in clinical tests. As for the widely held belief that buffered aspirin tablets cause less stomach discomfort than plain aspirin, available evidence indicates that this is not true. Clinical tests have recently shown that buffered aspirin causes as many ulcers and as much other gastrointestinal damage as plain aspirin.

Buffered aspirin solutions such as Alka-Seltzer are expensive, but some physicians believe that they may be the best way to take a single dose of aspirin. When aspirin is already in solution, the drug reaches the bloodstream more quickly than with a tablet that must first disintegrate and then dissolve. Since buffered aspirin solutions have much more buffering capacity than buffered tablets, they are much more effective in neutralizing gastric acidity, and they have been shown to cause less gastrointestinal bleeding than plain tablets. However, buffered aspirin solutions contain a great deal of sodium; they are not suitable for patients who must restrict their sodium intake, and continued long-term use of these solutions, as in treatment of arthritis, is probably not advisable for anyone.

Timed-release and enteric-coated aspirin

In timed-release aspirin preparations many small particles of aspirin are bound together in a capsule. In this form the absorption of aspirin into the bloodstream is delayed, and the presence of the drug in the body is prolonged. It has not been shown, however, that pain

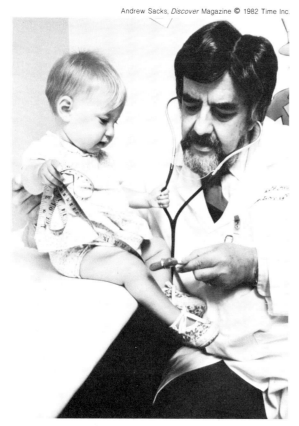

Recently an association has been discovered between aspirin administration in children and the development of Reye's syndrome, a potentially fatal disease.

relief from these preparations is also prolonged.

Enteric-coated aspirin tablets have a coating that does not dissolve until the tablet reaches the small intestine. They probably cause less bleeding than either plain or buffered aspirin tablets, but they may take a long time to produce a pain-relieving effect.

"More of the pain reliever that doctors prescribe most"

Some products, such as Anacin and Cope, contain 400 mg or more of aspirin per tablet, compared with 325 mg contained in the usual tablet of plain or buffered aspirin. Clinical tests indicate, however, that these higher doses of aspirin, which are likely to increase the incidence and severity of side effects, do not provide any detectable increase in pain relief.

Side effects

Aspirin has a double-edged effect that can cause serious bleeding from the gastrointestinal tract. First, the aspirin particles can cause bleeding by direct irritation of the stomach lining. Second, when aspirin reaches the bloodstream, it interferes with the function of platelets, which normally help control bleeding. Aspirin in solution may not cause irritation, but it can intensify

gastrointestinal bleeding that is already taking place. Patients who take aspirin regularly have been shown to have more than six times more ulcers and to require more than twice as many blood transfusions as otherwise comparable patients who do not take aspirin.

Much less commonly, aspirin can damage the kidneys. In rare cases even small amounts of aspirin can cause serious allergic reactions.

Aspirin versus acetaminophen

Acetaminophen is also an old drug, first used at the end of the 19th century. It has the same effect in relieving pain and lowering fever as the same dose of aspirin but has little anti-inflammatory activity and therefore is much less effective than aspirin for treatment of arthritis. The main advantage of acetaminophen (*e.g.,* Tylenol) over aspirin is that acetaminophen does not irritate the stomach and does not cause a bleeding tendency; therefore it is preferable for patients who cannot tolerate the gastrointestinal effects of aspirin and for those with bleeding disorders.

The main disadvantage of acetaminophen is the danger associated with overdosage in suicide attempts or accidental childhood poisoning. In overdose acetaminophen causes severe damage to the liver, which may not be apparent until several days after the drug was taken and then may be irreversible. In the United Kingdom acetaminophen (or paracetamol, as it is usually called in the U.K.) is more widely used than in the U.S., and it is a common cause of death by suicide. Aspirin poisoning is also potentially lethal, but it is easier to detect and much easier to treat.

Aspirin for children

Many different brands of aspirin are sold in smaller dosages for children. The standard children's tablet contains 80 mg of aspirin, compared with 325 mg in adult tablets. The number of tablets given to a child varies according to age and weight. Since some of these are flavored like candy, the greatest problem with aspirin in children has been accidental overdosage. Recently, however, an association has been discovered between aspirin usage in children and subsequent development of a serious disease called Reye's syndrome, with hepatitis and encephalitis that can be fatal. Although many children with Reye's syndrome have not taken aspirin and only a very small percentage of children who take aspirin develop the disease, the U.S. Public Health Service now recommends that aspirin not be given to children who might have influenza or chickenpox, the two diseases most frequently followed by Reye's syndrome. Since both influenza and the early stages of chickenpox may be indistinguishable from other types of respiratory infections, this admonition will probably lead to a sharp decrease in the use of aspirin to lower fever in children.

—*Mark Abramowicz, M.D.*

236

Special Report:

Solved: The Riddle of Thalidomide

by Joann Ellison Rodgers

In 1958 the sedative-hypnotic drug thalidomide was introduced in West Germany. Available without a prescription, it soon became that country's leading sleeping medication. It was also used by pregnant women to alleviate morning sickness. Thalidomide was sold, by prescription, in Portugal, Great Britain, Australia, New Zealand, and Canada. In 1960 a U.S. pharmaceutical company applied to the U.S. Food and Drug Administration (FDA) for permission to market thalidomide in the U.S., but medical officer Frances O. Kelsey refused to approve the application, citing inadequate information on possible side effects. Her decision proved to be prophetic.

Soon after the introduction of thalidomide, reports began to accumulate of an increased incidence of phocomelia, a birth defect in which the long bones of the arms, and sometimes those of the legs, are much shortened or even absent. Other defects included malformations of the gastrointestinal tract, eye, heart, and auditory canal.

In November 1961 West German scientists became the first to formally report that these defects were caused by thalidomide that women had taken during pregnancy. Their report described 150 infants born with phocomelic flipperlike limbs. In all, an estimated 6,000 thalidomide babies would be discovered. Helen Taussig, a well-respected Johns Hopkins University pediatrician who devoted her career to treating birth defects, was alerted to the threat by colleagues with overseas ties. She rapidly notified U.S. doctors and officials of the FDA and helped uncover serious weaknesses in experimental trials under way with thalidomide in the U.S. Thalidomide was removed from the world market in 1962.

In the four years that thalidomide was sold worldwide, only a few American women took the drug. One was a Phoenix, Ariz., television personality named Sherri Finkbine. Finkbine became a media celebrity when she underwent a widely publicized abortion in Sweden in August 1962 after failing in a month-long court battle to obtain the operation in the U.S. Swedish doctors confirmed that her fetus was deformed. Fink-

These West German children, born in the early 1960s to mothers who had taken the drug thalidomide, cope with their limb deformities. Klaus writes with the aid of a specially designed device for his shortened arm; Gabi, who has no hands, feeds herself by using her feet.

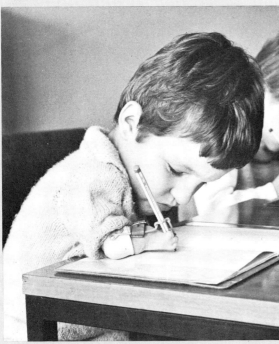
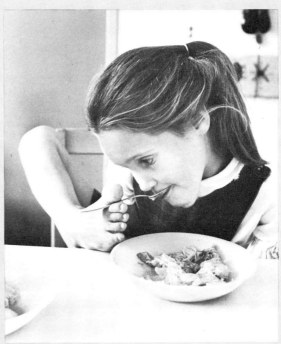

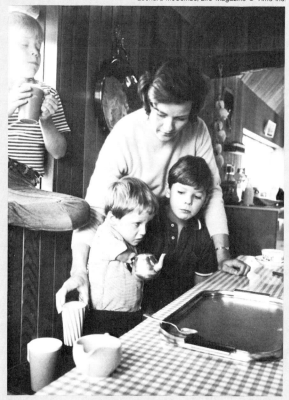

Thalidomide was taken by pregnant women, mainly in Europe, for four years before official reports of serious drug-induced birth defects in some 6,000 children emerged. This child is from Sussex, England.

bine and her husband later had a fifth child, a daughter, who was normal.

The publicity surrounding the Finkbine case and the narrow escape from mass disaster in the U.S. led to drastically tightened controls on drug testing and marketing. For an anxious public the worst seemed over.

The riddle of thalidomide solved

The fact that clinical trials had failed to reveal thalidomide's danger to the unborn left scientists uneasy. Moreover, it was not understood how the drug did its damage. Extensive tests on animals and humans had never uncovered the potential for teratogenicity, the ability to induce birth defects.

Now, more than 20 years after the first reports from West Germany, researchers have found answers to some puzzling questions about thalidomide's effects. The discoveries, published in the 1981 *Proceedings of the National Academy of Sciences,* have finally brought to a close a tragic chapter in the annals of drug marketing and testing. In the process they have also refocused attention on the shortcomings of tests used by the FDA and other regulatory agencies to assess drug safety, particularly for a pregnant woman and her unborn child.

The new research, fittingly, was conducted by a group of Johns Hopkins scientists from the departments of gynecology and obstetrics, pharmacology and experimental therapeutics, and pediatrics. The group was led by Stephen Spielberg and David Blake. In a series of studies they found that thalidomide slipped through drug safety screening tests because it behaves in a highly unusual way.

The compound, it appears, is not directly poisonous to living cells the way some drugs are. Instead, in order for thalidomide to do harm, its molecules require the presence of enzymes in the fetal or maternal liver, along with other natural products, to break down the drug into compounds called arene oxides. The arene oxides, which have been implicated in cases of animal chromosome damage since 1977, are the cause of the birth defects associated with thalidomide.

To prove their case against arene oxides, the Johns Hopkins investigators added the breakdown products, or metabolites, of thalidomide to specially prepared human white blood cells (lymphocytes) drawn from healthy volunteers. Not only did a subsequent assay reveal dead cells, it also enabled the scientists to precisely calculate the sensitivity of the cells to specific metabolites by counting the number of cells killed.

The metabolites themselves were obtained by mixing thalidomide with substances found in liver cells and with natural drug-altering chemicals made by pregnant animals. In effect, the experimenters created a test-tube model of how they suspected a female's body reacted to the tranquilizer. And the model turned out to be right on the mark.

The medical detective work that led to the model and the solution of the thalidomide puzzle grew out of studies dating back to 1967. These studies demonstrated that although rabbits and monkeys were sensitive to the effects of the tranquilizer, rats were not. Blake and Spielberg, along with co-researchers Gary Gordon and Venkataramn Balasubramanian, considered this an important clue because mammals, whether rats, monkeys, or humans, tend to have biological sensitivities that are more similar than different.

Analysis of the variations in the drug's effects on different species showed that thalidomide metabolites bind to rabbit and monkey (but not rat) liver cells and are able to dissolve in fat-protein complexes in those liver cells. The studies further identified several chemical by-products found in the urine of thalidomide-treated rabbits but not found in that of rats.

These results in turn led the team to suspect that thalidomide would produce arene oxides only under certain special conditions. That notion fit with what was known about thalidomide's preference for damaging only some fetuses and only at certain times during pregnancy. After more tests confirmed their early findings, the researchers discovered that it was possible to enhance the toxic effect of thalidomide on white blood cells by adding more liver-cell substances taken from pregnant rabbits. That enhancement did not take place if the liver substances were taken from pregnant rats. Indeed, the researchers could prevent thalidomide poisoning by adding enzymes known to interfere with those liver substances. Finally, analogues of thalidomide (drugs very similar in chemical design) performed the same way as thalidomide in the white blood cell tests, while two other drugs whose chemical structures were deliberately altered did not.

Applications to future drug testing

What is now known about thalidomide should lead to more accurate methods of testing other drugs for potential dangers to humans. It resoundingly confirms two principles of utmost importance in drug development and testing. First, the failure of a drug to cause damage in one species of animal is no guarantee whatever that it will not cause damage in another species. Second, current drug safety tests based on test-tube cell cultures do not necessarily reveal a drug's dangerous potential unless the drug's full biochemical breakdown cycle is investigated.

The thalidomide blood cell assay is one of many new tests the U.S. government is considering for inclusion in its expanded program of reproductive toxicity risk assessment. The program is led by a coordinating group of representatives from the FDA, the Consumer Product Safety Commission, the Environmental Protection Agency, the National Institute of Occupational Safety and Health, the Occupational Safety and Health Administration, and the Department of Agriculture. The goal of the group is to develop a bank of tests so sensitive and accurate that the likelihood of another thalidomide disaster will be greatly diminished.

At present, pregnant women are still being given drugs whose effects on their unborn babies are largely unknown. Studies suggest that eight out of ten women take prescription drugs during pregnancy; the average is four different drugs. Thus, in addition to the danger inherent in any one drug, there is the danger posed by drug interactions from both prescription and over-the-counter medications.

In some cases doctors may be lax in warning pregnant women about taking drugs and may prescribe too many of them. But the more important hazard is the glaring lack of information about the effects of drugs on the developing fetus. Because of ethical and legal problems, some 80% of all drugs on the market today have never been tested in pregnant women or approved by the FDA for that group. Pregnant women cannot be used as subjects in drug trials because of the possible danger to them and their unborn children; yet these are the two groups that this drug testing seeks to spare from harm. Moreover, human test subjects must give their consent before participating in drug trials—a provision clearly impossible for an un-

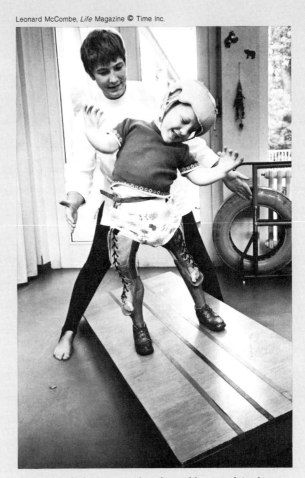

Only recently have researchers been able to explain the thalidomide tragedy. This knowledge should help prevent future birth defects that could be caused by other drugs.

born child. Testing of drugs in fetuses is a highly emotionally charged issue. Only a few states permit the use of aborted human fetuses to test the effects of drugs on the unborn. Yet fetal tissue is essential to such tests because animal studies—as the thalidomide case illustrates—do not always accurately reflect what happens in humans. Scientists need to know how drugs cross the placenta from mother to fetus and how the fetus absorbs and metabolizes drugs. And they need to know at what times in a woman's reproductive cycle an unborn baby is at risk. Drugs may damage a woman's egg supply long before she becomes pregnant or may, in a man, affect sperm just before conception, producing birth defects whose origins are nearly impossible to trace.

Solving the riddle of thalidomide has not eliminated the risk that other drugs pose to the unborn, but it has given scientists new insight and new strategies for reducing that risk in the future. In the meantime, women of childbearing age must still consider the avoidance of drugs to be the first line of defense against drug-related birth defects.

Special Report:

The Beta-Blocking Drugs
by Stephen E. Epstein, M.D.

Although the body's response to stress is complex, activation of the sympathetic (or adrenergic) system provides one of the major mechanisms through which rapid adaptations to stress are mediated. Two major arms of this system exist, consisting of a neural response and a hormonal response. The neural response to stress involves activation of sympathetic nerves, which release the chemical mediator norepinephrine locally to various organs and tissues. The hormonal response involves release by the adrenal gland of both norepinephrine and epinephrine into the blood, which delivers these hormones to all tissues and organs of the body. Norepinephrine and epinephrine, whether released locally or transmitted by the blood, then stimulate tissues to increased levels of activity as part of a generalized stress response.

The heart provides an excellent example of how the adrenergic system helps the body adapt to rapidly changing needs. Under resting conditions the heart beats 60–75 times per minute, ejects about 50% of the blood it contains, and pumps about five liters of blood each minute. During physical stress, release of norepinephrine and epinephrine cause the heart to work more vigorously and more rapidly such that during peak exercise the heart beats between 180 and 200 times per minute, ejects 70–90% of the blood it contains, and pumps more than 20 liters of blood each minute.

Norepinephrine and epinephrine contribute to the production of these changes by stimulating receptor molecules located on the cell surfaces of the organs that they activate. When these receptors are stimulated, a series of biochemical reactions occur leading to the typical organ response. There are two basic types of adrenergic receptors, termed alpha and beta. The muscle of the heart (myocardium) has few alpha receptors but has a rich supply of beta receptors. When its beta receptors are activated, the heart muscle responds by increasing its rate and the vigor of its contraction. The smooth muscle that lines blood vessels is well supplied with beta and alpha receptors. When stimulated, the beta receptors cause the blood vessels to dilate, whereas the alpha receptors cause them to constrict.

Effects of beta receptor blockade

In 1958 researchers synthesized the first of many compounds that are capable of blocking the stimulation of beta receptors by competing with epinephrine and nor-

epinephrine for available receptor sites. These drugs diminish the increases in heart rate and vigor of cardiac contraction that occur during physical or emotional stress, thereby decreasing the amount of blood pumped by the heart (cardiac output). Blood pressure levels are critically dependent on cardiac output, since blood pressure is a function of both the amount of blood pumped and the resistance to flow caused by the degree of constriction of blood vessels. Thus beta adrenergic receptor blockers not only slow heart rate but also decrease blood pressure as the result of lowering cardiac output.

In 1967 certain experimental findings suggested that two different subtypes of beta receptors existed. Like the blood vessels, the bronchioles (the tubes forming the passageway through which air is conducted into and out of the lungs) are lined with muscle that carry beta receptors. When these receptors are stimulated, dilatation ensues. In the case of the bronchioles, air passes more easily into and out of the lungs; in the case of the blood vessels, blood passes more easily into the capillaries and veins. If only one type of beta adrenergic receptor existed, then drugs capable of stimulating beta receptors of the heart would also be expected to stimulate beta receptors of the bronchioles and blood vessels. Some beta-stimulating agents, however, were found to be more potent in stimulating the heart, whereas others were found to be more potent in stimulating the bronchioles and blood vessels. To distinguish the two kinds of beta receptors, those that predominate on the cell surfaces of the heart were called $beta_1$ receptors, while those of the other type were called $beta_2$ receptors. *See* Table I.

Subsequently, beta-blocking drugs were developed that also had beta receptor specificity; that is, they were more effective in blocking $beta_1$ receptors than $beta_2$ receptors. Useful specific inhibitors of the $beta_2$ receptors have not yet been found. Among nonspecific beta-blocking drugs available for therapeutic use in the U.S. are propranolol (Inderal), nadolol (Corgard), and timolol (Blocadren). Specific inhibitors of the $beta_1$ receptors include metoprolol (Lopressor) and atenolol

Table I: Predominant type of adrenergic receptors present			
organ or tissue	*beta₁*	*beta₂*	*alpha*
heart	+	−	−
blood vessels	−	+	+
bronchioles	−	+	+

240

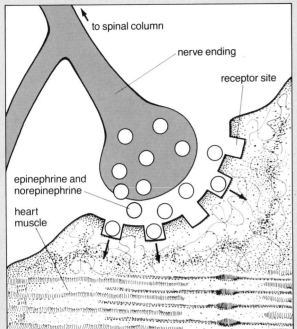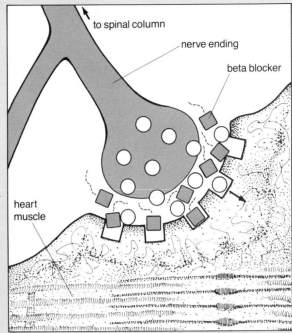

Part of the response of the sympathetic nervous system to stress involves release of the chemical mediators norepinephrine and epinephrine, which stimulate heart action by binding to beta receptor sites located on the cell surfaces of the heart muscle (left). Beta blockers counteract this effect by competing with epinephrine and norepinephrine for these sites, thereby reducing their availability (right).

(Tenormin). There are advantages to using a beta blocker that is more specific for the heart (beta$_1$ blocker). The main reason is that the major therapeutic effects of beta blockers are exerted through the blockade of the beta$_1$ receptors. No documented clinical advantage is gained from the blockade of beta$_2$ receptors. In addition, because some of the side effects of the nonspecific beta blockers are due to blockade of the beta$_2$ receptors, these effects are avoided when cardiospecific beta blockers are used.

Therapeutic actions of beta blockers

Angina pectoris. The heart is a working muscle and needs oxygen to satisfy its metabolic energy requirements. During physical stress, when the heart rate and contractile function of the heart increase, myocardial oxygen needs increase. These increased needs are met by an augmentation in the amount of blood delivered to the myocardium by the heart's coronary arteries. When coronary arteries are narrowed by atherosclerotic plaque, their capacity to deliver blood and oxygen to the heart muscle is compromised. Hence, when the heart's demands for oxygen increase, for example, during exercise, the blood vessels supplying the heart muscle may not be able to meet the increased needs. The situation that exists when the supply of oxygen is insufficient for tissue needs is called ischemia. The individual senses this imbalance as pain,

a common symptom of coronary artery disease that is termed angina pectoris.

One way of reestablishing the balance between the heart's needs for oxygen and the available supply of oxygen is to decrease its oxygen demands. The beta-blocking drugs achieve this effect by diminishing the increases in heart rate, vigor of contraction, and blood pressure that occur in response to physical stress. As a result the body is able to continue working at a given level of exercise demand, while the heart works less hard—ideally, at a level below that which would cause angina. The beta-blocking drugs work very well in this respect and are among the drugs most frequently prescribed for the control of angina.

Following acute heart attack. Recently it was demonstrated conclusively that administration of beta adrenergic blockers to selected patients significantly reduced deaths during the first year following acute myocardial infarction (heart attack). Table 2 summa-

Table II: Mortality in selected patients one year after acute heart attack			
drug	mortality rate without drug	mortality rate with drug	reduction in mortality
timolol	13.9%	7.7%	45%
propranolol	9.5%	7.0%	26%
metoprolol	8.9%	5.7%	36%

rizes the results of several studies involving different beta adrenergic blockers, which were given to heart attack victims who were felt to be candidates for this form of treatment. These figures are extremely encouraging, although administration of the beta-blocking agents still has not eliminated the problem of sudden death following heart attacks.

High blood pressure. There has now been wide experience attesting to the efficacy of the beta adrenergic blockers in the treatment of elevated blood pressure (hypertension). The precise mechanism by which these drugs lower blood pressure is not entirely known. However, it appears related to the blockade of the $beta_1$ receptor; this effect causes a decrease in the cardiac output, which in turn causes blood pressure to fall. Beta blockers are often used as initial therapy in the treatment of hypertension. In stubborn cases the drugs are employed in combination with other hypertension-reducing medications.

Other uses. The beta-blocking drugs have additional uses. One, timolol, has been found effective in lowering the intraocular pressure in patients with glaucoma, although the precise mechanism of action is not known. Reduction in pressure is achieved with a very low incidence of unpleasant local side effects, which are frequently present when other types of therapy are employed. Beta blockers have also been found useful in controlling some manifestations of psychological illness. For example, individuals with anxiety often develop tremors and palpitations, which may in turn contribute to maintaining or worsening their feelings of anxiety. Beta blockers, by decreasing the intensity of tremors and palpitations, can ameliorate to some extent the basic anxiety state. These drugs also have been used on occasion by lecturers, musicians, and actors to control symptoms of anxiety.

Side effects

As is the case with most drugs that have important therapeutic effects, patients taking beta blockers at times will experience troublesome and occasionally serious side effects. Some side effects are due primarily to inhibitory actions on the $beta_1$ receptor and others to inhibitory actions on the $beta_2$ receptor.

$Beta_1$ side effects. Patients with normal or near-normal heart function rarely will exhibit serious side effects due to the depressant effects that these drugs exert on the heart (by blocking sympathetic stimulation). However, in patients who have a weakened heart before therapy is begun, administration of beta-blocking drugs could further impair the pumping capacity of the heart. As a result, such patients may experience severe shortness of breath and fatigue and even accumulation of fluid in the lungs.

$Beta_2$ side effects. The beta adrenergic blockers can markedly increase the resistance to airflow through the bronchial passages of patients with asthma. These in-

dividuals have partially constricted air passages as a result of their asthmatic condition, and it is believed that circulating levels of epinephrine help maintain some degree of bronchial dilatation by stimulating the $beta_2$ receptors found in the muscles lining the air passages. Inhibition of the $beta_2$ receptors will thereby worsen the tendency to bronchial constriction. It has been shown that the $beta_1$-selective blockers have less tendency to produce bronchial constriction than the nonspecific beta-blocking drugs. Hence, $beta_1$-specific blockers are used most commonly in individuals who have asthma complicating their primary problem of angina or hypertension.

Some patients have a type of peripheral vascular disease involving constriction of the smaller blood vessels. One notable disorder of this type, called Raynaud's disease, is characterized by a sensitivity to cold such that fingers or toes turn progressively pale, white, and then purplish because of reduced blood flow to these tissues. Patients with such disorders often find that their symptoms become worse when they take beta-blocking drugs.

The responsible mechanism is probably similar to that which causes constriction of the bronchial passages. Epinephrine circulating in the blood maintains a certain level of dilatation of the smaller blood vessels located in the extremities. When the beta receptors of the blood vessels are blocked, this vasodilator influence is removed, and unopposed vasoconstrictor influences emerge. Again, it appears that this side effect is more likely to occur and is more pronounced when patients predisposed to this condition take a nonspecific rather than a $beta_1$-blocking agent.

Other side effects. Patients who are taking beta-blocking agents sometimes experience depression, poor memory, bad dreams, insomnia, fatigue, or impotence. Many of these symptoms are probably mediated by the central nervous system, and although not very common, they are not as rare as once believed. Although it is far from certain, some evidence exists suggesting that those beta-blocking agents that are water-soluble have a decreased tendency to produce these side effects than beta-blocking agents that are lipid-soluble (oil- or fat-soluble). This observation, if true, may find its explanation in the fact that water-soluble beta-blocking agents accumulate to a lesser extent in the brain than do lipid-soluble agents. Very recent research appears to have identified a minority of people who experience an exaggerated response to standard doses of the beta blockers because they lack an enzyme necessary for the breakdown and elimination of the drugs from the body. With continued use the drugs accumulate in the blood to levels that excessively reduce the heart rate, causing fatigue, dizziness, and fainting spells. It is possible that these people may still benefit from the beta blockers, but in dosages tailored to their particular response.

Emergency Medicine

A two-year-old boy is caught by his mother with several philodendron leaves in his mouth. A distraught woman takes an overdose of Valium and is brought to an emergency room. Several workers going into the hold of an unused barge to clean it develop shortness of breath and chest tightness; one man dies within minutes. All of these people have in common the fact that they have been poisoned.

A growing problem

Because of an increasingly heavy reliance on technology, poisoning, whether it be environmental, accidental, or intentional, is becoming a national emergency in the U.S. Today 5–10% of all ambulance transports, 10% of all emergency-room visits, and 5–10% of all medical admissions to hospitals are the result of poisoning. Between five million and eight million cases of poisoning are reported yearly. This figure may be only a fraction of the actual number of people poisoned who are unaware of the problem, not ill enough to report it, or ignorant of the fact that a network of agencies, the Emergency Medical Services Systems' Poison Control Centers, exists to help them.

Although anyone at some time may be exposed to a toxin, certain groups have a higher incidence of poisoning than others. For example, 59% of all cases of poisoning reported to the Food and Drug Administration (FDA) in 1979 were children five years of age or younger. Only 12% of those cases could actually be called toxic; *i.e.,* the patient had signs and symptoms of illness related to what was taken and required a visit to an emergency room or hospitalization. However, of the 41% of reported cases in persons over five years of age, about 52% were toxic. Whether these older people communicate their symptoms better or whether they take larger doses of a poison is not clear.

One reason for the high number of reported poisonings in young children is that they innocently take medicines that resemble candy; for example, vitamin tablets or baby aspirin. They also sample whatever looks interesting, such as plants, or things that smell good, such as perfume or furniture polish. Empty food containers inappropriately used for storing bleach, fertilizer, insecticides, paint, or other poisonous substances are unrecognizable to a preschool child for the lethal materials they hold. In people older than five, particularly teenagers and adults, drugs and medicines in various combinations (often in association with alcohol) are the leading toxic substances.

Developing a national strategy

For years people who were poisoned had to rely on their own doctors or their local hospital emergency rooms for advice and help. Unfortunately, these sources of aid were often as ill-informed as the patients about the toxicity of what had been taken and the manner in which it should be treated. One of the first efforts to deal with the growing problem of poisoning was the establishment in Illinois in 1953 of a poison center where poison-information specialists with special laboratory equipment attempted a scientific approach to toxicologic problems. Although the need for similar approaches in other states was evident, the gradual development of poison centers was hampered by a scarcity of trained staff, lack of funding, and poor communication between centers. No system existed

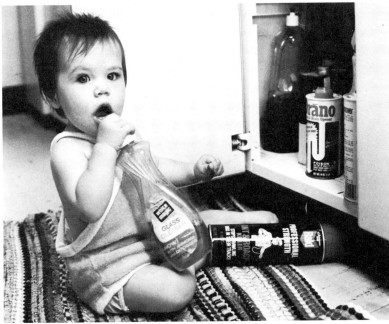

Brent Peterson, *Parade*

Of the seven million accidental poisonings reported to U.S. poison control centers in 1981, more than 80% involved children five years of age or younger. Most of these incidents took place while a parent was nearby. Small children are likely to put any substance into their mouths, even strong-smelling household cleaners and petroleum products.

nationally to coordinate the care of the poisoned patient; consequently, there was little improvement in the rising incidences of illness and death associated with poisoning.

In 1973 passage of the Emergency Medical Services Systems Act (PL 93-154) inaugurated the development of a national strategy to handle the emergency needs of the critically ill. Rather than the states themselves serving as the basic unit of organization, the U.S. was divided into 304 Emergency Medical Service (EMS) regions based in large part on preexisting health-care-delivery systems. Each EMS region was headed by a governing unit responsible for developing patient-care subsystems for particular problems; for example, multiple trauma, high-risk infants, burns, central nervous system problems, and toxicologic emergencies. Because of the high cost of setting up and running a poison center, the scarcity of trained poison specialists, and the relatively low number of actual patients, the toxicologic responsibilities of the EMS regions were combined into a suggested plan of 70 poison control regions. Model programs in San Diego, Calif.; Salt Lake City, Utah; Denver, Colo.; Boston, Mass.; and Nassau County, N.Y., pioneered the role that a comprehensive poison control center would play.

Poison control regions were defined with both geographic and demographic considerations in mind. Such natural boundaries as rivers and mountains as well as travel patterns within the area, governmental districts, and economic and trade patterns were considered. Also of major importance were the medical and educational resources already existing in the proposed region. In addition, the population base was evaluated. The ideal number of persons to be served by a given region ranged from approximately two million to about ten million, although maximum efficiency would probably be obtained with five million to six million. A population base of this size could be expected to generate about 300–400 calls per day to the center. This number of inquiries would provide the center with enough continuous experience to remain proficient in a variety of toxicologic problems, to develop meaningful treatment protocols, and to maintain the interest and motivation of the center's personnel. Defining regions in this manner also would allow urban and rural areas to share resources without overlap or duplication of services.

Poison control regions are organized using one of two basic models, called X and Y. In the X model a single centralized regional poison control center handles all calls both from the public and from health care professionals, arranges triage (sorting of patients and allocation of treatment for them) or referral, and follows up on calls received. The center is surrounded by many treatment facilities that provide care for the poisoned patient but have no information and consultation role of their own and are not responsible for developing protocols and programs for the area. Examples of the X

model are the San Diego Regional Poison System, the Massachusetts Poison System, and the Intermountain Poison System in Utah.

The other model is the Y model, in which a regional center is again the focal point for coordinating all programs in the region. In this model, however, there are also satellite poison control centers. Each satellite center receives calls for poison information and treatment protocols from the public and the local hospitals in its vicinity. Usually situated at a considerable distance from the regional center, this subcenter serves a population that does not necessarily identify either politically or geographically with the locale of the regional center. The Rocky Mountain Regional Poison System, for example, is based in Denver but has 26 satellite centers located in Colorado, Wyoming, Montana, and North and South Dakota and serves about four million to five million people.

Functions of a poison control center

A regional poison center has a multiplicity of functions. First and foremost it is a source of information about poisons. Always open, it provides free telephone access to comprehensive toxicologic information for the general public, such public services as police and fire departments, and health care professionals. In areas outside the center's local call zone an "800" toll-free number is publicized to permit free access to the center. The center itself is directly tied into its EMS region's hot line so that it can notify EMS ambulances of critical cases needing immediate transport and brief ambulance crews about any special treatment required en route to the emergency room. Using its expertise, the center's staff develops protocols for commonly encountered toxic syndromes (sometimes called toxidromes). These protocols can furnish a caller with consistent, easy-to-follow information for initial poisoning care. Prompt action based on accurate information may obviate the need to bring the patient to an emergency room. Health care professionals also are given standardized recommendations for case management.

Not only does a poison control center furnish treatment information, it develops treatment plans. It identifies hospitals located within its region by their ability to handle poison cases, since the choice of hospital may depend on the severity of the case or the support equipment and personnel needed for handling patients of a particular age group. Planning for treatment requires identifying regional ambulance, fire, or police transport systems to expeditiously transport patients to appropriate centers.

Furnishing poison information to callers for immediate needs is a limited form of education. Consequently, poison control centers offer a more structured and more extensive program of education for both health professionals and the public. The first group includes emergency-room physicians, critical-care nurses, para-

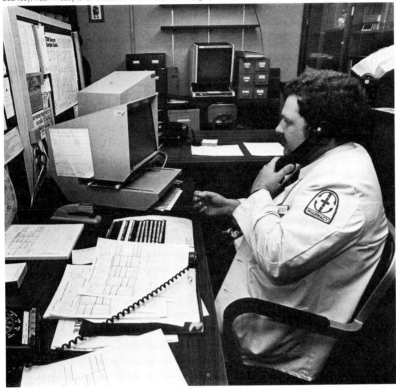

Always open, the regional poison control center is first and foremost a source of information about poisons. Calls to the center are taken by a poison information specialist experienced in toxicologic work. Microfiche data systems and a library of specialty publications assist the specialist in providing appropriate and up-to-date advice and support.

medics, and emergency medical technicians (EMT's). Conferences and seminars tailored for this audience stress first aid and general management techniques, but innovations and advances in toxicology are also featured.

The public must be included in poisoning education efforts since the best treatment for poisoning is prevention. Radio, television, and newspaper media are avenues for disseminating educational information regarding poisons. Special brochures left for distribution in drugstores and doctors' offices inform people of the existence and work of their local poison center and how to contact it. This literature also describes specific measures for preventing poisoning in the home. Simple precautions such as discarding old medications, not storing poisons in soda bottles or food jars, and keeping medications in containers with safety caps and well out of reach of toddlers can have a major effect on reducing incidents of poisoning. Talks and programs to parent and student groups, civic organizations, and legislative and industrial interest groups bring the staff of the poison center into direct contact with the people who use the center's resources and who are needed for its support.

The centers perform a data collection function, reporting to state and national agencies findings of cases brought to them. They compile statistics that result in profiles of toxicologic data. Research projects are often generated when clusters of cases or new toxic syndromes seem to be emerging. For example, one regional poison control center took calls from several area hospitals that had received children who were victims of a "nature salad" containing items picked in a forest by a well-meaning but poorly informed camp counselor. All of the children recovered, but the problems of plant misidentification leading to food poisoning and the toxic potential of some health foods (such as sassafras and herbal teas) that were highlighted by this "epidemic" generated several articles in medical journals and stimulated interest in local seminars on botanical toxins.

The poison control team

Because of the enormity of the task of protecting the public from toxicologic dangers, poison centers use an interdisciplinary team approach. Each staff member must bring to the job specific training or experience within the field of toxicology. Good interpersonal skills are also essential.

The director of a regional poison control center is usually a physician with specialization in internal medicine, pediatrics, or emergency medicine. Since the field of toxicology is expanding, many directors are now taking a certifying examination given by the American Board of Medical Toxicology.

The director of a regional center plays a dual role. As a clinician he provides direct patient care and serves as a consultant on hospitalized cases of poisoning. He is responsible for quality assessment and quality assurance through direct medical supervision of the staff as well as audits of poison cases handled by the center. He develops new protocols that will ensure consistent and rational treatment for poisoning victims. As a manager the director must set organizational goals while still maintaining an overall perspective of the national system. He must work with other directors to integrate programs, share ideas, and define national goals and priorities. The ability to negotiate governmental bureaucracy is needed to assure funding and legislative support for the center. Finally, enthusiasm and commitment are necessary to motivate the staff to strive for ever better patient care and to win public confidence.

The majority of poison control centers have no single funding source. All costs for establishing and maintaining a regional poison center, which at a conservative estimate can be a half million dollars for start-up and a quarter million for an annual budget, have to be met by support from numerous sources since many different agencies participate in the center's activities. The medical director, therefore, has the difficult job of gaining financial support from federal, state, and local governments, from regional EMS agencies, from medical institutions in the area, and from grants and donations provided by industry and individuals. The director needs to be a good fund raiser and financial manager to stay on top of escalating costs and precarious resources, for without his efforts the center would be unable to maintain itself.

Calls to the poison center are taken by a poison information specialist formally trained in nursing, pharmacology, medicine, or a similar field and experienced in toxicologic work. These specialists are the front-line people who function as the point of contact between the public and the poison center. Their communication skills and interpersonal abilities are of the utmost importance since they must be able to extract needed information from callers, who may be hysterical, hostile, or possibly very ill, and must give support and advice. They will ask for specific information from callers who are trying to identify a poison and its harmfulness. Using the references at the center and drawing on their own expertise, they can provide appropriate information on home treatment or advise interim measures to be instituted while transport to a medical facility is being arranged. Once a patient arrives, the poison specialist can continue to play an active role by providing information to the attending physician about the pharmacology of the toxin and the suggested treatment.

The poison information specialist participates actively in teaching physicians-in-training, medical students, and pharmacology students; in community poison-prevention programs; and in helping the medical director gather information for toxicologic research.

"All substances are poisons; there is none which is not a poison. The right dose differentiates a poison and a remedy." Although these words of the 16th-century physician Paracelsus are still true, because of the astronomical increase in the number of new substances being manufactured today, along with all potentially poisonous plant and animal material, no one specialist can hope to have all the answers in all situations. For this reason poison control centers maintain a list of specialty consultants on call 24 hours a day to provide the center's regular staff with expertise in very limited or specialized areas of toxicology. This extended staff may include veterinarians with interest in snakebites, entomologists with knowledge of insect venoms and stings, botanists who can help with plant or mushroom identification, chemists with an understanding of industrial chemicals, pharmacologists with skill in sorting out the complicated physiologic consequences of multiple drug overdoses, and subspecialty physicians (such as pathologists, neurologists, and nephrologists) who can lend insight into the actual clinical management of a critically poisoned patient. Many of these people are volunteers who donate their time and experience because they are stimulated by the challenges to their skills that toxicology provides.

Resources of the poison center

The poison control center is usually located within a hospital or in the immediate vicinity of one. Informational resources are normally kept at the center, but the laboratory, which does not need to be directly on site, may be situated elsewhere. Textbooks describing general and specific management of both acute and chronic poisoning play a major role at the center in defining appropriate care. Journals, manuals, case reports, foreign books, and old books (unfamiliar medicine or out-of-date compounds occasionally are ingested) are also included in the center's library. Microfiche data systems such as Poisindex and Toxifile are becoming increasingly popular. These computer-generated information files on consumer products are cross-referenced and continually updated by their publishers, thus making product identification easier for the poison information specialist. Most poison centers also maintain a comprehensive, updated file-card system issued by the National Clearinghouse for Poison Control Centers.

The institution with which the regional poison center is affiliated is either a medical school or a major teaching hospital. This kind of association permits the center access not only to the general medical library in the teaching institution but also to some of the on-line computerized systems available only in large libraries. One of these systems, Toxline, the National Library of Medicine's toxicology data bank, has subsystems that give information on occupational toxins and mutagenic and teratogenic substances.

Another benefit from the poison center's close affiliation with a medical institution is the presence of many experts who can consult with the poison center as the need arises and assist the center's staff in educational programs. Yet another benefit is the availability of sophisticated patient-care facilities that permit handling victims of rare or unusual poisonings or patients who require extremely difficult and complex treatment.

Some resources of the poison control center, although not nearby, do provide much useful information. Such federal agencies as the FDA, the Consumer Product Safety Commission, and the Environmental Protection Agency are frequently consulted. Many manufacturing associations or groups like the National Pesticide Telecommunications Network or the Chemical Transportation Emergency Center provide nongovernmental support and act as important sources of information.

The laboratory of a modern poison center is one of the major reasons such centers must be regionalized. Necessary equipment may cost hundreds of thousands of dollars, and the technicians running the tests need sufficient cases to maintain their techniques and skills. The director of the laboratory is usually a faculty member of a medical school, and the laboratory itself may be incorporated into the school's pathology, laboratory medicine, or pharmacology department. Alternatively, it may be affiliated with the city or state medical examiner's (coroner's) office. The technicians in the laboratory need to regard themselves as an integral part of the regional poison center since they can tell the poison information specialists what types of specimens are needed (*e.g.*, blood, urine, gastric contents, or body tissue). In turn they depend on clinical information to help them in narrowing the range of possible tests to be run and in interpreting test results. The better the rapport between the laboratory and the clinical staff of the poison center, the better will be the speed and accuracy of diagnosis.

Until the late 1950s most toxicology labs depended on chemical tests and reactions, thin-layer and paper chromatography, and spectrophotometers using ultraviolet, visible, or infrared light. Later, development of the gas chromatograph permitted separation of complex chemicals and mixtures of chemicals from body tissues and fluids. In the 1970s this equipment was further refined and combined into machines that not only could perform these tests but also had built-in computers to help analyze the data obtained. Today's toxicology laboratory—equipped with high-pressure liquid chromatographs; nuclear-magnetic-resonance, fluorescence, and atomic absorption spectrophotometers; and immunoassay techniques—lets the toxicologist identify poisons in minute quantities and with an accuracy unattainable in the past.

A positive effect

Recognizing that all three sides of the epidemiologic triangle—namely, host, environment, and agent—con-

tribute to every case of poisoning, poison control centers are starting to have an effect. For example, the poison prevention project in Rochester, N.Y., in the late 1970s was associated with a 60% reduction in hospital admissions for poisonings and a 40% decrease in poisonings treated in emergency departments in the Rochester area. Engineering efforts to create a safer environment, as mandated by the national Poison Prevention Packaging Act of 1970, have resulted in child safety caps, safety mechanisms to limit the dispensation of products from their containers, and single-dose drug packaging. Poisonings from products that switched to safety packaging decreased by 38% from 1973 to 1976 among children under five years, and the number of accidental deaths of children under five from aspirin, a safety-package-regulated product, declined 56% in 1977 over 1976. With the interest and effort that are now being put into the development of professionally run poison centers, the future is bright for saving lives.

—Mary Jane Koren, M.D.

Gastrointestinal Disorders

Recently introduced drugs that help the body achieve the normal but delicate balance between the aggressive activity of gastric juice and the natural resistance of the digestive system to that activity have contributed much to the effectiveness of modern treatments for peptic ulcer. On another front a successful large-scale clinical trial has crowned a decade of efforts to develop a safe and effective vaccine for hepatitis B, a serious viral infection of the liver. Additional highlights of gastroenterological research include progress in understanding the physical basis of irritable bowel syndrome and a suggestion that abnormal conditions in the stomach may allow the production of carcinogenic substances responsible for stomach cancer.

Modern peptic ulcer drugs

Peptic ulcer is a sharply demarcated loss of the inner lining of those parts of the upper digestive tract exposed to gastric juice containing hydrochloric acid and the digestive enzyme pepsin. The organs subject to ulceration consist of the lower esophagus, the stomach, the upper intestine (especially the first portion of the duodenum), and that portion of the small intestine adjacent to a surgically produced connection with the stomach. Peptic ulcers are believed to occur because of a decrease in the protective action of the mucus secreted by the epithelium, an increase in gastric secretion, or a combination of both. Drugs used to treat ulcers reduce the secretion of acid and pepsin, neutralize acid, directly protect ulcers from acid and pepsin, or help promote natural mucosal protection.

Antisecretory drugs. Certain drugs are known to block the stimulating action of histamine on the acid-secreting cells (parietal cells) of the stomach, resulting in a reduction in acid secretion. Use of these drugs, as well as of antacids, follows from observations that ulcer disease is very unusual in the absence of gastric acid and pepsin and that the activity of acid and pepsin is markedly decreased when the acidity of the stomach contents falls below a certain measured level (when the pH is above 3.5). In addition to cimetidine, which has had dramatic success as a treatment for peptic ulcer since its introduction in the late 1970s, other such histamine blockers (technically, H_2 receptor antagonists) have been developed. These newer drugs, ranitidine, for example, are more potent and longer acting than cimetidine and thus need to be taken less frequently for a similar therapeutic response.

A number of clinical trials in recent years have shown that both gastric and duodenal ulcers heal better after treatment with cimetidine than with placebo treatment. In addition, cimetidine is useful in preventing their recurrence, although many duodenal ulcers recur after treatment with cimetidine is stopped. Side effects are, for the most part, infrequent, but extended use (longer than one year) should be undertaken only under special circumstances since the long-term effects are still unknown.

Coating agents. In contrast to antacids, coating agents do not neutralize gastric acid; instead they heal peptic ulcers through a local effect. They are believed to bind to dead tissue at the base of ulcers and to form a protective barrier, shielding the ulcer crater from further effects of pepsin and acid.

Sucralfate is among the newest medications to be released for ulcer therapy. Chemically it is the aluminum salt of a sulfated disaccharide (a complex sugar). When sucralfate enters an acidic milieu such as the stomach, its consistency changes to that of a viscous, pastelike substance. Under such conditions sucralfate is negatively charged and binds to positively charged tissue proteins in the ulcer crater. Sucralfate also binds pepsin and bile acids (thought to be important in some aspects of ulcer development). Clinical studies have indicated that sucralfate is as effective as cimetidine in the therapy of duodenal ulcers, and the drug is undergoing extensive evaluation in the therapy of gastric ulcers. The overall incidence of side effects is similar to that of cimetidine.

Bismuth compounds (such as Pepto-Bismol) also coat ulcers and are thought to be effective in healing both gastric and duodenal ulcers. One especially promising compound in this group, tripotassium dicitratobismuthate, is not yet available in the U.S.

Agents that increase mucus secretion. Licorice gets its distinctive sweet taste from glycyrrhizic acid, which is the active principle of carbenoxolone, a drug that has been used in countries other than the U.S. to treat ulcer patients. Carbenoxolone increases the production, se-

Peptic ulcers occur in those parts of the upper digestive tract that are exposed to gastric juice and the enzyme pepsin. There is a loss of the lining of the digestive tract at the location of the ulcer.

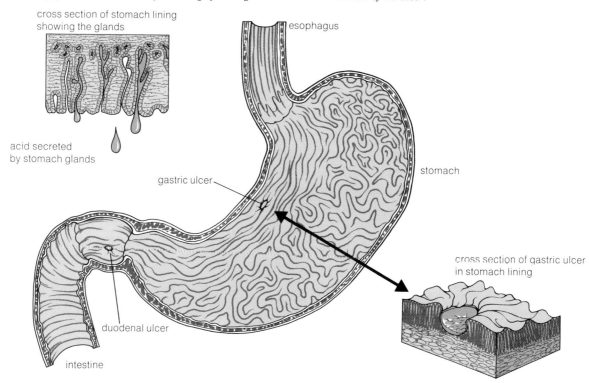

cross section of stomach lining showing the glands

acid secreted by stomach glands

esophagus

stomach

gastric ulcer

cross section of gastric ulcer in stomach lining

duodenal ulcer

intestine

cretion, and viscosity of mucus and strengthens the ability of the stomach lining to resist gastric acid. Clinical trials have demonstrated its effectiveness in healing both gastric and duodenal ulcers. Unfortunately, carbenoxolone has actions similar to those of the steroid hormone (mineralocorticoid) aldosterone; such serious side effects as sodium and water retention and hypertension occur.

Prostaglandins are derivates of arachidonic acid. The naturally occurring forms are rapidly inactivated within the stomach. However, a number of synthetic prostaglandin analogues (*e.g.,* 16,16-dimethylprostaglandin E_2) are effective against peptic ulcer when taken orally. Prostaglandins increase mucus secretion, stimulate gastric secretion of bicarbonate (an acid neutralizer), and increase blood flow to the gastric mucous membranes. Some prostaglandins also inhibit acid secretion and reduce pepsin secretion. These drugs are currently undergoing clinical evaluation for treatment of peptic ulcer in the U.S. and other countries.

Irritable bowel syndrome

Irritable bowel, or colon, syndrome is probably the most common gastrointestinal disorder in Western societies. Symptoms are often present for many years although they may be intermittent. The key features are alteration of bowel habits and abdominal discomfort or distention, particularly after eating, in the absence of a demonstrable cause. For victims in their middle years, especially, a specific cause for such symptoms should be sought before a diagnosis of irritable colon syndrome can be made by exclusion. Diagnostic tests that may be employed include flexible sigmoidoscopy, examination of the stools for blood or parasites, and X-rays of the lining of the stomach and intestines. It may be necessary to examine the inside of the stomach or colon using sophisticated flexible fiber-optic instruments. Occasionally computerized tomography or ultrasonography is used to search for a cause for the pain in the pancreas and other structures that are not readily visualized by other techniques.

Irritable colon syndrome is not an inflammation, and the terms spastic colitis or mucous colitis are totally inappropriate. It has no relationship to ulcerative colitis or other inflammatory bowel diseases, and it does not lead to cancer of the intestine.

Investigations of the physical basis of this disorder have concentrated on studies of the behavior of the colonic muscle, although neither cause nor cure has yet been found. The colonic musculature in victims of the disorder differs from that in normal individuals and shows a characteristic type of slow-wave activity that does not occur in other gastrointestinal disorders. After a meal in normal individuals there is an increase in electrical ''spike bursts'' from the musculature, which correlate with increased peristaltic movement of the colon (leading to evacuation). In persons with the syndrome the increase in electrical activity is not as pronounced. Normally the presence of consumed fat and protein in the duodenum stimulates the release of the hormone cholecystokinin, which prompts the gallbladder to release its store of bile salts, thereby aiding the digestion of fat. Individuals with irritable colon syndrome are more sensitive to this hormone and will experience abdominal pain. These patients often, but not invariably, exhibit particular personality traits. They tend to be overly methodical and conscientious and possess fairly rigid behavior patterns.

After exclusion of a specific cause by appropriate tests, management of these patients includes adequate reassurance and explanation about the nature of the disorder. Some patients may need supportive psychotherapy. Treatment to control symptoms must be individualized. For example, certain patients require medication or dietary manipulation to control diarrhea, while others need relief from constipation. For the latter group an increase in dietary fiber often is helpful. Some patients have an intolerance of lactose (milk sugar), which can promote diarrhea. For such people excluding lactose from the diet may help. Alternatively, the milk can be pretreated by adding an enzyme (lactase) derived from bacterial sources.

Current research efforts are directed at understanding the roles of dopamine and other neurotransmitters, enkephalins, and hormones (including cholecystokinin, gastrin, and glucagon) in the control of the neural and muscular elements of the colon. New techniques of studying the colon in the body are providing important clues about the relationship between such stimuli as psychological stress and eating and the electrophysiological responses of the muscle.

Hepatitis B vaccine

A recently developed vaccine against the virus responsible for hepatitis B has been shown in clinical trials to be effective and safe and has been made commercially available for medical use in the United States. The groundwork for active immunization against hepatitis B was laid by the work of Saul Krugman and co-workers at the New York University Medical Center from 1970 to 1973. They found that diluted blood serum capable of causing hepatitis B infection lost its infectivity when boiled for one minute but retained its antigenicity (the ability to stimulate an immune response). When used as a vaccine, the serum prevented or modified hepatitis B in 70% of vaccinated patients who subsequently were inoculated with infectious material. It was later shown that the serum contained large quantities of Australia antigen, or hepatitis B surface antigen (part of the viral protein coat), discovered by Baruch S. Blumberg in 1964. Maurice Hilleman at the Merck Institute for Therapeutic Research in Pennsylvania developed a more sophisticated vaccine, which consists of highly purified, formalin-inactivated surface antigen derived

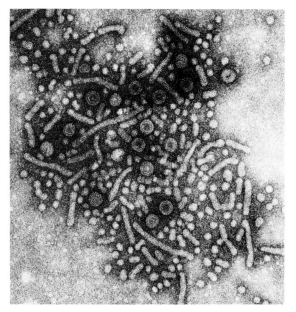 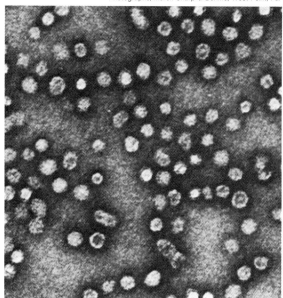

A newly formulated vaccine has been shown to be effective against the highly communicable hepatitis B virus (photomicrograph at left, larger round particles). The vaccine (photomicrograph at right) contains particles of Australia antigen, which stimulate antibody protection against the virus.

from the plasma of chronic carriers of the antigen. Extensive testing was first done in marmosets and chimpanzees, and its safety and ability to cause formation of antibodies was confirmed in a later evaluation using human volunteers.

In mid-1978 a large-scale field trial was begun in a group of male homosexuals who agreed to participate in a randomized, controlled study. The risk of hepatitis B infection is unusually high in this population, 20 to 30 times that of the general population. The vaccine trial was conducted with the cooperation of five clinics serving homosexual men in large cities across the U.S. The volunteers were required to have no serological evidence of ongoing or past hepatitis B infection. This was established by the absence in the subject's blood of viral surface antigen, antibody to surface antigen, and antibody to the viral core antigen.

Within two months of administration of the vaccine, 77% of the vaccinated persons had high levels of antibody against the hepatitis B surface antigen. This rate increased to 96% after the booster dose. During the next 18 months hepatitis B developed in only 1.4–3.4% of the vaccine recipients, compared with 18–27% of placebo recipients. No one with a detectable immune response to the vaccine developed evidence of a clinical attack of hepatitis or of viral infection in the bloodstream. Interestingly, a significant reduction of incidence was already seen within 75 days after vaccination. Since the incubation period of hepatitis B is relatively long (six weeks to six months), this observation suggests that the vaccine may modify early cases even before a strong antibody response has occurred. The vaccine was safe, and only 8% of the recipients reported a sore arm lasting one day.

Guidelines for use of the vaccine are currently being formulated. Initially it will be offered to certain high-risk groups, including hospital personnel (especially surgeons and those exposed to blood products), dialysis workers, and blood transfusion recipients in addition to male homosexuals. Patients undergoing maintenance hemodialysis are also exposed to infectious doses of the virus.

Development of the vaccine and the proof that it prevents hepatitis B represent an extemely important advance in the control of this devastating and widespread disease. The number of cases of acute hepatitis B in the U.S. is approximately 100,000 per year, with a fatality rate of 1–2%. The total number of carriers is estimated to be about 800,000 persons in the U.S. and 200 million throughout the world. The majority of carriers show no symptoms, but many eventually develop chronic active hepatitis, a severe form of destruction of the liver that can eventually lead to cirrhosis. The architecture of the cirrhotic liver is markedly deranged, with a substantial increase in fibrous tissue (scarring), and the delicate biochemical functions performed by the normal liver may be substantially altered.

The hepatitis B virus has been incriminated as the single most important cause of primary hepatocellular carcinoma, an extremely common disease in Asia and Africa. It is therefore reasonable to hope that mass immunization programs against infection with hepatitis B virus may ultimately reduce the incidence of this form of liver cancer.

250

Cancer of the stomach

The incidence of stomach cancer varies considerably from region to region throughout the world, allowing study of the environmental and genetic factors in its causation. For example, the incidence rates in Japan for men and women are 60 and 39 per 100,000, respectively. In marked contrast, the incidence in the U.S. has dropped sharply over the past 40 years to the present figure of 8 per 100,000 for white males. Interestingly, studies of Japanese immigrants to Hawaii and their offspring have shown a decreasing incidence compared with native Japanese.

It is suspected that diet may be important in the causation of stomach cancer. N-nitroso compounds, or nitrosamines, are possible causative agents. An increased incidence of gastric cancer is found in those whose stomach lining is unable to produce acid as a result of chronic inflammation or atrophy. Under such circumstances, the stomach can become populated with bacteria that accelerate the endogenous formation of nitrosamines. In addition, these bacteria reduce dietary nitrate to nitrite, which can react with various dietary constituents to form nitrosamines. Although there is no definite proof that these compounds cause cancer in humans, the circumstantial evidence is substantial, and no animal species has been found to be resistant to their carcinogenic effects.

In the U.S. the increased availability of refrigeration may have contributed to the decline in stomach cancer by helping to reduce the bacterial content of food and thus the production of nitrite from nitrate. Ascorbic acid (vitamin C) also has been shown to inhibit the nitrate–nitrite reaction, and it has been speculated that rising use of this compound in the U.S. may also be a contributory factor.

— Bernard Levin, M.D.

Glandular and Metabolic Disorders

It is now an acknowledged fact that diabetes is not a single disease. Rather, it is a series of related metabolic and endocrine disorders having two aspects in common: poor regulation of the blood sugar level, leading to a chronic rise in circulating blood sugar, and inadequate insulin action due either to poor or absent production of insulin or to a lack of proper action of insulin in the tissues. Further research will undoubtedly identify various forms of diabetes according to their causative mechanisms. The causes must be ascertained for each form so that appropriate forms of treatment can be developed.

The majority of diabetics, 85–90%, have the less severe adult-onset form, type II. This type can usually be controlled through diet. Type I diabetes, the juvenile-onset form, affects 10–15%; this severe type must be controlled by daily subcutaneous injections of insulin. Patients who develop diabetes early in life are more likely to have trouble with complications of their disease; complications often take years to develop, and a person whose diabetes becomes active late in life may be spared them altogether.

Two possible predictors

It has been known for many years that diabetes has a familial component, and much research has been done to try to determine if it is possible to predict which persons will develop diabetes in later life. The complicated causation of the disease has made precise predictions difficult.

In February 1982 the results of an interesting study were reported in the *Journal of Clinical Endocrinology and Metabolism.* The study followed 52 women, most of whom were overweight, a factor known to be associated with diabetes. Researchers found that women whose excess weight was found primarily in the upper body were eight times more likely to develop diabetes than those with excess lower-body fat. This finding was linked to the type of fat cells present: in women with excess upper-body weight, the individual fat cells were found to be greatly enlarged but with a decreased number of receptors on the cell surfaces through which insulin is able to bind to the cells and perform its function in the body's metabolism. In response to the lack of receptors the body produces an excess of insulin. In women with excess lower-body weight the fat cells were of normal size with an adequate number of receptors; there were simply more cells. This finding also helps to explain why it is often easier to lose weight in the upper body—the enlarged cells shrink to normal size. It is more difficult to shrink or eliminate normal-size lower-body fat cells.

Another kind of predictor may indicate which children with type I, juvenile-onset diabetes are at greatest risk for complications. If a child with apparently normal joint and muscle function cannot press his fingers together for their full lengths palm to palm (in a prayerlike posture), this stiffness may signal that complications are beginning to occur. Treatment in such children should be adjusted to fine-tune the insulin supply; this adjustment, it is now thought, can prevent the destructive, disabling complications due to blood-vessel and nerve degeneration.

Degenerative complications of diabetes

The chronic complications of diabetes can be divided into two groups on the basis of their immediate causes. The first group involves progressive damage to organ systems. The second group (discussed below) involves damage through atherosclerosis (hardening of the arteries).

Progressive damage to nerves (neuropathy), to the small blood vessels of the retina (retinopathy), and the blood vessels of the kidney (nephropathy) are often

Photographs, courtesy, Obesity Research Center, St. Luke's-Roosevelt Hospital Center

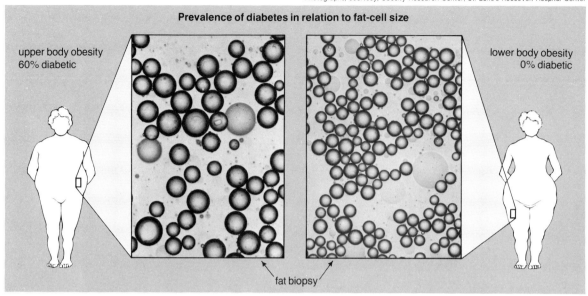

Prevalence of diabetes in relation to fat-cell size

upper body obesity
60% diabetic

lower body obesity
0% diabetic

fat biopsy

In a six-year study of 52 women, it was recently found that those with excess upper-body weight had large fat cells with fewer insulin receptors, while those with excess lower-body weight had numerous normal-sized fat cells with more receptors. The former group was found to be more likely to develop diabetes.

seen in diabetics. Observations of patients and recent experimental data derived from diabetic animals point very strongly to the theory that the damage to small blood vessels and nerves is inflicted by high blood sugar levels.

When the blood sugar rises above 150–180 mg/100 ml (milligrams of sugar per 100 milliliters of blood), a glucose molecule is chemically added to a host of different proteins in the blood and within the cells (glycosylation). It is surmised that these glycosylated proteins change their chemical and biological properties over time, leading to the overgrowth of collagen and other connective fibers. In time the walls of the small vessels become thickened and nonfunctional, resulting in microscopic aneurysms (ballooning), local bleeding, and tissue destruction. The intensity of this process seems to be governed by the amount of excess blood sugar and by an as yet unknown genetic factor that makes an individual susceptible to the process.

The most frequent complication of diabetes is neuropathy. This is a lesion occurring in the peripheral nerves, most commonly in the nerves serving the sensory and motor functions of the legs and arms. The sheaths and substance of the nerves are progressively damaged, resulting in severe pain and movement disabilities. When the nerves supplying the skin are affected, there is a loss of sensations (touch and perception of heat, cold, and pain). Therefore, when an injury to the skin occurs, it may not be noticed and treated. Wound healing is poor in diabetics, so that severe ulceration and infection are common even after slight injuries. If the blood supply is also restricted, the situa-

tion may lead to irreversible injury requiring amputation. Hence, diabetics must be careful to keep their feet and legs meticulously clean and dry. They must avoid injuring the skin (for example, by scratching insect bites or when trimming the toenails).

Less frequently the nerves serving internal organs are affected, producing what is called autonomic neuropathy. This may manifest itself as a disorder of the stomach or intestines or as a dysfunction of the urinary bladder. In male diabetics it is common to see erectile impotence.

As with the other diabetic complications the strict regulation of the blood sugar level seems to be the best means of prevention and treatment. Common analgesics are effective in helping control the pain of neuropathy. For male impotence surgical treatment may bring the solution through the installation of implants to produce erection.

While the glycosylation hypothesis of the cause of the complications is as yet only a theory, it derives its support from the fact that one can reverse the process in diabetic animals by pancreatic transplants but not by treatment with daily injections of insulin. The difference between these two forms of treatment lies in the fact that a good transplant of insulin-producing beta cells (β cells) from the pancreas provides a normal insulin secretion pattern, which keeps the blood sugar values between 80 and 150 mg/100 ml at all times. This is difficult or impossible to achieve with a regime of intermittent insulin injections.

An important advance in the monitoring of diabetics' blood sugar was announced in 1982 with the develop-

252

ment of an easy-to-use test that the diabetic can administer to himself at home to determine if his insulin dosage needs adjusting. Two or more times a day the diabetic obtains a tiny drop of blood by pricking his finger and places the drop on a test strip, which changes color according to the blood sugar level. The patient checks the results by comparing the color with a reference strip. The test is more accurate than similar tests that sample sugar levels in urine. The test is considered especially valuable for patients whose blood sugar levels tend to fluctuate substantially.

The search for an artificial pancreas

Because of these considerations the research effort into automatic and semiautomatic insulin delivery systems has been greatly intensified. Insulin cannot be taken orally because it is a protein and would be digested before it could reach the bloodstream. Injections, even given several times a day, are not an adequate substitute for the constant regulation that the pancreas supplies. What is needed is an artificial pancreas that would monitor blood sugar levels and deliver insulin to the body as needed.

Many such systems have been devised and are undergoing extensive tests. The most elaborate of these devices consists of a sensor that continuously measures the blood sugar of the patient. These measurements are relayed to a computer, which activates a syringe for the accurate delivery of the amount of insulin that will normalize the blood sugar. This artificial pancreas is the fully automatic, so-called closed-loop system; that is, it is self-regulating according to need. It is a most useful research tool but is unsuitable for routine use because it is not portable and is quite complex in its operation. The more practical machines are battery-driven syringes that are set to deliver a precalculated amount of insulin continuously. Before meals the patient can set the syringe to inject an added amount in order to take care of the rise in blood sugar produced by the meal. Such an apparatus is a semiautomatic, or open-loop, system. The device is compact, can be worn easily by the patient, and has proved to be of much value in selected test cases.

It is easily understood why, at present, the open-loop syringe is not yet fit for general use. It is only of value when used by individuals who can be relied upon to keep their dietary regime meticulously, to monitor their blood sugar levels six to ten times per day, to understand how to operate the syringe pack for delivery of precise amounts of insulin, and to be sensitive to low blood sugar levels. This last characteristic is of great importance since in the absence of premonitory signs of low blood sugar levels, severe and dangerous hypoglycemia can occur. The patient must be aware at all times of the amount of physical work he is doing since labor and exercise add to the power of insulin to lower the blood sugar level. At present, data are being care-

fully gathered on the best use of the open-loop systems. These will undoubtedly lead to improvements in procedure and to the development of syringes with fail-safe mechanisms that will allow more general, less supervised use.

Pancreatic transplants

The ideal therapeutic method for the severe type I diabetic would be the successful transplantation of healthy beta cells in sufficient amounts to supply insulin on demand. The great problem, of course, is in preventing the recipient's immune system from rejecting and destroying the transplanted cells. Recent work has demonstrated that the recipient can successfully stave off rejection for considerable periods of time if care is taken to purify the β cells from any contamination with donor lymphocytes, white blood cells that incite antibody production and thus hasten rejection. Another major difficulty is to identify a reliable, safe, and efficient source of supply of human β cells once a rejection-free technique is found to be both feasible and practical.

It is not possible to predict the time in years before research into these problems will bear fruit. It now appears that computerized syringe devices may come into general use before the successful establishment of a safe β cell transplant technique.

Atherosclerotic complications

The second major set of late complications of diabetes are the consequences of premature and severe hard-

A wearable insulin pump, still in the experimental trial stage, allows diabetics to inject appropriate amounts of insulin as they are needed.

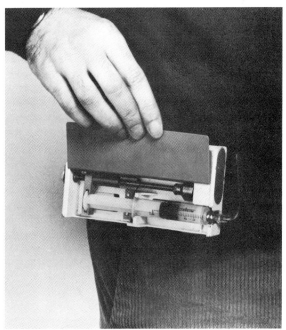

Bill Aller—The New York Times

Glandular and metabolic disorders

ening of the arteries (atherosclerosis). The arteries throughout the body are affected, in particular the coronary vessels of the heart and the arteries supplying the circulation to the legs. The incidence of coronary occlusion is three to five times more frequent in diabetics than in individuals of the same age who are not diabetic. Very often the blood supply of the legs is chronically diminished, a condition that manifests itself by difficulty in walking, cramping pain on exertion, changes in the color of the skin, and poor healing of wounds with an increased tendency to infection.

The acceleration of atherosclerosis is due to a variety of factors that are related to the cellular and chemical mechanisms operative in the process of hardening of the arteries—which occurs in most individuals whether or not they are also diabetic. This process is thought to consist of the following sequence: injury to the delicate lining of the arteries, the vascular endothelium; the accumulation of blood platelets at the point of injury; the entry of lipid (fatty material) into the layers of the arterial wall; the formation of a lipid-laden plaque, or atheroma, due to the proliferation of special fat-filled cells; thickening of the artery wall and narrowing of its channel; and obstruction to flow and clot formation. Factors that tend to aggravate the situation are partly genetic; others are due to such environmental situations as dietary excess, smoking, and stress. In the diabetic two aspects are present in addition, high blood sugar and insulin in excess. In the presence of a ready supply of glucose, insulin accelerates the formation of fat within the arterial wall.

It is evident that the aim of good treatment is to eliminate causative factors such as smoking and dietary excess, to maintain low blood sugar values, and to avoid insulin excess. Consistent exercise is very helpful in the control of blood sugar and in easing the need for excess insulin.

Diet and exercise

The type of diet prescribed for diabetics has come full circle since the late 18th century, when a high-fat, low-carbohydrate diet was recommended. At present the majority viewpoint favors the employment of a diet based primarily upon the proportionate intake of the three following food groups. Carbohydrate intake (in terms of calories) should represent 50–60% of the diet, protein intake 15%, and fat intake 35%. Diabetics are advised in addition to avoid simple sugars or foods cooked with them. The meals should be calorically equivalent from day to day so that the uniform insulin dosage will be neither too low nor too high for the body's demands.

Within the last ten years it has been found advantageous to add dietary fiber, generally in the form of bran and fibrous fruits and vegetables. This is done because fiber slows up the rate of carbohydrate breakdown and absorption by the intestinal tract. Thereby sugar excretion and blood sugar content are lowered. The comparatively low fat intake is in line with good practice in the prevention of atherosclerosis and coronary disease—a very important principle in the therapy of a diabetic.

Since the vast majority of diabetics are overweight (especially those individuals with type II diabetes), the total caloric intake should be adjusted to allow for the achievement and maintenance of ideal weight. This is also important for type I, insulin-dependent individuals since insulin promotes the making and deposition of fat and has a tendency to increase appetite. The maintenance of appropriate weight is the single most important factor—in addition to the regulation of the blood sugar itself—in guiding the treatment of the diabetic.

European clinicians of the 19th century observed that diabetics who performed hard physical labor were able to control the amount of sugar in their urine (which reflects the blood sugar level) better than the group that was generally sedentary. Soon after insulin came into use in the 1920s, it was shown that young diabetics who exercised in school or on the playing field would frequently experience episodes of low blood sugar, so that their need for insulin decreased. In other words, muscular exertion acted like insulin in lowering the blood sugar.

In recent years clinical and experimental observations have clarified some of the mechanisms by which muscular exercise tends to lower the sugar content of the blood. A muscle produces, when it is active, a material that speeds up the entry of sugar into tissues. Secondly, exercise increases the rate by which insulin is absorbed and gets into the tissues. Thirdly, exercise increases (by an unknown mechanism) the number of insulin receptors on the cells. The consumption of blood sugar then increases, and control of the diabetic metabolism improves. Thus an important aspect of treatment is the pursuit of a program of regular exercise in addition to the appropriate regime of diet and insulin or oral medications that help lower the blood sugar level.

Aging and diabetes

The frequency of diabetes increases with age, rising between the ages of 40 and 70 years. Thereafter the incidence of diabetes declines, as does the severity. Very few elderly patients require the administration of insulin. They can be quite satisfactorily treated by diet and oral agents. Meticulous normalization of the blood sugar level becomes less important to a diabetic who is first diagnosed in his seventies. Complications are not likely to be a problem—they take time to develop, from 5 to 15 years.

The aged diabetic must also guard against comparatively low blood sugar levels and the effect these have on the energy supply of the heart and of the brain. It has been demonstrated that oral antidiabetic medication in the elderly may cause hypoglycemia from doses that do not produce such an effect in the younger patient. It has also been observed that a healthy person, when he ages, will show blood sugar values that are in the main higher than those exhibited during adulthood and through middle age. For all these reasons there is a danger of overmedication and of unnecessarily rigorous dietary restrictions that may cause other nutritional problems in the elderly.

—Rachmiel Levine, M.D.

Gynecology and Obstetrics

Although gynecological research has made huge strides in recent years, there are still many aspects of female physiology and reproductive function that are not completely understood. Menstruation and its effects on women is one; through the centuries this mysterious event has given rise to a vast body of myth and misinformation, much of which persists into the 20th century. Most recently, the psychological effects of premenstrual tension have been reexamined now that the physiological basis is better understood. Another subject being reexamined is the frequency of cesarean section and the circumstances under which it is being employed. A new technology finding gynecological applications is the surgical laser, which may soon become the method of choice in treating certain medical conditions.

Until recently, premenstrual tension was steeped in myth and misunderstanding.

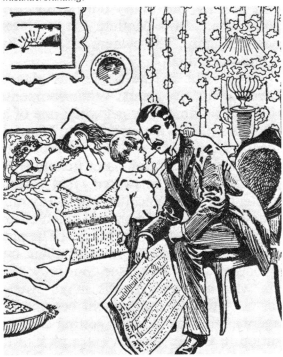

"What makes Mama so cross?"

The San Francisco Call, 1898

Premenstrual tension

For centuries women have been perceived as being the victims of their menstrual cycles. A comment made in a 1970 interview by U.S. physician Edgar Berman, then a member of the Democratic Party's Committee on National Priorities, is still widely quoted, to the effect that menstruating women cannot be trusted to make important decisions while "under raging hormonal influences." The same argument was used to deny women the right to vote and to bar them from higher education. Innumerable similar comments have been made regarding the impact of premenstrual tension (PMT) on the behavior of women, including its contribution to violent crime.

There has always been great debate about whether there is such a thing as premenstrual tension and, if so, whether it is physiological or psychological in origin or both. Numerous studies by medical as well as social scientists seem to support the position that there are a few women who have severe symptoms from PMT and many who have minor difficulties. Furthermore, certain of these symptoms appear to be hormonal in origin, while others seem to be the result of cultural and emotional factors. However, there is no indication that premenstrual tension seriously afflicts all women.

A large number of symptoms have been included in the overall description of the premenstrual tension syndrome. These occur, in varying degrees of intensity, in 30–50% of women and are more common as women grow older and have more children. In general, a particular woman will tend to have the same complaints each month, but they may vary in severity. All of the symptoms usually disappear when the menstrual flow begins each month.

Symptoms of premenstrual tension fall into several general categories. Certain of these are probably related to the elevated levels of estrogen and progesterone normally found in the body during the second half of the menstrual cycle, following ovulation. Included in this category are enlargement and tenderness of the breasts and a sense of heaviness in the pelvis that is accompanied by backache and urinary and bowel symptoms resulting from increased pelvic vascular congestion.

Other frequently reported complaints may be due to increased fluid retention (edema) in body tissues, perhaps caused by the increased production of aldosterone, a hormone that causes the retention of sodium and water by the kidneys. Weight gain, abdominal bloating, and swelling of the ankles may be produced by this mechanism. Edema of brain tissues may account for a whole constellation of mental symptoms: irritability, inability to concentrate and solve problems, agitation, restlessness, depression, sleeplessness, lethargy, fatigue, nervousness, dizziness, fainting, headaches, and temper tantrums.

Support for the hormonal theory of causation comes

Sarah Putnam

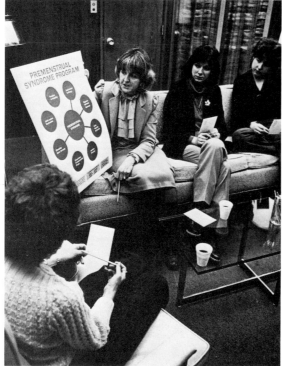

Counseling and medication are now available for women who suffer from severe premenstrual tension, which may include psychological as well as physical changes.

from the observation that many women report an amelioration of their premenstrual symptoms when they start to use oral or injectable contraceptives, both of which suppress ovulation. In addition, diuretics appear to help individuals who retain excessive amounts of fluid, and sedatives and tranquilizers are of value for those who are hyperactive and emotionally disturbed.

Another line of research has produced a number of recent investigations that seek to evaluate the impact of cultural factors on the events of the menstrual cycle. In one such study, when women were asked to record their symptoms daily, there were cyclic variations only when they knew that the study was concerned with menstrual patterns. The same results were obtained in women who had undergone simple hysterectomies that left their ovaries intact. Similarly, careful and detailed measurements of intellectual and physical performance have also often failed to show a correlation with the different phases of the menstrual cycle. In one study, women who were told that their menses were about to begin developed symptoms, whereas women at the same stage of their menstrual cycles who were told that their periods were a week or more away had significantly fewer complaints.

It has also been found that there are major variations in the symptoms reported by women in different cultures. American women complain most often of bloat-

ing and less often of headache; the opposite pattern is found in other countries: Japanese women have very few symptoms of any sort. Even within the same country, premenstrual complaints differ among the various racial, social, and religious groups. Finally, it is hard to rule out learned behavior—symptoms being expressed as a self-fulfilling prophecy, representing what women have been told to expect by their mothers, sisters, and friends.

Late in 1981 two British women were acquitted, one of murder and the other of the threat of murder, based upon their testimony that they were suffering from severe PMT. These cases are reminiscent of similar ones some years ago in France and have sparked considerable medical and legal conflict. It has been cautioned that PMT may become an all-purpose excuse for violence by women, despite the fact that it has never been conclusively proved that PMT is a cause of aggressive behavior.

Feminists fear that these cases may help to reinforce the idea that women are endocrinologic cripples. Others have pointed out that women commit only 10% of violent crimes and that men's hormonal patterns and behavior also exhibit marked cyclicity. The best outcome of this publicity about PMT would not be that it would result in an excuse for extremes of behavior but rather that it would encourage further research into this long-debated question to bring the subject out of the realm of speculation and into the purview of scientific investigation.

Cesarean section

A cesarean section (c-section) is the surgical removal, after 28 weeks of gestation or longer, of a fetus with its placenta and fetal membranes through an incision in the abdominal and uterine walls. It is undertaken when normal, vaginal delivery is not feasible or would threaten the life or well-being of either the mother or the fetus or both. For example, if the mother's pelvis is so small relative to the size of the baby's head (cephalo-pelvic disproportion) that vaginal delivery would be either very traumatic or impossible, a c-section should be done. The same is true if labor does not progress normally because of ineffective uterine contractions (uterine inertia). Cesarean section is also indicated in the case of placenta previa. If the placenta is in an abnormal position and will be delivered ahead of the baby, a normal birth will be difficult or impossible; there is also a major threat to the mother of serious, possibly fatal, hemorrhage. If a woman has had one cesarean section in the past, many physicians will require that subsequent deliveries also be by c-section because of the fear of uterine rupture during labor, a dangerous situation for both mother and baby. However, if the problem that mandated the first operation does not recur with subsequent pregnancies, vaginal delivery is sometimes attempted under close supervision.

Other indications for cesarean section are the prolapse of the umbilical cord into the vagina and abnormal positions of the fetus in the uterus; *e.g.,* breech (feet or buttocks first) or transverse, in which a shoulder, arm, or other part of the trunk presents first.

Another frequent indication is the development of fetal distress. Until fairly recently fetal distress was usually diagnosed by changes in the fetus's heart rate, particularly during labor. Today, fetal distress that develops before the onset of labor can often be detected by finding a progressive decrease in the levels of a maternal hormone, estriol. This hormone must be followed carefully when a high-risk mother (such as a diabetic) is approaching term. During labor fetal monitoring can frequently pick up early signs of danger. When changes occur either before or during labor that suggest that the well-being of the baby is becoming compromised, delivery (either vaginally or by c-section) must be promptly effected. Earlier and more accurate detection of fetal distress has significantly improved the outcome of these pregnancies.

The debate over the frequency of c-sections. In recent years the number of cesarean sections has risen steadily, particularly in those under the age of 20. In 1970 the rate was 5.5% of all deliveries; by 1979 it had risen to 16.4%—one out of every six; and in 1980 it remained stable at 16.5%. In some hospitals, however, the rates were as high as 40%. Several factors have combined to produce this continuous rise. First, babies presenting in abnormal positions are now almost always delivered by c-section. Second, a woman whose pelvis is just barely adequate for normal delivery would previously have had birth assisted by a low or mid forceps (when the fetus's head is partially descended through the pelvis). Today such a woman would usually have a c-section. Third, babies in distress are less apt to be delivered vaginally. Fourth, as more women have c-sections, the number of repeat sections, of necessity, will also continue to rise. Finally, malpractice suits are becoming progressively more common and their settlements progressively more expensive, particularly where fetal damage is concerned. The period of liability in such cases now extends for many years, until the child becomes of age (18–21 years). Therefore, doctors are less and less willing to run any risk from prolonged labor and vaginal delivery when it might later be claimed that fetal damage could have been avoided by the use of c-section.

As the cesarean rate has continued to rise, concern has been expressed by both doctors and their patients that perhaps not all of these operations are really necessary. It has been suggested that some of them are really being done for the convenience of the doctor or the patients. Questions have also been raised about the effects of an increased number of c-sections on maternal and infant morbidity and mortality.

In order to respond to these concerns and to answer

National Center for Health Statistics

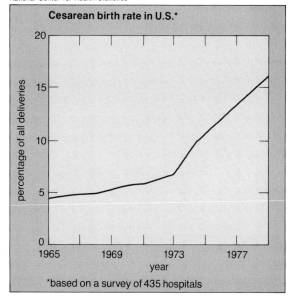

these questions, a number of studies have been carried out. It appears unlikely that convenience is a major factor in the increased use of cesarean section. Much more important are the various medical and legal considerations.

There is no doubt that, overall, cesarean section is more hazardous than vaginal delivery. The present maternal mortality rate associated with cesarean births varies from 4 to 8 per 10,000, which in one series is 26 times the mortality rate with vaginal delivery. Morbidity rates are also somewhat higher, as would be expected with the substitution of a surgical procedure. Any surgery inevitably carries with it a slight increase in certain risks owing to the operation per se and to the anesthesia required for its performance. Infections, sometimes serious, may be a complication.

As far as the baby is concerned, the effects seem to be predominantly positive. Perinatal mortality rates stayed about the same during the 1950s and early 1960s. Studies since then have shown a rapid and continuous decline in mortality coincident with improved prenatal care and the development of better techniques for handling complications during pregnancy and delivery as well as during the period immediately after birth. The rate reached a record low of 12 per 1,000 live births in 1980. A major part of this improvement has been ascribed to the increased use of cesarean section.

Many obstetricians believe that babies are better off being born by cesarean section than going through the trauma of a long and difficult labor and vaginal delivery. This is particularly true for infants weighing less than 2,000 g (4.4 lb), where perinatal mortality rates are significantly lower when c-sections are performed. However, despite the overall drop in mortality, there is

257

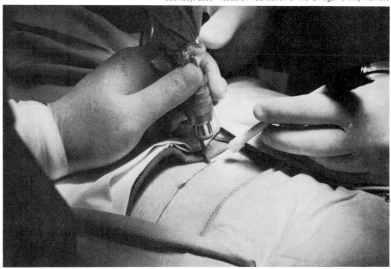

Courtesy, Laser Research Foundation of the Omega Fertility Institute

Surgical lasers are being used with increasing frequency in treating gynecologic disorders. One important benefit of laser use is a reduction in scarring, so that the functioning of delicate internal structures is not obstructed.

insufficient evidence thus far to prove that the increased use of cesarean section has significantly reduced the frequency of neurological problems or has improved levels of mental performance in those babies who have survived.

New uses of lasers

Laser is an acronym for light amplification by stimulated emission of radiation. The laser beam is a form of light energy that is coherent (all of its radiation is in phase) and of the same wavelength. When focused on a small pinpoint area, the laser beam can reach very high temperatures. In addition to having multiple uses in industry, space technology, and telecommunications, for more than two decades lasers have played an increasing role in medical practice.

Surgical lasers are constructed using a ruby crystal in the form of a rod or either argon or carbon dioxide gas in a glass cylinder. The argon beam is used in retinal surgery because it can pass through the fluids of the eye to the retina without being absorbed en route. The carbon dioxide laser, on the other hand, is used when absorption of energy is desired. Body tissues are 80% water; since the beam is absorbed by anything containing water, the laser can selectively destroy areas that are diseased, the cells actually being vaporized by the beam.

The carbon dioxide laser was developed in 1965. Its first reported use in gynecology occurred in 1973, when laser treatment of cervical erosion (destruction of the surface cells) was described. Since then, multiple applications have been found for this new therapy.

Lasers have several advantages over conventional surgical methods. First, because of the beam's precision, it can be utilized so as to destroy only abnormal cells, leaving normal tissues intact. Since the light can be bent, it can destroy tissues that cannot be reached

with a scalpel. Second, the laser seals off small blood vessels so that it is not necessary to clamp and tie them as the surgery proceeds. Thus anesthesia and operating times are decreased, there is less risk of infection, and recovery time is reduced. Finally, healing after laser surgery does not produce scarring, a very important factor in delicate procedures where scar tissue may interfere with functioning after healing.

Following the observation that the laser was valuable in the clinical management of cervical erosions, doctors began to use it in the treatment of dysplasia and cervical intraepithelial neoplasia (CIN), both potentially precancerous lesions. Instead of needing hospitalization to have surgery under general anesthesia, certain women with CIN (or with premalignant conditions of the vulva and vagina) are now often treated in a gynecologist's office under local anesthesia with a high level of success. Since precancerous cervical lesions are becoming increasingly common and are being seen in younger and younger women, laser treatment may be one way of helping to prevent the subsequent development of true malignancies.

Applications to venereal infections. Condylomata acuminata (venereal warts) have plagued women for centuries. Originally believed to be caused by some form of venereal disease such as syphilis or gonorrhea, it has now been shown that these warts are actually a viral infection transmitted by sexual intercourse. The virus found to be responsible for these lesions is the human papilloma, or papova, virus; it attacks the vulva, vagina, cervix, and perianal area. The warts may be small, localized lesions or may be very extensive, involving major portions of the lower reproductive tract.

Venereal warts are very troublesome, producing pain and tenderness, itching, and an irritating, foul-smelling discharge, particularly when they become infected. The lesions tend to spread, especially during pregnancy, when they may actually become so large that they prevent vaginal delivery. In addition, babies born to infected women have been found to develop both laryngeal and genital lesions due to the virus they acquired during birth.

Prior to laser therapy venereal warts were treated by local medications such as podophyllin and 5-fluorouracil cream; autoimmune vaccines; destroying the unwanted tissues with electricity or by freezing them with an ultracold liquid gas; surgical removal; or, most often, a combination of these methods. Venereal warts in pregnancy have posed a particularly difficult problem, since podophyllin and 5-fluorouracil have been found to be toxic to the fetus. Treatment with the laser beam, on the other hand, can be done during pregnancy.

Laser therapy has produced a high rate of cure of venereal warts, up to 100% in some reported series, even with extensive lesions. In addition, it does not cause severe scarring, as was the case with prior forms of surgical therapy. With laser treatment the recurrence rate has dropped to approximately 5–10%, a considerable improvement over many of the older methods of treatment.

Another viral infection, one that has now reached epidemic proportions, is caused by herpes simplex I and II. This too is a sexually transmitted disease (STD) which attacks the lower genital tract. The infection produces painful ulcerations and tends to recur. In addition to causing debilitating symptoms, this disease is now believed to play a major role in the development of cervical cancer. Moreover, the virus also attacks unborn babies, often killing them *in utero* or leaving them extensively and severely damaged after birth.

To date, no cure has been found for this very dangerous and destructive disease, although a new drug, acyclovir (Zovirax), was approved by the Food and Drug Administration (FDA) for the symptomatic relief of herpes in the initial infections. Lasers have also been used to treat herpetic lesions. It has been found that the laser beam will give women pain relief and will eliminate the herpesvirus from the lesions, making them noninfective. However, since the virus continues to grow elsewhere in the body, the majority of patients suffer repeated attacks of the disease.

Lasers for infertility. Infertility is now seen with increasing frequency beause of two clinical conditions, venereal disease and endometriosis. The increase in the first case is related to the changes in sexual mores and behavior (coitus beginning at an early age and with many sex partners) and the second, to the postponement of childbearing.

There are more than a dozen infections of the reproductive tracts of both men and women that fall into the STD category. In the female they frequently result in damage to the uterus, ovaries, and fallopian tubes. When these infections become overwhelming, they often can be cured only by the surgical removal of all the pelvic reproductive organs, leaving the patient both sterile and castrated. In the case of less severe infections the tubes may become permanently blocked by adhesions and scar tissue.

Endometriosis is a disease in which endometrial tissue, which normally lines the uterine cavity begins to grow outside the uterus, usually in the pelvic area but occasionally elsewhere in the body. This condition is quite common in young women and is frequently asymptomatic. As women grow older, however, the disease frequently spreads, producing pelvic pain, especially on intercourse and during menses. This tissue responds to the hormonal signals regulating menstruation, so it also breaks down and bleeds each month. With more extensive involvement of the pelvic organs, infertility is often the result.

Both of these diseases can sometimes be treated medically, the first with antibiotics and the second with hormones. Frequently, however, surgery must be performed to free the tubes and ovaries from adhesions and scar tissue. This requires meticulous care, with delicate dissection to avoid damaging the remaining normal tissues. Microsurgical methods have previously been used, but lasers seem ideally suited for these reconstructive procedures because of the precision of the laser beam, the control of bleeding and infection, and the lack of postoperative scarring. It is still too early, however, to be sure whether or not overall success rates will be substantially improved by the use of the laser.

Further applications. One of the newest applications of laser surgery is the cauterization of the lining of the uterus in order to control abnormal bleeding. A visualizing instrument, the hysteroscope, is passed into the uterine cavity. A small optical fiber, which serves as flexible pathway for the laser beam, is placed through the scope, and the laser is turned on. The laser beam destroys the abnormal tissue responsible for the bleeding. It has been suggested that this procedure may someday replace hysterectomy as the primary form of treatment for excessive bleeding due to benign (noncancerous) causes.

It is not yet clear exactly what role laser therapy will play in obstetrics and gynecology in the future. The laser is an expensive piece of equipment, and its safe and effective use requires special training. Physicians who work with lasers must acquire new surgical skills and knowledge about the indications and contraindications for this new form of surgical intervention. Almost 500 physicians have now received training in laser techniques. It is unlikely that the laser will completely replace other older procedures, at least not in the immediate future. However, the development of laser technology clearly offers a new and exciting approach to the treatment of many problems faced daily in the practice of obstetrics and gynecology.

— *Elizabeth B. Connell, M.D.*

Special Report:

Endometriosis

by James A. Merrill, M.D.

Endometriosis is a common disorder of adult women. Its severity and the amount of discomfort and disability it causes vary widely from case to case. Although endometriosis was described as early as 1860, the disease did not receive clinical attention and scientific investigation until the 1920s.

What is endometriosis?

The endometrium is the soft, spongy tissue that lines the cavity of the uterus and is shed during menstruation. In endometriosis this tissue is found growing outside the uterus. The displaced endometrial tissue usually is responsive to the hormone variations of the menstrual cycle and undergoes the same cyclical changes as the endometrial tissue in the uterus. Menstrual-type bleeding is an important symptom of this disorder. Endometriosis is often self-limiting and may regress following removal of the ovaries or cessation of ovarian activity following menopause.

The nature of this disorder defies categorization. Endometriosis has some characteristics of malignancy as well as characteristics of inflammation but in fact is neither. It is not infectious, not a response to a pathogenic organism, and it is not a congenital abnormality. The precise mechanism of development has engaged the minds of many investigators and scientists.

Most lesions of endometriosis are limited to the pelvic area. The ovary is the most common site where this tissue is found; usually both ovaries are involved. The next most common site is the surface of the peritoneum, the glistening membrane that lines the pelvic cavity and covers the uterus and fallopian tubes. Endometriosis may occur in the space between the upper vagina and the rectum. Much less commonly, endometriosis involves some other portion of the body, including scars, intestines, and even such rare locations as the lung and spinal canal.

Most commonly, endometriosis appears as multiple small hermorrhagic spots surrounded by scar tissue. Occasionally actual blood-filled cysts are present. The hemorrhage and the blood-filled cysts result from menstrual-type bleeding that occurs in these areas each month, and the scarring is a response to the presence of the blood. There may be nodules of fibrous tissue, and adhesions, bands of fibrous tissue that form in response to injury or inflammation, are often present.

Who gets endometriosis?

The exact incidence of endometriosis is difficult to determine because the disorder exists in many patients without causing symptoms, and the diagnosis is made with accuracy only by identifying the lesions during surgery. There is great variation from one hospital to another in the reported incidence. It is possible that endometriosis is present to some extent in 20% of adult women who have gynecological difficulties. However, endometriosis is a *significant* finding in only about one-third of patients in whom it is discovered.

Since the biologic behavior of endometriosis is unpredictable, the diagnosis is difficult. There are no laboratory tests that are of particular value, and X-rays and ultrasound are not helpful. A *clinical* diagnosis established on the basis of symptoms and physical

In order to make an exact diagnosis of endometriosis, the internal structures must be examined. This is usually accomplished through the use of a laparoscope, a viewing instrument that can be inserted into the abdominal cavity through a small incision.

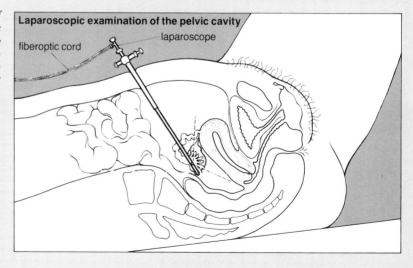

Laparoscopic examination of the pelvic cavity

laparoscope

fiberoptic cord

examination is often in error. An *exact* diagnosis can be made only by visualization of the lesions. This may be accomplished directly with external lesions or by exploratory operation or laparoscopy. Laparoscopy is a technique commonly employed in women with complaints of pelvic pain or infertility. The organs of the pelvis are examined with the aid of a small telescope inserted through the wall of the abdomen. The diagnosis is also made as an incidental finding during surgery for other reasons.

Active endometriosis is found most commonly in women between the ages of 30 and 40; its occurrence in women under 20 is rare. Because endometriosis is usually responsive to the cyclic hormones of the ovary, the disorder usually regresses following artificial or natural menopause. However, there are cases of endometriosis that become active and symptomatic following the menopause.

Endometriosis often is described as a disease of career women. The typical patient is said to be a young woman who is well educated, highly motivated, and an achiever. She is well groomed and fastidious. There are also several studies that report a hereditary tendency to the development of endometriosis.

Many gynecologists believe that endometriosis is more prevalent among high-income white patients than indigent nonwhite patients. It has been suggested that this is accounted for by late marriage and late child-bearing in the higher-income groups. Others have questioned the reliability of these impressions, and at least one report shows equal incidence rates in black and white patients and no differences based on social or economic status. In a study of 646 patients with proved endometriosis, it was found that these patients married and became pregnant just as early as comparable patients without endometriosis. It is likely that nonmedical factors account for the variations in incidence—well-educated, affluent patients may be more likely to seek help for their troublesome but not intolerable minor complaints.

It is often stated that endometriosis improves during and following pregnancy. However, it is impossible to document this impression, and there have been cases in which there was active growth during pregnancy.

What causes endometriosis?

The exact cause of endometriosis is unknown. At present, it seems likely that no one theory satisfactorily explains all cases of endometriosis, and that this interesting entity may arise from a combination of influences. The disorder is found only in women whose uteruses are exposed to the sex hormone estrogen, either from their own ovaries or by administration of estrogen supplements. It is rare or nonexistent in the absence of menstruation.

Many observations and experiments support the idea that fragments of menstrual endometrium, by one

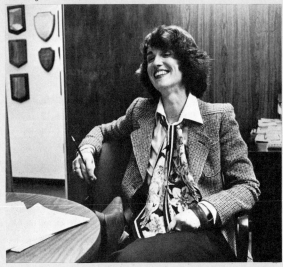
Jean Boughton—Stock, Boston

Active endometriosis is often found in young career women who have never been pregnant. Because exact diagnosis is difficult, its true prevalence is unknown.

means or another, are transported to various sites in the pelvic cavity and endometriosis develops from them. The most likely route of transportation is the retrograde flow of menstrual fragments from the uterus through the tubes to the ovaries and into the pelvic cavity. Menstrual fragments may also be transported through lymphatics and blood vessels. Such vascular transportation is necessary to explain the rare locations of endometriosis at sites far distant from the uterus. Precisely how transported menstrual fragments cause the development of endometriosis is controversial. Although the growths may simply be formed by tissue that transplants itself at the new site, there is evidence to support the theory that menstrual discharge induces a transformation of tissue into endometrial tissue at the various sites.

What problems does endometriosis cause?

The symptoms of endometriosis are extremely variable, and the frequency and degree of symptoms are poorly related to the extent of the disorder. Many patients, even those with extensive disease, have no symptoms at all and are totally unaware of their disorder. On the other hand, many patients with small lesions appear to be disabled.

Pelvic pain is the most significant symptom of endometriosis. This characteristically takes the form of pain or cramps occurring during menstruation, but not all pain with endometriosis is related to menstruation. Pain may be constant or intermittent. Pain during sexual intercourse is common. The hemorrhage and degeneration that occur in areas of endometriosis are the most frequent cause of pain.

Irregular, excessive, or prolonged uterine bleeding is

the presenting symptom of patients who have endometriosis (the symptom that brings them to seek medical help) almost as often as is pain. The cause is uncertain.

The rare sites of endometriosis produce interesting situations. For example, patients have complained of periodic blood in the urine when endometriosis is present in the bladder. Other patients have coughed blood during menstruation when endometriosis involved the lungs or the bronchial tree. Periodic pain, swelling, and bleeding have been observed in patients with endometriosis in an abdominal or vaginal scar.

Infertility may bring a patient with endometriosis to her physician. It is impossible to determine a true incidence of infertility in patients with endometriosis or the frequency with which endometriosis exists in women who are infertile. Endometriosis has been reported in 8–30% of infertile women. Further, it is difficult to explain exactly how endometriosis may interfere with fertility. In some cases the fallopian tubes are distorted or obstructed by scar tissue and adhesions, but in many the tubes are open and the ovaries regularly release an egg. Currently, there is active investigation into the possible relationships between endometriosis and altered fertility. It is probable that substances are produced that interfere with normal transportation of sperm and ova. Despite the difficulty in assigning a specific mechanism, endometriosis is associated with at least relative infertility. It is equally clear that many patients have extensive endometriosis with no alternation of their fertility whatsoever.

True malignancy has been reported to occur in endometriosis, but it is extremely rare, appearing in less than 0.1% of patients who have endometriosis. In almost every case the diagnosis of cancer arising in endometriosis has been established in the laboratory after examination of a surgical specimen and has not been a preoperative diagnosis.

How is endometriosis treated?

The treatment of endometriosis is influenced by knowledge that it is predominately a disease of women of childbearing age, that infertility is often a presenting complaint, that the diagnosis is often made at surgery done for other reasons, and that it often exists in patients who have no symptoms or perceived problem. Since endometriosis is responsive to the hormones of the ovary, removal of the ovaries usually will result in relief of symptoms. Removal of the uterus alone may often improve symptoms. Obviously, such treatment can be recommended only for those patients who have completed childbearing. For young patients treatment should be designed to produce maximum relief of symptoms with a minimum of interference with childbearing function; in many cases treatment should actually increase fertility.

In general, treatment options are observation and relief of symptoms, surgery, and hormone therapy. En-

dometriosis need not be treated in every patient in whom the diagnosis is made. Education, observation, and mild analgesia are effective in many patients and should be the initial management of young patients whose symptoms are not severe or incapacitating. Reassurance that a life-threatening or health-threatening process does not exist is often helpful.

Surgery is often done, either as a result of misdiagnosis or when symptoms are severe, incapacitating, or acute. Surgery also is indicated if symptoms become worse and if infertility persists and no cause other than endometriosis can be found. The extent of the surgery will depend upon the extent and location of the endometriosis. If a patient is symptomatic and is approaching the menopause or has no desire to bear children, the operative procedure usually consists of removal of the uterus, both tubes, and both ovaries, together with all areas of endometriosis that can safely be removed. It may be impossible to remove all of the endometriosis without causing undue injury to normal organs and tissues. In such situations symptoms usually are relieved even though there are residual areas of endometriosis. Giving cyclic synthetic estrogen to patients who have had the uterus and ovaries removed will not aggravate endometriosis in most cases.

When endometriosis exists in patients who are complaining of infertility, all options are open to consider as therapy. A significant problem exists in comparing results of different treatment modalities because different test series contain patients who have different degrees of involvement of the pelvic structures. For this reason, researchers have now started to employ anatomic classification systems for describing the location, extent, and severity of endometriosis. While most investigators have shown a relationship between the extent of the endometriosis and success of pregnancy following treatment, some have found no relationship between extent of endometriosis and the duration of infertility or extent of disability. Further, relief of symptoms and correction of infertility appear unrelated.

For infertile patients with very mild endometriosis, a careful search should be made for other causes of infertility. If none is found there may be no advantage in treating the endometriosis. Recent reports have indicated that success, measured in terms of pregnancies, may be similar with or without active treatment.

With all but mild endometriosis, surgery is an effective method of therapy for infertile patients. Such surgery involves removal of all areas of endometriosis while the uterus and at least one tube and ovary are preserved. Sometimes release of adhesions and reconstructive surgery on the tubes is also done. The exact procedures will vary depending upon the extent of endometriosis. The results of such surgery are generally good, with relief of symptoms. The disease may progress, however, when there is residual endometriosis and continuing ovarian function. The recurrence rate is

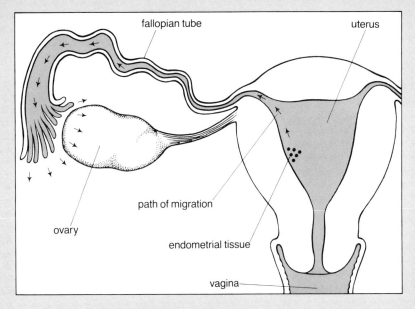

fallopian tube

uterus

path of migration

ovary

endometrial tissue

vagina

It is thought that endometriosis develops when pieces of the uterine lining migrate out of the uterus via the fallopian tubes and become transplanted, often on the ovaries.

10–13%. The average reported pregnancy rate following surgery is 50%, but rates as high as 87% have been reported. Most pregnancies occur within the first year following surgery.

Since endometrial growth is highly responsive to ovarian hormones, it is natural that hormone therapy has been advocated. A variety of sex hormones have been used, and each has enjoyed a measure of success. There are few comparative studies between hormone and surgical therapy and, unfortunately, none of them has carefully employed the same classification system. Therefore, comparisons of the two methods of treatment are difficult at best.

Essentially all of the synthetic progestins in combination with the estrogens have been used in doses that cause "pseudopregnancy," months of absence of menstrual bleeding. Low-dose progestin-estrogen contraceptives are given in a continuous fashion starting with one tablet daily. This dosage is increased by one additional tablet daily if breakthrough menstrual bleeding occurs. Treatment is continued as long as nine months. Symptomatic improvement has been reported in 85% of patients. Subsequent pregnancy has been reported in 30–47% of infertile patients. Unfortunately, a significant number of patients treated with this pseudopregnancy complain of nausea, restlessness, swelling, irregular menstrual bleeding, and excess weight gain. Improvement in the endometriosis following therapy persists for varying intervals, but in many cases the findings and symptoms return.

The need for operation after pseudopregnancy is reported in 11–51% of patients. Improvement is often overestimated when compared with surgical findings. Some gynecologists feel that there is no evidence that synthetic progestin-estrogen actually cures endometriosis and that the use of such agents should be considered a temporizing measure for selected cases and occasionally may be helpful prior to surgery.

The therapeutic effect of a new synthetic androgen hormone, Danazol, is being studied extensively. This drug interferes with the pituitary hormones that drive and control the hormonal function of the ovaries. Therefore, such treatment is analogous to induction of a state of pseudomenopause. Danazol is given daily in multiple doses and causes cessation of menstruation. In patients with mild disease, treatment usually extends for three to four months, with moderate disease, six to eight months, and with severe disease, longer than eight months or until physical examination reveals that there is improvement. The medication is expensive and is likely to cost over $100 per month. Symptoms can be expected to improve in 70–100% of patients. Unlike pseudopregnancy, the improvement is prompt and may occur within the first month of administration. Overall pregnancy rates for infertility patients are approximately 50%, which compare favorably with pregnancy rates following surgery. For successfully treated patients most pregnancies occur in the first year following treatment. At one year after treatment, however, endometriosis recurs in 23% and at three years after treatment, in 39%. Acne, hot flashes, swelling, weight gain, excessive body hair, and muscle cramps are occasional side effects. Danazol largely has superseded the use of pseudopregnancy as the preferred medical therapy.

Medical treatment with hormones interrupts the cyclic release of an ovum, so patients cannot become pregnant during the course of treatment. For this reason and because the medication may be expensive, treatment should be started only after an accurate diagnosis and should not be prescribed on the basis of clinical impression only.

Health Care Law

On the surface, having access to medical records may seem an easy issue to the typical patient. The patient is paying for the medical service; the record is written about the patient; and the record is available to others who make decisions about the patient's care and future on the basis of its contents. It therefore seems only fair and reasonable that patients should have access to their own medical records.

The opposite view seems equally logical to many physicians and hospital administrators. The record is the physician's working notes generated to help in the care of the patient; it is filled with medical jargon and speculation, which may be unintelligible and frightening to the average person; it is written on paper owned by the doctor or hospital and stored in a safe and secure manner by the doctor or hospital. Under these circumstances it seems right and proper to conclude that the medical record is the physician's property and should be viewed by the patient only with the physician's permission.

Patient access to medical records

Up to the early 1970s the law was heavily weighted in favor of physicians and hospitals who wished to keep records from patients. The only effective way for patients to gain access was to commence a lawsuit. But all that is changing; now the assumption is that the patient is entitled to access, and the physician who does not comply is out of step with both health care law and modern medicine. What brought this dramatic change about, and what does the future hold?

What is contained in a patient's record? There are now about a billion visits annually in the United States to doctors' offices and hospitals—each one either generating a new record or adding to an existing one. At the turn of the century approximately 90% of all medical services were directly delivered by physicians; today fewer than 5% of all health-care providers are physicians. In the typical hospital only one-third or less of a patient's record will be created by the attending physician. Access is thus open to many persons other than the physician.

Even though the variety among medical records is kaleidoscopic, there is little dispute about the primary purposes for which they are kept. In the private physician's office they are generally maintained to document the patient's history, condition, and treatment; to aid in continuity of care; and to provide a record for billing. The Joint Commission on Accreditation of Hospitals (JCAH) interprets the purposes of the medical record in the hospital as: (1) a basis for planning patient care and for continuity in the evaluation of the patient's condition and treatment; (2) documentary evidence of the course of the patient's medical evaluation, treatment, and change in condition; (3) documentary evi-

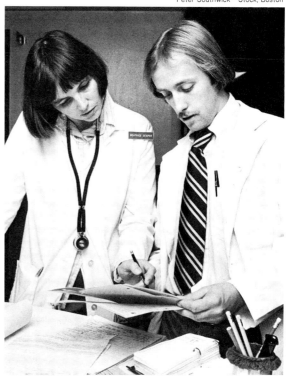

Today many members of the health care team in addition to the primary physician have access to the information contained in a typical hospital patient's chart.

dence of communication between the responsible practitioner and any other health professional contributing to the patient's care; (4) protection of the legal interests of the patient, hospital, and practitioner; and (5) a data base for use in continuing education and research.

Of course, all of these rationales can be applied to some extent to records kept in the private office or clinic as well. With growing governmental involvement in financing and auditing medical care, the purposes of the medical records are likely to continue to expand. And as new uses for the medical record appear, former uses are falling into disfavor. For example, even though it is usually appropriate to have a complete history of the patient in the record, it is inappropriate to include personal criticisms (*e.g.,* this patient is "fat and sloppy"; "shabbily dressed again today"; or "I love her perfume") in a patient's record. Such statements not only unfairly color the attitude of the patient's next medical caretaker who views the record but also lead to concealment of the record from the patient simply for fear of embarrassment. Such comments should also not be included in the medical record because the record may be viewed by many third parties during its lifetime, and even casual comments may be used against the patient by schools, employers, insurers, or governmental agencies. Facts about a patient (*e.g.,* "speech is slurred, eyes bloodshot," and so forth) rather than conclusions from these observations that may not be true (*e.g.*, "patient is an alcoholic") are appropriately recorded.

Who "owns" the record? Today there is an increasingly sophisticated view of ownership. The general rule is that the owner of the paper on which the medical record is written is the "owner" of the record. But ownership of a medical record is a limited, not an absolute, right and should be considered primarily custodial in nature. Possession of the record is governed by many other statutes (*e.g.*, state licensing statutes) and contracts (*e.g.*, Blue Shield contracts) as well as by the interests of the patient himself in the contents of the medical record. Providers have custody of records and strong interests in them, but patients have interests that are usually strong enough to give them a right of access to the information contained in the records.

Legal measures: toward change. Part of the change that is occurring today involves state legislatures and courts, which are acting to help patients gain access. In every state patients can obtain their records by filing a suit against the provider, usually alleging negligence, and subpoena the records for use in developing the case. At present in at least nine states the patient is given an additional statutory right to inspect his hospital record without resort to litigation. In some states the statute applies only after discharge, while in others no such distinction is made. Statutes in some other states also have limitations on psychiatric records. In Colorado, for example, psychiatric records need not be disclosed if, in the opinion of an independent third-party psychiatrist, such disclosure to the patient "would have significant negative psychological impact upon the patient." Other states limit the types of records that are available. For example, in Minnesota access to "laboratory reports, X-rays, prescriptions, and other technical information used in assessing the patient's health condition" is specifically excluded. In still other states, such as Tennessee and Mississippi, the patient must show "good cause" before he has a right to view the record, but what is meant by this term is not specified in the statute.

Instead of requiring access to the records themselves, Florida law requires only that "reports" made of physical and mental examinations and treatments be made available to the patient. Many other states have more limited statutes that either provide for access under certain circumstances or require the patient to obtain access to records through an attorney, physician, or relative.

Access is guaranteed by judicial decisions in other states, such as Illinois, Nebraska, New York, and Texas. The general theory of the case law is that "the fiducial [trust] qualities of the physician-patient relationship require the disclosure of medical data to a patient or his agent on request" and that patients have a right to access to their own records based on a "common law right of inspection." Other courts have mentioned "today's positive attitude towards openness and against bureaucratic concealment."

State medical licensing boards are also beginning to recognize the importance of patients having access to their medical records. New York in 1977 and Massachusetts in 1978 required their licensees to make such records, or a summary of the relevant data in them, available to patients upon request. On the federal level (*e.g.*, Veterans Administration facilities) the Privacy Act of 1974 requires direct access under most circumstances, and the Privacy Protection Study Commission, established by that act, has recommended that "upon request, an individual who is the subject of a medical record maintained by a medical care provider, or another responsible person designated by the individual, be allowed access to that medical record including an opportunity to see and copy it."

This recommendation is significantly broader than one made more than five years previously by the Department of Health, Education, and Welfare's Medical Malpractice Commission, which recommended that "states enact legislation enabling patients to obtain access to the information contained in their medical records through their legal representatives, public or private, without having to file a suit." And in 1980 the Occupational Safety and Health Administration issued regulations that guarantee workers in most companies access to any medical information that is kept on them by company physicians.

None of these changes has come easily. In almost every case the legislature, agency, or court involved had to grapple with two questions: the mental state of patients who seek to see their medical records and possible harmful effects of reading their records.

Who wants access?

Some view the "record-seeking patient" as sick, manifesting a basic distrust in the health care system. Perhaps the best example of this attitude was published in *The New England Journal of Medicine* in January 1980. Four psychiatrists at Boston's Peter Bent Brigham Hospital interviewed the 11 out of 2,500 patients at the hospital who, in a one-year period, asked to see their medical records. It is doubtful that anything of general usefulness can be learned about patients who read their records in an uncontrolled, nonblind, clinically impressionistic study of those few persons who, for whatever reason, buck a system that routinely fails to inform them of the right to access to their records. Nonetheless, the authors concluded that such patients had a variety of personality defects, usually manifesting themselves in mistrust of and hostility toward the hospital staff.

An accompanying editorial by psychiatrist Don R. Lipsitt noted that in a setting where trusting patients are not routinely told of their right to record access, it seems reasonable to assume that only the least trusting or most angry would ask to see their records. To locate the source of this mistrust in the patient's personality or in the stress of illness or hospitalization is to forget that "the doctor-patient relation cannot be understood simply in terms of the patient's side of the equation." For example, it would seem that the ten women who asked to read their charts "to confirm the belief that the staff harbored negative personal attitudes toward them" were correct in their belief; the psychiatrists labeled them "of the hysterical type with demanding, histrionic behavior and emotional over-involvement with the staff." While they stopped short of defining a new psychiatric disorder of "record-seeking" neurosis, the authors do not view patient access to medical records as an activity that should be encouraged.

Nor are they alone in this belief. At Beth Israel, Boston's most progressive hospital in terms of informing patients of their rights, although all patients are clearly informed of their right to access to medical records in a pamphlet given to them (usually before they enter the hospital), actual exercise of this right is discouraged by the following recommendations in the pamphlet:

As a general rule we do not recommend that you review your medical record in the midst of a Hospital stay because, while you are an inpatient, your medical record is incomplete; it serves as a worksheet for your physicians and nurses rather than as a clear-cut listing of the pertinent medical facts of your case. During your hospitalization we urge you to direct questions to your physicians and your primary nurse, but if you still wish to see your record you have a right to do so.

Can access be harmful to patients?

Perhaps it will be years, if not decades, before physicians are comfortable with patients seeking to see their records. But the argument that an ignorant patient is a happy patient is unpersuasive—especially when the patient wants specific facts. Patients who *ask* to see their own medical records are not "less anxious" when refused than they would be if access were provided. In fact, every study that has been done supports the conclusion that patient access to medical records is a positive step and poses no threats to their health care.

In one study in Burlington, Vt., for example, staff physicians in the Rehabilitation Medicine Service at the Medical Center Hospital of Vermont routinely gave patients copies of their records. Of 103 patients surveyed, 88% registered moderate to enthusiastic interest in their medical records, 60% asked for clarification, and 50% made minor corrections in their records.

An Australian study at the Royal Melbourne Hospital provided open access to records for patients in the Clinical Research Unit. While some believed before the study that the hospital setting "might worsen anxiety," this concern was not borne out, and the results indicated positive patient acceptance. The primary problems patients had with the records involved medical abbreviations, vocabulary, and physicians' handwriting. The study also had some therapeutic payoffs. In two cases patients with chronic debilitating diseases expressed their unfounded fear that they had cancer only after reviewing their records. This provided an opportunity for the physician to discuss this belief with them. In another case a pregnant woman found a mistake in her blood type; an unnoted but medically very important Rh incompatability existed. Similar positive results were reported from a study in a psychiatric unit at Valley General Hospital in Renton, Wash., where inpatients were permitted to read their records at will. In another study at the Given Health Care Center in Burlington, Vt., 8,000 patients were given copies of their complete office records. Of these 93% felt that the process reduced their anxieties about their health.

The standardization of methods of record keeping and the increasing practice of allowing patients access to their records may result in an improvement in the quality of the records. Personal, subjective statements are being replaced with objective data and observations. In the computerized system pictured at right, a doctor retrieves information about a patient.

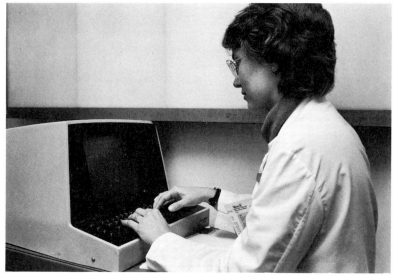

Moreover, in places where access is available, no adverse reactions have been reported. In Massachusetts, for example, patient access to hospital records has been mandated by statute since 1946 without reported incident. And the Privacy Study Commission, hearing from all federal agencies that had adopted access policies under the Privacy Act of 1974, found that "Not one witness was able to identify an instance where access to records has had an untoward effect on a patient's medical condition." Finally, a two-year study (1976–78) at the outpatient department of Boston's Beth Israel Hospital concluded not only that physicians' fears about liberal patient access to records were unwarranted but also that the access policy made the relationship between patients and professionals "more collaborative."

Some physicians have even suggested giving all patients carbon copies of their records as soon as they are made. The advantages of this system would include: (1) increased patient information and education; (2) continuity of records as patients move or change physicians; (3) an added criterion on which patients may base selection of physicians; (4) improvement in the doctor-patient relationship by making it more open; (5) an added way for physicians to monitor quality of care; and (6) increased responsiveness to consumer needs. Such proposals deserve serious consideration, as the burden of proof is now on those who deny patients access to their records to demonstrate other than self-serving reasons for this policy.

But might disclosure of medical records be harmful to the physician? This possibility is considered likely by some, but the general policy of open access is likely to create far fewer potential problems than a general rule of denying patients access to their records. The late Michael J. Halberstam, a highly respected cardiologist-commentator, unequivocally advised against patient access, arguing that "the chart is none of the patient's business." He further advised concealing mistakes from patients (at least those that do not seem to have caused any serious damage) and suggested this is not a conspiracy of silence but "merely the instinctive tact and acumen of people who work together toward the same goal."

Such policies tend to perpetuate the public's view that health care providers are trying to hide something from them, lead to cynicism about the potential for peer review, and increase the likelihood that a lawsuit will be filed primarily for the purposes of gaining access to medical records. There is some evidence that a policy of open records does change the content of the records themselves; the changes are usually improvements in records, such as deleting personal opinions and replacing them with objective data.

If the patient has a statutory right to the record, there is nothing that can legally prevent the patient's access as provided in the statute. However, inherent in the law is the notion of reasonableness. It may be reasonable for a hospital to suggest that the patient's physician be present while the patient inspects the record. On the other hand, it is unreasonable for the hospital to require this in most circumstances. For instance, it is unreasonable for a hospital to deny the patient access to records if the patient must make a treatment decision and needs the information to do so. Any delay in allowing the patient access would be judicially evaluated in light of all of the surrounding circumstances. A hospital or physician may likewise not make it difficult or impossible for the patient to exercise the right by imposing an exorbitant charge for copying.

Some state statutes provide, and common sense dictates, that if the physician has good reason to believe that access to the record will be harmful to the patient, access may be denied. But this is not to be treated casually—the physician must be reasonable in this belief and should be able to document the belief on the basis of objective evidence. The patient should also be given the opportunity to challenge such a decision or to designate another person to receive the information for him. And if the record contains information received by others, including members of the patient's family, in confidence, it may be proper to withhold these portions of the record.

Record access will continue to be controversial for many physicians for a long time, and special rules may still need to be worked out regarding some categories of psychiatric patients and teenagers. But the general trend today is toward direct consumer access to all kinds of records: credit, life insurance, education, police, and so forth. Medicine is behind the times in this regard, and the law is nudging it, sometimes not gently, to catch up.

—George J. Annas, J.D., M.P.H.

Heart and Blood Vessels

To sustain life, the human heart must function every second of every day. Stopping it for only six seconds inevitably causes unconsciousness, and stopping it longer than three to five minutes usually causes irreversible brain damage. For the heart muscle, or myocardium, to beat continuously, it must receive a constant supply of energy, mostly in the form of oxygen, from the blood. Although other organs can function for various periods of time without oxygen, the heart cannot; thus it is called an obligatory aerobic organ.

Oxygenated blood is transported to the heart muscle by vessels called coronary arteries, which traverse the surface of the heart before penetrating the myocardium and delivering their precious load. Flow through normal coronary arteries increases as the work of the heart is augmented, thereby increasing myocardial oxygen supply to meet the workload. Heart function thus remains normal. When blood flow is impaired, either by fixed obstructions in the coronary arteries caused by atherosclerosis (hardening of the arteries) or by dynamic obstructions produced by spasm of muscle in the arterial wall, the balance between oxygen supply and demand is disturbed. Ischemia is the name applied to the situation that develops when blood flow cannot satisfy the energy requirements of heart muscle.

In general, ischemia can occur in two ways. In the first, the work of the heart increases—for example, during exercise—leading to an increase in oxygen needs. If a coronary artery is narrowed, blood flow may increase but not enough to supply the heart with the required amount of oxygen. The patient is made aware of the presence of ischemia by the development of chest pain, or angina pectoris. The pain continues until exercise is stopped, myocardial oxygen demands decrease, and myocardial blood flow again becomes adequate to meet the reduced requirements. Alternatively, coronary flow can decrease because of the development of a blood clot (thrombus) or of a spasm of a coronary artery, either of which can partially or totally occlude the artery. Under such conditions the patient will experience angina while at rest.

Ischemia of a portion of the heart muscle has various outcomes. If the ischemia is short-lived, angina comes and goes with shifts in the balance between oxygen supply and demand. Although a patient may experience several ischemic attacks each day, if they are brief, the structural integrity of the heart muscle usually remains intact. If ischemia is prolonged, the chance that myocardial damage may occur is increased. The amount of damage depends on the duration of an ischemic attack, on the amount that blood flow is reduced, and on the amount of muscle that is jeopardized by the reduced flow. When the heart muscle is actually damaged so that tissue death occurs, the event is called a heart attack, or a myocardial infarction.

Based on this understanding of myocardial ischemia, it seems reasonable that anginal attacks and myocardial infarctions can be prevented or aborted by maintaining or restoring the balance between myocardial oxygen supply and demand. This goal can be accomplished by increasing blood supply, reducing myocardi-

al work, or both. There are several currently used approaches, some very new; these include: (1) controlling angina medically by reducing heart work, or augmenting blood flow, (2) controlling angina by dilating narrowed coronary arteries nonsurgically, and (3) reducing the damage that occurs during the course of heart attacks by dissolving clots that have blocked coronary arteries.

Medical treatment of angina pectoris

Medical treatment of ischemia has focused on the use of several classes of drugs to reduce the oxygen demands of the heart. One group, called beta adrenergic receptor blockers, or beta blockers, block the effects of the sympathetic nervous system in stimulating the heart, thereby reducing the frequency and vigor of the heartbeat. Blood pressure is also reduced. Each of these actions leads to a decrease in the work of the heart. Drugs belonging to this category are propranolol (Inderal), metoprolol (Lopressor), nadolol (Corgard), atenolol (Tenormin), and timolol (Blocadren). Nitrates are another group of drugs that reduce the oxygen requirements of the myocardium, mainly by their capacity to dilate blood vessels. In so doing, they reduce blood pressure and thereby lower the stresses encountered by the heart when it contracts and ejects blood. Because nitrates can also dilate coronary arteries, it is possible that, in addition to reducing oxygen requirements, they may also enhance oxygen supply. Nitroglycerin and isosorbide dinitrate are the best known agents in this category.

Recently another group of drugs has become available in the U.S. for treating angina pectoris. These drugs are called calcium channel blockers, or calcium antagonists. Diltiazem (Cardiem), nifedipine (Procardia), and verapamil (Calan, Isoptin) are representatives of this group. The calcium ion helps to regulate the activity of most of the cells of the body. In most organs such regulation is controlled by the movement of calcium within cells, and the immediate availability of extracellular sources of calcium is not necessary. The cells of the heart muscle and of vascular smooth muscle, however, are exceptions to this situation; they depend

Various actions of the beta blockers and calcium channel blockers on the heart and blood vessels are compared. The drugs in the latter group are not entirely interchangeable; each exerts its own unique combination of effects.

Cardiovascular effects of beta and calcium channel blocking drugs				
	heart rate	blood pressure	myocardial contractility	myocardial blood flow
beta blockers	strongly lowers	lowers	reduces	reduces, or has little effect
calcium channel blockers				
verapamil	lowers	strongly lowers	reduces	increases
nifedipine	raises		increases	
diltiazem	has little effect		has little effect	

on extracellular sources of calcium for their continuous functioning. The calcium channel blockers do not actually "antagonize" calcium in the sense of directly opposing its regulatory effects. Rather, they interfere with calcium flow across cell membranes and thus reduce the availability of extracellular calcium to the internal components of cells. These calcium channel blockers may also have other effects on calcium flow; they may enhance calcium transport out of cells or affect the movement of calcium between structures within cells. Although many agents are called calcium channel blockers, the various medications do not share all of these actions and thus are not entirely interchangeable.

A common action of this group of drugs is relaxation of the smooth muscle in the walls of arteries, especially in the small arteries (arterioles) that serve as the chief regulators of blood flow and blood pressure. They accomplish this action by virtue of the fact that changes in the inside diameter of arterioles result in profound changes in the resistance to flow; when arterioles contract, resistance to flow increases and flow thereby falls. Dilatation of these vessels leads to opposite effects on resistance and flow. The calcium channel blockers, by relaxing the smooth muscles that regulate the interior size of the arterioles, are potent vasodilators and reduce blood pressure by lowering peripheral vascular resistance.

This same mechanism may lead to dilatation of coronary arteries and a resulting increase in coronary blood flow. Such an effect would be particularly important when frank coronary spasm or lesser degrees of coronary constriction are present. Through their action on calcium flow, some of these drugs can also slow the heart rate as well as reduce the vigor with which the myocardium contracts. The decreases in heart rate, blood pressure, and myocardial contractile function all reduce the oxygen needs of the heart, while dilatation of coronary arteries can enhance the oxygen supply to the myocardium.

Although the calcium channel blockers can thus exert beneficial actions, excessive decreases in blood pressure, heart rate, or contractile effort can lead to serious adverse effects. As with all drugs, the dosage of calcium blockers must be carefully regulated to achieve maximal benefits. Less serious side effects also occur, but only infrequently do they necessitate discontinuation of the medication.

Because the beta adrenergic blockers and the calcium channel blockers have similar actions, it is expected that their combination would produce synergistic actions and thereby more effectively control symptoms of angina pectoris than could be achieved by either drug alone. This, in fact, has proved to be the case. Nevertheless, just as the beneficial effects of their combination are synergistic, so too are their capacities for producing the complications mentioned above.

Photographs, courtesy, Douglas R. Rosing, M.D.

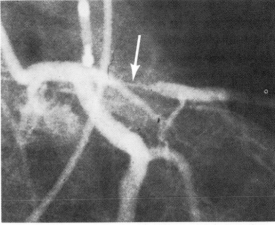

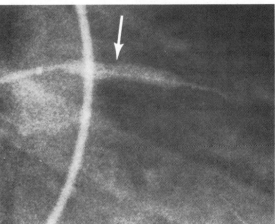

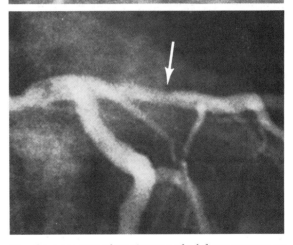

The above sequence of arteriograms of a left coronary artery partially blocked by atherosclerotic plaque charts the progress of balloon angioplasty in opening the vessel. (Top) Tight constriction, indicated by arrow, has severely reduced blood flow through the left anterior descending artery. (Center) A balloon catheter tip, at the arrow, has been inserted in the center of the narrowed region and inflated. (Bottom) After dilatation and removal of the catheter, blood flow through the reopened artery, at the arrow, is clearly improved.

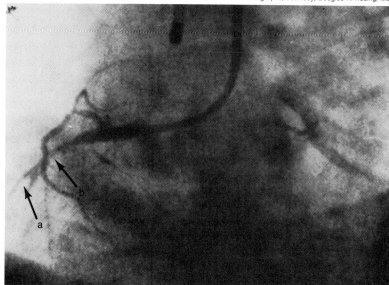

Arteriograms of the right coronary artery of a patient experiencing an acute myocardial infarction illustrate the effect of direct infusion of the clot-dissolving enzyme streptokinase. Before treatment (right), artery is completely blocked by a blood clot (a); a preexisting partial occlusion due to plaque deposits is also present (b). After infusion of streptokinase (opposite page), former site of clot is completely clear (a), although the atherosclerotic narrowing remains (b).

Balloon dilatation of the coronary arteries

A new, nonoperative therapeutic approach called percutaneous transluminal coronary angioplasty has been developed for persons afflicted with coronary artery disease to help relieve the ischemia caused by reduced blood flow to heart muscle. Its concept is deceptively simple: a tiny balloon is inflated within the narrowed area of the coronary artery in order to dilate it and thereby improve flow. In practice, the balloon, which is located on the tip of a long plastic tube (catheter), is inserted through the skin (percutaneously) into an artery and advanced into the diseased coronary artery. The catheter is manipulated so as to place the balloon in the middle of a region that has become partially occluded by atherosclerotic plaque. When the balloon is properly positioned, it is inflated, thereby compressing or fracturing the plaque and opening the vessel. The actual mechanism by which the narrowed artery is opened is still uncertain, but it probably involves several different processes including compression of the obstruction, stretching of the outer components of the vessel wall, and fissuring of the atherosclerotic plaque with a resulting reduction of the scar during healing.

The initial description of transluminal angioplasty was published by Charles Dotter and Melvin Judkins in 1964. These investigators, however, did not employ the technique to dilate coronary arteries, nor did they use a balloon. They used a set of percutaneously inserted catheters of increasing size to compress atherosclerotic narrowings located within arteries supplying the legs. A relatively high incidence of bleeding and blood clots occurred, and it was not until 1973 that Andreas Grüntzig of the University of Zürich developed the balloon-tip catheter system to open narrowings in blood vessels supplying the legs. At this point the early

and long-term results of this technique for peripheral arteries began to compare favorably with those of surgery. In 1976 Grüntzig developed a miniaturized balloon catheter for use in the coronary arteries, and in September 1977 coronary angioplasty was first performed in a patient.

Since then several thousand such procedures have been performed around the world. Results at the present time indicate that about 60–70% have been successful in increasing the inside diameter of the coronary artery by at least 20% and that with more experience and better selection of patients the success rate may reach 80%. When the inside diameter of a coronary artery is reopened to at least 50% of normal, the patient almost always experiences a marked improvement in symptoms. The most common reason for failing to dilate a narrowing is an inability to pass the balloon across a tight narrowing; in about 10% of patients a narrowing is traversed by the balloon but will not dilate because of its rigidity.

The complication rate from balloon angioplasty has been low. Fewer than 1% of patients die during or shortly after the procedure, and in about 6–8% of patients the condition is made worse, necessitating emergency coronary artery bypass surgery. In view of this potential complication angioplasty should not be performed unless an operating room and surgical team are readily available. In experienced centers other complications such as myocardial infarction are uncommon.

Follow-up of patients indicates that the artery continues to open, by at least 20%, in about 10% of patients during the first six months following the procedure, but narrowing returns in 15–25% of cases. Recurrence of significant narrowing usually appears in the first four months after dilatation and is almost always heralded

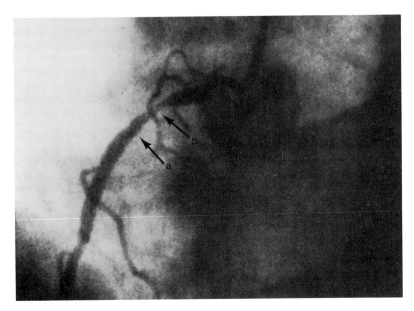

by the reappearance of angina pectoris. A second or even third attempt at dilatation is indicated for such people, since the narrowing can almost always be re-opened and made to remain so. Long-term success of coronary angioplasty is still being evaluated, and only a few patients have been followed for more than three years. However, the fact that some patients are pain free and show good results on X-ray examination at three years is encouraging.

Presently, certain general guidelines for performing angioplasty are recommended. First, patients should be candidates for coronary bypass surgery. Second, the diseased vessels should be so located that suc-cessful dilatation of one or two lesions would be ex-pected to lead to significant improvement. Third, the narrowing or narrowings should be discrete and close to the origin of the coronary artery and should not form a complete blockage; furthermore, only one significant narrowing should be present per vessel. If these guide-lines are followed, it is estimated that fewer than 10% of patients presently undergoing X-ray visualization of the coronary arteries because of findings suggestive of coronary artery disease would be candidates for this procedure. As more is learned about coronary angio-plasty, the role it should play in treating patients with coronary artery disease will be better defined and pos-sibly further expanded.

Dissolving clots during heart attacks

One intervention being used to prevent or reduce the death of heart muscle during heart attacks is the infu-sion of agents designed to break up blood clots (throm-boses) in arteries. In about 90% of patients with an acute myocardial infarction who arrive at the hospital within six hours after the onset of symptoms, the attack has been shown to be caused by total occlusion of a

coronary artery. Atherosclerotic plaque usually ac-counts for only part of the obstruction; in about 90% of the occluded arteries a fresh clot is also present. As a result of these observations, patients arriving at spe-cially equipped hospitals within three hours of the on-set of a heart attack are being taken to the catheteriza-tion laboratory to identify the coronary artery blocked by thrombus. Attempts are then initiated to break up or dissolve the clot.

The drugs used to break up clots are enzymes called thrombolytic agents, and the two currently employed clinically are streptokinase, derived from bacteria, and urokinase, obtained from human urine. These agents most commonly are infused with a catheter directly into the coronary arteries. Since this approach is quite com-plicated, requiring emergency catheterization and spe-cially trained teams of physicians, nurses, and techni-cians on call around the clock, studies are being conducted to determine whether simple intravenous infusion of thrombolytic agents are as effective as in-tracoronary infusion. In studies in Europe and the U.S., where thrombolytic agents were infused directly into the blocked coronary artery, the occluded vessel was partially or totally opened in at least 75% of cases. Oc-clusion recurred, however, in as many as 30% of pa-tients. This is not a surprising finding, for in half of the patients undergoing thrombolysis at least a 50% ob-struction remains at the site of the dissolved clot.

Thrombolytic agents can be helpful in salvaging heart muscle only if they are administered before irre-versible damage has taken place. Thus, a major factor in determining which patients are good candidates for this treatment is early arrival at the hospital—ideally, less than six hours after the onset of symptoms.

Although present evidence suggests that successful thrombolytic treatment at the time of a heart attack increases blood flow to ischemic tissue and helps preserve heart function, it is not known definitively whether lives are saved. A recent study carried out in Europe, however, provided encouraging preliminary evidence. Streptokinase administered intravenously to patients with acute myocardial infarctions resulted in a 50% reduction in deaths over the first six months after the infarction, compared with patients receiving placebo (no active drug).

In addition to these potential salutary effects, however, significant complications can develop during the procedure. They include hemorrhage and irregular, sometimes chaotic, heart rhythms that may end in death. Although there is a temporal relation between the treatment and these complications, it is not always clear that these events are true complications of the thrombolytic therapy; with the exception of hemorrhage they may occur despite treatment, rather than because of it.

Due to the potential complications of thrombolytic agents, the lack of controlled studies comparing intravenous and intracoronary administration, and the absence of long-term investigations comparing patients treated with thrombolytic agents with those treated by conventional means, it is still not clear (1) exactly which patients should receive the treatment; (2) how the treatment should be administered; and (3) what other procedures, such as coronary angioplasty or coronary bypass surgery, should be performed after a clot is successfully dissolved. Investigations presently being conducted should provide some answers to these questions.

— Douglas R. Rosing, M.D.,
and Stephen E. Epstein, M.D.

Kidney Diseases

Chronic renal failure is failure of the kidneys that ordinarily cannot be reversed by therapy. By contrast, acute renal failure is a short-term, generally reversible illness, the course of which is defined in weeks or, rarely, in months. Currently public attention is focused on the treatment of chronic renal failure, with emphasis on treating patients in the last stages of the disease, but acute renal failure is also a major health problem, with high incidences of morbidity and mortality.

Causes of acute kidney failure

Acute renal failure commonly results from one of two sets of circumstances. In the first the victim suffers an illness that temporarily reduces the blood supply to the kidney. Illnesses of this type include conditions as diverse as myocardial infarction, *i.e.,* a heart attack, which causes a drop in blood pressure; bleeding peptic ulcer, which lowers blood volume in the body; and severe burns, which cause a loss of blood plasma through the injured skin.

The second circumstance occurs when toxic substances interfere with normal kidney function. These substances can be drugs used therapeutically, like antibiotics, or actual poisons. For example, in recent years a group of new drugs known collectively as nonsteroidal anti-inflammatory agents has been developed to treat pain in general and arthritis in particular. These drugs act by inhibiting the production of prostaglandins. Prostaglandins are naturally occurring substances in the body that, among other effects, help maintain blood flow in the kidney, particularly when such flow is threatened. Consequently, if prostaglandins are inhibited, renal blood flow will also be reduced, and if kidney function is already impaired, the reduced blood flow may bring on acute renal failure. Kidney function may be impaired if the person has been using diuretic drugs or has an inflammatory disease of the kidney called glomerulonephritis. Under these circumstances the stage is set for an anti-inflammatory drug to inhibit prostaglandin production. The patient will usually recover, however, when the drug is stopped in order to permit blood flow to the kidney to resume normally.

Apart from these causes of acute renal failure, loosely known as acute tubular necrosis, diseases that affect the other structural parts of the kidney or an obstruction to the urinary stream may also cause renal function to decrease suddenly.

Whatever the cause, reduction in kidney function can range from clinically undetectable loss to complete cessation. If failure is mild, it may not be recognized until it has been present for several days. On the other hand, if it is severe, symptoms caused by the buildup of toxic substances in the blood may quickly become obvious. In some patients with mild acute renal failure, contrary to what might be expected, urine output is increased rather than reduced because the kidney's ability to concentrate the urine has been lost. When acute renal failure is severe, however, urine output may virtually cease completely. In such a case, substances that normally are filtered by the kidneys are retained in the bloodstream; these include urea, creatinine, phosphate, and other, still unidentified substances that cause the complex symptoms observed in patients with acute renal failure. Depending on the severity of the condition, the patient may become lethargic, stuporous, or even comatose unless therapy is provided.

Modern therapy for acute kidney failure

With the widespread availability of dialysis, the patient's survival is not related directly to the failure of the kidneys themselves but to the nature of the underlying injury or disease. In addition to frequent and even daily dialysis, basic therapy consists of providing only the amount of fluid needed to account for losses from the body (including sweat losses and exhaled water vapor), a high intake of calories, and correction of electro-

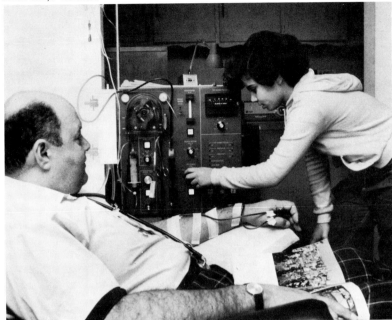

Dialysis for chronic kidney disease is expensive—the U.S. government's share of the bill was forecast at $900 million for 1982 and could total $2.2 billion for 1983. The average cost of maintaining a patient in a dialysis center is $24,000 per year. For those who have acquired equipment for dialysis at home, the cost is about $15,000 a year. In the U.S. chronic renal failure is the only catastrophic disease for which the federal government provides fully funded treatment.

lyte disturbances. Dialysis with the artificial kidney requires access to the circulation, which is often gained by a catheter placed in the subclavian vein underneath the collarbone. This catheter may be left in place for weeks until there is no further need for dialysis, with strict attention paid to sterility.

Since infection and gastrointestinal bleeding are two major causes of death from acute renal failure, much attention is also devoted to preventing these complications. Moreover, since most patients with severe injury are unable to eat, intravenous nutrition becomes an important part of therapy. The so-called hyperalimentation solutions used for this purpose contain high concentrations of sugar in the form of dextrose, amino acids, and certain salts. A great deal of attention is also paid to the patient's respiratory tract in order to provide adequate ventilation and drainage of bronchial secretions and to the skin to prevent bedsores. Successfully treating such patients requires the cooperative effort of physicians, nurses, physiotherapists, respiratory technicians, and many laboratory personnel. In milder cases of acute renal failure, peritoneal dialysis may be sufficient to prevent toxic substances from accumulating in the bloodstream. This technique, which depends on the diffusion of toxic substances through the membrane lining the abdominal cavity, is less efficient than hemodialysis but does not require access to the circulation. Patients who survive acute renal failure usually experience no long-term consequences once kidney function has returned to normal.

To prevent renal failure in elderly patients or in those with vascular disease who are to undergo major surgery, a high blood volume must be maintained before and during surgery. Urine output must also be kept high, sometimes by using diuretic drugs during surgery.

When patients are seen very early in the course of renal failure, the use of diuretics may alter the course of the disease favorably. For this purpose a new class of calcium-blocking drugs is being investigated for their potentially favorable metabolic effects on the kidney. These drugs are currently used widely to treat forms of heart disease, particularly angina, and to control cardiac arrythmias.

Acute renal failure is a very expensive illness both in economic and in human terms. It would not be unusual for a patient who develops acute renal failure after receiving multiple injuries in an automobile accident to incur hospital expenses of $50,000. Of more concern is the cost to human health and life from this illness. Despite modern methods of therapy, and probably because older and sicker patients are now being treated more vigorously, more than half of all patients with severe acute renal failure die. Wartime experience in Korea and Vietnam led to significant improvements in methods of therapy, but there have been few advances in recent years. Consequently, new and better means of reducing the severity of acute renal failure will have great value.

Federal funding for chronic renal failure

Chronic renal failure, a generally permanent condition, is the only catastrophic disease in the U.S. for which the federal government provides fully funded treatment (through the end-stage renal disease program, or ESRD). Public Law 92-603 (1972) extended Medicare coverage to all individuals with this disorder, regardless

273

of their financial need. By 1974 about 9,000 patients were being treated at a cost of $228 million. By the end of 1981 the cost of the program exceeded $1.2 billion, and about 68,000 people were receiving care.

Before 1972, treatment had been rationed because of the expense of dialysis and kidney transplantation. Although 40% of patients were on home dialysis, which is cheaper, in the absence of local financial support, the cost of treatment was still beyond the reach of all but the rich. Those who received treatment had to pass through selection committees or were treated on a first-come, first-served basis. Once the green light was given to treat people with end-stage renal disease regardless of age or income, the number of dialysis patients treated at centers increased substantially, and in most parts of the country the percentage of home dialysis patients decreased. During this period there were only small increases in the number of patients who received transplants, and by 1980 the percentage of patients on home dialysis had declined to about 12%.

Concurrently dialysis became a very lucrative business, and by the end of 1981 profit-making organizations were performing more than 30% of all dialysis treatments in the U.S. In the earlier years there had been discussions in the press concerning the ethics of physicians benefitting financially from facilities that provided medical care to patients, but the lack of apparent problems—and possibly financial considerations—have caused this controversy to disappear. For-profit companies have defended their facilities on the basis of their operating efficiency and their contributions through the payment of taxes.

At the time the ESRD program was established, home dialysis patients were required to pay 20% of the

cost of the equipment they used, even though it was in the public interest that they be treated at home; moreover, they were not reimbursed for equipment maintenance. In addition, they had to pay 20% of the cost of their supplies. Another deterrent to home dialysis was that physicians were not enthusiastic about it. Not until June 1978 did Congress pass a bill that encouraged home treatment by providing incentives for patients on home dialysis. Public Law 95-292 stated that the maximum practical number of patients who were medically, socially, and psychologically suitable for home dialysis should be so treated. It took approximately two more years before the regulations to implement this provision were published.

Effects of limiting reimbursement

During all the years since the ESRD program began, facilities were paid 80% of their costs or a limit of $138 per treatment, whichever was lower, unless an exception (rather freely granted) had been deemed justified by higher costs. Free-standing facilities, that is, those not related to hospitals, in general were able to make large profits when reimbursed at this level, whereas many hospitals had to seek an exemption because of their higher costs. In-hospital dialysis averaged $159 per treatment. Part of the higher costs that hospitals incur reflect higher overheads because of the method of allocating indirect costs in hospitals. Nevertheless, many in-hospital dialysis units operate inefficiently, and their exaggerated costs could hardly be justified.

Because of the growing expense of the ESRD program, both the Jimmy Carter and Ronald Reagan administrations attempted to set a limit on reimbursement. Before leaving office the Carter administration

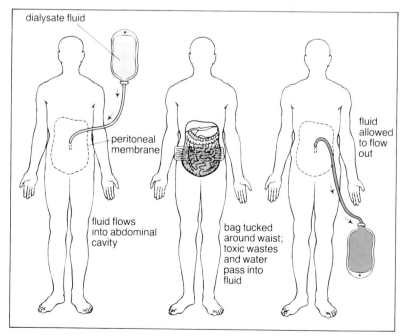

Continuous ambulatory peritoneal dialysis, or CAPD, is an alternative to hemodialysis that the patient, once trained, can carry out on his own. The process involves introducing a dialysate fluid into the abdominal cavity. Wastes from the bloodstream pass through the peritoneal membrane and into the fluid. After a few hours the fluid is drained out by gravity and replaced with a fresh supply. This procedure is not suitable for all patients.

recommended a single rate of reimbursement for both hospitals and free-standing facilities, which would either force hospital units to become more efficient or, in effect, exclude them from providing dialysis services. Because Congress was concerned that a single rate might further reduce the use of home dialysis (since hospitals generally provide this form of treatment), the Department of Health and Human Services was directed to develop separate composite rates for hospitals and free-standing facilities. In February 1982 the proposed regulations appeared in the Federal Register. Under the new proposal dialysis centers would be paid at a fixed rate for each patient whether treatment was done at the center or at home. Because the cost of a home dialysis treatment averages less than $100, centers would have an incentive to promote home dialysis as well as to increase their efficiency. Hospital-based facilities would receive $132 per treatment, and free-standing facilities would get $128. Variations on these bases would depend on wage indexes derived from countrywide differences in labor costs. Although physician reimbursement would be reduced substantially, the same payments would be made whether dialysis was carried out in the patient's home or in either type of center. According to this plan, physician reimbursement would be identical whether the patient was seen about 13 times a month, as is typical of in-center hemodialysis, or once a month, as in home dialysis.

One of the disturbing side effects of the proposed regulations is that, because home dialysis is being stongly encouraged, the easiest techniques of performing this form of treatment are likely to be undertaken. Since continuous ambulatory peritoneal dialysis (CAPD) is easier to teach and to learn, more people may follow the current trend and adopt this form of home dialysis rather than the more difficult hemodialysis treatment. In addition to the obvious possibility that many patients who are unsuitable for CAPD will be forced into this form of therapy, hospital units may be put in a position of choosing between survival and their ethical obligations to their patients. Many physicians believe that CAPD is untested and that too few long-term morbidity and mortality figures are available. In Europe only about half the patients who begin CAPD therapy are still receiving it at the end of a year. In Canada, however, where CAPD is much more popular than in the U.S. or Europe, survival figures are considerably more encouraging.

The future of ESRD
Organizations involved in intense discussion over the future of the ESRD program include such patient organizations as the National Association of Patients on Hemodialysis and Transplantation; the National Kidney Foundation; the Renal Physicians Association, representing nephrologists; the American Hospital Association; and others. Among those dialysis units not funded

by Medicare programs, the most important are represented by the Veterans Administration, which is responsible for approximately 50 centers and 25 satellite facilities that treat more than 1,500 patients in centers and more than 1,000 at home. Approximately 10% of the transplants being performed in the U.S. are done in Veterans Administration hospitals.

One major criticism by nephrologists of the government's approach to ESRD is that few pertinent figures are available about the results of the program to date. In order to institute the proposed regulations the Department of Health and Human Services performed a cursory audit of only 110 facilities from the approximately 1,200 that operate in the U.S. Using deflated dollars to compute the average benefit payment, the audit found that no actual cost growth had occurred per patient since 1973. The increase in the cost of the program was due entirely to the increase in the patient population.

One of the most important costs occurs when the patient is in the hospital. No information is available on the admission of patients to a hospital from units that have reduced standards of efficiency, nor is adequate information available on admission rates of patients treated with various modalities of dialysis. It is theoretically possible that the cost savings that appear so attractive for free-standing facilities or home dialysis may be misleading and that the actual total cost for these alternatives may be as great as or greater than that of in-hospital facilities.

Recent attempts have been made to reduce the cost of dialysis by encouraging application of established techniques for reusing dialyzer filters. California has passed a law that mandates that dialyzer filter reuse be performed under controlled conditions and by certified technicians. There is little doubt that dialyzer filters can be reused safely with quality control and that this is an acceptable method for containing costs. Increasing use of reused dialyzers, however, will have an adverse effect on manufacturers faced with a shrinking market for their equipment.

Keeping ESRD patients alive
The future of treatment for the ESRD patient is uncertain. It appears likely that many hospitals will no longer be able to continue treating their patients and will have to either send them to more successful free-standing units or place many of them on home dialysis. From an optimistic point of view, it is possible that some patients who previously had not been considered candidates for transplantation or home dialysis will now be seriously evaluated for these therapies.

Although the problems of the survival of kidney transplants have not been solved, promising new therapies to prevent rejection are being developed; for example, the immunity-suppressing drug cyclosporin A is now close to being marketed. More patients are surviving the transplantation operation and subsequent treatment but without much corresponding improvement in the success of the transplant itself. Consequently, more patients than in earlier years are reentering dialysis, with the ironic effect of maintaining or increasing the overall cost of the treatment program.

The success of the ESRD program has been a mixed blessing. It has been very successful for patients because it has transformed an invariably fatal illness and has enabled substantial numbers of people to remain alive. Unfortunately, the rehabilitation of those in the program has been poor. Most patients are not engaged in rehabilitation programs and are not working gainfully. Between 35 and 40% could be considered disabled. However, the average age of patients in the program is over 50, and many live in areas with widespread unemployment. Hypertension is now being treated more efficiently, a gain that should eventually result in less renal failure due to this cause. Unfortunately, chronic renal failure that occurs as the result of glomerulonephritis and diabetes currently cannot be prevented. ESRD has certainly produced valuable information about the problems associated with providing catastrophic health insurance to the population generally and to groups of patients who suffer from other costly diseases.

A major question that will have to be answered in the next few years is how far society is prepared to go to keep people alive. At what point does compassion have to give way to practical considerations? In particular, how could the large amount of money currently being spent on a small fraction of the chronically ill be more usefully spent? Only when these larger issues are resolved will the financial problems caused by use of the "half-technology" of dialysis be of historic interest.

— *Nathan W. Levin, M.D.*

Lung Diseases

Collectively, pneumonia and influenza are the sixth most common cause of death in the U.S. Among the many agents responsible for pneumonia, that caused by material aspirated into the lungs is discussed below. New drug therapies for influenza rely on the antiviral properties of agents that reduce both the morbidity and the mortality of this difficult and pervasive disease.

Aspiration pneumonia

A 1946 report described an often fatal form of lung injury in 66 pregnant women who during labor, anesthesia, or delivery aspirated (inhaled) acid stomach contents into their airways. Since known as Mendelson's syndrome, this injury is now considered a subgrouping under the larger designation aspiration pneumonia; that is, inflammation of the lungs caused by the presence of foreign particles or chemicals in the trachea, bronchi, and smaller respiratory passages. Aspiration

pneumonia can be a devastating problem among those at greatest risk: the elderly, the weakened and disabled, the neurologically compromised, the sedated and narcotized, and even those who sleep normally but deeply. The aspiration syndromes can be classified most simply by the type of material that is aspirated into the lungs. Three main categories are recognized.

The first type results from aspiration of inert and nontoxic substances such as water—drowning is an extreme example, a more common one is the coughing and sputtering of a person who has trouble swallowing. Also in this category are gastric contents that are free of bacteria and not strongly acidic, as may be aspirated during simple regurgitation, and blood, which may be inhaled during an epileptic seizure if the tongue is bitten. In the average individual these substances usually cause little direct lung injury, but they can lead to impeded respiration if the airway obstruction is major, as in the "café coronary," or obstruction of the windpipe by food. Unless the volume or particle size of the aspirated material is excessive or the oxygen deprivation is sustained, recovery typically follows vigorous coughing or other mechanical relief of obstruction. Infection complicates such aspiration infrequently, but in the elderly, who have lessened gastric acidity and diminished gut motility, bacteria from the alkaline bowel may enter the gastric contents. If an elderly person inhales his stomach contents, he may suffer lung infection from intestinal organisms.

The second category is aspiration of toxic or highly acidic materials, such as gastric hydrochloric acid, bile, animal fats, alcohol, mineral oil, or corrosive medications. Within seconds such "chemical" pneumonias injure the delicate gas-exchanging membranes of the lung's small air sacs and mimic the wet lung (pulmonary edema) of heart failure. In many instances secondary bacterial infection of the damaged tissue is then the final cause of illness and death. Pregnant women in labor may aspirate material of either the first or second type, depending upon whether their stomachs contain solid food, buffered acid (if they have consumed milk), or fasting acid (from not having eaten for a time previously). A woman may retain a meal for hours, as the mechanical activity of her stomach ceases when she goes into labor.

The third category of aspiration pneumonias involves bacterial material in the lungs from the mouth and throat. In this case bacterial infection is primary. Depending upon the type and virulence of the bacteria, these patients may develop simple bacterial pneumonia, necrotizing pneumonia ("gangrene" of lung), lung abscess (with foul-smelling sputum), or suppurative pleurisy (empyema), a dangerous inflammation in which pus collects around the lungs. Primary bacterial aspiration pneumonia is more common in the elderly and in weakened persons of any age, and it is often associated with disorders of consciousness, seizures, alcoholism, laryngeal dysfunction, or respiratory muscle paralysis.

Dormant nests of organisms in the gums may be the source of disease-causing bacteria. In fact, for this reason individuals with poor dental hygiene are at far greater risk of lung-damaging forms of aspirated infection than those without any teeth. In addition, the character and potency of the infection are influenced by the type of bacteria that is inhaled. In the hospital the patient may encounter altered bacteria that have been affected by antibiotics.

In essence the course and prognosis of all aspiration pneumonias depend on the extent of airway obstruction or damage to lung tissue; the degree of impairment of oxygen supply to critical organs; the presence of infection, whether primary or secondary; the development of bacterial infection of the blood; and shock. Aspiration of any of the materials of the three categories is an emergency.

Certain widely used therapies are standard, others experimental or controversial. Cleansing of the mouth and throat, body postures conducive to drainage, and suctioning help to clean the airways and reduce imme-

diate damage. Flexible catheters can suck out sticky fluids and some particulate material, but obstructing food is better extracted using the rigid bronchoscope. The bronchoscope is an instrument that is passed into the bronchi; it is equipped with a light that enables the physician to inspect the bronchi as well as remove foreign bodies from them. Oxygen can be delivered through the nose or, for more critical need, directly by a tube inserted into the trachea. Mechanical support of ventilation is used to correct insufficient spontaneous breathing. Low blood pressure and shock are controlled with intravenous fluid resuscitation.

Antibiotic therapy becomes important if there is evidence of infection; the appropriate drug is determined by analyzing material from the lungs. The early use of antibiotics "prophylactically" after aspiration is controversial. Many lung specialists believe that early administration of antibiotics does not prevent infection and may promote invasion of the injured lung by antibiotic-resistant ("opportunistic") bacteria. In many cases preventive drugs needlessly expose the patient to antibiotic side effects that can be more serious than the disease itself. Similarly, the use of corticosteroid (anti-

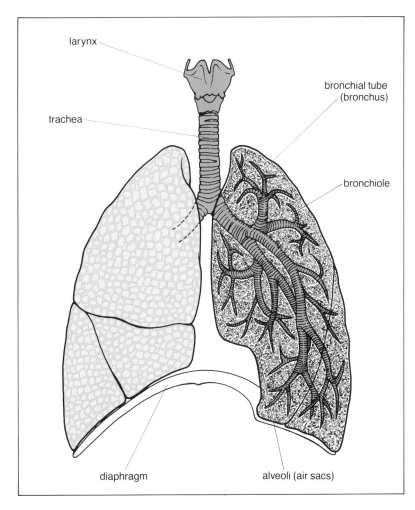

larynx

trachea

bronchial tube (bronchus)

bronchiole

diaphragm   alveoli (air sacs)

Aspiration pneumonia is inflammation of the lungs caused by inhalation of foreign material into the airways. The seriousness of the condition depends on the amount of the material inhaled and its nature—whether it is inert or toxic or contains infectious agents.

Lung diseases

inflammatory) agents is discouraged. It is possible that the prompt and brief use of corticosteroids may prevent the full-blown immediate inflammatory response to chemical injury, but no evidence establishes convincingly that these drugs reduce complications or improve survival; indeed, many believe that they impede and delay healing. The use of pulmonary lavage—actual washing out of areas of lung through a controlled system for irrigation and suction—is still under investigation; it, too, may actually be harmful.

Preventive measures are essential for individuals at high risk of aspiration. Patients with less than full consciousness must be observed closely and fed carefully. The beds of comatose patients should have the feet raised above the level of the head; this gravitationally protects the patients' airways against secretions and regurgitation, as do the careful maintenance of prophylactic tube airways and the choice of intravenous over stomach-catheter feeding (the latter often impairs the integrity of the sphincter between the stomach and esophagus).

When emergency surgery must be done on a patient who has food in his stomach, regional anesthesia should be considered, if possible. The likelihood of aspiration can be diminished by inserting a breathing tube while the patient is conscious. This can be followed by rapid induction of general anesthesia, simultaneously using a pressure maneuver at the neck to momentarily close off the esophagus. The stomach can be mechanically drained by tube and its acid contents neutralized with buffers. These adjunct procedures have proved highly effective when there is sufficient and properly trained staff to perform them. The patient may actually be more at risk during recovery from anesthesia, when staff vigilance may be relaxed.

For the pregnant woman the risk is far greater with emergency delivery. The upright "birthing chair," currently enjoying a revival, helps protect the woman in labor against gastric aspiration. Experience gained through home deliveries and birthing clinics emphasizes that patients who are fully able to cooperate and who have received little or no sedation have the added advantage of a diminished risk of aspiration.

Drug therapy for influenza

Year after year influenza epidemics cause a vast amount of suffering and death. The factor that makes influenza difficult to control is the ability of the influenza virus to undergo genetic variation, so that a vaccine developed for one strain is useless against a slightly different strain. These changes are relatively few among the influenza B and C viruses, but the ease with which genetic variants emerge from the population of A viruses—those that can quickly spread from population to population into a worldwide epidemic—repeatedly circumvents established immunity and permits reinfection of persons previously exposed to virus strains of the

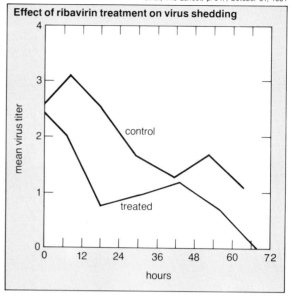

Adapted from "Ribavirin Small-Particle Aerosol Treatment in Influenza," Vernon Knight *et al., The Lancet,* p. 947, October 31, 1981

Effect of ribavirin treatment on virus shedding

Ribavirin is an antiviral agent that has shown promise in the treatment of influenza. In a test involving college students who took the drug via an aerosol, the treated students showed a dramatic and rapid decrease in virus titer (a measure of virus shedding) as compared with untreated (control) patients.

same subtype. Furthermore, the A strains appear to be the only influenza viruses with a range of natural hosts that include in addition to man other animals such as birds (wild and domestic), horses, and swine; the larger the host population, the greater the chance for genetic variation of the virus.

During epidemics the mortality from influenza and its complications is significant among the high-risk population, and the illness it causes takes a high economic toll, causing absenteeism from work and school and a burden on the health care system. Vaccination with inactivated virus vaccines, which has been the practice for over 35 years, is the method of choice for influenza types A and B (type C is of no importance to humans) and is estimated to be 60 to 90% effective. The public, however, is not uniformly persuaded that the benefits of the vaccine exceed its complications.

The effectiveness of the vaccine may be compromised by idiosyncratic responses to the influenza antigens in the immune systems of the elderly, the very young, the debilitated, the chronically ill, and those with heart, lung, or metabolic disorders—the very high-risk group most in need of protection. Even among normal individuals the question of vaccine ineffectiveness occasionally arises, as in a report from a residential school in England in which the cumulative attack rate for influenza in the period from 1970 to 1976 was found to be the same for vaccinated and unvaccinated students. The beneficial effects of successful vaccination are not immediate since antibody levels reach their peak in 7 to 14 days in primed subjects (those with prior exposure to that influenza antigen) and not for up to five weeks in unprimed subjects; this delay may be significant during outbreaks of disease. Other reasons for vaccine underuse are unavailability of vaccine, inappropriate content of virus in a given year's vaccine, and fear of adverse reactions.

In contrast with the growing choice of antibiotic agents effective against bacterial infections, the number of antiviral drugs for the treatment of man is quite small. However, research in molecular virology has begun to identify specific viral functions that can be chemically interrupted without damage to the cellular mechanisms of the host. These drugs have immediate antiviral activity and do not blunt antibody response to vaccine. Three of these agents deserve wider attention in influenza therapy.

Amantadine, licensed in 1967 but little used, is an effective preventive agent when administered for the duration of an influenza epidemic, usually about six weeks. It can also be given for one to two weeks after vaccination, to protect during the lag while antibodies are being produced; given throughout the entire season, it prevents influenza about as well as vaccine. The drug is taken orally once a day and is absorbed through the gastrointestinal tract. Since amantadine is excreted exclusively through the kidneys, reduced dosage is required when used for patients with impaired renal function. About 5% of those receiving the drug experience mild transitory side effects, in particular insomnia, dizziness, and other central nervous system symptoms. The drug is active against all influenza A subtypes but not against influenza B. Even when started at the time of influenza virus infection, amantadine can prevent or mitigate symptoms.

Amantadine is also effective therapeutically against type A influenza. The drug reduces symptoms, halves the duration of fever, speeds recovery, and reduces often fatal complications, such as primary influenzal viral pneumonia and secondary bacterial pneumonia. Mass amantadine administration may prevent a devastating outbreak of influenza in the concentrated high-risk setting of a long-care hospital or nursing home. Among amantadine-treated patients there is a marked reduction of those shedding virus and in the quantity of virus shed, further slowing the spread of disease. Studies show that the reduction in pulmonary function caused by influenza is more rapidly reversed in those receiving amantadine. Evidence suggests that for optimal protection vaccine should be received in the fall and amantadine administered in the winter.

Rimantadine, a drug closely related structurally to amantadine, is widely used in the Soviet Union but has not yet been licensed by the Food and Drug Administration for use in the U.S. Research to date has revealed that as an antiviral agent it seems prophylactically and therapeutically the peer of amantadine;

furthermore, it has virtually no toxicity. This is clearly an advantage for prolonged prophylactic use in patients who have not yet contracted the disease. It seems likely that when it is approved for use in the United States, rimantadine will become the drug of choice in influenza A prophylaxis and therapy.

Ribavirin is a synthetic drug structurally similar to drugs used in cancer chemotherapy. It was described in 1972 and was reported to have antiviral activity against herpes simplex, vaccinia (cowpox), and both A and B types of influenza. In clinical tests, however, orally administered ribavirin failed to prevent experimental influenza in volunteers and was inconsistently therapeutic for naturally infected patients.

During a recent outbreak of influenza A among college students in Texas, selected patients were treated by inhalation of ribavirin in the form of an aerosol. In this form the drug was deposited directly upon the respiratory surfaces. Judged against a control group receiving a saline aerosol, the ribavirin-treated students showed rapid recovery with highly significant reduction and duration of fever, amelioration of systemic illness, and disappearance of influenza virus from respiratory secretions. Therapy was begun within 24 hours of symptoms, and a total of 23 hours of ribavirin aerosolization was carried out over an interval of three days by the use of a face mask to administer the medication.

The compressed-air generator and aerosol system used by this group is easily adapted to transmit a continuous flow of small particles for up to 24 hours. In laboratory animals this method showed aerosolized ribavirin to be effective against influenza strains A and B, even when treatment was delayed for as long as five days after virus inoculation. Moreover, a combination of ribavirin and amantadine, both given by aerosol, increased the effectiveness of the therapy. Tolerance of ribavirin is excellent; no toxicity has been reported, and recovery from clinical viral influenza appears to be prompt and without complications. The investigators in Texas consider ribavirin aerosol treatment distinctly superior to therapy with amantadine alone, both in clinical response and in suppression of virus shedding, and they found that ribavirin did not reduce the treated patients' antibody response. Their equipment can be easily adapted for use in hospitals and nursing homes, and their therapy may be the best choice for influenzal viral pneumonia.

— L. Fred Ayvazian, M.D.

Neuromuscular Disorders

The last few years have seen a major breakthrough in understanding the cause of myasthenia gravis and in its treatment. This breakthrough has resulted from advances in basic sciences that have revealed lessons of importance to the understanding of clinical diseases of the neuromuscular system. The use of animal models

Neuromuscular disorders

has resulted in improved understanding and treatment of polymyositis, a chronic, relatively common neuromuscular disease.

Myasthenia gravis

Myasthenia gravis (MG) can appear at any age, though typically it affects women in their twenties and thirties and men in the later decades of life. The incidence in females exceeds that in males by about two or three to one. The typical case is a woman in her twenties who begins to complain of fatigue and weakness. She may note that her eyelids tend to droop at the end of the day and that she develops double vision at this time. Gradually these symptoms become more pronounced, and she also develops weakness of her voice and has trouble swallowing. There may also be weakness of her arms and respiratory muscles. Characteristically, this weakness is made worse by repeated effort and exercise but is improved by rest. After a few months or years, her condition may deteriorate to such an extent that she becomes unable to breathe and swallow and may need a respirator to help support life. The condition often goes through periods of relapses and remission, usually without any known reason. There is an increased instance in MG patients and their families of a number of other chronic diseases, including diabetes, pernicious anemia, rheumatoid arthritis, and thyroid

disorders, all of which are sometimes grouped as the autoimmune diseases. Autoimmune diseases share a common characteristic; they are thought to be the result of a malfunctioning in which the immune system, the body's defense against invading organisms and other foreign material, begins to attack the body's own cells, causing progressive damage to a number of types of tissue.

Steps leading to a breakthrough. One feature of myasthenia gravis that was recognized at the time that the neuromuscular disorder was first described was the development of muscle fatigue after exercise. This fatigue means that an MG patient cannot contract muscles he wishes to use.

The contractions of muscle fibers are controlled by motor nerves. The impulse governing movement travels along the surface of the motor nerve cells as a minute electrical charge; when it reaches the end of the nerve it stimulates the secretion of tiny amounts of a chemical, acetylcholine, which is known as a neurotransmitter because it forwards information from the nerve. The nerve and muscle fibers are separated by a microscopic gap called the neuromuscular junction. The acetylcholine crosses the junction and attaches to the muscle fiber through receptors that are present on the surface membrane of each muscle cell. If enough acetylcholine is received, chemical changes occur that

Patients with myasthenia gravis are unable to initiate muscle movement. Drooping of the eyelids is one of the early problems (left). With the administration of drugs called anticholinesterases, there is in many patients a marked improvement in muscle control.

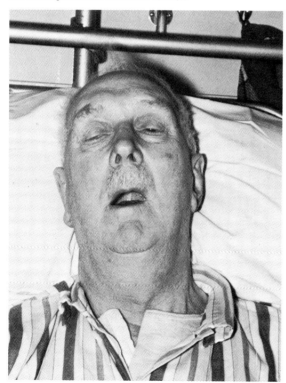 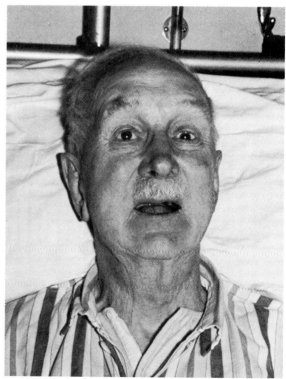

Photographs, courtesy, Walter G. Bradley, D.M.

lead the muscle to contract. A minuscule but measurable amount of electrical activity takes place as small ions (positively or negatively charged atoms) move into the muscle cells. After acetylcholine has acted, it is destroyed by an enzyme, acetylcholinesterase, which breaks it down into simpler compounds that can be reused by the body.

About 1930, researchers became interested in the action of curare, an arrow poison used by South American Indians to paralyze animals they hunt. Animals poisoned with curare show marked fatigue; they are unable to move their muscles. It was soon discovered that certain drugs called anticholinesterases inhibited the breakdown action of acetylcholinesterase, prolonging and intensifying the action of acetylcholine. These drugs could partially overcome the effect of curare. This observation led to the use of anticholinesterases in MG, with dramatic improvement in many patients. The improvement in muscle strength proves that MG is not due to the destruction of muscle but is related to some functional abnormality of the interaction between the nerve and the skeletal muscle.

In the 1960s electrophysiological studies of muscle biopsies from patients with MG demonstrated that the voltage produced at the neuromuscular junction by the release of acetylcholine was much reduced compared with normal levels. It was initially concluded that this indicated that an insufficient amount of acetylcholine was released from the nerve to act upon the muscle membrane. However, recent advances in the basic sciences of electrophysiology, membrane biochemistry, toxicology, and immunology have led to a breakthrough in our understanding of myasthenia gravis. It is now known that in this disease it is the muscle membrane receptors for acetylcholine that are immunologically damaged.

Studies of the venom of a number of snakes have demonstrated that the venom contains chemicals that produce a neuromuscular blockade somewhat similar to that of curare. One such toxin (alpha bungarotoxin) from the venom of the multibanded krait, a poisonous tropical snake, was found to bind very specifically to the neuromuscular junction. Scientists interested in the membrane receptor for acetylcholine made use of this specific binding of alpha bungarotoxin to obtain purified specimens of the acetylcholine receptor. They also made use of the recognition that the electric organs of such fish as the electric eel and the electric ray are composed of highly specialized stacks of neuromuscular junctions with high concentrations of the acetylcholine receptor. Homogenization of these electric organs released the acetylcholine receptor, which was able to be purified by binding to alpha bungarotoxin. In order to study further the acetylcholine receptor protein, rabbits were immunized with this protein so that they would produce antibodies against it. Generally, immunization of rabbits with a foreign protein produces no untoward

effect, but these particular rabbits developed a paralytic syndrome very similar to human myasthenia gravis. This syndrome has been called experimental autoimmune myasthenia gravis. Detailed investigation of this animal model has allowed a virtually complete understanding of the mechanism of production of the human disease.

The pathogenesis of myasthenia gravis. Acetylcholine receptors are concentrated at the normal neuromuscular junction to receive acetylcholine released from the nerve endings. Normally, there are three to four times as many receptors and three or four times as much acetylcholine released as necessary to activate the muscle fiber. Therefore there is a large margin of safety for neuromuscular transmission. In human myasthenia gravis, however, there are antibodies in the bloodstream against the acetylcholine receptors. The antibodies reach the neuromuscular junction, bind to the acetylcholine receptors, and damage that area of the muscle fiber membrane. In a few cases these antibodies may actually block the receptor. Damage to the membrane and to the receptors results in a lowering of the number of receptors at each neuromuscular junction and therefore a loss of the safety factor. Thus, in muscles that are totally paralyzed, though a normal amount of acetylcholine is released, it will not activate the muscle fiber. In less severe cases the muscle may be able to contract a few times, but thereafter the muscle fatigues and becomes paralyzed.

The role of the thymus gland in causing myasthenia gravis is still an enigma. About 15% of patients with MG have a tumor of the thymus called a thymoma. For more than 40 years it has been known that removal of the thymus gland improves patients with MG. In some cases the disease goes into complete remission, and in others there is considerable alleviation of symptoms. The thymus gland is a repository of lymphocytes, white blood cells important to the immune system. It has recently been discovered that the thymus gland also contains a small number of cells that are very similar to skeletal muscle fibers and have acetylcholine receptors on their membranes. This suggests the possibility that some damage to the thymus gland might induce an immunological reaction against the acetylcholine receptor. Such damage might be induced by a viral infection or might result from an imbalance between the very complex normal control mechanisms of the immunological system. Both these possibilities are also being actively considered in research to discover the causes of all the autoimmune diseases and the collagen-vascular disorders, in which alterations in the blood vessels and collagen (connective tissue) cause damage to many organs of the body. Some recent evidence has raised the possibility that the thymus gland may secrete a substance that aids in the damaging effect of the acetylcholine receptor antibodies on the neuromuscular junction.

Treatment of MG. As a result of the breakthrough in understanding the cause of myasthenia gravis, the ability to treat the disease has advanced dramatically. The use of anticholinesterase drugs and removal of the thymus gland (thymectomy) have already been mentioned. Recognition that MG is an autoimmune disease has allowed therapy to be directed against this immunological response. Immunosuppressive treatment includes high doses of anti-inflammatory corticosteroids such as prednisone and of cytotoxic drugs that inhibit the proliferation of lymphocytes, which produce antibodies. The use of both of these types of drugs has dramatically reduced the severity of MG in many patients. In others it has been possible to remove the antibody from the plasma by a process of plasma exchange (plasmapheresis). In this process, small volumes of the blood of a patient are taken into a machine like a centrifuge, and the red cells are separated from the plasma. The red cells are then resuspended in normal plasma and reinfused into the patient's veins. In this way it is possible to wash away the antibodies. However, the abnormal lymphocytes continue to produce acetylcholine receptor antibodies, so that immunosuppressant therapy and further episodes of plasmapheresis continue to be required.

The overall effect of the new treatment is a dramatically reduced number of patients who are severely paralyzed. Many such patients once required artificial respiration to help their breathing. It is now possible to produce dramatic improvement in virtually all of these patients. Inconvenience and side effects of treatment are still important, however. Research is actively continuing to find a way to permanently prevent the abnormal production of the acetylcholine receptor antibody and thus to cure the disease.

Polymyositis

Polymyositis is a relatively common chronic neuromuscular disease which is frequently confused with muscular dystrophy. The fact that polymyositis improves with treatment makes it very important to separate these two conditions.

Polymyositis affects both sexes of all ages and may develop either in a rapid fashion or very chronically. In about a quarter of the cases there is associated inflammation of the skin of the face, hands, and trunk; in these cases the term dermatomyositis is applied. In about a quarter of the cases there is an associated autoimmune collagen-vascular disorder, such as rheumatoid arthritis, scleroderma, or systemic lupus erythematosus. In about another 10% there is an underlying cancer that seems to be responsible for the polymyositis, since removal of the cancer may bring about remission of the polymyositis. Thus it appears that there may be several different diseases coexisting in the condition we currently call polymyositis or that several different conditions can precipitate a common autoimmune

process damaging the skeletal muscles.

A typical patient is a woman in her thirties who becomes aware of a rash on her cheeks and knuckles and then notices that her arms are becoming weak when she tries to carry heavy objects. She may eventually notice some difficulty in climbing stairs because of leg weakness. Over a few months the symptoms reach the stage that necessitates medical investigation. In some patients muscle weakness and soreness are mild, but other patients can have such severe muscle weakness that they are confined to bed and have difficulty breathing and swallowing.

Laboratory findings. In order to make a diagnosis of polymyositis, it is necessary to undertake detailed laboratory investigations. The most important of these is the removal of a piece of muscle for examination under a microscope. Since polymyositis is a patchy process, fairly large muscle biopsies are usually taken from at least two muscles. Typically, the muscle is seen to be inflamed, with lymphocytes scattered in collections between the muscle fibers and in cuffs around blood vessels within the muscle biopsy. The muscle fibers themselves show signs of damage, including necrosis (tissue death) and degeneration. The degeneration of muscle fibers releases their enzymes into the bloodstream; a high level of such enzymes, including the enzyme creatine kinase, supports the diagnosis of polymyositis. It is now possible to undertake studies of the electrical events occurring during muscle contraction using electromyography—an investigation that demonstrates that muscle fibers have been damaged in muscles affected by polymyositis.

The cause of polymyositis. The most important questions that remain to be answered are the cause of the diffuse inflammation of muscles in polymyositis and how it can be treated. It has been recognized for many years that many patients with this disease also have other collagen-vascular disorders such as rheumatoid arthritis, scleroderma, or systemic lupus erythematosus, conditions now thought to be due to an abnormality of the control of the body's immune system, with consequent development of antibodies and immunoreactive lymphocytes that attack the body's own cells. Evidence from recent studies indicates that a similar process exists in patients with polymyositis. The lymphocytes in the bloodstream of patients with polymyositis have been shown to be abnormally sensitive to the proteins of skeletal muscles. When exposed to such proteins, the lymphocytes become active and divide rapidly. In tissue culture, the lymphocytes of patients with polymyositis appear to seek out and adhere to skeletal muscle fibers, which they destroy by releasing poisons termed lymphokines. Lymphocytes from the blood of normal individuals do not exhibit such excessive reaction to skeletal muscle proteins. A few persons with polymyositis also have antibodies in their blood against muscle proteins.

An occasional patient with a viral illness like influenza develops muscle pains, weakness, and inflammation very like that seen in polymyositis. A small number of patients with typical polymyositis have been found to have structures that look like viruses when their muscle biopsies have been examined under the electron microscope. This finding suggests that viral infection of the muscle might cause the inflammatory disease.

Animal models have played an important part in advancing our understanding of polymyositis. Some of the common viruses like coxsackie virus can infect muscle in animals, producing muscle destruction and inflammation very similar to polymyositis. This supports the suggestion that virus infections cause the human disease. Immunization of an animal with the muscle of a different animal produces an inflammation of the skeletal muscles very like polymyositis (experimental allergic myositis). It has been shown that several different muscle proteins can produce this reaction.

The question that still remains is what causes the autoimmune process to begin. It is possible that a viral inflammation of the muscle releases muscle proteins, against which the patient becomes immunized. Alternatively, antibodies against the virus may crossreact with some protein in the muscles. The third possibility is that the condition is one in which there is loss of control of the body's immune system, with the development of clones of lymphocytes reactive against muscle.

Treatment. For 20 years it has been known that high-dose corticosteroid therapy can suppress the inflammation in polymyositis, with consequent improvement in muscle weakness. Immunosuppressant drugs, which inhibit the division of cells like the lymphocytes, have been used from time to time, and recently it has been proved that these drugs definitely benefit patients with chronic polymyositis. With the rapid increase in our understanding of immune responses and their control, it is possible that treatment of polymyositis will improve dramatically in the next few years.

Plasmapheresis has not proved to be highly successful in treating patients with polymyositis, probably because antibody activity is relatively slight in this disease. However, by lymphopheresis, a process similar to plasmapheresis, it is possible to separate and remove the lymphocytes from the bloodstream while retaining the red cells and plasma. Lymphopheresis has been shown to be effective in some autoimmune diseases. In the future it may be possible to render this lymphopheresis process more specific by removing only lymphocytes that are reactive against muscle proteins.

An alternative approach that is beginning to be studied in experimental animal models is to manipulate the control mechanisms of the immune system. In the future it may, for instance, be possible to turn off the abnormal lymphocytes in such a disease by immunizing the patient with a protein that has been slightly altered.

Alternatively, it may be possible to kill the abnormal lymphocytes by injecting patients with small amounts of the muscle protein against which the lymphocytes are reactive after the protein has been linked to a cytotoxic agent such as radioactive iodine. Though these treatments are at present restricted to the realm of future research, advances in the understanding of immune control are likely to be of major benefit to patients with polymyositis.

—Walter G. Bradley, D.M.

Orthopedics

Scoliosis is the term given to a lateral curvature of the spine, a condition that afflicts more than 2% of youngsters in their early teens. Scoliosis has been with mankind since antiquity, yet the cause of the most common form is still unknown. However, treatment of scoliosis has developed to the degree that the person with this condition can live an active and normal life. Scoliosis can occur alone or in association with over 100 different diseases. This deviation in the normally straight vertical line of the spine can, however, be subdivided into three major groups: paralytic, congenital, and idiopathic (meaning the cause is unknown).

The earliest reported cases of scoliosis were probably paralytic and caused by poliomyelitis. It is likely polio produced the "hunchback" and the deformed court jesters that have been immortalized in plays and operas through the ages. With the development of polio vaccine in the mid-1950s and its widespread use, scoliosis secondary to polio has nearly disappeared from the United States, although it is still common in other parts of the world. In the U.S. today cases of paralytic scoliosis are usually associated with a specific congenital nerve or muscle disease. The spinal curvature develops because of muscle imbalance or a generalized weakness that causes the spine to collapse under the weight of the head, arms, and chest.

Congenital scoliosis results from an abnormal development of the bones of the spine, which occurs even before the mother knows that she is pregnant. Because congenital scoliosis occurs during such an early embryotic stage, the unknown mechanism that produces the defect may also affect other organs such as the kidneys or heart. After birth the abnormal bones may grow slowly or rapidly, but owing to their misshape and to their abnormal growth potential they produce spinal curvature as they grow; there is great variability in their behavior, and it is impossible to predict when an abnormal bone segment that has been dormant will suddenly start to produce a deformity. As a result, regular evaluation of patients with congenital scoliosis is mandatory during the growth years.

The most common type of scoliosis in the U.S. is of unknown etiology (idiopathic). It affects children and teenagers who are otherwise completely healthy and

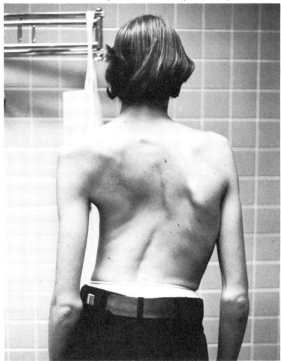

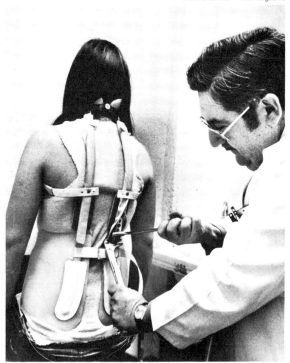

Severe scoliosis, or curvature of the spine (left), causes pain and may interfere with the functioning of the lungs and other internal organs. For a curvature that affects the thoracic (chest area) spine, the Milwaukee brace (right) is a corrective device that is commonly used to minimize the defect.

normal in every respect. Because medical science does not have an explanation for the development of the curvation, much folklore about possible causes has evolved. Specifically, it is known that scoliosis does not result from improper diet, carrying school books on one shoulder, or sleeping in an inadequate bed.

Minor curvatures

In some cases the diagnosis of scoliosis does not imply a problem. Long-term studies from many countries indicate that minor curves in an adult often are not serious or disabling, nor do they cause cosmetic concern. An adult with a minor curve can have as strong and healthy a back as anyone with a straight spine. There are no limitations on any activities because of minor scoliosis, and the chance of having back pain is no greater than in the general population. A woman with a minor curve encounters no additional risk in pregnancy or delivery.

If scoliosis is not recognized until it has become more severe, the outlook is not so favorable. The degree of deformity may be such that a rib hump, chest asymmetry, or waist imbalance is cosmetically unacceptable. More serious are severe curves in the midsection of the spine, the thoracic spine, which may reduce lung capacity and respiratory endurance. Severe curves in the lower section of the spine, or lumbar spine, may be associated with back pain. Thus, minor

degrees of scoliosis are trivial, but the more severe curves are associated with unpleasant sequelae.

Curves progress from mild to severe most frequently during the time of the teenage growth spurt. Since treatment of mild to moderate spinal curves can prevent the development of severe scoliosis, many communities have instituted school screening programs. The purpose of these is to detect children who are at risk for later progression to more serious curvatures as well as children who may currently need treatment. Although it has been questioned if scoliosis screening is cost effective for society as a whole, the individual whose scoliosis might otherwise have been undetected has clearly gained by this procedure.

Population studies have shown that about 3% of sixth- to eighth-grade children have minor curves that will be identified in school screening programs. In the vast majority of children these minor curves will not progress. About one-fifth of the children identified in screening will need treatment; the challenge to specialists is in determining who will and who will not progress.

A few facts are known about the risk of progression. Girls have a five to seven times greater risk of progression than boys. The presence of an older child or parent with a significant curve seems to increase the likelihood of a curve's becoming worse. Caucasians have a higher risk than do blacks. Despite what is known about these general risk factors, for any one child with a small curvature the future is absolutely unknown. Thus, the prudent treatment of the immature individual is close observation to follow the natural history of the curve and then immediate intervention if the curve at any time begins to worsen.

Moderate to severe curves

The proved treatments for scoliosis are bracing and surgery. Bracing can be either supportive or corrective. In a teenager who has little growth remaining, a brace will stop the advance of a progressive curve. In a young child with paralytic disease, a brace may keep the curve from progressing rapidly to allow growth of the trunk before surgery. These applications could be considered supportive. In a preteenager who is just beginning the adolescent growth spurt, a brace can actually produce an improvement in the curvature. Because the brace is begun at an earlier age, the individual will wear it several years longer than the older patient but gains better results. Thus, in these patients the brace can be considered as actually corrective.

Surgery is indicated when the curve is progressing beyond brace control or when the curve is not recognized until the degree of curvature is too great for brace application. Surgery is designed to provide some correction of the curve and to make the spine solid by adding additional bone. Once the curve has become solid, it will not progress. Thus, surgery treats scoliosis by producing a rigid portion of spine.

In addition to these proved means of treatment, a number of nonverified treatments exist, usually endorsed by enthusiastic proponents. These include exercise programs and various forms of biofeedback. Of current interest is electrical stimulation of the muscles of the ribs and flank. Although much initial enthusiasm has developed about this and other newer therapies, the early results on the average are not as good as bracing, and long-term effects are not known.

Treatment for paralytic scoliosis. The child with a nerve or muscle disease that leads to scoliosis will ultimately need a spinal fusion. Because the long-term stability of the spine is dependent on the strength of the solid bone developed, fusion in both the front (anterior) and hind (posterior) sides of the spine may be indicated.

Motion of the spine occurs at the posterior joints between each vertebra, much like joints elsewhere in the body. Some motion also occurs anteriorly where the discs and the thick ligaments join the vertebral bodies. In a posterior fusion the lining of the joints (cartilage) is removed and bone packed into the space. This grows into both sides of the joint and produces a solid bar of rigid bone. In an anterior fusion the spine is approached from the side and the disc totally removed. Bone is packed into the disc space, which grows in a similar fashion into a very solid bar of bone. Obviously, having solid bone both anteriorly and posteriorly pro-

vides greater strength than either alone. Therefore, the decision in paralytic disease for a single or combined approach is based on a determination of long-term needs for strength.

The fusion is accomplished by the packing of bone, which results in the ultimate growth of new bone in the previous joints. This is the most critical step in the surgical treatment of scoliosis, and the ultimate success or failure is dependent on a perfectly solid fusion. Publications in the lay press have often ignored this aspect of surgery and have instead focused on describing the metallic implants that may be an additional part of the surgical procedure. Metallic implants are used to gain correction of the curve and to provide stability while the bone is growing and solidifying. Many such implants have been devised. The standard implant for posterior fusions is a set of steel hooks and rods known as Harrington rods. These attach with the small hooks around the flat plates of bone projecting from the vertebral arches (laminae) and joints of the posterior portion of the spine. The most commonly used rod fits in the concave portion of the curve; it corrects by distracting or lengthening. Harrington rods can also be placed on the convex side of a curve, in which case they correct by compression. The original version of the Harrington rod was designed in 1958; thousands are implanted successfully every year.

Recently, a method of wiring each vertebra to an L-shaped rod (known as the Luque rod) has received a great deal of attention. This system has the advantage of providing greater stability and has its most generally

The internally implanted Harrington rod helps to stabilize the spine after surgery for scoliosis. It eliminates the need for wearing a heavy, restrictive body cast.

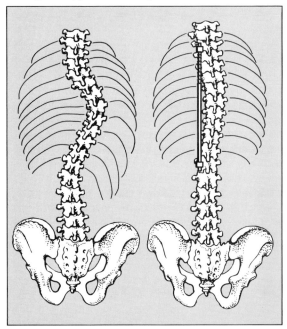

accepted application in paralytic scoliosis. Its long-term role in other forms of scoliosis has not yet been determined.

There are also a number of metallic instrumentation systems for surgeries involving the anterior portion of the spine. The most commonly used system (Dwyer) consists of a set of titanium screws and cables that attach and compress bodies of the vertebrae on the convex side of the curve. For technical reasons these usually span a shorter portion of the curve than do the posterior Harrington rods.

Although surgery is the definitive treatment in paralytic scoliosis, bracing is sometimes used to delay a fusion operation until a child is older. The reason for undertaking bracing is that the spine does not grow in the area of a solid fusion. This means that after a long fusion at a very young age, the child would end up considerably shorter than if the surgery were delayed. Usually some compromise between ideal height and control of the curve is required.

Treatment of congenital scoliosis. The basic problem in congenital scoliosis is unequal bone growth due to the abnormal structure of the bones. The treatment is nearly always surgical but with a different goal than in other forms of curvature. Treatment takes advantage of the fact that a solid fusion will stop the growth of the abnormal vertebrae. The aim of the fusion in congenital scoliosis is to stop the imbalanced growth in the area of the congenital anomaly. Because the forces generated by bone growth are very powerful, this may occasionally require both anterior and posterior fusions. Since stability is not a problem, implants are used much less frequently in treating congenital scoliosis than in treating other types.

Treatment of idiopathic scoliosis. The ideal approach to the progressive curve caused by idiopathic scoliosis is detection while the curve is still small and treatable with a brace. This will result in a mobile spine with completely normal function, even though the person will always have a minor curve. For scoliosis of the thoracic spine the so-called Milwaukee brace is usually used. This is the oldest of the currently used braces and therefore the one with which most physicians have the greatest experience. Its disadvantage is a high metal neck ring that encases the neck and is of cosmetic concern to many teenagers. There are a number of newer braces available today that seem to be equally effective for low (lumbar) curves; the appropriate selection is generally made by the physician and orthotist (brace specialist).

A great fear that many children and parents have is that wearing a brace may force inactivity and separation from peers. Teenagers wearing braces have participated in many sports, including baseball, cheerleading, ballet, and horseback riding. While having to wear a brace for a few years may be a nuisance and a frustration to wearers and parents alike, it need not

represent an overwhelming psychological burden or a period of invalidism.

Surgery in idiopathic scoliosis is reserved for those teenagers who are discovered too late for bracing, for the occasional brace failure, or for adults who develop pain or respiratory symptoms. The technique and instrumentation systems are the same as those described for paralytic scoliosis. Combined anterior and posterior surgery is done much less frequently than in paralytic scoliosis.

Surgery in the adult is most often indicated for pain relief. The curve causes the joints in the posterior column of the spine to be abnormally aligned. This, in turn, leads to excessive force on the joints and to a form of degenerative arthritis. The natural reaction of the body is to build up new bone in the arthritic area, which may lead to a narrowing of the opening in a vertebral arch (foramen) through which the spinal cord nerves exit, causing pain by compression.

In the adult the postoperative incidence of complications is greater and the results less gratifying than in the teenager. The bone graft takes longer to grow solidly, and the probability of obtaining a solid fusion with a single operation is less. The cosmetic correction is usually minimal. Pain relief, however, is usually substantial and sufficient to justify the surgery.

—*Wilton H. Bunch*, M.D., Ph.D.

Physical Fitness and Sports Medicine

Better to hunt in fields, for health unbought,
Than fee the doctor for a nauseous draught.
The wise, for cure, on exercise depend;
God never made his work for man to mend.

John Dryden's 17th-century beliefs, entertained by a minority over the years, have never been more commonly held than they are today in many Western countries, particularly in the United States. Aerobic dance classes pack in energetic men and women of all ages; athletic shoe sales flourish; and San Francisco now braces for the annual trans-city passage of 50,000 runners in the Bay-to-Breakers race, which 20 years ago attracted scarcely 100. The increased involvement of women in sports has been particularly marked in recent years; "unsuitable" sports, such as soccer and long-distance running, are now recognized as perfectly suitable for many women. Children have taken naturally to greatly increased exercise opportunities, often encouraged by parents and teachers. Finally, ground has been gained even by the elderly, as witnesses to the over-80 pole vault competition at the World Veteran Games can confirm.

There are several points to note. Our improved fitness levels result almost entirely from increased participation in vigorous leisure-time activities, not from enhanced popularity of the few remaining physically demanding occupations; we have to create our own exercise today. The most popular exercises—walking, running, swimming, and cycling—tend to be accessible, reasonably inexpensive, and at least moderately vigorous, or *aerobic.* It is clear that many of the new exercisers have become personally convinced that regular exercise improves the health, efficiency, and appearance of their bodies and does something for their minds, too. Most seem to have joined the movement as a result of contact with other converts or via the popular written word. The exercise explosion in the United States of the 1970s was certainly not the result of massive exercise promotion campaigns by our major health agencies.

The question arises: Are these exercisers the enlightened vanguard of a new, health-promoting lifestyle? Or are they the misguided adherents of a temporary aberration, a fad that will pass as we soon slip back again into the comfortable step-saving ease of the 1950s?

Rewards and costs of fitness

Habitual aerobic exercise leads to a state of physical fitness, in which structural and metabolic changes have occurred in the body, in comparison with the sedentary state. The heart becomes larger and expels more blood with each beat, and the resting heart rate decreases. The lung capacity increases, and exercised muscles become more efficient and develop higher concentrations of the energy-generating enzymes. This combination of events can lead to the extreme fitness of the Olympic athlete, but many men and women now attain and enjoy the rewards of more modest fitness levels. The fit person can more easily and enjoyably perform many activities demanding muscular stamina—furniture moving, climbing steps, and sex—than can the sedentary, deconditioned individual. The annual vacation is often more enjoyable for the year-round exerciser, who has acquired the built-in stamina required to climb mountains, go cross-country skiing, or take long hikes in the wilderness.

There is a general impression, albeit poorly researched, that the fit individual does better when stressed by illness or accident. Few people train with the object of better withstanding such unexpected and challenging happenings, but almost certainly the greater cardiac reserves of fit individuals can make the difference between survival and death in extreme circumstances.

In Western society today the length and quality of our lives particularly depend upon our experience with the chronic diseases, especially coronary heart disease. The fit person appears to have a distinct advantage here, too, according to the pioneering epidemiological studies of Jeremy N. Morris, who studied London civil servants from 1968 to 1970, and the more recent studies of Harvard and University of Pennsylvania alumni,

conducted by Ralph S. Paffenbarger. In these prospective studies a large group of men initially provided information on their physical activity habits and were then followed for many years during which the occurrence of heart attack and death from heart attack was documented. In both studies the most active men went on to suffer the least number of heart attacks and coronary deaths, even when allowance was made for other factors commonly accompanying the active life-style, such as leanness. In other words, high levels of physical activity seemed to confer an independent protective effect against heart attack.

It is only fair to list some costs associated with maintenance of physical fitness. Some sports, such as American football and downhill skiing, involve well-known injury hazards, but these sports also tend to be the less beneficial, nonaerobic type. Risk of automobile injury is clearly increased for those walkers, runners, and cyclists who frequent crowded roads, and suitable precautions should be observed. Almost all aerobic sports involve some risk of muscle, joint, or tendon injury through overuse; these are usually minor in the noncontact sports and can be minimized by preventive measures. Heat exhaustion is a potential hazard for all vigorous exercisers during hot weather, and adequate hydration is essential. Finally, all fitness-promoting activities require time, which might otherwise be devoted to other pursuits. Therefore, a personal judgment must be made, weighing these costs of physical fitness against the growing catalog of potential rewards.

Weight control and caloric intake

Perhaps the most visually obvious characteristic of regular exercisers is their leanness. This has been established scientifically in numerous studies showing the relatively low body fat content of cyclists, runners, tennis players, and other strenuous exercisers. Although beset with frequently made assertions in the popular press to the contrary, many men and women have discovered that regular exercise indeed is a good way to lose weight and to maintain their newly acquired figures. Since exercisers are usually lean, it is often believed that they must eat rather little; the blunting of appetite has been considered one of the benefits of exercise. For the dedicated exerciser, the reverse is the case. The runner regularly putting in 70 mi per week in training for a marathon consumes about 1,000 cal per day more than a similar but nonexercising, sedentary individual. The lower-level exerciser will also increase his daily caloric intake but in most cases to a less noticeable extent.

These facts relate to an interesting finding from several large population studies; generally speaking, fatter people eat less than thinner people. Although this may seem unjust to some, and it certainly is contrary to traditional views of gluttony, it makes sense when the activity factor is considered. Frequently, lean people are very active and eat heartily, while fat people are inactive and eat rather little. The moral for those who wish to eat well but remain slim is clear. The public health implications are also apparent. Large numbers of people in Western society are overweight by any standard, and obesity carries health penalties—e.g, any tendency to hypertension or diabetes is worsened. The solution to the problem, as presented in extremely popular diet books and magazine articles, invariably revolves around tricking the unwilling overweight subject into eating less. The variety of ingenious and exotic techniques used for this purpose is nothing short of amazing. Yet all these approaches sound the same clarion call: Eat less!

There are several disadvantages to the "eat less" approach to obesity prevention, apart from the obvious one that most people like to eat, and so relapse and re-gain of weight are almost par for the course. One problem is that many obese people already eat so little that further restriction of food may easily lead to inadequate vitamin and mineral intake. Again, low caloric intakes, often with low fiber contents, combined with little physical activity, lead to constipation; and further reduction of food intake can only worsen the condition. A final possibility is that the so-called appestat—the mechanism located in the brain that should nicely regulate an individual's regular food intake in relation to his or her energy expenditure—may function more precisely when food intake is high rather than low. This would account for the relative ease with which very active people maintain a desirable weight, while the sedentary tend to practice "the rhythm method of girth control."

The operation of the eat-more, weigh-less principle was observed in a one-year training study conducted recently by the Stanford Heart Disease Prevention Program in which 48 sedentary, middle-aged men took part in a progressive running program. At the end of the year, those men who had lost the most weight were those who had *increased* their caloric intake the most. Of course, they were also the men who did the most running.

No fewer than five prospective population studies have shown that caloric intake is a predictor of future heart death. Individuals who died were reported to have had lower caloric intakes than those who survived. (The former group was surveyed many years before death.) This is probably a reflection of the more sedentary life-style of the low-caloric-intake group, but it does provide further evidence that weight control by exercise is preferable to weight control by further reduction of an already low caloric intake. Of course, caloric restriction should be used in some cases as therapy for obesity; however, in most cases it probably should not be recommended as a desirable permanent feature of the modern life-style.

Exercise, cholesterol, and heart disease

It has long been known that the cholesterol count, the concentration of cholesterol in our blood plasma, predicts risk of developing coronary heart disease in the future. A number of early investigators examined the cholesterol level in the blood of vigorous exercisers and found it to be little different from that of average, sedentary people. Cholesterol, an important water-insoluble lipid substance, is carried in the blood as part of minute lipoprotein particles, which are spherical and composed of protein, cholesterol, fat (triglyceride), and phospholipid. These particles are not all identical; they belong to three families with names reflecting their densities: relatively large very-low-density lipoproteins (VLDL), intermediate size low-density lipoproteins (LDL), and small high-density lipoproteins (HDL). Most of the cholesterol making up our total cholesterol count is borne on LDL and HDL. It has been known for many years that high levels of LDL are atherogenic (producing degenerative changes in the walls of arteries) and predict future coronary artery disease. More recently it has been found that high levels of HDL predict *low* rates of future heart disease, and these small, dense particles may actually protect the walls of the arteries from disease.

Of course, this interesting finding has led to a search for circumstances associated with low levels of LDL and high levels of HDL—the lipoprotein prescription for healthy arteries. When the blood plasma of very active people, for instance, long-distance runners of both sexes, was reexamined for lipoprotein distribution, it was found that a rather "average" total cholesterol count concealed relatively low LDL levels and high HDL levels, compared with levels in sedentary controls; this might suggest that a long way down the road enhanced physical activity may confer on the exerciser the additional benefit of delayed or absent coronary artery disease, heart attack, and coronary death. As yet, however, this particular association must be viewed as a speculative one.

This cross-sectional finding has prompted longitudinal studies in which lipoprotein changes are followed as sedentary individuals are persuaded to become fit. The Stanford training study mentioned earlier suggests that a minimum of a mile per day of jogging (or probably an equivalent energy expenditure in other aerobic activities) is required for a period of at least nine months before significant beneficial changes in lipoproteins can be expected. Although such amounts of exercise would have been regarded as improbably excessive for sedentary Americans only a few years ago, many millions of people of all ages are now exceeding this level, with a modest expenditure of time.

Loss of body fat almost invariably accompanies the sedentary person's progression to fitness. Work is in progress to attempt to disentangle the salutary effects on lipoproteins and heart disease risk of weight loss on the one hand and of increased physical fitness on the other. The interesting possibility exists that weight loss by dieting (without increased exercise) may have quite different physiological and health consequences in comparison with an equal amount of weight loss by increased exercise (without dieting).

Other advantages of fitness

Growing numbers of additional health advantages are now attributed to the active life-style. The strength of the scientific evidence supporting these attributions varies widely, and in some cases very little research has been devoted to the particular issue. Nonetheless, active people often see in their activity a strong defense against an array of bodily ills.

Cigarette smoking. Aerobic exercisers seldom smoke, and when they do, the level is usually low. It might be thought that this reflects among these exercisers an estrangement from vice in all its forms. Studies indicate, however, that a considerable proportion of men and women exercisers are in fact ex-smokers, and that their present alcohol consumption is very similar to the national average. They appear to have selectively rejected smoking. The serious health penalties of smoking—lung cancer, emphysema, and coronary heart disease—are now so well established that it is unnecessary to dwell upon them. Although it is seldom specifically pointed out, the association of the active life-style with avoidance of smoking is one of the clearest and most welcome health benefits.

Bone density. Exercise retards the mineral loss from bones—a loss that is known to accompany the aging process. An active life allows us to arrive at later middle age with denser bones and so should help to prevent

"You should try race walking. It's better for you than running. It's good for your cardiovascular system, and at the end of fifteen minutes, your glands excrete a juice that will make you happy."

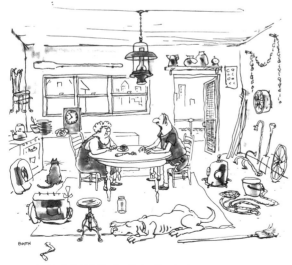

Drawing by Booth; © 1982 The New Yorker Magazine, Inc.

or postpone the fractures commonly resulting from osteoporosis (bone thinning in postmenopausal women and in elderly men).

Constipation. Exercise has long been recommended as a treatment for constipation and, indeed, very active individuals seem seldom to be afflicted. A recent survey of 335 men and women members of the Fifty Plus Runners' Association indicated that this irritating problem is virtually unknown among this active group.

Sleep. Regular exercise seems to improve sleep patterns, provided the activity is not performed too soon before bedtime.

Mental outlook. A striking feature of the exercise explosion of the past decade has been the interest—perhaps preoccupation—with the mental, psychological, even spiritual aspects of vigorous exercise. To the question, "Why do you regularly swim, or cycle, or jog?" the most common reply is, "Because I feel better when I do." Or, for less positive individuals, "Because I feel terrible if I don't." The so-called runner's high describes a pronounced euphoria reported to descend upon runners after they have covered ten or more miles. There is evidence that exercise promotes the release of opiatelike substances, notably the endorphins, from the brain. Possibly these substances may be responsible for the spectrum of pleasurable and stimulating sensations so commonly reported by the frequent exerciser. This research area is likely to be pursued in the coming years.

The early pioneering work of psychiatrist Thaddeus Kostrubala, at first regarded with considerable skepticism, introduced the use of vigorous exercise, usually running with a therapist, into the psychological treatment armamentarium. It seems clear that in some instances group exercise sessions may have results as good as or better than those obtained with conventional drug treatment for some depressed and even some schizophrenic individuals.

Post-heart attack. Exercise programs, particularly those involving walking, calisthenics, and jogging, are now routinely recommended for the rehabilitation of victims of uncomplicated heart attack. A fit body is particularly important for the owner of a damaged heart. As a result of such programs, for instance, that of pioneer Terrence Kavanagh of the Toronto Rehabilitation Center, some postcoronary individuals are physically fitter than they have ever been at any other point in their lives. A small but growing group of postcoronary patients have completed marathon races. The degree of rehabilitation achieved by such runners and the sense of return to the healthy world must exceed in curative power the effects of anything that ever came out of a medicine bottle or syringe.

Temporary conclusions about aerobic exercise

The past decade has seen great changes in attitudes toward and practice of aerobic exercise as a means of disease prevention. Although there are costs associated with regular exercise, on balance the health benefits far outweigh them. Health areas especially likely to benefit from the renewed interest in exercise are prevention or postponement of coronary heart disease, weight control, and mental health. Regular physical exercise is particularly associated with that most valued attribute, vigor.

Physical fitness should now be the birthright of both sexes at all ages. It is particularly important to encourage good exercise habits in children, especially through enlightened school programs. Aerobic activities should be particularly stressed, with a minimum of 40 minutes of reasonably strenuous, continuous activity on three or four occasions per week being recommended for normal, healthy people. The vigorous use of the legs and other major muscle blocks for as little as 2 to 3% of a 168-hour week would almost certainly greatly benefit the health of the vast majority of the population.

It seems most unlikely that the increased physical activity that has occurred in recent years is a temporary fad. Rather, the fad will probably be seen historically as that strange period of some 60 years during which Western societies unaccountably moved away from all unnecessary activity, lured by the automobile and the television set. The new exercise behavior is likely to

Runners, compared with sedentary persons, have shown higher levels of protective high-density lipoproteins and lower levels of disease-promoting (atherogenic) low-density lipoproteins.

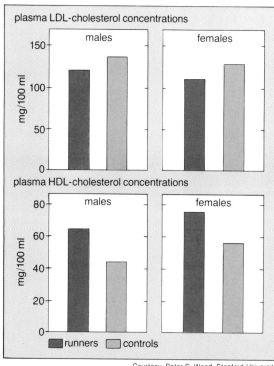

Courtesy, Peter D. Wood, Stanford University

persist because it too is seductive as well as self-rewarding; there is rapid feedback to the exerciser of a variety of pleasurable sensations that promote long-term adherence.

The late John Knowles said, "The next medical breakthrough is the patient taking responsibility for his own health." The exerciser appears to have partially achieved this breakthrough and is pioneering the new preventive medicine.

— Peter D. Wood, Ph.D., D.Sc.

Preventive Medicine

The routine health examination has become an annual ritual for a significant percentage of the adult population in the United States. Each year millions of Americans feel compelled to seek medical attention, not for specific symptoms of disease, but for assurances concerning their general state of health. Implicit in this activity are two assumptions: first, that the totally normal checkup assures one of being in good health; second, that disease, if discovered on routine examination, can be treated more effectively than if it were diagnosed after symptoms developed. Proponents of the periodic examination claim that these are exactly the benefits enjoyed by those who have had these examinations. Unfortunately, there is little evidence that the annual physical, as it is now performed, achieves either of these goals.

Nevertheless, the periodic health examination is now more popular than ever. It is, in fact, the most common reason people go to doctors, accounting for 7.2% of all office visits. The health care industry has created automated screening centers to expedite the procedure. With such limited information available regarding its efficacy, how then has it become so popular? The answer can be found at least in part by tracing its development over the past 80 years.

The evolution of the regular checkup

By the turn of the century, medicine in the United States had made significant advances. Primarily through public health measures, the prevalence of many communicable diseases (for example, cholera, smallpox, and typhoid fever) had been greatly reduced. The causes of greatest morbidity and mortality no longer were infectious in nature but were chronic ailments such as heart disease, kidney disease, and cancer. At the same time, new insights into pathophysiology of various disease states led to greater diagnostic capabilities.

With newly acquired diagnostic skills, physicians began to uncover physical defects in apparently healthy individuals. Examinations during World War I detected significant impairments in some 15% of draftees. Life insurance companies, particularly Metropolitan Life, developed programs of periodic examination, and they, too, found physical defects in asymptomatic individuals. Major corporations began to provide examinations for their employees in an attempt to prevent the spread of infectious disease within factories. Proponents of the periodic health examinations began to claim that the early discovery of these physical defects would prevent the later development of serious diseases. They claimed, in fact, that life itself could be prolonged through periodic checkups.

But a problem arose with the widespread acceptance of these conclusions. It is important to look at the types of diseases that were uncovered. The military, for example, found many cases of foot problems, decreased visual acuity, and venereal disease. Life insurance companies discovered a prevalence of problems associated with the eyes, ears, nose, and throat. The early treatment of these relatively minor ailments was no doubt important and in many cases probably resulted in improved health. However, that the incidence of the major killers—cardiac disease, cancer, and kidney disease—would be reduced in those examined was never substantiated. It was the failure to review critically the early reports that set the stage for increasing public and professional acceptance of the periodic health examination as a general means of early disease detection.

Despite this lack of data medical organizations such as the American Medical Association (AMA) began to promote the concept of periodic health examination. Articles in the medical literature soon appeared explaining the appropriate ways to perform such examinations and claiming that they would forestall serious illness. In 1923 the National Health Council and the U.S. Public Health Association supported a nationwide campaign to publicize this view, using the slogan "Have a Health Examination on Your Birthday." The goal was for ten million Americans to have examinations during the first year. The premise underlying these checkups was that preclinical states of disease, if detected early, could be treated easily and perhaps eradicated. But the problem with this assumption was twofold: first, since the technology had not been developed for screening occult cancer and heart disease, examinations were not capable of detecting the major causes of mortality. More importantly, if the examination did uncover these diseases, there was no effective therapy available at that time to treat them. For example, even hypertension, a disorder commonly seen in the asymptomatic individual, at that time could not be managed because effective drugs had not yet been developed.

The Great Depression was associated with a decrease in interest in the periodic health examination. However, after World War II, industry, which had always played a major role in preventive health measures, began to promote the health examination for management. While there were no specific health haz-

ards associated with management jobs, it seemed "good business" for a company to maintain the health of members of this group because of the pivotal roles they played. The examination was looked on as a fringe benefit for the executive and as a boon to the company; detection of disease would lead to rapid treatment and return to work instead of later detection, long invalidity, and loss of services of a valuable employee. Each corporation developed its own format for executive health examinations. Some relied heavily on laboratory tests, and others emphasized the history and physical examination. It was therefore difficult to compare results. The varied approaches again reflected the lack of evidence of effectiveness of any particular scheme. In fact, to this day there has never been a well-designed study showing that executives undergoing these examinations have benefited in terms of reductions in morbidity and mortality.

Around 1950 the practice of performing screening tests began to proliferate. Screenings were meant to sort out in a rapid manner those likely to have a disease from those who were not. Those individuals with positive tests would then be referred to physicians for diagnostic follow-up. In contrast to periodic health examinations, so-called multiphasic screening could be performed with limited physician involvement and at reduced costs. Common screening tests included chest X-rays for detection of tuberculosis, blood tests for the diagnosis of syphilis, and electrocardiograms for the uncovering of heart disease. This approach, although less costly and more technically advanced than standard examinations, met with significant resistance from the medical profession. For one thing many of the early screening tests were neither sensitive nor specific—e.g., they often missed disease when it was present, and when they indicated disease they were wrong. The electrocardiogram, for example, is normal in over a third of patients with symptomatic heart disease. It has even less diagnostic value in the asymptomatic patient. The electrocardiogram is thus an extremely poor device to screen for heart disease, independent of the cost and the manpower required to perform it. But ten years after the introduction of periodic screenings no study had shown conclusively that participating persons lived longer or had less illness than nonparticipants. By 1960 most of the early screening tests had been abandoned as ineffective by most experts.

Are periodic health exams warranted?

There is increasing awareness in the medical profession today that an annual checkup does not accomplish the goal of early disease detection. The grandiose claims of life extension have been replaced by the realization that many patients will have a major health disaster in the interim between the dates of scheduled examinations. The rising costs of health care today and the lack of a rational approach to preventive health measures have led to a critical reevaluation of the periodic health examination.

In 1976 a major undertaking was initiated by a group referred to as the Canadian Task Force on the Periodic Health Examination and comprised of an international group of distinguished scientists and clinicians. Their purpose was to ascertain whether early detection of 78 major preventable conditions would be beneficial and to develop a rational scheme for periodic health examinations. Around the same time at least three similar endeavors were also undertaken in the U.S. by groups, including the American Cancer Society (ACS). The ACS findings resulted in a major revision of recommendations on cancer-related examinations. Although there were differences in some of the specific recommendations that emerged from such studies, the tailoring of examinations to the needs and risks of various age groups was a unifying concept.

The Canadian Task Force, in reviewing each potentially preventable condition, focused on the overall effectiveness of available treatments or preventive measures, the burden of suffering caused by the conditon, and certain characteristics of the early detection procedure to be used. In deciding whether a particular condition should be a candidate for regular examinations, ratings were established. Class A meant there was good evidence that a condition should be included in periodic health checkups; class E meant there was good evidence that the condition should be excluded. The effectiveness of treatment was also rated. Grade I indicated that there was evidence from well-designed studies of the merits of treatment; grade III (the lowest) indicated that evidence regarding treatment was based on the convictions of some respected experts but not on properly performed studies.

The Canadian results, based largely on a comprehensive survey of the worldwide medical literature, were not surprising. They clearly showed that scientific evidence on the merits of the periodic health examination concept was substantially lacking. In fact, treatments were graded III for a majority of conditions. Nevertheless, there were a few recommendations strongly advocated by the task force. These were called health protection packages and were aimed at various age groups. The recommendations for the person under 30 were significantly different from those for the person over 45, reflecting the fact that the greatest risk of acquiring specific medical disorders occurs at specific stages in life.

Colonic cancer, for example, is the second most common cause of cancer death in the United States. However, the risk of colon cancer starts to increase at age 45 and continues to increase with progressive aging. The Canadian recommendation thus was that screening for occult blood in the stool should begin at age 45 and be repeated yearly. Hypertension is another disorder that occurs more commonly in the older population. However, owing to its frequency in the younger population, the relative simplicity of screening for it, and the benefits derived from its early detection, the task force recommended that blood pressure screening begin at age 16.

The task force recognized as well that the periodic health examination also affords the setting for providing important information, such as counseling the patient about the potential hazards posed by excessive alcohol consumption, smoking, overeating, and failure to use seat belts. A further recommendation was for immunization against influenza for adults 64 and older and for diphtheria/tetanus boosters every ten years beginning at age 16. Chest X-rays, electrocardiograms, urinalysis, and blood chemistries were not generally recommended. In fact, the only X-ray considered beneficial was a mammogram for women over the age of 50.

The future of regular checkups

Perhaps the most important result of the Canadian Task Force's documentation (and that of other recent studies) was in directing physicians' practices and future research. In the 80 years since the introduction of the periodic health exam public enthusiasm for getting regular (yearly) checkups has steadily increased. Moreover, a recent survey in the U.S. found that 14% of office visits to an internist include an electrocardiogram and 39% a clinical laboratory test, despite scant evidence of their value for the patient.

From now on the potential value of these examinations should be determined only after careful study of each specific test and screening method. Physicians for the first time have some concrete information to guide them in providing preventive health care. While the perfunctory annual examination is not a valuable tool in early disease detection, there are several screening tests that appear to be effective in uncovering early, treatable diseases. It is hoped that future research will provide new methods of screening that will lead to a periodic health examination capable of reducing the ravages of cancer and heart disease.

Recently a number of physicians groups in the U.S. have urged new approaches. The American College of Physicians recommends that each internist develop an individualized plan for each patient. The Council on Scientific Affairs of the American Medical Association in 1982 conducted its first review in 35 years of the AMA's policy on physicals. The recommendation is for fewer, more cost-effective exams. Finally, it is obvious that physicians will have to reevaluate their practice habits as more is learned about preventive medicine. Probably they will need to tailor their provision of health care toward *selective* approaches (determined in large part by the patient's age and sex) rather than *routine* annual checkups for all.

—*Mitchell H. Charap, M.D.*

Special Report:
Benefits of Moderate Drinking
by Thomas B. Turner, M.D.

In ancient Greece the influential Athenian statesman Eubulus wrote, "Three bowls [of wine] only do I mix for the temperate; one to health, . . . the second to love and pleasure, the third to sleep." Only in the last two decades, however, have modern investigations supported the concept of favorable health effects from moderate drinking. It cannot be ignored, of course, that alcoholism and misuse of alcohol are enormous problems the world over. The problems posed by the excessive consumption of alcohol must be recognized universally as a major threat to the public health.

Findings concerning beneficial effects obviously need to be viewed in perspective to assist the individual in making an informed choice about his own use of alcohol. The favorable relationships concern particularly the risk of coronary thrombosis, relief of stress, use of alcohol by the aged, and even the nutritional attributes of some types of alcoholic beverages.

Basic to an understanding of the issues involved is an appreciation of the central importance of the *quantity* of alcohol consumed. For convenience the terms light, moderate, and heavy drinking, which convey a general quantitative notion of consumption, are used; more precise definitions are given later.

The body's metabolism of alcohol

Ethanol, or alcohol, as it will be termed, is a product of the fermentation of carbohydrates, mainly from fruits or grain, by enzymes present in yeast or bacteria. Absolute prohibition of alcohol use is therefore an impossibility, since it can be made easily in any home. A small amount of alcohol ($\frac{1}{2}$ to 1 oz [1 oz = 30 ml]) is, in fact, produced daily within the body in the human intestinal tract.

Ingested alcohol is absorbed from the stomach or upper intestinal tract into the bloodstream and carried to the liver, where it is metabolized by the enzyme alcohol dehydrogenase (ADH) to acetaldehyde and by aldehyde dehydrogenase (ALDH) to other breakdown products, then to carbon dioxide (CO_2) and water. What are known as blood alcohol levels (BAL) peak in 20–40 minutes after consumption of an ordinary drink. If a second drink is taken half an hour later, BAL reaches a higher peak with more prolonged disappearance. Absorption from the stomach is slower and BAL lower when alcohol is taken in the form of wine or beer than in more concentrated form; absorption is also slower when taken with food. Because of these variables only an approximate relationship between

amount ingested and peak blood levels can be established.

Size of drink in relation to body weight is the most important variable, however. Yale University physiologist H. W. Haggard and his associates in 1941 made observations on BAL in 112 volunteers, male and female, after one drink containing 22 g (1 g = 0.035 oz) of alcohol, the amount in 2.3 oz of 80-proof spirits. (The term proof refers to a measure of the proportion of pure alcohol in spirits, the strength indicated by a number that is twice the percent by volume of alcohol present, so that 100-proof represents 50%, 80-proof, 40%, and so forth.) Blood levels varied inversely according to body weight. The largest persons, 176–246 lb, showed average peak levels of 0.04% (40 mg/100 ml); the middle-weight group, 143–174 lb, 0.05%; and the smallest persons, 103–140 lb, 0.056%. After a meal the highest BAL was 0.03%. The reading for the same amount of alcohol in beer on an empty stomach was 0.03%. Doubling the amount of alcohol in a single drink did not quite double the BAL. Age and sex were not significant variables. These findings were confirmed in substance by the Swedish physiologist Leonard Goldberg in 1963 and in studies in Canada in 1973.

Acute and chronic effects may result from consumption of alcohol at levels of one gram per kilogram of body weight and over (*i.e.,* more than 8 oz of spirits for a 175-lb person). It is estimated that 10% of the drinking population either imbibes chronically to excess or occasionally, as in "binges." It is these individuals who not only endanger their health but account for the alcohol-related tragedies that give alcohol a bad name. Like automobiles and fire, alcohol must be used responsibly. The factors that promote transition from moderate to excessive drinking in a minority are poorly understood and have received too little research attention.

Presumed healthful effects of alcohol

The moderate use of alcohol carries a minimum risk of ill health and, as noted above, recent scientific studies have shown several possible *beneficial* effects occurring with measured, moderate intake. Some of these presumed salubrious effects involve the following:

Coronary heart disease. Myocardial infarction, commonly due to narrowing and obstruction of one or more arteries that supply blood to the heart, is one of the prime causes of death or partial disability in persons between the ages of 40 and 60, especially men. In

1964 in a study of 464 men with this condition treated in the Kaiser-Permanente health care system, cardiologist Arthur Klatsky and his associates found that the proportion of moderate drinkers averaging one or two drinks daily was significantly lower than the proportion of abstainers when compared with controls matched for race, age, and sex. When conditions that predispose to heart attacks, such as diabetes, hypertension, heavy smoking, and obesity, were considered, the result was the same. This study appears to have demonstrated then that while regular moderate use of alcohol did not eliminate this type of heart attack, its use was associated with a reduced risk.

Similar findings have been reported subsequently by at least eight other groups of investigators from such diverse locations as Massachusetts, Florida, Illinois, Hawaii, Scotland, New Zealand, Israel, and Yugoslavia. In each study the difference between moderate drinkers and nondrinkers was statistically significant. In several studies this seemingly favorable effect of alcohol extended to those who averaged more than two drinks a day, but as alcohol intake increased, the incidence of other disabling conditions also increased, eventually negating the advantage.

While the association of moderate alcohol use with a lower incidence of coronary thrombosis does not prove a cause-and-effect relationship, two related types of observations suggest that alcohol may play a protective role. At the turn of the century a Boston internist, Richard Cabot, noted that alcoholics coming to autopsy tended to have a lesser degree of arteriosclerosis than other autopsied persons of the same sex and age. During the next four decades similar observations were reported from Chicago, New York, and, again, Boston. More recently (1977) pharmacologist J. J. Barboriak

and his associates at the Medical College of Wisconsin, Milwaukee, analyzed the degree of coronary artery involvement in 909 nondiabetic male patients who underwent coronary arteriography in two hospitals over a period of four years. They correlated the findings with the patients' drinking and smoking habits—the two sets of determinations being made "blind." Among groups matched for age and smoking, "coronary occlusion scores" showed consistently unfavorable readings for abstainers and those who averaged less than 20 g of alcohol daily, compared with those drinking more than that amount.

A physiological explanation of these findings may lie in the results of studies on different fractions of blood cholesterol. An excess of low-density lipoprotein (LDL) cholesterol is associated with increased deposition of cholesterol-derived plaques in the arteries, while high-density lipoprotein (HDL), which varies inversely with LDL, transports cholesterol more effectively and reduces the likelihood of arterial cholesterol deposits.

The next step in this unfolding story was the observation, reported from many clinics in North America, Europe, and Australia, that alcohol consumption raised HDL levels. The association is more striking in males, but it is also observed in females; women, however, tend to have normally higher HDL levels than men, especially in the premenopausal years. Exercise is also known to raise HDL levels.

Relief of stress. It has been conjectured that the long popularity of alcoholic drinks rests primarily on its action in relieving the stress of daily events. It is a beverage used by millions the world over because it gives pleasure and relaxation. It has been difficult, however, to test the stress-reduction hypothesis either through controlled trials or sociologically oriented investiga-

In addition to the increased sociabilty that drinking brings, modern investigations have recently suggested that moderate drinking can have beneficial effects on health as well.

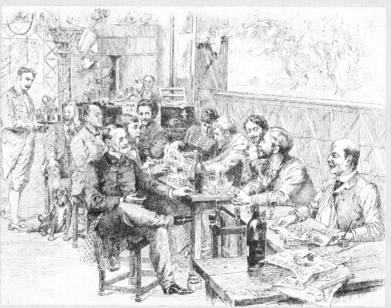

tions. British psychiatrist Griffith Edwards in a well-designed study in 1972 looked at 306 men belonging to different London socioeconomic suburban groups, concluding that the relief of stress and anxiety constituted a major component of the urge to use alcohol, with the enhancement of social interaction being another major component.

In a laboratory setting galvanic skin conductance response has been employed as a physiological measure of stress. With this method, which detects very minute alterations in electrical resistance of the skin, associated with the sympathetic nervous system, it has been shown, for example, that sudden emotional responses cause large and rapid increases in conductance (a phenomenon commonly measured by the lie detector). Thus, experiments have been devised in which stress is induced by external factors such as exposure to heat or to unexpected loud noise. The level at which these stresses created alarm was considerably raised by one or two drinks.

In 1978 Rutgers University psychologist T. R. Lipscomb and his associates devised an ingenious method of creating stress based on social interaction of the sexes, specifically involving unrequited attention and rejection. As determined by heart rate, skin conductance, and certain verbal tests, the experiment showed that stress had in fact been created; it was then observed to be ameliorated by small amounts of alcohol.

The results of these rather meager experiments are supported by much work in animals placed in various stressful situations, but to what extent stress in animals under those conditions resembles the ordinary stresses of life to which human beings are so frequently subjected is debatable. Nevertheless, the experimental evidence, together with accumulated common experience, indicates that alcohol in moderate amounts does appear to have a tranquilizing effect on anxiety and stress.

Alcohol and the aged. Recent controlled studies show that small amounts of alcohol taken once a day, especially in social settings, significantly improve the quality of life of the institutionalized elderly. The effects seem to be both physiological and psychological, but whether relief of stress is a major component of the effect is not clear. Leaders in this field have been Brian L. Mishara and Robert Kastenbaum, clinical psychologists, working mostly in homes for the elderly in Massachusetts. Others, too, have conducted studies of a similar nature. Most clinical trials in this area have followed a generally similar pattern. Groups studied have been residents of either nursing homes or retirement housing, with participation on a voluntary basis. Usually there is a pretest period in which various physical and psychological tests are performed. A period of four to six weeks follows in which all participating members of a group are given either an alcoholic drink, usually wine or beer, or a nonalcoholic drink before the evening meal. The groups then are reversed in respect to the type of drink; this is followed by a no-drink period for all participants. Physiological and psychological tests are performed blind by observers; that is, they do not know whether the group is receiving an alcoholic or nonalcoholic drink. Frequent observations of group behavior by nurses and attendants are also made.

The outcome of these studies has been that the groups receiving alcoholic drinks were consistently judged to be more tractable, capable, and possibly more contented than when receiving the nonalcoholic beverages. The consumers of alcohol also showed less need for tranquilizing medications. Moreover, no incident of subsequent excessive drinking was noted. The results of one study involving a group of 34 senile men were particularly striking. After two months of access to a drink in the evenings, not only was the general attitude of the patients better but certain measurable physical indexes had improved. For example, the number of incontinent men dropped from 26 to 9; those requiring physical restraint to prevent falls from chairs decreased from 26 to 4; and the number of ambulatory patients rose from 7 to 25.

Medical practitioners of a previous generation were generally aware of the beneficial effects of small amounts of alcohol, one to two drinks, in the aged, but under the constraints of prohibition the practice was largely discontinued in the U.S., with tranquilizing drugs often being substituted in more restless persons. The rationale of alcohol use has now been put on a firmer medical basis.

Nutritional aspects of alcohol use. Alcohol, alone, yields seven calories per gram. Since an ordinary drink contains approximately 15 g of alcohol, the caloric contribution to the diet from the alcohol would be about 105 cal. The caloric contribution is similar to that derived from carbohydrates. Very heavy drinkers, however, seem to have some poorly understood mechanism of metabolizing alcohol in which the full caloric contribution is not made.

Most alcoholic drinks, except spirits diluted with water, contain other food elements. A 12-oz bottle of beer, for example, has a caloric value of about 140 derived from alcohol, carbohydrates, and a small amount of protein. It also contains minerals such as potassium, magnesium, and calcium; metals—zinc, chromium, copper, and manganese—in trace amounts; and the vitamins thiamine, riboflavin, niacin, and pyridoxine in small amounts. All alcoholic beverages are virtually devoid of fat and cholesterol; beer is low in sodium, compared with many foods. Wines, too, contain other food elements besides alcohol, with a total caloric value of about 85 in a 3.5-oz serving of table wine. Because of the smaller volume, the actual amount of minerals and vitamins in a one-drink portion of wine is less than in malt beverages.

It is estimated that alcohol accounts for about 8% of

The party begins.

2 drinks later.

After 4 drinks.

After 5 drinks.

7 drinks in all.

Although moderate drinking may be harmless, the evils of heavy drinking are a pervasive and chronic problem. This public interest advertisement from a liquor manufacturer seeks to help educate the public to learn to drink responsibly and sensibly, and in particular not to drive after drinking.

the total calories in the typical adult diet in the U.S. Clearly there is no reason to use alcoholic beverages from a purely nutritional standpoint; if used, however, they constitute a nonfat contribution to total caloric intake. Obviously, for persons attempting to reduce caloric intake significantly, alcohol consumption would not be beneficial.

Longevity. Apart from the impact on the quality of life, data are emerging to suggest that the moderate use of alcohol may contribute on balance to longevity. Raymond Pearl, a Johns Hopkins University biologist and biostatistician, in a study of a Baltimore population in the 1920s, observed that moderate steady drinkers exhibited somewhat lower rates of mortality and greater expectation of life than did persons who did not drink. Although the differences did not reach statistical significance, Pearl concluded from that and other studies that moderate drinking did not increase the overall risk to life.

More recently Arthur Klatsky and his associates in California have reported on the ten-year mortality rate among 8,060 persons grouped according to drinking patterns and controlled for various risk factors. Overall mortality was lowest among those averaging two drinks or fewer a day; rates among abstainers and those averaging three to five drinks were significantly higher; former alcoholics were not included. The rate

for those averaging six or more drinks was the highest. Somewhat similar findings were reported in 1980 by A. R. Dyer, a specialist in community medicine, in Chicago and in 1981 by epidemiologist M. G. Marmot and associates in London. It can be concluded with assurance at the present time that regular moderate consumption of alcohol does not increase the overall risk to life; accumulating data seem to suggest a health-enhancing effect from one to two drinks a day.

What are the upper limits of "moderate" drinking?

To be useful as a guide to drinking patterns, the amount of alcohol consumed must be related to the body weight of the individual. The common practice in bars and restaurants of making all drinks the same whether the person weighs 110 or 180 lb puts responsibility squarely on the individual. For example, an airplane serving of spirits commonly contains 1.6 oz of 80-proof (40% alcohol), or 15 g of ethanol.

In an effort to develop simple guides to moderate drinking, a group at Johns Hopkins University have recorded what they considered to be upper limits of the total daily amounts of alcohol that could be termed moderate; the limit was set at an average of 0.7 g per kg body weight for any three-day period, with an absolute limit of 0.8 g for any 24-hour period. Shown in the

296

table is the application of the formula to persons of various weights and to different beverages.

These limits were derived from consideration of various types of data, including the following: (1) a review of alcohol intake data in patients with chronic illnesses attributable to alcohol; in most instances, the individual had been consuming more than 100 g of alcohol daily, and nearly all had been consuming more than 80 g, although as a rule no estimates of body weights were available; (2) a Swedish study of eight men in their twenties given 0.9 g per kg body weight of alcohol daily over a period of five weeks, which was preceded and followed by an alcohol-free period of six weeks; no adverse clinical or laboratory changes were noted; (3) the introduction of an arbitrary safety factor based on the data cited in the two above studies; and (4) health data derived from moderately drinking physicians followed for 20 to 30 years by internist Caroline B. Thomas and associates at Johns Hopkins.

It must be emphasized that the figure of 0.7 g per kg is an upper limit and not one to be regarded as a daily target; moderate drinkers consume considerably less on the average. While the limits might seem high, calculation will reveal that they are readily approached if alcohol is taken at lunch and again before dinner.

As an easy method of determining a personal upper limit for different types of beverage, the following formula can be used: for 80-proof spirits bare-body weight in pounds is divided by 30 to arrive at the proper number of ounces of beverage. Thus for 120 lb, 4 oz would be the upper limit; for 150 lb, 5 oz. For beer drinkers body weight is divided by 3; thus a 120-lb person would have an upper limit of 40 oz of beer; a 150-lb person, 50 oz. For table wine body weight is divided by 9; one who weighs 120 lb can have 13 oz; one who weighs 150 lb, 16.5 oz.

The evidence suggests that excessive alcohol intake in whatever form can be damaging to health. Most excessive drinkers, however, tend to gravitate to the more concentrated drinks—*i.e.,* spirits or fortified wines. Simple logistics of intake and urinary output operate against excessive use of the more dilute beverages such as beer. M. H. Brenner of Johns Hopkins in 1982 showed positive correlations between national and regional per capita consumption of spirits and certain health effects such as liver cirrhosis but considerably weaker correlations with consumption figures for the more dilute beverages.

Moderate drinking: daily upper limits								
body weight		grams ethanol	spirits*		wine		beer	
kg	lb	0.7 g/kg	oz	ml	oz	ml	oz	ml
70	154	49	5.2	153	18	532	48	1419
80	176	56	6.0	177	20	591	53	1567
90	198	63	6.7	198	23	680	60	1774
*80-proof								

There are obviously important cautions and caveats. One must avoid the foolish indiscretions that sometimes attend moderate drinking. Situations in which loss of balance or inattention may occur (*e.g.,* climbing ladders, boating, operating certain machinery, driving cars, and so forth) obviously pose a risk factor. The studies of Leonard Goldberg in Sweden (1963) indicated that in moderate drinkers impairment of various reflex activities did not begin until a blood level of 0.06% had been reached, and in most persons the threshold was higher, in some exceeding 0.10%. At the same time, impairment as determined by various laboratory tests was consistently observed at lower peak blood alcohol levels in persons who were normally abstainers or used alcohol only occasionally.

The safety of drinking moderately during pregnancy has not been settled. Some experts look to the apparently healthy generations of Europeans, exposed *in utero* to small daily amounts of alcohol. Recently, studies of the so-called fetal alcohol syndrome, well publicized in the U.S. in the past few years, leave little doubt that *excessive* drinking by pregnant women increases the risk of damage to the fetus. Whether moderate alcohol intake poses a risk to the unborn child is not absolutely clear. It is known that maternal infections, use of various drugs, and heavy smoking are associated with increased risk of fetal damage; most studies of the effect of moderate alcohol consumption have not been adequately controlled for these factors. Judgment must therefore be reserved at this time, but most experts currently think it best for pregnant women not to drink. Acting U.S. Surgeon General E. N. Brandt in 1981 recommended that until the situation is clarified, all women abstain from alcohol during pregnancy.

Reasonable conclusions

Recent studies indicate that the regular moderate use of alcohol is associated with a decrease in the risk of myocardial infarction and the development of atherosclerosis as compared with abstinence; other findings suggest that it may also enhance the quality of life, especially in the aged. It should be understood that these are statistical associations that do not prove a cause-and-effect relationship or suggest that each individual is necessarily benefited by the moderate use of alcohol. Common sense dictates that no one should interpret these findings as a sole reason for using alcohol. What they do clearly reveal is that alcohol used moderately and sensibly does not lead to ill health or to a shortened life.

It is not fully understood why some persons go well beyond the range of moderate drinking and become abusers or alcoholics; in this sense moderate drinking for a few may pose a health hazard. What can be stated with assurance, however, is that if one who wishes to drink adheres to the practice of moderation, no harm from alcohol is likely to ensue.

Special Report:
Sleep: How Much Do We Need?
by Lynne Lamberg

"Get eight hours of sleep every night." Most people have received this advice from parents, teachers, or family doctors. Although advice on sleep habits is easy to come by, scientists have yet to establish both what it is that sleep does and whether a fixed amount is necessary to obtain the supposed benefits.

In the past two decades sleep researchers have begun to penetrate the mysteries surrounding the subject of sleep. In order to treat disorders such as insomnia (difficulty in getting to sleep), narcolepsy (uncontrollable sleepiness), and sleep apnea (frequent pauses in breathing during sleep), researchers have monitored the sleep of thousands of "normal" and "abnormal" sleepers, recording brain activity and alterations in bodily functions. In addition, researchers have examined the subjects' own attitudes about sleep and their assessments of their physical and mental well-being after varying amounts of sleep. More than 60 medical centers, universities, and teaching hospitals now have clinics for treating sleep disorders and for doing research into the nature of sleep, and the number is expected to reach 100 by 1985.

The researchers agree that the need to sleep is an inborn trait. Most people do, indeed, spend between seven and eight hours of each day sleeping, for a total of some 220,000 hours in an average lifetime. Even people living in isolation in caves or windowless research facilities with no clocks or other clues to time of day, who may go to bed and get up whenever they wish, sleep about one-third of the time.

Whether sleep and dreaming are viewed as a period of gentle refreshment and preparation for a new day or as a continuation and transformation of psychological events, it is agreed that sleep is needed by everyone.

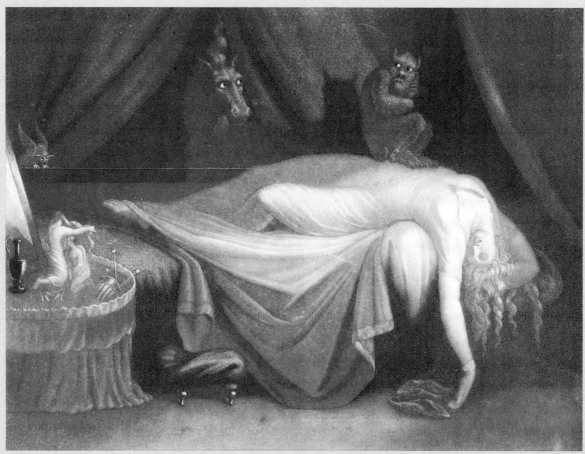

"Short sleepers"

While reports of persons who never sleep circulate from time to time, no such case has ever been verified. Sleep researchers at the Royal Edinburgh Hospital in Scotland recently reported their study of a man who claimed he had not slept for ten years, blaming his sleeplessness on a traffic accident that left him momentarily unconscious. He had not worked since the accident and continued to receive disability benefits. He agreed to be observed in the sleep laboratory if he could be accompanied by his wife. The first night he did not sleep. The second, he slept 20 minutes. The third, he again did not sleep. By the fourth day, his speech was slurred and rambling and he looked disheveled. That night he and his wife talked loudly through the early hours; he then got out of bed to walk around. He finally fell asleep at 6 AM and slept until 8:30 AM, when his wife awakened him. He insisted he must have been cured by an injection. He was a natural "short sleeper" who had profited from this condition.

Although everyone seems to need sleep, some people can get by on very little. A 70-year-old nurse is one of the most extreme cases of short sleep on record. She had slept only an hour daily since childhood, she told sleep researchers at Bedford College in London. In the sleep laboratory, she averaged only 67 minutes a night five nights in a row. She did not nap and was not sleepy at other times. The existence of satisfied short sleepers demonstrates that the amount of sleep people need is widely variable.

While most adults average 7 to 8 hours of sleep per night, about one in every 20 persons usually sleeps under 6 or over 9 hours in every 24. However, only one person in 100 regularly gets less than 5 or more than 10 hours of sleep a night; 5 to 10 hours is considered the "normal" range. Differences in the number of hours people sleep, like differences in height or intelligence, represent individual variations.

Age and sleep

One important factor that affects the amount of sleep people get is age. Newborn babies spend an average of 16 to 18 hours out of every 24 in sleep; sleep is parceled out into six to eight periods. However, some normal, healthy babies may sleep as many as 22 hours or as few as 5. The newborn baby's seemingly random periods of waking and sleeping swiftly adjust to its parents' schedule. By only three months of age, a baby typically stays awake the longest in the late afternoon and early evening. By the time the baby is six months old, it usually sleeps the longest at night. Dispensing with the 2 AM feeding occasions parents considerable relief, for they then can get a longer stretch of unbroken sleep themselves.

By age two the average child sleeps about 12 hours a day, with most of it coming at night and the remainder in a single nap. Still, three out of four two-year-olds waken at least once during the night. By age four most children abandon naps. A six-year-old as a rule sleeps about ten hours a night. The amount of time spent sleeping gradually declines until puberty; a 14- or 15-year-old sleeps an average of seven to eight hours a night, the same as most adults.

Children aged 6 to 12 tend to go to sleep and get up at about the same time on weekdays and weekends. By contrast, adolescents often follow very different schedules during the school week and on weekends, when they go to bed later and sleep longer than on weekdays. Extra sleeping on weekends may be an attempt to recover sleep lost during the school week. However, there also may be a true increase in sleepiness during the rapid growth that takes place during adolescence. Stanford University studies indicate that children aged 10 to 13 rarely experience daytime sleepiness or fall asleep in the classroom. However, among 500 college students surveyed, one in four admitted sleeping in class. Even when older adolescents are permitted to sleep as long as they wish at night, some are still sleepy during the day.

Most American adults also sleep longer on weekends than during the week, a fact that suggests they may not be getting as much sleep as they need for full alertness. Studies show that most American adults are chronically sleepy, as indicated by the rapidity with which they fall asleep during the day. The Multiple Sleep Latency Test, developed at Stanford, measures sleep latency, or the time it takes to fall asleep. Individuals are given the opportunity to fall asleep five or six times at two-hour intervals during the day, but not permitted to sleep longer than ten minutes at a time. On this test college students and middle-aged adults take about ten minutes to fall asleep. By contrast, preadolescent children do not fall asleep at all.

Sleep researchers stress that it is not "normal" to fall asleep in meetings or concerts or while watching television, despite the fact that such behavior is quite common. William Dement, a pioneer in sleep research who is director of the Stanford Sleep Disorders Clinic, suggests that such behavior indicates that a person is not getting enough sleep. Extreme daytime sleepiness also may indicate disorders of sleep, such as narcolepsy, which may make a person fall asleep suddenly in the midst of some activity, or sleep apnea, which involves numerous pauses in breathing during sleep.

The ability to sustain sleep usually declines gradually with age. The older people get, the more likely they are to wake more often and stay awake longer during the night. The elderly do not seem to need less sleep or to get less sleep; they simply spread their sleep out by napping during the day. On the Multiple Sleep Latency Test persons in their sixties and older fall asleep in an average of only five minutes, demonstrating extreme sleepiness. Particularly in the very elderly there often is a lack of daytime alertness.

When young and middle-aged adults get as little as an hour more sleep than usual, their performance on tests of addition and memory improves. The same cannot be said for many elderly persons, who prove unable to sleep longer even when they wish to do so.

Other factors affecting sleep needs

Although sleep commonly is thought necessary for rest and restoration of body and mind, differences in daytime physical or mental activities do not account for differences in the amount of sleep an individual needs. People who work principally with their hands, for example, do not need more or less sleep than those who work mainly with their minds. Conditioned athletes as a rule do not need more or less sleep than spectators; the weekend athlete often mistakes physical fatigue and the desire to rest for a need for additional sleep.

Work and family demands affect the amount of sleep people get. A Harvard Medical School study found that lawyers were more likely than doctors to sleep eight or more hours a night. The lawyers also were more likely to rate the pressure in their work as high and their practices as less satisfactory. The researchers suggested that the lawyers might be compensating for their job stresses by sleeping more.

Cultural habits also may play a role. Mexican adults sleep more than American or English adults, thanks to the customary midafternoon siesta. Mexican adults get the same amount of sleep at night as adults of other nationalities.

Psychiatrist Ernest Hartmann, director of the sleep laboratory at the Lemuel Shattuck Hospital in Boston, surveyed variable sleepers; that is, persons who said they consistently needed more sleep at certain times and less at others. He found that the majority of a group of 500 variable sleepers needed more sleep when they were ill, performing extra physical work, or under mental stress. They needed less sleep when they were experiencing few changes or stresses in their lives or were engaged in some pleasurable pursuit.

Most people recognize that no fixed number of hours of sleep is necessary on any given night. A person can stay up to meet a job deadline or watch over a sick child and still function the next day. One may forgo sleep under pleasant circumstances such as a high school prom or in the excitement of the night before Christmas. Most people sleep for somewhat different lengths of time from night to night, going to bed when they want to but getting up when they have to.

Going without sleep

Going without sleep, even for days on end, is not life-threatening, nor does it, as once was popularly believed, trigger madness. A 17-year-old student stayed awake for 264 hours—11 days—as a research project for a school science fair. The last 90 hours were spent in the company of sleep researchers. The youth con-

versed well and played games with dexterity until the conclusion of the project and suffered no ill aftereffects. *The Guinness Book of World Records* says the longest recorded period of wakefulness, 449 hours (18 days, 17 hours), was achieved by Maureen Weston of England in a rocking-chair marathon in 1977.

Sleep researchers now realize that no one goes entirely without sleep. Most people, after about 72 hours without sleep, start to experience brief sleep episodes, known as microsleeps. Eventually, and even under painful circumstances, longer sleep becomes irresistible. In animal experiments, even when rats were crowded together in cages they managed to sleep by hanging by their upper teeth from the wire mesh on top of the cage.

The effects of going without one's accustomed sleep are of particular interest to the military; during wartime, combatants may have to be alert 24 hours a day. Studies at the Walter Reed Army Medical Institute show that soldiers given encouragement and support were able to stay awake and to perform well for 72 to 98 hours. After going without sleep for several days, most people are able to feel normal again after sleeping only their usual amount, plus perhaps an hour or two.

People with hectic lives sometimes view sleep as a waste of time and wish they could give it up. In a study at the Naval Health Research Center in San Diego and the University of California at Irvine, four couples reduced their sleep gradually over a four- to six-month period. Three couples began the study as eight-hour sleepers and reduced their sleep by one to two hours. One couple began as 6.5-hour sleepers; although they reduced their sleep during the study, at its conclusion they reverted to their original pattern. Six years later the eight-hour sleepers still were sleeping less and professed satisfaction with the lesser amount. While it appears that it is possible for a person to reduce the amount of sleep he regularly gets and to remain at a lower level, the long-term implications for the sleeper's health are not yet known.

Researchers are concerned about the effects of manipulating the body's customary requirement for sleep and of shortening sleep. One large-scale study raised the issue of whether sleeping considerably less—or more—than average could, in some instances, shorten a person's life. A research group at the Veterans Administration Medical Center in San Diego reviewed statistics gathered by the American Cancer Society on the habits of more than one million people, who were followed for six years. They found that people who on the average slept either less than seven hours or more than 7.9 hours were more likely to have died by the six-year follow-up. Additionally, they found that people who reported using sleeping pills "often" were about 50% more likely to have died than those who reported "never" taking sleeping pills. However, in a report published in the *Archives of General Psychiatry* in Janu-

Photographs, Christopher Springmann

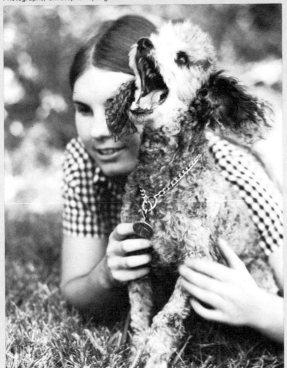 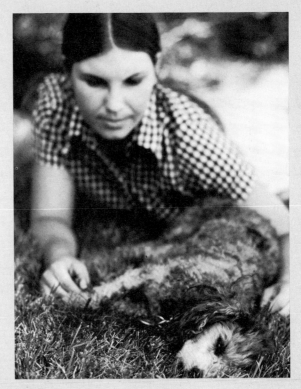

Narcolepsy is a condition in which the uncontrollable desire to fall asleep may come at any time. Researchers at the Stanford University Sleep Disorders Clinic are studying the behavior of narcoleptic animals in order to unravel the mysteries of this potentially dangerous condition.

ary 1979, the researchers cautioned: "It would be a mistake to conclude that long or short sleep or sleeping pills cause deaths." Further research into this association is in progress.

The search for satisfying sleep

Specialists in the field of sleep disorders occasionally are consulted by people seeking treatment for insomnia who complain that they are able to sleep only six hours a night. Such persons sometimes turn out to be natural short sleepers who have the mistaken belief that eight hours of sleep are necessary for health. Parents of a short-sleeping child may worry that their child is not getting enough sleep. On the other hand, parents of a long-sleeping adolescent may equate sleeping late with laziness and may fret about too much sleep.

The only criterion for assessing how much sleep anyone needs is a simple one: How does he or she feel and act during the day? Lack of interest and motivation frequently is tied to lack of sleep. With introspection, most people can readily tell the difference that an hour more or less of sleep would make in their lives.

In a quest for better sleep, many people regularly take sleeping pills. Sleep laboratory studies of prescription medications used as sleep aids show that these drugs typically lose their efficacy in about two weeks as the body develops tolerance to them. Sleeping pills are most useful for occasional troubled nights—during hospitalization or after lengthy air travel, for instance. The most widely prescribed sleeping medications are benzodiazepines, especially flurazepam (Dalmane). As of mid-1982, antihistamines, which cause drowsiness, were the most common ingredients in sleep aids that could be bought over the counter. Such products, however, were expected to undergo a major reformulation in 1982 following a U.S. Food and Drug Administration review.

Getting enough sleep is not the only determinant of how fit a person feels the next day. The number of awakenings during sleep also is critical; the more awakenings, the more likely a person is to rate his sleep as poor. The quality of sleep also depends on how long a person takes to fall asleep at the beginning of the night or to fall back asleep when awakened. Other qualitative factors include experiences that disturb sleep but usually are more obvious to a bed-partner; these include periodic muscle movements or such difficulty breathing that the sleeper must gasp for air.

Anyone who is experiencing difficulty sleeping at night or staying alert during the day should see a physician; a referral to a sleep specialist may be indicated. A list of such specialists may be obtained from the Association of Sleep Disorders Centers (P.O. Box YY, East Setauket, N.Y. 11733).

Skin Disorders

One in every three cancers is a cancer of the skin. Skin cancers develop each year in about 400,000 people in the United States alone. Because most are highly visible, they can be recognized and treated early in their course. Over 95% of skin cancers are cured, a rate that surpasses that for all other cancers. Although relatively few people die from cancer of the skin, these growths, like many other problems that involve the skin, may cause significant disfigurement and even disability. Recent advances in knowledge about skin cancers and their treatment include better understanding of the way they arise, stronger evidence of the role of ultraviolet radiation in causing the majority of skin cancers, earlier identification of people prone to these cancers, and the development of more effective methods of both treatment and prevention.

Types of skin cancer

The skin, by weight, is the largest organ of the body. Most skin cancers originate in the outer skin layer, the epidermis, a tissue thinner than a sheet of paper. The cells of the epidermis are among the most active in the body, replacing themselves every 30 days. In the epidermis, cells are arranged in layers. Most cell division takes place in the lowest, or basal cell, layer. In the next and thicker squamous cell layer, final steps take place in the manufacture of keratin, the skin's scaly, outermost protective coating. Intermingled with basal and squamous cells are melanocytes, the cells that make pigment. Clumps of melanocytes in fair-skinned persons are easy to see; they are called freckles.

Cancers of basal and squamous cells are the most frequent types of skin cancer. Melanomas, derived from melanocytes, are far less common, representing only about 3% of all cancers of the skin. Like other cancers, skin cancers involve disorderly and unchecked cell growth. Fortunately, most basal and squamous cell cancers do not break away from the primary tumor and spread through the bloodstream or lymphatic system to other parts of the body, a process known as metastasis. Melanomas are more likely to metastasize, and they are responsible for about two in three deaths from skin cancer, or about 5,000 deaths in the U.S. every year. Hence, for melanomas in particular, early recognition and treatment are crucial.

Basal cell cancers account for 70% of all skin cancers. Ultraviolet light from excessive exposure to the Sun is regarded as the most common cause of basal cell cancers. Most occur on parts of the body that are almost constantly exposed to the Sun: the face, the tips of the ears, and the backs of the hands. These cancers are more common in southerly regions than northerly ones. They occur more often in persons with light complexions, particularly blondes or redheads who easily sunburn. They are rare in blacks. Further,

these cancers are most frequent in sailors, farmers, construction workers, and others who spend considerable amounts of time out of doors.

A basal cell cancer usually appears as a small raised lump with a shiny or pearly surface which forms a depression in the center as it grows. These lumps may seem harmless because they are painless and do not bleed, but if left untreated they may invade deep into adjacent tissue, even into bone, and cause extensive tissue destruction. They almost never metastasize.

Squamous cell cancers occur less often than basal cell cancers, but they grow faster and have a greater potential to destroy tissue, metastasize, and cause death. Like basal cell cancers, squamous cell cancers also occur most often on Sun-exposed parts of the body. In addition, they are more likely than basal cell cancers to appear on covered parts of the body, particularly at sites of chronic damage, such as areas near long-term leg ulcers, old burn scars, or radiation treatment. The lower lip is another frequent location in persons who have had excessive chronic exposure to the Sun, particularly if they also have been pipe smokers and as a result have had long-term contact with heat and tobacco tar.

Malignant melanoma has gained considerable notoriety because of its rapid rate of increase as well as its danger. The incidence of melanoma has recently been described as a "virtual epidemic," having doubled from the 1950s to the 1980s. This increase does not simply reflect better recognition of the disease or altered definitions or even more thorough reporting. Since 1960 in the United States, the rate of increase of deaths due to malignant melanoma has been second only to that of cancer of the lung.

Melanomas are usually black or brown in color but sometimes are no darker than the surrounding skin. About half of the time, they arise from preexisting moles; the rest appear on previously normal skin. The average adult has about 20 moles, but no more than one mole in a million becomes a melanoma. Removal of moles is unnecessary unless they undergo alterations. Everyone should be alert to changes in moles or the appearance of dark brown or black growths on the skin, particularly those that bleed. Such growths should be examined by a physician. In many cases a biopsy or removal of the growth will be required, as the distinction between a benign mole and a malignant melanoma can be made only under the microscope.

The rise in melanomas is thought to result from increased recreational exposure to the Sun, the wearing of thinner clothes, and changing atmospheric conditions. Pollutants have damaged the ozone layer of the upper atmosphere, permitting an increased amount of ultraviolet light to reach the Earth's surface. Melanomas are eight to nine times as common in Caucasians as in blacks and are most common in people with fair skin, blue eyes, and light-colored hair who sunburn

Courtesy, National Institutes of Health   Henri Dauman

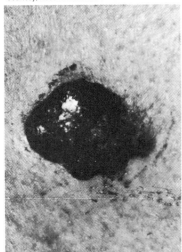

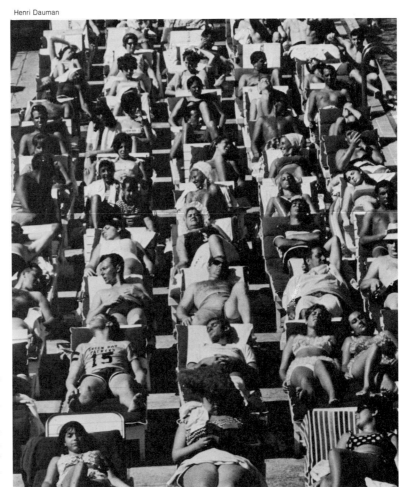

*Malignant melanoma is a potentially
fatal skin cancer that appears as a
small, dark patch on the skin. The
incidence of melanoma has risen
dramatically from the 1950s to the
1980s; it is thought that the rise is due
to increased exposure to the Sun and
the thinning of the protective ozone
layer of the upper atmosphere.*

easily and spend a considerable amount of time out of doors. The closer people live to the Equator, the higher their rate of melanoma. New melanomas appear in 15,000 people in the United States each year, a rate of 6 per 100,000, compared with a rate of 18 per 100,000 in Sun-drenched Australia. The parts of the body on which melanomas have increased most rapidly in the past two decades are the back for men and the legs for women; in some cases these body areas have received more Sun exposure as fashions have become more scanty. Although this evidence suggests that exposure to sunlight plays a strong causative role in melanoma, other factors, such as occupational exposure to chemicals or other substances and an inherited tendency for the disorder, also appear to be involved.

Researchers at the National Cancer Institute and the University of Pennsylvania recently found that certain families are predisposed to develop melanoma. Perhaps 10% of persons with melanoma are members of such families. The recognition of these families may allow the identification of family members who have early melanoma or who are at higher risk of developing melanoma. These individuals tend to have large numbers of moles, usually more than 100, and unlike most people, they may continue to develop new moles as adults. Sometimes these moles are large, two centimeters (¾ of an inch) or so across. They often are raised in the center and have irregular outlines. If a biopsy is obtained and viewed under a microscope, these moles have a distinctive appearance; studies indicate that they are unusually susceptible to malignant transformation. Because some of these atypical moles also have been found in persons with melanoma who have no family history of the disorder, they may prove to be a biological marker of increased risk.

It is unusual to find pigmented moles present at birth; most appear during childhood and puberty. Moles, particularly large ones, that are present from birth are more likely than most other moles to develop into melanomas. Medical debate continues over whether all congenital moles should be removed; certainly such moles should be examined periodically.

Other cancers of the skin

There are other less common types of skin cancer. Among these are mycosis fungoides, which starts as

303

itchy patches on the skin and later spreads to lymph nodes and internal organs. It is a disorder of T cells, one type of white blood cell. In most cases treatment in its early phases with radiation or anticancer drugs is beneficial.

Kaposi's sarcoma is an uncommon tumor of blood vessels, generally seen in older men of Eastern European origin. In such patients the course usually is slow, and response to treatment with radiation or anticancer drugs is good. Recently, however, this cancer has appeared with abnormal frequency among young homosexual men; in many of these cases the course of the disease has been rapid and sometimes fatal. It is not known what is causing this increase, and many factors are being investigated. One hypothesis is that infections that are common in homosexuals may be lowering their immunity, making them more susceptible to this form of cancer. The earliest signs of Kaposi's sarcoma are bluish-red or brown swollen areas resembling bruises or moles.

Noncancerous alterations of the skin

Although the possibility of skin cancer is the main reason for concern about growths appearing on the skin, most skin growths are neither cancerous nor irritating and do not need to be removed. Those listed below generally appear in midlife and increase in numbers with aging.

Actinic keratoses appear as reddish or pink, scaly, slightly irritating, nonhealing patches, usually restricted to chronically Sun-exposed parts of the body. Actinic keratoses are especially common in persons with fair skin who have spent excessive time in the Sun. They are on the border between benign growths and skin cancer. Although fewer than 1% actually become malignant, they do have the potential to do so. Because of this factor, their unsightly appearance, and their tendency to be irritating, they often are destroyed or removed.

Seborrheic keratoses are tan to brown crusted growths, ranging from a few millimeters to a few centimeters in size, with the appearance of being stuck onto the surface of the skin. They are most common on the back and chest. Seborrheic keratoses never become cancerous.

Lentigines often are called liver spots although they have nothing to do with disorders of the liver. They also are tan to brown in color but, unlike seborrheic keratoses, are not elevated above the surface. They are most common on Sun-exposed parts such as the face, backs of the hands and arms, and, in women, the lower legs. They never become cancerous.

Angiomas are bright red raised bumps, ranging in size from that of a pinhead to that of a rice grain. They most commonly appear on the upper part of the trunk. They seldom become irritated or bleed and never become cancerous.

Treatment for skin growths

Arriving at the diagnosis may require a biopsy. Since several techniques can be used to treat both benign and malignant skin growths, with possibly differing medical and cosmetic results, the choice must take into account the nature of the tumor and its location.

The most direct approach to treatment is cutting out the growth (excision). Melanomas almost always are treated by surgery. The thickness of a melanoma at the time it is removed is a good predictor of the patient's chances for long-term survival; the thinner the tumor, the brighter the prospects. Earlier diagnosis of melanoma probably accounts for today's improved five-year disease-free survival rate of 60–80%, compared with 25–40% in the 1950s.

Squamous cell and basal cell cancers also may be destroyed by an electric current and scraped away, a surgical technique known as electrodesiccation and curettage. In addition, destruction of tumors may be accomplished by cryosurgery, a technique in which the tumor is frozen, using solid carbon dioxide (dry ice) at −70° C or liquid nitrogen at −200° C.

Chemotherapy utilizes chemicals termed antineoplastics that are applied to the skin. These drugs do not penetrate deeply and are effective only for premalignant actinic keratoses or for skin cancers that are confined to the epidermis or slightly below it. The use of such drugs is justified when the growths are superficial and numerous, as these drugs must be used for weeks to be effective.

Radiation therapy is effective in destroying basal cell and squamous cell cancers; furthermore, it is painless. However, because a portion of normal skin must be included in the treated area and reaction to the radiation, including scarring and even additional skin cancers, may develop at the site 20 or more years later, radiation usually is reserved for elderly patients for whom complications decades later will not be a concern. It is also used for certain widespread types of skin cancer such as mycosis fungoides and Kaposi's sarcoma.

Preventing skin cancer

Skin cancers are most commonly initiated by ultraviolet light. This light can also cause fine wrinkling and other signs of aging of the skin. While the Sun is the primary source of such light, opportunities for year-round exposure have been increased by the recent institution of suntan salons; more than 2,000 now exist in the U.S. Ultraviolet rays also come from fluorescent lighting widely used in industries and schools. The U.S. Food and Drug Administration has estimated that 5% of an office worker's total exposure to ultraviolet light comes from such lights. Tanning is the body's natural response to injury induced by ultraviolet light; melanocytes produce more pigment and the keratin layer thickens. However, this protection is only partial; the amount of light that leads to tanning also injures cells.

According to a report from the National Academy of Sciences released in April 1982, a 5–9% reduction in stratospheric ozone—and, as a result, a rise in skin cancer—is expected by late in the next century if production of chlorofluorocarbons (used as propellants in some aerosol sprays and in refrigeration systems) remains at 1977 levels. Ozone is a form of oxygen making up a layer about 15 mi above the Earth; it blocks considerable amounts of harmful ultraviolet light from the Earth's surface. Chlorofluorocarbons destroy ozone. The Academy's report estimates that for every 1% decrease in stratospheric ozone, there will be a 2–5% increase in basal cell skin cancer and a 4–10% increase in squamous cell skin cancer. Since the likelihood of developing melanoma involves contributing factors in addition to sunlight, the impact of a decrease in ozone on melanoma rates is not clear. Many U.S. companies have found replacements for chlorofluorocarbons in household products.

Because people such as farmers and ranchers who work in the Sun are at increased risk of developing skin cancer, interested groups, notably the American Cancer Society, have conducted surveys to detect premalignant and malignant skin lesions in such people. Rural clinics have identified lesions in as many as 20% of the people examined. Such people should try to decrease their exposure to sunlight and should report skin changes to their physicians.

People who burn easily in the Sun can lessen their risk by staying indoors between 10 AM and 2 PM, when the rays are most intense. On the beach a Sun-sensitive person should wear a sunblocking chemical and a broad-brimmed hat and use a beach umbrella. Improved sunblocking chemicals now on the market provide substantial protection from the damaging effects of ultraviolet light. The efficacy of a sunblock can be estimated by using the SPF number (Sun Protection Factor) on the package; the higher the number, the greater the protection. An SPF of 10, for example, means that skin protected by the sunblock can take ten times more exposure without burning than an area to which the preparation has not been applied. Sunblocks should be reapplied frequently since most are washed off by swimming or perspiration.

—Stanford I. Lamberg, M.D.,
and Lynne Lamberg

Stress

The United States' latest and longest war continues to plague thousands of Vietnam veterans. Of the 2,769,000 American military personnel who served in Vietnam, 57,692 died in the war, 303,704 were wounded, and many more suffered psychological damage. Researchers estimate that as many as 500,000 to 700,000 Vietnam-era veterans still require help in adjusting to the emotional conflicts the war wrought.

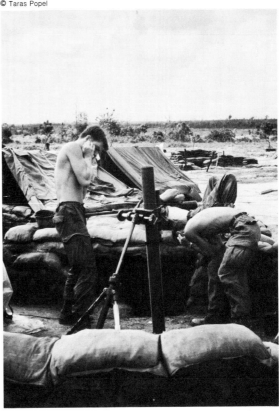

Many of the 2,769,000 American military personnel who served in Vietnam returned home to face physical and psychological problems.

Unique aspects of the Vietnam war

The Vietnam war was unique. All war exposes combatants to danger, loss, helplessness, destruction, and despair, but the Vietnam war was fought in the context of political confusion, disillusionment, and deceit. It inflicted trauma beyond the grisly realities of combat. The Vietnam war differed from other U.S. wars in four crucial respects:

1. Lack of unit morale. For Vietnam veterans there was minimal unit morale and identification. After training, replacement recruits, rather than being transported as a group, were shipped separately to Vietnam aboard various commercial jetliners. In Vietnam servicemen joined and left units one at a time. The soldier was keenly aware that a tour of duty lasted only a year, and he became devoted to his own survival rather than to the victory of his unit.

2. Turmoil at home. Unprecedented antiwar sentiment and lack of home support for the war caused sorrow and confusion among the troops in Vietnam. Many servicemen in Vietnam began to feel the war made no sense on any level. This purposelessness fostered distrust of all authority and of society itself. Upon returning home, the combat-weary veteran discovered that many people thought that the only heroes

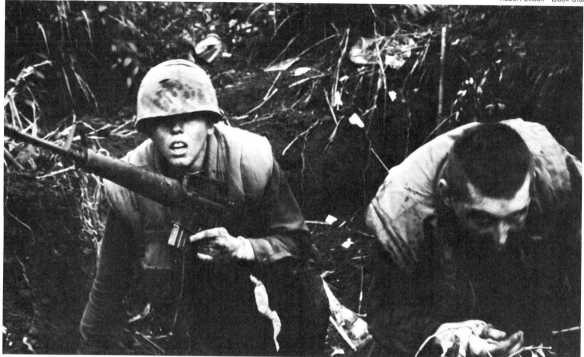

Young military recruits in Vietnam suddenly found themselves in an alien country where nothing seemed familiar and where it was impossible to tell friend from enemy.

of the Vietnam war were those who fled across the Canadian border to avoid the draft. The returning soldier was left with only a sense of loss and disillusionment.

3. Nature of the war. The lack of an all-out attempt to win the war frustrated the serviceman. Hard-won territory was given up voluntarily, only to be fought for again and again. There were no front lines. The enemy's use of women, children, and old people made it impossible to distinguish friend from foe. Infants in baby carriages were wired with booby traps; young boys tossed hand grenades; women who worked as smiling maids during the day carried Viet Cong weapons at night. There was no safe haven from the war: the trails were booby trapped; the roads were mined; restaurants and movie theaters were blown up; the United States embassy in Saigon was repeatedly attacked.

4. Abrupt transition. The return home was abrupt, almost surreal—plucked out of their year-long hell, set down in commercial airliners, and whisked back home, combat veterans went from foxhole to front porch in 36 hours. For the Vietnam veteran there was no gradual comedown, no psychological decompression, no welcome party upon return.

Posttraumatic stress disorder

Although most Vietnam veterans have learned to cope fairly well with their war experiences, at least a half million Vietnam veterans continue to suffer the disturbing effects of psychological damage. In 1980 the third edi-

tion of the *Diagnostic and Statistical Manual of Mental Disorders* (*DSM-III*), an official publication of the American Psychiatric Association, defined this suffering as posttraumatic stress disorder (PTSD).

PTSD is characterized by nightmares about the war, mental flashbacks during which the veteran feels as if he is back in Vietnam, and startle reactions—at the sound of a loud noise the Vietnam veteran falls to the ground. The Vietnam veteran with PTSD is edgy, irritable, easily depressed, and has difficulty relating warmly to other people. He drifts from job to job, and his marriage is a shambles. Wives of Vietnam veterans frequently report that their husbands awake screaming in the middle of the night. Sometimes the veteran may strike out at his wife when he becomes angry.

Many of the 7,500 women who served in Vietnam also report difficulties. Nurses were immersed in the absurdity of war. Time and time again they had to hold the hand of a dying young man who was not quite old enough to shave regularly. Nurses who served in Vietnam cannot get feelings of hopelessness and bitterness out of their minds. They remain cool and aloof, emotionally numb.

There may be a time lag between experiencing a traumatic event and suffering the emotional consequences of the stress. When an individual is exposed to trauma, there is an initial reaction of numbness that may go on for several days, weeks, or even months. As the human mind tries to work through the significance of the trauma, nightmares, startle reactions, and flash-backs occur.

The delayed reaction found in the Vietnam veteran suffering from PTSD reflects society's view of the war. Many veterans report that when they returned home they felt alienated. No one wanted to hear about the war, not even their families. They began to drift off alone, drinking and becoming involved with drugs. Vietnam veterans account for 55% of veterans receiving outpatient care for drug dependence. In 1970 Vietnam veterans made up 13% of veterans classified as having alcohol problems; in 1977 the percentage had jumped to 31%. More recently, as society has become more open about the Vietnam war, veterans have begun to talk about their problems for the first time. The problems have always been there, but no one listened, no one talked.

Causes of stress disorders in veterans

There is nothing new about psychological trauma caused by fighting in a war. After the Civil War it was called nostalgia; after World War I, shell shock; after World War II, battle exhaustion; after Korea, battle fatigue. Studies have shown that no matter how stable an individual might be, with sufficient trauma he or she will develop a stress disorder.

In a relatively stable individual repeated severe trauma may be only one cause for the development of PTSD. In some individuals the war may reactivate childhood emotional problems. For example, a soldier in Vietnam who had difficulty relating to his father developed symptoms of PTSD soon after he was forced to shoot an old man. In other individuals severe emotional conflicts may have already been present prior to

the war; exposure to combat simply unmasked the psychological symptoms. A few veterans seem to have persistent symptoms because of some perceived benefit that disability brings. For example, a veteran may be resistant to treatment because he does not want to give up his disability rating. Another individual's symptoms may continue because they allow him to cling to his mother.

Impaired emotional growth also contributes to the persistence of PTSD symptoms. The average age of the soldiers was 19.2 years; the war interrupted the normal psychosocial development of many Vietnam soldiers. During late adolescence and young adulthood most young men and women are developing stable, enduring personality structures. Normally, the young adult frees himself of parental control, learns responsibility, and begins to recognize his abilities as well as his limitations. For many young Americans the Vietnam war interrupted this developmental process, producing a confused sense of self. These Vietnam veterans are now entering middle age, perhaps losing their hair and going through many physical mid-life changes, but emotionally they are still teenagers.

Techniques of treatment

The U.S. Congress has recently become responsive to Vietnam veterans' needs. A nationwide network of "storefront" counseling centers have been established, consisting of 131 four-person teams distributed among all 50 states. Each of the teams has one professional who is either a physician, psychiatric nurse, psychologist, or social worker; two technicians with special training; and one clerical assistant. Concentrated in the urban centers with the largest veteran populations, this

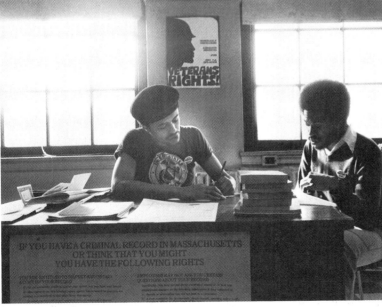

Vietnam vets have recently begun to tell their stories. They have formed support groups to help with jobs, health problems, and the lingering difficulties of adjusting to the stresses of combat.

Tyrone Hall—Picture Group

outreach program has three basic aims: (1) to reach the veteran in a nonclinical setting; (2) to provide readjustment counseling for those veterans with marital and work difficulties; and (3) to refer individuals with severe emotional difficulties to Veterans Administration hospitals for more intensive therapy. There are many treatment techniques for posttraumatic stress disorder, but it should be noted that none of them has been systematically studied.

During and immediately following World War II and the Korean conflict, so-called supportive techniques were widely used for troubled soldiers. Individuals suffering from stress reactions were withdrawn from active combat and given a period of rest and support. For individuals with adequate personality development or those who experienced minor stress, supportive psychotherapy was sufficient for recovery. Unfortunately, studies of World War II veterans have shown that symptoms of stress disorders afflict some individuals for a lifetime unless more intensive psychotherapy is administered.

The sedative Amytal Sodium (the so-called truth serum) was widely used during and immediately following World War II to treat soldiers suffering from stress disorders. Psychologists conducted interviews or therapeutic sessions while patients were under the influence of the drug. Subsequent studies have shown that in most cases Amytal Sodium interviews were insufficient to allow complete recovery from all the symptoms of a stress disorder. Other medications, including antidepressants, antianxiety agents, and antipsychotics help to diminish some of the symptoms of PTSD, but they do not completely alleviate the problem.

Behavioral techniques have been used to help diminish dreams and flashbacks associated with PTSD. The individual is first taught to relax. After a satisfactory level of relaxation is achieved, the patient is shown a set of anxiety-evoking images, each slightly more troubling than the preceding one. When the individual begins to feel tense, he is again relaxed, and the images are presented once again in a step-by-step fashion. Gradually he learns to tolerate memories that were once acutely disturbing.

In working with individuals suffering from PTSD, Mardi J. Horowitz, director of the Stress Research Unit of the Langley Porter Psychiatric Institute in San Francisco, found behavioral patterns that characterize a general stress response syndrome: (1) the initial realization that a stressful event has occurred, accompanied by an emotional "outcry"; (2) a phase of denial and numbness; (3) oscillation between emotional numbness and intrusive-repetitive thoughts of the trauma; and (4) either psychological retreat (regression) or the gradual acceptance of the traumatic event.

According to Horowitz the phase of emotional numbness is an attempt by the psyche to suppress unpleasant memories of the traumatic event. The denial phase eventually breaks down, however, and nightmares, flashbacks, and unpleasant memories haunt the veteran. With time the oscillation between denial and intrusive memories eventually leads to acceptance of the traumatic events. Some individuals are unable to come

An added bitterness that afflicts veterans of the Vietnam era is the refusal of their country to acknowledge the veterans' experience—there were no triumphant parades for these returning soldiers. The Vietnam war is widely viewed as a huge mistake that should be swept under the rug and forgotten.

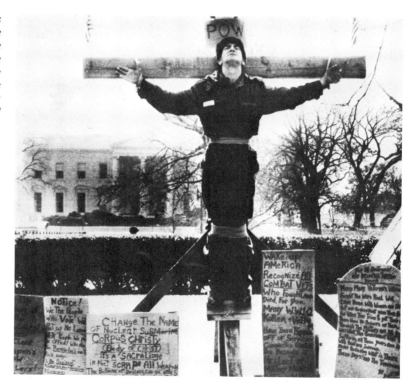

to grips with the traumatic memories and exist in a chronic regressive state manifested by low self-esteem and social isolation. These unfortunate individuals become nonproductive drones, a financial drain on society, and a burden to their families.

Individual psychotherapy helps the Vietnam veteran express, organize, and control his feelings and thoughts concerning the war. The psychotherapist helps the Vietnam veteran understand and work through the meaning of the trauma so that the veteran's self-image and interpersonal relationships are improved. The therapist accomplishes this task by empathetically listening to and clarifying the combat veteran's experiences.

In the early 1970s, partially as a response to military psychiatry's failure to initiate an active treatment program for Vietnam combat veterans, informal groups evolved as a special method for dealing with stress in Vietnam veterans. These "rap" groups were formed to talk about the war in a general debriefing process. The meaning of the war, intense examinations of political issues, reflections of value systems, and the examinations of the self in relation to cultural values were all part of the discussions.

What has been learned from rap groups is now being applied in more formal group settings in Veterans Administration hospitals and community mental health centers across the United States. These groups focus on the existential problems of the war as well as on individual maladaptive behavior.

The major goal of group therapy is to help the veteran find personal meaning for his military experience. The veteran begins to realistically assess the good and bad aspects of his war experience and gradually puts them into perspective. The individual confesses, experiences emotional pain, and gradually clarifies his role in the war. The group gives social support that renders each member's suffering meaningful. In addition, members help each other gradually understand that self-inflicted pain must stop—that they must get on with the process of daily living. As the individual's self-esteem improves, he once again begins to love and work effectively.

—J. Ingram Walker, M.D.

Surgery

In 1982 approximately 750,000 persons in the U.S. suffered a stroke. About 250,000 of the victims died, making this disease the third leading cause of death in the United States. Eighty percent of stroke deaths occur in persons over age 65; the remaining 20% of stroke victims die during their most productive years. However, the full impact of this disease is seen in the fact that it incapacitates far more people than it kills; it is the leading cause of disability in the United States. There are approximately 2.5 million stroke survivors,

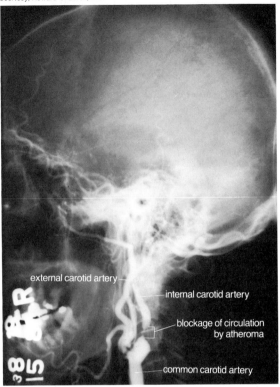

external carotid artery

internal carotid artery

blockage of circulation by atheroma

common carotid artery

Many strokes are caused by blockage of the carotid arteries due to arteriosclerosis. A common site for this problem is the point at which the artery divides into two branches. In this X-ray a fatty plaque has nearly closed off the blood flow.

but only about 30% ever resume normal productivity. A stroke, or apoplexy, or cerebrovascular accident, as it is sometimes called, is most commonly caused by a lack of blood supplying a particular area of the brain. This is what happens when a critical artery carrying blood to the brain becomes blocked with a fat-laden arteriosclerotic plaque called an atheroma. A new surgical technique, carotid endarterectomy, holds great promise for potential stroke victims. The technique involves opening the artery and removing the atheroma, thus ensuring adequate blood supply to the brain.

The vital carotid arteries

Most organs can survive if they are deprived of their blood supply for a period of time, but this is not so with the cells in the brain. So great is their demand for blood and oxygen that they receive 20% of the total output of blood from the heart and consume 20% of oxygen that is breathed. Not only does the brain require a great deal of oxygen but its demands are constant. The brain is unable to do without oxygen for more than four minutes at most. Beyond this, damage to the brain is permanent.

As many as 40 to 60% of all strokes are caused by arteriosclerosis of a segment of one of the carotid ar-

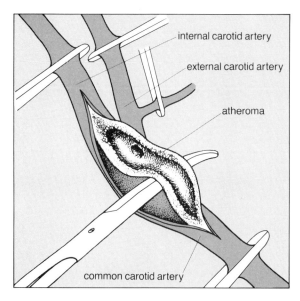

For some patients surgery may offer new hope for preventing devastating strokes. The surgeon opens the blocked carotid artery and removes the fatty plaque, restoring circulation.

teries, which supply most of the blood to the brain. The most common site of trouble is the point in the neck where the carotid artery divides into two branches, the internal carotid division going directly to the brain and the external branch supplying part of the face with blood. Exactly why the problem so often occurs here at the bifurcation is a matter of considerable debate.

The American Heart Association reports that for a first stroke originating as a result of a block in the carotid arteries, there is an initial mortality of 20% within five years; within a two-year period, 60% of the survivors will have a second stroke. Eventually 50% of these individuals will succumb to a recurrent or second stroke as a result of an atheroma in one of these critical neck arteries. When this occurs, any form of therapy short of physically removing the arteriosclerotic obstruction simply will not help.

Heeding the brain's warning

Fortunately, many people receive a warning before a major stroke in the form of a "mini-stroke," or TIA, transient ischemic attack. It is an episode that is usually accompanied by slurred speech, numbness or weakness of a hand or foot, or a temporary visual disturbance. In most instances, the attack lasts only minutes and does no permanent damage. However, one in three persons experiencing a TIA will have a stroke within five years, many within months. It is patients in this group who can be saved from a devastating, permanent stroke by carotid endarterectomy.

As many as 85 to 95% of patients sustaining a TIA can be completely spared an impending, life-threatening stroke. Clinical strategy in eliminating or reducing

the risk of a stroke centers around identifying those patients who are candidates for a vascular surgical procedure that can remove the offending lesion before permanent brain damage occurs.

Before surgery is undertaken, the status of the carotid arteries is assessed. In some cases the physician can pick up sounds of diminished or obstructed blood flow by listening to the arteries through a stethoscope. Dye injected into the arteries enables any narrowing or obstruction to be detected by X-rays; this test, angiography, is quite reliable and informative but is expensive and requires hospitalization, and it carries a definite risk to the patient—serious complications occur in about 1% of patients tested. Other, noninvasive tests, including ultrasound imaging and tests of the circulation that supplies the eyes, are also currently in use.

Patients in whom angiography has shown significant (50% or more) narrowing of a carotid artery and who are under 70 years of age are considered good candidates for carotid surgery. Persons in this age group are better able to tolerate surgery and have been shown to be more likely to have a stroke after a TIA. Early surgery also removes the need for lengthy drug therapy.

The surgical procedure

Surgery consists of exposing the carotid artery in the neck at its point of branching. Following this an incision is made in the wall of the artery over the diseased portion containing the arteriosclerotic plaque. If necessary, at this point a temporary shunt (a small plastic tube) may be placed in the opening above and below the obstructed area so that blood may continue to flow in an adequate supply to the brain while the vascular surgeon works. The obstructing arteriosclerotic lesion is removed from the wall of the artery. The incision in the artery is then closed with a fine suture after the temporary shunt is removed.

The risk from this operation is minimal, and the results following surgery have been extremely gratifying. The vast majority of patients are completely relieved of their neurological symptoms. One study of 131 patients undergoing endarterectomy at the Johns Hopkins Medical Institutions showed that 129 achieved full functioning after the operation. An interesting aspect of the surgery is that many patients report noticeable improvement in intellectual ability and other aspects of mental function that had been assumed to be lost due to the aging process.

The success of this operation in preventing stroke has led surgeons to apply this therapy to patients who have already experienced a stroke. If the stroke has been minor, and no substantial permanent damage has been done, the patient may be a candidate for preventive endarterectomy. Even patients who have recovered but have sustained some damage may be spared a second, more devastating stroke by surgery.

—Howard C. Baron, M.D.

Special Report:
Surgeries for Obesity
by Joann Ellison Rodgers

Hippocrates observed nearly 2,400 years ago that "persons who are naturally very fat are apt to die earlier than those who are slender." The trouble is, of course, that for many people getting very fat is a great deal easier than staying slender. Morbidly obese individuals have failed on every diet—including near-total starvation. Morbid obesity can be defined as a body weight twice or more the desirable level defined by life insurance standards. This level of overweight presents a serious health hazard, even in young persons. For example, the mortality rate of grossly obese men aged 25 to 34 is 12 times higher than that of normal-weight peers.

As a result, during the last 20 years thousands of morbidly obese persons have submitted to various types of drastic procedures in an attempt to lose weight. Some have had their jaws wired shut for months while they subsisted on liquids. An estimated 200,000 have undergone intestinal bypasses, in which the surgeon first disconnects the stomach from the top of the small intestine, then attaches it to the bottom.

Jejunoileal bypass

The jejunoileal bypass shunts the food taken in past the jejunum and ileum, which make up 90% of the small bowel, the principal site of food absorption. Without absorption nutrients cannot reach the bloodstream and add to weight. The appeal of intestinal bypass rests on the fact that a quick and substantial weight loss is virtually guaranteed. Theoretically, a patient who has a bypass can overeat and still lose weight.

Pioneers in the intestinal bypass field, after two decades of follow-up, have now declared the procedure to be dangerous. Many bypass patients eventually develop severe complications of the kidney and liver. Up to 5% of patients die of complications, 25% require more surgery to reverse the bypass, and fewer than 20% have an overall satisfactory outcome in terms of both weight loss and safety. A significant proportion lose bone strength because their bodies cannot absorb calcium or retain vitamin D. Even among the most successful cases, anemia, vitamin deficiencies, and profound weakness remain constant problems.

The long-term health record of bypass patients is so poor, in fact, that physicians attending the 1981 meeting of the American College of Surgeons heard recommendations that it be completely abandoned. They were also warned to rigidly supervise those who had had intestinal bypass in the past in order to prevent death and disability.

Stomach reduction procedures

Fortunately for those whose lives are at risk because of their weight, surgical researchers have recently developed what so far appears to be a safer and better operation. Called gastroplasty (stomach shaping), stomach partition, or stomach stapling, the most widely used version of this operation consists of using special staples to divide the stomach into two sections with a narrow connecting outlet. The upper portion is much smaller than the lower portion. A variant of this procedure is the gastric bypass, which creates a small stomach pouch at the upper end of the stomach and reattaches the small intestine to this pouch. As with intestinal bypass and all surgical approaches to obesity, this procedure is an extreme one and is performed only on severely obese individuals who cannot lose weight by more moderate, conventional means.

The stomach partitioning is permanent, and patients undergoing the operation feel full after just a few bites of food. Unlike intestinal bypass patients, gastroplasty and gastric bypass patients must drastically limit their food intake so as not to overfill and stretch the pouch. A typical meal, for example, might consist of two small cubes of meat, a half-tablespoon of vegetables, and half a dumpling. Liquid is avoided altogether at most meals because just a few ounces fill the stomach. Overfilling and stretching the stomach can have serious consequences.

Despite the vastly reduced meal size and the risk of the operation, gastric surgery is currently considered the surgical procedure of choice for rapid, long-term weight loss in individuals at least 100 lb over ideal weight. For this group, heart, blood vessel, and other complications of morbid obesity pose greater risks to life and health than the operation. These individuals are at high risk of death by age 45 or 50. Further, the lost weight appears to be unwanted fat rather than vital muscle or protein.

Informal surveys suggest that 50,000 gastric surgery operations for weight loss have been performed in the United States. Refinements in technique have produced an 85% long-term success rate among patients properly selected and operated on by experienced surgeons. The same group has had few side effects and a death rate of less than 1%.

A study of 41 morbidly obese patients, conducted by Boston researchers affiliated with the Massachusetts Institute of Technology and Harvard University, found that while weight loss was rapid within the first year after gastric bypass, there was no liver damage or protein deficiency over the two-year study period. The patients in this group included 10 men and 31 women with an average age of 34 years. All had long histories of failure to lose weight with diets and drugs. Before surgery the patients weighed an average of 287 lb. The average weight loss within 12 months after the operation was 90 lb. In addition, most of the patients continued to lose weight over the ensuing 18 months.

The ideal surgical approach to morbid obesity has yet to be found. New versions of older procedures and entirely new procedures are in various stages of development. Edward E. Mason, professor of surgery at the University of Iowa College of Medicine, who pioneered the gastric bypass approach in 1966, has recently introduced a gastric bypass refinement in which a plastic mesh collar is fitted around the artificial opening made in the stomach wall through which food passes. The plastic collar strengthens the part of the surgically created pouch that takes the most stress. Surgeons are hopeful that the reinforcement will stop the pouch from stretching so easily.

In one of the newest techniques surgeons hope to achieve the same goal as gastric partition—vast reduction of stomach size—without staples or the need to cut into the stomach itself. Developed by Daniel Bereson, a surgeon at New York Medical College in New York City, the operation uses an inflatable balloon implanted in the abdomen to compress the stomach—the procedure is called balloon gastroplasty. The pressurized balloon distends the upper abdomen, giving a sensation of fullness. It also squeezes the stomach, reducing its capacity to hold food. The amount of compression, moreover, can be adjusted at any time or eliminated completely by injecting or removing the salt solution used to fill the balloon. The solution is sent through a tube connected to the balloon and inserted just under the skin of the abdomen. The technique has been tested in animals and in man, with mixed results. It is still considered to be experimental.

The behavioral component

The treatment of gastroplasty patients includes psychotherapy and behavioral modification that attempt to reform a lifetime of poor eating habits. John D. Halverson, associate professor of surgery at Washington University School of Medicine in St. Louis, Mo., has studied hundreds of gastroplasty patients and found that without psychiatric support, many will continue to eat too much. Whatever "satiety" factor is missing in the morbidly obese is not restored by a trip to the operating room. They must still learn to be aware of signals of satiety. Gastroplasty and gastric bypass patients who eat carelessly and fail to follow a strict diet and exercise regimen destroy the effects of the surgery either by stretching the stomach, tearing out the staples, or stretching the opening through which the food goes out of the stomach.

The emphasis on self-discipline may make gastric bypass therapy less appealing than intestinal bypass to the obese patient whose self-image and self-confidence have been shattered by repeated loss of control at the dining table. But the surgeons and psychotherapists who work with the patients claim that the behavioral component may be the most important factor in the long-term success of this treatment.

Emphasis on self-discipline works to correct the sense of failure and helplessness that the morbidly obese feel, restoring incentive to take charge of their lives and health. Diets and other treatments that promise these patients that they will lose weight without expending any effort to control their appetites may seem ideal, but in fact they make the patients feel like children who are unable to cope with adult responsibility.

It is popularly believed that the obese are lazy and weak and have no real desire to lose weight. The willingness of hundreds of thousands to undergo surgery would seem to contradict that belief. In the case of gastric surgery, which requires a lifelong commitment to severe dietary restrictions, there is little evidence to support the moral judgments often aimed at the obese. Physicians are careful to select for surgery only those who are willing to admit they need psychological as well as physical help.

In the past, surgical treatment of obesity has generally been viewed as a last-ditch therapy and one aimed more at an embarrassing social problem than a medical need. However, once such surgery is perfected it could become a well-accepted treatment for a disorder that not only causes psychological and financial distress but destroys health.

World Medical News

The 1982 edition of the *American Alpine Journal* consists of 366 pages of detailed reports of hundreds of notable climbs performed during the past year all over the world: Japanese on the west face of K2 in the Himalayan Karakoram; Americans on the Central Tower of Paine in Patagonia; Americans on Anyenaquen deep in central China; Yugoslavs on Dhaulagiri in Nepal; and more Americans, this time failing, on the vast, previously unclimbed, and horrendous Kangshung face of Mt. Everest.

Among the pictures of spectacular sunsets and dawns, of ropes and giant icicles draped down overhanging cliffs, of dotted lines tracing routes up gigantic faces is a picture showing a shaggy, ice-flecked profile, apparently breathing through a large tube, with big gloves gripping two levers attached to that tube. Beyond and far below one can dimly discern peak upon peak stretching into the distance. The legend to the picture reads, "Chris Pizzo taking alveolar gas samples on Everest's summit, October 24, 1981."

The American Medical Research Expedition

To any climber it is a reasonable ambition to get to the summit of Mt. Everest, but phrases such as alveolar gas samples are meaningless, and scientific instruments may seem intrusive on the summit of Everest, of all holy places. To the average physician it is incomprehensible that anyone should wish to sample alveolar gases on top of Everest—a spot so conspicuously hard to achieve and, once reached, so cold, windy, lonely, and dangerous. Yet to those few high-altitude physiolo-

gists who often climb to do research, this picture represents a logical, if spectacular, use of one of nature's most exotic laboratories.

Both the climber and the physician would be surprised to learn that the initial impetus for climbing, at the end of the 18th and during the first part of the 19th centuries, came largely from scientists. The photograph of Pizzo is in fact in the great tradition of physiologic investigations in the mountains. This tradition was established by the Swiss scientist Horace-Bénédict de Saussure, who established a high-altitude scientific station on Mont Blanc in 1788, and was continued by many notable physiologists—among them the Italian Angelo Mosso and the German Nathan Zuntz on Monte Rosa at the beginning of this century and the Scot John Scott Haldane along with Americans C. G. Douglas, Yandell Henderson, and E. C. Schneider on Pikes Peak in Colorado before World War I.

In August 1981, 21 climbers including 14 scientists, 10 of whom were physicians, took part in the American Medical Research Expedition to Mt. Everest, which was financed in part by the U.S. National Heart, Lung, and Blood Institute, the American Lung Association, and the National Geographic Society. Pulmonary physiologist John West, who is professor of medicine and physiology at the University of California at San Diego, led the 1981 expedition—the first climb of Everest having physiologic research as its primary object. As a climbing physiologist West was uniquely qualified to lead this expedition. He had been a member of the Silver Hut expedition—one of a group of scientists who spent the winter of 1960–61 at 5,800 m (19,000 ft) in the Himalayas. Either as a scientist or as a guinea pig

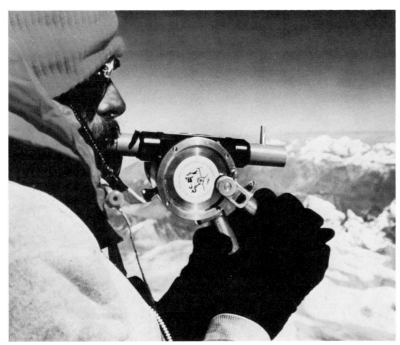

Chris Pizzo, a member of the American Medical Research Expedition, is shown taking aveolar gas samples on Mt. Everest's summit, Oct. 24, 1981.

Courtesy, American Medical Research Expedition to Everest

for his colleagues, West had already carried physiologic observations to some of the highest altitudes yet achieved, including tests at 7,830 m (25,700 ft) on Makalu, which is 23 km (14 mi) from Everest.

West's American Medical Research Expedition to Everest consisted of men with impressive records in high-altitude climbing and all deeply involved in low-oxygen, high-altitude physiologic investigations. The results of their studies will gradually appear in numerous articles in the scientific literature. The photograph of Chris Pizzo already mentioned was part of a preliminary report by West, a sketch of what turned out to be a very impressive list of achievements—not least of which were the establishment of a variation on the Hillary-Tenzing route; the placing of five men on the summit, two of them, Chris Pizzo and Peter Hackett, being physicians; the close and harmonious cooperation between "climbers" and "scientists"; and finally the safe return of all members of the expedition.

Summit experiments

What is so physiologically interesting about carrying out tests on the summit of Everest, the very highest point on Earth, 8,848 m (29,028 ft) above sea level? After all, Sir Edmund Hillary and Tenzing Norgay climbed the mountain as far back as 1953, and that was over 30 years after the first of many determined expeditions to attempt the mountain. In 1924, on the second British expedition, Col. E. F. Norton climbed to 8,580 m (28,150 ft) without the assistance of bottled oxygen, ending up only 268 m (878 ft) below the summit. Despite scores of attempts, this altitude was not exceeded without the use of supplementary oxygen until 1978, 54 years later, when suddenly each of the three highest mountains in the world, Everest, K2—8,611 m (28,250 ft), and Kangchenjunga—8,598 m (28,208 ft), were climbed without the benefit of oxygen. This immensely long gap suggests that these peaks lie not merely at the geographic but also at the physiologic limit achievable by climbers.

This physiologic extreme is further emphasized by extrapolation of measurements of maximal oxygen consumption made by numerous investigators on numerous mountains lower down. The value of these measurements, which reflect the amount of oxygen burnt up by the body in a minute of maximal exercise, falls steadily as height increases above an altitude of about 1,500 m (5,000 ft). If the average curve, falling with increasing altitude, is extended, it reaches the value of oxygen consumption when the climber is completely at rest, and this seems to happen at around 8,500 m (28,000 ft). In other words, it is probable that at the summit of Everest one would expect even those who did best at altitude to be at their maximal oxygen uptake even if they were resting, let alone clambering up those last few hundred meters over steep, treacherous ground, buffeted by high winds and encumbered by heavy clothing and climbing equipment.

West wanted to find out a number of facts about the summit of Everest, some of them extraordinarily basic. For example, from earlier work done by Griffith Pugh, who had been on the first successful expedition to Everest in 1953 as well as on the Silver Hut expedition, it seemed likely that the barometric pressure was not 235 mm Hg, which is what one would predict from the standard altitude-pressure calculations, but 250 mm Hg—the increase of 15 mm Hg being an essential ingredient for an unaided climber. The exact pressure was unknown. Stemming from this prediction were others of more physiologic and therefore medical interest. If the barometric pressure at the summit of the mountain was 250 mm Hg, then the partial pressure of oxygen in the air must be about 52 mm Hg, since oxygen constitutes 20.9% of the air. In arterial blood at rest the pressure of oxygen could then be calculated as 25 mm Hg (compared with a value of about 90 to 100 mg Hg at sea level). West went further and predicted that on mild exercise (less than that needed to reach the summit) the oxygen pressure in arterial blood would fall to less than 20 mm Hg.

Oxygen is an absolutely essential fuel; without it we would die in a few minutes. Diseases causing oxygen deficiency (hypoxia) at sea level are common. Yet these predicted values in healthy climbers at the end of their tether are far lower than those seen in patients critically ill because of oxygen lack due to heart or lung problems at sea level (e.g., emphysema) and are near or below those generally assumed to be incompatible with life. For these two reasons, one can see how important it is to understand how oxygen works and the effects of very low oxygen levels upon the human body, in this case, the bodies of otherwise exceedingly fit men operating at their limits.

At the summit of Everest the barometric pressure was indeed found to be 250 to 253 mm Hg and not 235 mm Hg—just as West had predicted—the temperature being "relatively balmy" at −8.8° C (16° F). Samples of expired air were taken to be analyzed, their composition reflecting the partial pressures of oxygen and carbon dioxide in the blood. (Reports are yet to come.) Meanwhile, continuous electrocardiograms were recorded to give information on heart rate and rhythm as well as on the degree of oxygenation of this aerobic, constantly exercising organ. Measurements of breathing during climbing to the summit (certainly maximal exertion by any standard) were also made, Pizzo and Hackett breathing through small turbine flow meters while the flow was recorded on tape.

Tests at lower levels

Farther down the mountain there was also intense scientific activity by this group in addition to the complicated and exhausting tasks of setting up camps, fixing ropes, and waiting out storms, which are so much a feature of every large Himalayan expedition. The base of Everest, at 5,400 m (17,700 ft), is the aim of numerous organized groups of tourists who ordinarily "trek" there in a few days from Lukla, a small dirt airstrip at 2,800 m (9,200 ft). The trail is gentle and safe, becoming progressively more barren and more spectacular as height is gained. It peters out in the rubble beneath the huge Khumbu icefall, at the foot of which lies the base camp, the place where the walking stops and the real climbing starts. At base camp, studies were done on Sherpas (skilled climbers living in the high valleys of eastern Nepal, who usually accompany expeditions) and on Westerners. Here blood changes associated with acclimatization were examined as well as the reasons for the increased breathing observed at high altitudes, both during waking and sleeping.

The mountain as laboratory

West's group's investigations extend the work of other groups, including one that did a number of physiologic investigations at 4,300 m (14,100 ft) at the tiny village of Pheriche, just a few miles down the trail, three years before. At the main laboratory (6,300 m; 20,700 ft) in the great West Cwm, above an icefall, Frank Sarnquist, one of the physicians with West's group, conducted psychological tests on his colleagues to see whether lack of oxygen affected memory, mood, or manipulative skills. Similar though inconclusive investigations had been done by Sarnquist on American physicians, including Peter Hackett, on Mt. McKinley in 1981. Also at the main laboratory, sleep studies confirmed and extended observations made by others that at high altitude breathing during sleep becomes very irregular and as a result the oxygen levels in the blood may fall to very low levels—a phenomenon that has important implications for patients at sea level. Intestinal absorption was also examined in an attempt to understand why all climbers lose weight at high altitude no matter how many calories are consumed, and numerous studies on blood and body metabolism were conducted. A surprising finding was that maximal work capacities measured on a stationary bicycle were much higher than expected and during the exercise blood oxygen levels fell very dramatically.

The recent expedition had hoped to measure maximal oxygen uptake not only at sea level and at the main laboratory but also at Camp V at 8,050 m (26,400 ft), actually above the South Col, one of the great shoulders of Everest where the final camp of expeditions is usually placed. The ferocity of the wind was such that the special science tent, though carried to Camp V, could not be pitched, and the stationary bicycle manhandled to this extraordinary altitude therefore could not be used. However, tests of blood acidity to test predictions about the optimal state of acidity for maximal oxygen transport were completed, as were sleep electrocardiograms on three climbers. All these specimens

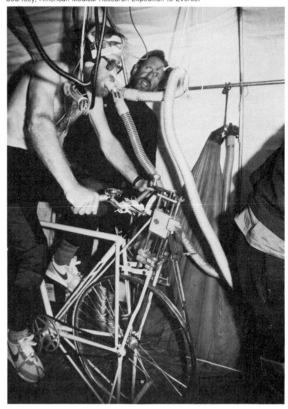

Expedition leader John West tests the heart and breathing rates of fellow climber Steven Boyer at Camp II, pitched at 6,300 meters (20,700 feet).

and recordings have yet to be analyzed in the United States, a process that will take months.

West has described in a matter-of-fact way an extraordinary piece of research. In the face of cold, tremendous gales, icefalls, avalanches, and extreme altitude, a vast amount of delicate scientific machinery was carried up the mountain (and down again) in addition to the food, the fuel, and the mountaineering equipment that any expedition requires. Simply existing at these altitudes and in these conditions where preparing a meal or defecating can tax climbers to the limit, and it is nothing short of remarkable that these men ran generators, slept covered with electrodes, took careful observations, undertook all the laboratory chores, and showed the discipline and good humor necessary for this ambitious project.

Why go to all this trouble? Not "because it is there," nor for individual glory, but because Everest is a unique laboratory for studying the effects of extreme lack of one of our most essential fuels. Further understanding gleaned from this mission and others in the future cannot fail to benefit those countless millions who will suffer debilitating heart and lung ailments causing lack of oxygen at sea level.

—*Drummond Rennie, M.D.*

Special Report:
Mental Health in China
by Lewis Bernstein, Ph.D., and Rosalyn Bernstein

In recent years the People's Republic of China has opened up considerably, becoming more knowable to foreigners. A substantial amount of information about medicine and health care in general has emerged. By comparison, relatively little has been reported on mental health. For the most part, what is known about mental health has been gleaned by groups of mental health professionals who have been privileged to visit psychiatric facilities in that country. American visits have been sponsored by agencies of the U.S. government or organizations concerned with health care and education. The groups generally confer with psychiatric personnel and visit mental health and mental health-related facilities during two- to three-week tours.

Several recent reports by American journalists who have lived in China for a number of years have accused the Chinese of manipulating the foreigner's view of their country. For example, Richard Bernstein, a *Time* magazine correspondent based in Peking since 1979, has observed that the Chinese often go to great lengths to keep foreigners from having unsupervised encounters with the Chinese people and with their institutions.

Obviously, the tours of mental health facilities for Westerners provide only a limited view. So brief an exposure to a vastly different culture cannot give a complete picture. It does, however, permit a direct view of at least some current psychiatric practices in several localities and discussion of mutual professional problems with Chinese colleagues.

Evolution of Chinese mental health practice

With the victory of the Communist revolution in 1949 after years of war and turmoil, great changes began to occur in every phase of Chinese society. Of the numerous public health problems facing the new government, mental illness was not at first given high priority. However, early nationwide attention to the elimination of the problems of prostitution, venereal disease, and opium addiction in itself reduced mental health problems.

American missionaries and others living in China before the revolution as well as Chinese physicians describe psychiatric care prior to 1949 as primitive and cruel. Psychiatric hospitals did exist in some of the major centers of population, but the estimate of the total number of beds for a population nearing a billion ranged from only 1,000 to 6,000. This scarcity of beds meant that most of the seriously ill psychiatric patients

went untreated. For those who did enter hospitals, treatment was largely a matter of custodial care and physical restraint. Abuse and isolation were common. Little is known of the care in the countryside, where the great majority of the Chinese population has always resided.

In 1952 growing concern about problems of mental health led to the establishment of the Chinese Society of Neurology and Psychiatry (affiliated with the Chinese Medical Association in Peking). Prior to the start of the Cultural Revolution in about 1966 all medical schools had initiated courses in psychiatry. There was considerable interest in psychiatric research, and care in psychiatric institutions was humanized; physical restraints and isolation were no longer widely used. Efforts were made to spread mental health care throughout China by bringing rural medical personnel to the medical schools for brief periods of training and by sending trained personnel from the medical schools to the countryside for lectures and demonstrations. By 1957 there were 20,000 psychiatric beds, approximately one bed per 50,000 people.

The Cultural Revolution, the movement launched by Chairman Mao Zedong (Mao Tse-tung) during the late 1960s, amounted to a revitalization of revolutionary values and a repudiation of "bourgeois" cultural influences in all spheres of life. At this time there was a shift away from developing interest in Western medicine toward an emphasis on combining traditional Chinese methods (in particular, acupuncture and herbal medicines) with those Western concepts deemed appropriate for Chinese society. Mao's saying was: "Let the past serve the present and the foreign serve China." This basic approach continues today in current psychiatric practice and research.

From reports of both visiting foreign and native Chinese mental health specialists, it is apparent that progress in improving the status of psychiatric care has resumed since the end of the Cultural Revolution. The mental health system is still small; there are only 88 psychiatric hospitals in 25 provinces in a country of about one billion—nearly a quarter of the world's population. Nonetheless, as an example of the progress, in 1973 a delegation sponsored by the National Academy of Sciences reported that the 1,000-bed Shanghai Psychiatric Hospital staff had 61 psychiatrists and 216 nurses. In 1981 another group visiting the same hospital, still with the same bed capacity, found that the professional staff had increased to 130 psychiatrists,

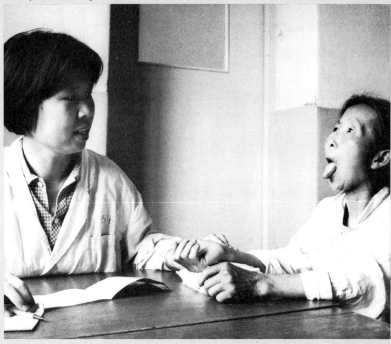

In China the term mental illness is reserved for only the severest cases. Many disorders that are considered to be psychosomatic or neurotic in the West are thought to be of physiological origin and thus are treated in medical settings—often in commune clinics.

315 nurses, and 52 psychiatric technicians.

The use of insulin shock in the treatment of certain schizophrenias and electroshock therapy for severe depressions (often effective, though not well-understood, treatments) had been discontinued during the Cultural Revolution but has been reinstituted. Psychiatric research has been resumed in the major teaching hospitals. Research efforts are now redirected toward finding practical solutions to mental health needs. At the Institute for Mental Health at Peking Medical College in 1981, studies were being conducted to compare the efficacy of Western drugs with Chinese herbal medications in the treatment of schizophrenics. In another study 800 brain-damaged schoolchildren will be followed for 18 years; each of three different groups will receive either Western drugs, herbs, or placebos. There are various ongoing epidemiologic studies for the joint purposes of increasing understanding of causation of mental disorders and assigning appropriate staff to treat various psychiatric problems. Psychiatric journals, suspended during the Cultural Revolution, are again being published. National conferences are being held, and postgraduate training courses are being offered.

The role of the political system

In looking at any aspect of Chinese society the political system in China must be understood as all-important. The collectivist philosophy expects all Chinese people to serve the nation. Thus it is assumed that even those with mental disorders can become productive members of society if given a sympathetic environment,

proper education, and, if necessary, "reeducation." The sympathetic environment encompasses the provision of food, housing, education, and medical care for all, albeit at minimal levels.

All society, whether in city or country, at home or at work, is organized in groups and committees. Therefore, everyone belongs to a social unit in the neighborhood or commune and at work. These units play an active part in each individual's life. U.S. social worker Ruth Sidel, who has made several visits to China and has published a number of reports on health care there, describes these neighborhood and work organizations as a "total community support system that encourages people to see themselves as part of a total structure, inspires them to participate actively in that social structure, and comes to their aid in times of stress." Family problems, for example, become the concern of the neighborhood committee. When an individual develops a psychiatric problem, care begins with the local committee's efforts to help. First, there is an attempt to reeducate the disturbed person. If this fails, the next step is to ensure that the person receives treatment at a clinic in the neighborhood or on the commune. The local clinic is likely to have a physician or a "barefoot doctor" (roughly equivalent to U.S. paramedics or nurse practitioners) who has had at least some exposure to psychiatric concepts and methods. As a last resort, the patient will be referred to a psychiatric hospital, where he and his family receive further education about the nature of the illness. Treatment involves not only medical staff but recovered or recovering patients who encourage the new patient in his efforts to understand and overcome his illness. In addition, any other individuals who may play key roles in the patient's life—friends, co-workers, neighbors, and so forth—join in "study" sessions at the hospital. This community involvement in psychiatric problems prompted psychiatrist Arthur Kleinman and sociologist David Mechanic to comment in a report summarizing their U.S.-government-sponsored three-week visit in 1978: "Mental illness in China is not a confidential relationship between patient and doctor. It is a social issue involving the home, the workplace, and the production brigade."

Unique aspects of mental health care

The Chinese ways of meeting the demands of the mentally ill are in many ways distinct. The Chinese do not subscribe to the beliefs of Freud. They do not use many treatment methods that are standard in Western nations—e.g., psychoanalysis, hypnosis, behavior therapies, or psychodrama. It is noteworthy that psychologists and social workers do not participate in the provision of mental health care in China. Social work is unknown, its functions assumed by the local committees and nurses with psychiatric training. Psychology was not recognized as either a field of study or a profession during the Cultural Revolution. Psychology courses and degrees are currently being reinstituted in the universities, but there is no evidence today of psychologists actively engaged in mental health practice. An American group visiting China in 1981 reported meeting only one psychologist, who had trained only to the master's level and was working at the Shanghai Psychiatric Hospital doing limited psychological testing.

It must be emphasized that the term mental illness is reserved in the People's Republic for only the severest cases—for problems that have not been resolved by reeducation or treatment in local clinics. The terms mental illness, psychosis, and schizophrenia are used almost synonymously. Neurotic disorders (such as anxiety neuroses, phobias, depressions, and hysteria) and psychosomatic illnesses (such as hypertension, ulcers, and migraine headaches) are considered physiological and are included under the rubric neurasthenia. In the U.S. the diagnosis of neurasthenia was formerly used to characterize a group of neurotic symptoms such as easy fatigability, vague pains, insomnia, and loss of appetite. The Chinese apparently define neurasthenia literally; i.e., as a debility of the nerves. Consequently, most of these patients are treated in medical or neurologic settings rather than in psychiatric ones, and they receive primarily herbal mixtures or acupuncture or both.

Although there are no available national statistics, the reported incidence of mental illnesses in the large urban centers is about 7 per 1,000 population. This statistic includes all psychoses, cases of severe retardation, and cases of epilepsy. (In the West epilepsy is recognized as a physical and not a mental illness.) Patients diagnosed as schizophrenic constitute the largest number of psychotic and hospitalized patients and therefore are the primary concern of Chinese psychiatrists.

In their current treatment of schizophrenia traditional methods (acupuncture and herbal mixtures) continue to be used as well as Western drug therapy, chiefly chlorpromazine. Chlorpromazine (Thorazine) is a major tranquilizer that usually brings about a decrease in psychotic thinking and a reduction in the bizarre behavior associated with schizophrenia. Dosages of chlorpromazine tend to be lower than those customarily given in the U.S.; it is claimed that the Parkinsonian symptoms such as tremor, shuffling gait, and drooling, common side effects in U.S. patients treated with major tranquilizers, are rarely experienced by Chinese patients. Several other Western drugs (e.g., lithium, used in the treatment of manic-depressive disorders, and haloperidol, another tranquilizer used in the treatment of schizophrenia) are being used at some hospitals but not extensively. Therapy for schizophrenia, for the most part, appears to be based on specific symptoms rather than on the disease itself. For example, a patient with auditory hallucinations will receive a different herbal mixture than one with visual hallucinations.

Chinese herbal preparations come from roots, barks, leaves, flowers, fruits, and seeds. The physician writes a prescription detailing the amount of each herb and indicating the method and the frequency of its use. Most commonly, one or several medicinal herbs are cooked in water, the residue is discarded, and the brew is kept for drinking. For psychiatric disorders the most frequently used herbal remedies are quince, mandarin citrus, gardenia, hemp, ginger, ginkgo, and milkwort. Although several institutes of materia medica in China are attempting to identify the effective constituents of herbal medicines, most have not, as yet, been adequately evaluated. It may take many years before the 5,000 varieties of medicinal plants can be subjected to Western-type controlled studies. However, Chinese health professionals are of the opinion that herbal preparations will continue to be used because the Chinese people and most physicians believe there is empirical evidence of their efficacy.

All patients are expected to participate in some form of work within the hospital as they begin to recover. Jobs for male patients range from maintenance of the hospital and its grounds to production work arranged for on a subcontract basis by local factories—for example, packaging detergent or pasting labels on cardboard boxes. Women patients work on production lines assembling dolls; they also sew and embroider. The work arrangement simulates as closely as possible real work on the outside.

The form of psychiatric care most comparable with

Western individual or group therapy is referred to as heart-to-heart talks. In these the patient, working individually with the psychiatrist or nurse, or in a group with other patients, is encouraged to discuss his problem, analyze its meaning, and develop "more correct" thinking about it. For example, a paranoid patient, who had accused fellow workers of talking about and plotting against him, learned through these heart-to-heart talks that he had misunderstood the situation at work because of his concern that his performance was not considered as good as that of others.

The usual length of stay in the hospital is two to three months, with an occasional patient remaining up to a year; 85% are discharged as improved. Patients who cannot be returned to the community may be sent to sanitoria, often associated with large factories and state industries, which are large hospitals for the treatment of all types of chronic illness. If they have not recovered after several years, they are returned home to be cared for by family.

One of the most impressive aspects of the mental health program in China is the posthospitalization care. Before the patient leaves the hospital, professional staff visit both home and workplace. Hospital personnel are already familiar with the patient's social network. His job, which has been held for him during illness (and his pay continued), and conditions at work are reviewed. Plans are made for changes that will help the patient return to the community with the least possible stress, including, if necessary, a change in job. Patients also return to the hospital for outpatient visits as needed and also to spend time with new inpatients, encouraging them in their efforts to recover. In short, the psychiatric patient in China is never left to fend for himself. He is not discharged from the hospital until a workable plan for his aftercare has been developed. In sharp contrast, recent publicity about practices in some areas of the U.S. presents a shocking picture of still-sick individuals, released from overcrowded mental hospitals, who become inner-city vagrants.

A Chinese reform school

Certain psychiatric problems of concern in Western countries are virtually unknown today in the People's Republic of China, notably sexual deviance and drug and alcohol addictions. Juvenile delinquency, however, remains a problem. In June 1981 Chinese authorities for the first time permitted a group of Western mental health professionals to visit one of the 11 Shanghai juvenile reform schools. The school is divided into two separate institutions at some distance from each other: 250 boys in one, 50 girls in the other. These uncontrollable teenagers are admitted on agreement between parents and teachers. There are no court referrals. Their offenses were described as theft, gang-fighting, gambling, and sexual activity before marriage (a legal offense in China). The causes of the delinquen-

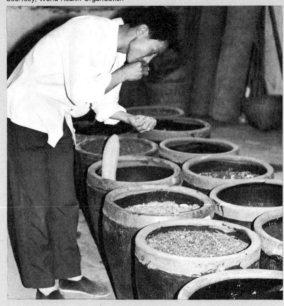

A hospital worker examines herbal preparations, which are used in conjunction with Western tranquilizers in the treatment of schizophrenia.

cy are thought to be the poor examples set by some adults, poor parenting practices such as physical abuse, and the disruptive effects of the Cultural Revolution, when many schools were closed.

The program in the reform school, which is usually of a year's duration, is strongly influenced by the political ideology, which expects all members of society to be law-abiding and to conform to socially productive standards of behavior. Corporal punishment is forbidden. During the first period in the school (about three months), students examine publicly the reasons for their "mistakes" and engage in "self-criticism." Students are encouraged to believe that they can improve and achieve success. Some reform school graduates who have made important contributions to society return to lecture other students; a graduate who is now a factory manager returned as a teacher in 1981. While the children are at the institution, factory or neighborhood committees work with the parents, teaching them how to handle the youngsters when they return home.

The second phase of the program involves part-time academic work and part-time (three hours a day) manual labor. Political study is a major portion of the academic program, but students also engage in typical high school subjects: languages, mathematics, music, history, sciences, and so forth. In the manual labor portion (designed to instill a "love for work") boys might assemble bicycles and large cardboard boxes; girls might sew garments for infants from scraps of cloth. The jobs derive from a consignment arrangement with a local department store. The students are paid one yuan (approximately 60 cents) per day.

319

In the third phase of the program students return to their homes and to their community schools. If their behavior is good, they remain in the community. If not, they return to the reform school. If repeated trials at home fail, they eventually go to prison. Statistics indicate that of 250 students who had completed the program since the school reopened in 1979, 70% were doing very well, 15% were performing acceptably, and 15% were repeaters. If these statistics are to be taken at face value, the Chinese seem to have greater success in handling juvenile delinquency than can be claimed in Western societies. Possibly the reform school programs are reinforced by the prevalent social controls in the society at large.

Emphasis on small families

In no area of Chinese life is there greater consensus than the need for population control. Official policy not only makes premarital sex a crime but encourages delayed marriages and highly favors one-child families. The first child entitles the family to a government grant for its support. If the first child is in any way defective, equal support will go to a second child, but the parents are strongly encouraged in all situations to avoid a second pregnancy for five years. If a second child is born to a family in which the first was normal and healthy, the family receives only half the subsidy. If a family has a third child, not only do they receive no subsidy but they incur the loss of certain allowances. Mothers who have had a third child are strongly encouraged to undergo sterilization by tubal ligation.

The above facts about population control are not irrelevant to the mental health situation in the People's Republic of China. If it is valid to assume that experiences in childhood are a major determining factor in adult mental health, future psychiatric problems of nonbiological origin may be minimal. The limitation of size of family means that each child is highly valued. Children are cherished, and fathers are as involved in parenting as mothers. This love is in evidence everywhere; on the perpetually crowded streets parents and grandparents of infants and toddlers encourage foreign strangers in a beguilingly friendly way to pay attention to their children. In the nursery schools visitors are entertained with dance and song ("Jingle Bells," sung by the children in English, is a favorite even in June!). Visitors become instant "aunties" and "uncles" and partners in group dances. Children generally strike observers as poised, confident, and well-behaved. Their upbringing appears to be kind but firm. Conformity is expected and highly rewarded.

Important questions

This ever present emphasis on conformity, the strict social controls, and the crowded conditions in which the Chinese live and work raise important questions in the minds of visiting mental health professionals. From a Western point of view the daily experience of most Chinese citizens could be seen as highly stressful, considering the high degree of repression that is required to maintain constant acceptable behavior. Prolonged repression often is recognized as a catalyst for breakdown of one form or another—antisocial acts, various neurotic reactions, or psychosomatic illnesses. Chinese authorities maintain that the incidence of such problems is very low. Yet of the major physical illnesses in the adult Chinese population, hypertension (high blood pressure) is the most prevalent—a condition in which stress is often a predisposing factor. Do these seeming contradictions mean that the relationship between stress and illness is not recognized? Or do cultural differences, involving different expectations, mean genuinely different reactions?

These questions and others are typical of those asked by visiting professionals. From the reports of various delegations that have visited China during the past ten years, it is obvious, too, that with minor variations all the visits are markedly similar. The same facilities tend to be on each group's itinerary. Tours are limited to two to three weeks. Itinerary changes or additions are usually discouraged. One delegation reported its request to observe nonteaching psychiatric units, knowing that these existed in areas close to the ones on their scheduled tour. Yet they were told that such institutions were "too distant." They were also taken on four- and five-hour trips to visit model production brigades when similar brigades were within walking distance of their hotels. Are visitors being allowed to see only what the Chinese want them to see? Or is it administratively easier to have foreign groups visit the same places?

If Chinese professionals sometimes seem defensive or unwilling to discuss some aspects of their institutions and mental health programs, they must get credit for having overcome enormous obstacles in achieving even minimal care for the psychiatrically ill. Richard Wyatt, chief of the adult psychiatry branch at the National Institute of Mental Health in the U.S., has recently reported, "The Chinese have a long tradition of respect for others and for the family. Their system strikes me as better, at least for the mentally ill in society. . . . I sense they have a jump on us in integrating their mentally ill." It is clear even from limited observations that intervention begins at an early stage of mental illness, that there is good posttreatment, and that continuity of care is provided for the mentally ill. Unresolved problems are many, of course.

For Western observers it may be that language barriers and discussion through translators impair communication, as do the sometimes hurried conditions of a study-tour visit. In spite of the many unanswered questions and the often frustrating lack of opportunity for in-depth study, most professional visitors find even brief tours highly rewarding and genuinely enlightening.

320

Health Education Units

The following articles on important medical topics and health-related concerns are meant to be instructive and practical. It is largely through general health education that individuals can maintain and enhance their physical well-being. While the units emphasize the activation of the layperson's sense of responsibility for his or her own health, their purpose is to inform, not to prescribe.

Contributors

Howard C. Baron, M.D.
Raynaud's Phenomenon; Varicose Veins; Phlebitis
Attending Vascular Surgeon, Cabrini Medical Center, New York City; Associate Professor of Surgery, New York University School of Medicine.

William A. Check
Vasectomy
Free-lance medical and science writer, Atlanta, Ga.

Sidney Cohen, M.D.
Irritable Bowel Syndrome
Chief, Gastrointestinal Section, Department of Medicine, Hospital of the University of Pennsylvania, Philadelphia; T. Grier Miller Professor of Medicine, University of Pennsylvania School of Medicine.

Steven G. Economou, M.D.
Hernias
Jack Fraser Smith Professor and Associate Chairman, Department of General Surgery, Rush-Presbyterian-St. Luke's Medical Center, Chicago.

Alvin N. Eden, M.D.
Middle Ear Infections; Scarlet Fever and Strep Throat; Hypertension in Children; Infant Nutrition
Chairman and Director, Department of Pediatrics, Wyckoff Heights Hospital, Brooklyn, N.Y.; Associate Clinical Professor of Pediatrics, New York University School of Medicine, New York City.

Charles J. Gudas, D.P.M.
Common Foot Problems
Director, Podiatric Education and Training Program, Department of Surgery, Section of Orthopedics; The University of Chicago Hospital and Clinics.

Rose Kushner
Coping with Mastectomy
Executive Director, Breast Cancer Advisory Center, Rockville, Md.; Member, National Cancer Advisory Board.

Lynne Lamberg
Hangover
Free-lance medical writer, Baltimore, Md.

Joann Ellison Rodgers
Breast-feeding; Labor; Genital Herpes
National Science Correspondent, Hearst Feature Service, New York City.

Lionel J. Schewitz, M.D.
Hysterectomy
Attending Obstetrician and Gynecologist, Lake Forest Hospital, Lake Forest, Ill.; Attending Obstetrician and Gynecologist and Assistant Professor, Rush-Presbyterian-St. Luke's Medical Center; Lecturer, Northwestern University Medical School, Chicago.

Rolf F. Ulvestad, M.D.
Motion Sickness
Motion sickness researcher and otolaryngologist in private practice, Minneapolis, Minn.

Title cartoons by John Everds

Contents

Middle Ear Infections

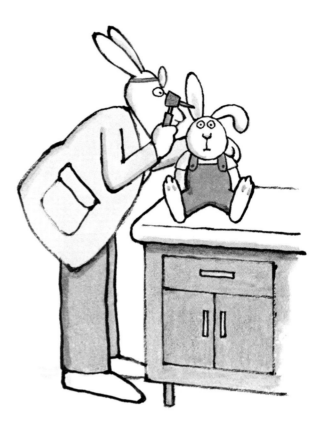

Otitis media, or inflammation of the middle ear, is one of the most common childhood infections. It can affect children of all ages, including infants. Because of the frequency of these infections and the complications that can develop, especially hearing loss, it is essential that parents be familiar with the signs and symptoms and the various methods of treatment. Treatment of otitis media is a complicated and controversial subject. At present there is no consensus among doctors as to optimal treatment and how best to prevent complications.

The middle ear and the eustachian tube

Otitis media is defined as an infection or inflammation of the middle ear cavity, the area located just behind the eardrum. Physicians have known for many years that otitis media affects some children while others are seldom involved. Most authorities now believe that the reason for this is related to the eustachian tube, which extends from the space in back of the nose to the middle ear cavity. Studies have shown that children who are prone to recurrent episodes of middle ear infections usually are found to have poorly functioning eustachian tubes. These studies also have shown that the group of children who have no (or very few) attacks of otitis media have eustachian tubes that function normally.

In order to understand the mechanisms involved in the development of middle ear infections, it is necessary to learn something about the eustachian tube and how it works. It has two main functions related to the middle ear. The first is ventilation of the middle ear in order to equalize the air pressure there with atmospheric pressure and to replenish the oxygen that has been absorbed. With a normally functioning eustachian tube the air that goes into the ear through the tube keeps the eardrum air pressure in balance with that of the air that enters through the outer ear canal.

The second function of the eustachian tube is drainage of fluid and mucus out of the middle ear cavity into the nasopharynx. If the tube becomes obstructed or does not function properly, the fluid is trapped in the the middle ear cavity. This causes a hearing loss if the fluid remains behind the eardrum.

Upper respiratory infections and allergies are two common conditions that interfere with eustachian tube

function and therefore lead to middle ear inflammation and infection. When a child with a normal eustachian tube swallows, the tube opens and any accumulated fluid and mucus drain out. However, when a child with a malfunctioning eustachian tube swallows, the tube fails to open, and the fluid remains trapped inside the middle ear cavity. This fluid acts as an excellent medium for bacterial multiplication. Bacteria from the back of the nose travel up the eustachian tube directly into the middle ear cavity and multiply and grow in the trapped fluid. As a result the fluid becomes thick and purulent (filled with pus).

An allergic child often develops swelling in the back of the nose. This condition leads to obstruction of the flow of air through the eustachian tube and results in the accumulation of clear fluid in the middle ear cavity. With a poorly functioning eustachian tube the fluid cannot drain out, and the trapped fluid can easily become infected with bacteria and become purulent. A recent study conducted at the University of California Medical Center at San Diego demonstrated that nasal obstruction due to allergy results in a negative shift in the middle ear pressure which produces an effusion (fluid accumulation) that is characteristic of one form of otitis media.

Enlarged adenoids also might cause obstruction of the eustachian tube, but there is no consensus among physicians as to the exact role of adenoids in the devel-

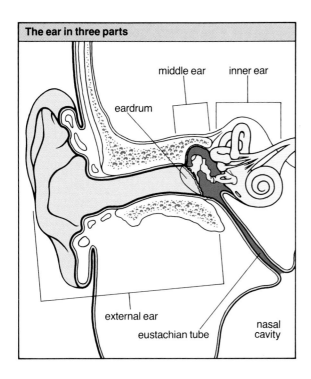

middle ear   inner ear

eardrum

external ear

eustachian tube   nasal cavity

opment of middle ear problems. A number of studies are attempting to determine whether or not the removal of adenoids is a useful procedure in the treatment of recurrent middle ear infections. The current consensus, then, is that children with poorly functioning eustachian tubes who develop frequent upper respiratory infections or who suffer from respiratory allergy are most susceptible to frequent and recurrent middle ear problems.

Frequency of middle ear infections

Investigations have shown that by five years of age more than 50% of all children have already had at least one episode of middle ear infection. Surveys of practicing pediatricians have reported that except for well-baby and routine child-care examinations otitis media is the most frequent reason for office visits. The statistics related to recurrence rates are especially interesting. About one-half of the children who had one episode of middle ear infection before one year of age averaged six or more middle ear infections during the next two years.

Some studies have suggested that all children can be divided into three broad groups in relation to otitis media: one-third never develop otitis media; one-third have an occasional episode; and one-third have frequent recurrent infections. The last group is believed to have eustachian tubes that do not function normally.

Otitis media can occur at any age, including the newborn period. The highest incidence of such infections is between six months and two years of age. After a child is two years old, the incidence at first decreases but

then starts to increase between five and six years of age. This takes place at the time the child usually enters school, when there is increased exposure to other children and so the greater likelihood of catching viral and bacterial respiratory infections. Middle ear infections are less commonly seen in children who are seven years of age and older. Most of the cases are reported during the winter months, when the frequency of respiratory infections increases.

There have been conflicting reports as to sex differences in the occurrence of middle ear infections. One study that was conducted in Boston concluded that boys had significantly more episodes than girls. However, the results of other studies do not agree. These investigations found no difference in incidence between boys and girls. The Boston study also showed that white children had significantly more episodes of otitis media than black children. This difference is not readily explained. Among possible reasons may be differences in the anatomy of the eustachian tubes between whites and blacks and the fact that higher economic groups, predominantly white, report episodes of illness more frequently than do less affluent people.

There are many complicated methods of classifying otitis media. This discussion will be limited to the two types seen in children most frequently, acute purulent otitis media and serous or secretory otitis media, sometimes called otitis media with effusion. The signs and symptoms as well as the complications and treatment are different for each type.

Acute purulent otitis media

In acute purulent otitis media the middle ear cavity is filled with pus, and there is possible abscess formation. Children suffering with this infection are quite ill. The symptoms include severe earache; fever; irritability, often with persistent crying; weakness; and headache. Many of these children also have accompanying nausea, vomiting, and complete loss of appetite. In babies the fever may be very high. The thick purulent material within the middle ear cavity increases the pressure against the eardrum, causing severe pain. A physician examining a child with acute purulent otitis media will find that the eardrum is red and bulging. If the pressure continues to increase, it can result in rupture of the eardrum. The pus then drains out through the ear canal. When this happens, the excruciating pain caused by the pressure on the drum quickly subsides.

Many studies investigating the causes of acute purulent otitis media have been conducted. It has been proved by analyzing the thick fluid in the middle ear that this condition is almost always due to a bacterial infection. *Streptococcus pneumoniae* and *Hemophilus influenzae* are the two most frequently isolated bacteria from the fluid, while the third most common is *Streptococcus pyogenes.*

The results of studies of the bacteriology of otitis

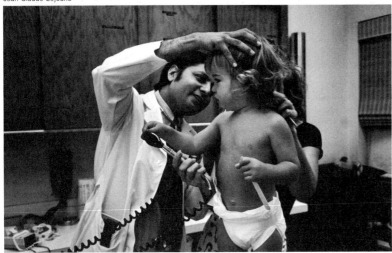

Middle ear infection (otitis media) is a common problem in infants and young children. Such infections should be carefully treated, as one serious complication is permanent loss of hearing.

media in children from Sweden, Finland, and the United States were all similar. *Streptococcus pneumoniae* was the most frequent cause of all, and it was also demonstrated that *Hemophilus influenzae* is infrequently seen in children over eight years of age.

A number of antibiotics including ampicillin and amoxicillin are effective in treating these infections. The child's physician decides which specific antibiotic to use and for how long it should be given. The consensus of most pediatricians is that a full ten-day course of antibiotic therapy is required. In most cases a child's condition improves soon after the start of the appropriate antibiotic. If the organism is sensitive to the antibiotic chosen, the fluid in the middle ear becomes free of bacteria 90–95% of the time. A small number of children do not improve with antibiotic therapy and continue to have pain and fever. If such is the case, it may be necessary to drain out the thick purulent fluid so as to relieve the symptoms caused by the increased pressure. Despite proper antibiotic therapy some of these children are left with fluid in the middle ear that does not drain out or become absorbed.

Serous otitis media

Serous otitis media is much more difficult to diagnose than the acute purulent form. Usually there are very few associated signs and symptoms, and so the diagnosis is often delayed or never made. Serous otitis media is characterized by watery fluid in the middle ear cavity that produces little or no pressure on the eardrum and therefore is not associated with pain. As stated above, it can develop after a child has been adequately treated for acute purulent otitis media. It has been estimated that about one out of every four children with acute purulent otitis media is left with some clear, sterile fluid behind the eardrum.

The most important complication of serous otitis media is the hearing loss that may result. It is considered

the most common cause of loss of hearing in school-age children. The problem may not be recognized until a teacher in school notices that a child is inattentive and has difficulty in hearing. The child is then examined by a physician and found to have serous fluid behind the eardrum. Often the eardrum is difficult to see because of wax obstructing the physician's view through the otoscope. There are other methods and techniques available besides the usual examination through an otoscope that are now available for the examining doctor in order to determine whether or not fluid is present. One method is called tympanometry, the insertion of a probe in the external ear canal that both presents and measures the sound pressure level of a tone. In this way the acoustic impedance of the

In some cases of serous otitis media it may be necessary to remove fluid from the middle ear and to surgically implant a ventilating tube in the eardrum.

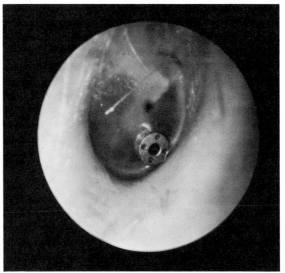

middle ear as a function of ear canal air pressure can be assessed. Another method involves the use of a pneumatic otoscope, an instrument in which a rubber suction bulb is used to test the reaction of the tympanic membrane. The child's physician will decide if and when these specialized techniques are indicated, and he may refer the patient to an otologist or otolaryngologist for the tests. The longer the fluid remains in the middle ear cavity, the greater is the likelihood that it will cause decreased hearing. This makes it important for every child treated for acute purulent otitis media to be reexamined after the treatment is completed in order to make certain that the middle ear cavity is free of fluid. As was explained earlier, those children with poorly functioning eustachian tubes are at greatest risk. Eustachian tube dysfunction associated with allergies or with frequent upper respiratory infections is the combination of factors that is most likely to lead to serous otitis media.

The treatment of serous otitis media is complicated, difficult, and controversial. When there is no associated hearing loss, the consensus is to treat conservatively and not to intervene surgically. Some physicians believe that the use of decongestants or antihistamines reduces the swelling and allows the clear fluid to drain out of the middle ear cavity through the eustachian tube. But others do not agree. They claim that decongestants and antihistamines are not effective and believe that the best method of treatment is no treatment at all. In time, they maintain, the middle ear fluid resorbs or drains and gradually becomes replaced by air, a process that usually takes between one and three months.

Treatment of serous otitis media with an associated hearing loss is a real and difficult problem. There have been a number of recent reports describing hearing difficulties that have been attributed to prolonged and repeated episodes of serous otitis media during the first three years of life. This has resulted in a more aggressive approach to the problem by many physicians.

The consensus among both otolaryngologists and pediatricians at present is to intervene surgically when a child with serous otitis media is found to have significant hearing loss over a period of many months or when the child has had a history of recurrent and frequent episodes of serous otitis media with associated hearing loss. The fluid in the middle ear can be drained out either by means of a surgical incision in the eardrum (myringotomy) or by a myringotomy followed by the insertion of small ventilation tubes, called tympanotomy tubes, into the eardrum. These tubes are believed to help keep the middle ear cavity free of fluid. These surgical procedures should not be performed after only one or two episodes of serous otitis media because associated with them are complications and risks, such as psychological trauma, anesthesia risk, secondary infection, and eardrum scarring. Some otolaryngologists recommend removal of the adenoids to prevent recurrent episodes of serous otitis media, claiming that enlarged adenoids obstruct the eustachian tube. As mentioned earlier, researchers are attempting to determine whether adenoidectomy is a useful procedure.

Complications

The complications of middle ear infections have decreased dramatically in recent years. With the use of appropriate antibiotics many potentially serious complications, including mastoid infection, brain abscess, and meningitis, have been almost entirely eliminated. However, physicians continue to be confronted with hearing loss owing to the persistence of serous fluid in the middle ear cavity following treatment of the acute purulent otitis media. In order to protect a child adequately, it is essential that the diagnosis of acute purulent otitis media be made early so that appropriate treatment can be instituted as soon as possible. It therefore is imperative that a physician be consulted when otitis media is suspected. If the diagnosis is unduly delayed, successful treatment is more difficult and may result in chronic ear problems.

It also is necessary to have a physician recheck the ears after treatment is complete to determine whether or not fluid remains in the middle ear cavity. Longstanding hearing loss may impair a child's speech, language, and cognition. Therefore, all preschool-age children should have their hearing tested, especially those who have had histories of recurrent ear infections, recurrent respiratory allergy attacks, or frequent upper respiratory infections.

Middle ear infection in children remains one of the most poorly understood and complicated problems facing both the physician and the parents of the affected children. The key to preventing possible complications is to maintain a high index of suspicion so that an early diagnosis can be made and proper treatment instituted without delay.

—*Alvin N. Eden, M.D.*

Scarlet Fever and Strep Throat

Scarlet fever is an acute infectious disease that is caused by bacteria called group A hemolytic streptococcus. It can affect people of all ages but is most often seen in children. It is called scarlet fever because of the red skin rash that accompanies it. This infection can now be easily treated with appropriate antibiotics, and the potentially dangerous complications that may follow can usually be prevented. Before the advent of antibiotics, scarlet fever was indeed a dangerous, serious illness, but this no longer is the case.

Any discussion of scarlet fever of necessity must include streptococcal tonsillitis and pharyngitis as well—that is, streptococcal inflammation of the tonsils and throat, also called strep throat. Streptococcal tonsillitis and streptococcal pharyngitis are nearly identical to scarlet fever, except that there is no rash. The particular group A hemolytic streptococcus that causes scarlet fever infects the throat and gives rise to a specific antigen called the erythrogenic ("redness-producing") toxin that is responsible for the rash. All the following information about scarlet fever also relates to the other group A hemolytic streptococcal infections that occur without the rash.

Characteristics of the infection

Scarlet fever is rarely seen during the first two years of life, begins to increase in incidence gradually thereafter, and reaches a peak incidence just before the adolescent period, being most common between 6 and 12 years of age. Scarlet fever is more common in temperate areas than in tropical, hotter areas. In the United States strep throat is seen more frequently in the North, with an especially high incidence in the Rocky Mountain states. It is endemic in most of the large cities in the temperate zone of the United States.

The main sources of the streptococci are discharges from the nose and throat of patients with the disease or people who are carriers of the bacteria. It has been shown that people who carry streptococci in the nose are a particularly frequent source of transmission, usually by droplet spray, such as results from sneezing or coughing. The bacteria can also be transmitted indirectly by contact with contaminated objects or the unwashed hands of a person who is attending a patient with the disease. Food-borne epidemics have been reported from contaminated milk, ice cream, and eggs.

The incubation period of scarlet fever ranges between one and seven days. The disease usually begins

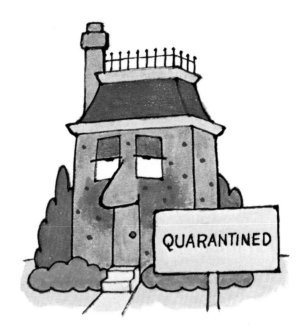

with the sudden onset of fever, vomiting, and severe sore throat. Along with these symptoms the child usually develops a headache, chills, and weakness. Between 12 and 24 hours after the onset of the fever, the typical scarlet fever rash appears. Occasionally the child complains of severe abdominal pain. If a child develops streptococcal tonsillitis without the scarlet fever rash and has this combination of vomiting and abdominal pain, the illness can easily be mistaken for a case of acute appendicitis.

In the typical case the temperature rises to 103° F (39.5° C) or higher. The child with scarlet fever has a red and sore throat. The tonsils are enlarged, reddened, and covered with patches of matter that has oozed from them. The glands under the angles of the jaw become swollen and tender. The tongue changes in its appearance as the disease progresses. At the start the tip and edges are reddened and the rest of the tongue has a whitish appearance. By the third or fourth day the white coat has peeled off, and the tongue then develops the typical red "strawberry" appearance.

The rash of scarlet fever, which appears shortly after the fever, has been described as a "sunburn with goose pimples." The skin is covered with tiny red spots that blanch on pressure and has a rough sandpaperlike texture. This scarlet rash usually covers the entire body except for the area around the mouth, which remains pale. One of the most characteristic features of the rash of scarlet fever is the desquamation, or peeling, that occurs at the end of the first week. The desquamating skin comes off as fine flakes like bran. The hands and feet are usually the last to desquamate, not until the second or third week after the onset.

Most cases of scarlet fever can be diagnosed just by the typical signs and symptoms. However, strep throat without the scarlet fever rash is more difficult to diagnose. The throat culture is the most useful and most important confirmatory test. The group A hemolytic streptococci can be isolated from the throat or the nose and the results of the culture determined after 24 hours of incubation. Since it is important to determine whether the throat infection is caused by a streptococcus, more and more physicians are obtaining throat cultures whenever streptococcus is suspected. Another helpful laboratory result would be an elevated white blood count. Blood samples can also be drawn and analyzed for antibody levels to various of the toxins that the streptococci give off. These tests are usually not required for diagnosis.

Treatment

Although a number of antibiotics are effective in the treatment of group A streptococcal infections, penicillin still remains the drug of choice. This form of therapy is consistently followed by a rapid reduction of the fever and improvement in well-being. The penicillin can be given by injection or by mouth. The aim is to maintain an adequate blood level of penicillin against the bacteria for *at least ten days of treatment.* The danger is that often, after the child is feeling better, the parents stop the treatment too soon, after three or four days. Therefore, there will be occasions when the doctor will decide to give the penicillin by injection. Various long-acting penicillin preparations maintain adequate blood levels for at least the crucial ten-day period, so one injection is all that is required. For children who are allergic to penicillin there are a number of other antibiotics that are equally effective, for example, erythromycin or a cephalosporin. A recent study carried out in the department of pediatrics of the University of Texas Health Science Center, Dallas, demonstrated that penicillin by mouth, long-acting penicillin by injection, cephalodroxal (cephalosporin), and erythromycin are equally effective in the treatment of strep throat in children.

Possible complications

The prognosis for a child who is adequately treated for a streptococcal infection is excellent. Recovery is rapid, and the early complications of the spread of the infection are almost always prevented. The late complications, especially acute rheumatic fever, can usually be prevented by prompt antibiotic therapy, providing the full course of treatment is administered.

The early complications generally occur during the first week of the illness. The infection may spread, inflaming the middle ear, the sinuses, or the lymph nodes in the neck. A rare early complication is bronchopneumonia. Even rarer are osteomyelitis (infection of the bone), mastoiditis (infection of the mastoid processes, bony areas behind the ears), and septicemia (blood poisoning). If the child is adequately treated, such complications rarely develop.

Of great importance are the two serious late complications, rheumatic fever and acute glomerulonephritis. As yet the cause of these late complications is unknown. The accepted explanation is that they are due to a hypersensitivity reaction to the bacteria or to some of their by-products. The onset of these complications after the initial infection varies from one to two weeks for glomerulonephritis and two to four weeks for acute rheumatic fever. They may follow a mild streptococcal infection just as often as a severe one.

Rheumatic fever is a relatively uncommon but serious complication. The incidence is said to be about 3% after a case of strep throat that is inadequately treated and less than 1% after full treatment. Rheumatic fever is rarely seen in children under three years of age. Since rheumatic fever often causes damage to the heart, it is extremely important that any child with a streptococcal infection be correctly diagnosed and adequately treated.

Rheumatic fever can be serious. It causes swelling and pain in the joints, especially the knees, elbows, ankles, and wrists, and a red skin rash. These usually clear up with no aftereffects. More ominous is inflammation of the heart, including the pericardium (the sac enclosing the heart), the heart muscle, inner lining, and valves. The inflammation causes malfunction of the heart valves, so that the heart must labor to perform adequately. After the infection has subsided, scar tissue may appear on the valves, preventing them from opening and closing properly. In time, heart failure can occur as the malfunctioning worsens.

A more common late complication is acute glomerulonephritis, infection of the capillaries in the glomeruli, which are tufts of tiny blood vessels in the outer cortex of the kidneys. A child who develops acute glomerulonephritis has fever, blood in the urine, puffiness in the face, and, occasionally, high blood pressure. However, in most cases the prognosis for full recovery is excellent. There is no consensus at present as to whether or not a child who is adequately treated for a streptococcal infection will be less likely to develop this late complication.

The diagnosis of scarlet fever still strikes fear in the hearts of many parents. In the preantibiotic era this illness was extremely serious, often causing long periods of illness, many dangerous complications, and even death. Children with scarlet fever used to be immediately isolated and quarantined, and entire schools and neighborhoods panicked when a case was discovered. But with the advent of antibiotics the entire picture has changed. Today most cases of acute rheumatic fever can be prevented if the parents promptly contact their physician whenever their child has a sore throat and high fever and if they are conscientious in following their physician's orders.

—Alvin N. Eden, M.D.

Raynaud's Phenomenon

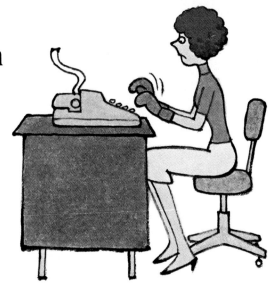

There are several circulatory disturbances that manifest themselves by color changes in the skin of the hands, even though no evidence of an organic disease can be found. Such disturbances are considered "functional" vascular diseases. The most common functional vasospastic disease (characterized by spasms of the blood vessels) was first described in the mid-19th century by a Parisian physician, Maurice Raynaud. Now known as Raynaud's phenomenon, this circulatory disturbance affects the hands, especially the fingers. There are in fact two distinct medical entities that can bring about similar transient skin-color changes and other symptoms in the digits of the hands due to spasm of the small arteries. One entity is called Raynaud's phenomenon; the other, Raynaud's disease. Unlike Raynaud's disease, Raynaud's phenomenon is always a secondary symptom caused by a disease or some form of trauma. The most common cause, however, is Raynaud's disease itself, which is of unknown etiology, or cause.

Characteristics of the phenomenon

Raynaud's phenomenon is the transient constriction of the small arteries in the extremities, resulting in intermittent changes in the color of the skin of the digits, the change being most marked in lighter-skinned persons. Typically, the involved fingers blanch on exposure to cold, then turn a bluish color, and soon thereafter turn bright red. During the time when the blood vessels are constricted in spasm, from a few minutes to several hours, the digits become cold and numb, and the hand often becomes wet with perspiration. The return of reddish color to the skin indicates the return of normal blood flow. Along with it comes pain, tingling, occasional swelling, and a rise in skin temperature. Initially, the attacks may involve only one or two fingers of one hand, but with time both hands become involved. Raynaud's phenomenon affects women far more frequently than men—the incidence is five times greater in women. It rarely occurs before puberty or after the age of 40, but it may appear at any age.

The primary causes of Raynaud's phenomenon are Raynaud's disease and occupational trauma. The latter occasionally occurs in individuals who develop vascular symptoms in their hands and fingers as a result of their trade; for example, from working with tools that require a squeezing action or when the hand is subjected to blunt trauma from vibrations. Workers who use jack-

hammers or drills powered by compressed air are typical of those who develop this problem. Raynaud's phenomenon is also occasionally seen in pianists and typists, whose fingers are subjected to repeated sharp thumps. The worker who acquires Raynaud's phenomenon through one of these avenues must either cease the activity that is causing the trauma or modify the operating techniques to lessen the effects on his or her hands. Some patients have had to change their occupations.

There are rarer causes of Raynaud's phenomenon. One is from intoxication following the ingestion of ergot, a fungus occasionally found on rye and certain other cereals. Ergot poisoning has generally been caused by the ingestion of ergotized grains or certain pharmacologic agents, primarily used in the treatment of migraine, that contain ergot. It produces serious vasospastic manifestations in the digits of the hands and feet. Another rare cause is arterial disease in which the arteries become blocked, or occluded. Among these diseases are arteriosclerosis obliterans, or hardening of the arteries in which the passages of the small arteries become totally blocked, and thromboangiitis obliterans (Buerger's disease), an inflammatory disease of the small arteries of the hands and feet. Finally, there is a miscellaneous group of diseases that have been known to bring about Raynaud's phenomenon. The most common of these are systemic diseases affecting the connective tissues, including scleroderma, lupus erythematosus, and rheumatoid arthritis.

Treatment of individuals who are susceptible to attacks of Raynaud's phenomenon consists primarily of protection from exposure to cold. Tobacco smoking is known to produce spasm of the small arteries and should be avoided. Mild sedation and the use of drugs that relieve arterial spasm play a role in the therapy.

Certain drugs derived from *Rauwolfia,* a genus of plants of the dogbane family, and used in the treatment of hypertension will often decrease the severity and frequency of the attacks associated with Raynaud's phenomenon.

Raynaud's disease

Typically, Raynaud's disease starts with an episode of color changes in the fingers, similar to that seen in Raynaud's phenomenon, in a young woman following exposure to cold. Less frequently the toes may be involved. Generally, several fingers of *both* hands are involved in the episode, which consists of the same color alterations that are seen in Raynaud's phenomenon. As the disease progresses over time, all that is necessary to produce a typical episode is the exposure of one hand to cold water or cold air. An emotional crisis will also trigger the symptoms. In severe cases ulceration or even gangrene of the fingertips can result.

The diagnosis of Raynaud's disease is relatively easy to make if Raynaud's phenomenon has been present for two or more years in both hands and was brought on by exposure to cold or emotional stimuli, and if the presence of any other recognizable disease that might cause the phenomenon to appear has been ruled out. Further evidence is the presence of an ulcer or of gangrene, usually limited to small areas of the skin over the tip of the digits.

The primary therapeutic objective in a patient with Raynaud's disease is to make the digital arteries less responsive to spasm. Factors that are known to produce spasm should be minimized or eliminated, if possible. Exposure to cold temperatures, perhaps the most common triggering circumstance, should be avoided. Warmly lined gloves and boots should be worn whenever exposure to cold is anticipated. Immersion of the hands in cold water should be avoided as much as possible. When periodic exposure to cold air, even that of a household refrigerator, is necessary, fleece-lined gloves should be kept handy and donned in the kitchen. And, of course, avoidance of stress is recommended to minimize emotional triggering of symptoms.

Although a direct correlation between tobacco smoking and the progression of this disease cannot be established, smoking should be avoided because it is known to constrict the peripheral blood vessels. It is imperative to stop smoking if ulcers or gangrene of the tips of the fingers has developed.

There are a number of pharmaceutical agents that cause temporary relaxation of the smaller arteries, thus decreasing the responsiveness of these vessels to external stimuli. These drugs fall into several different categories, those that block nerve stimuli that cause spasm of the smaller arteries and those that cause the smaller arteries to dilate by acting directly on the muscles of the artery wall. There is another group of thera-

peutic agents that may be effective in treating vasospasm because of their ability to bring about temporary dilation of the small blood vessels in the extremities. In this category are certain alcoholic beverages. Often the routine, moderate use (one to two ounces per day) of a beverage such as whiskey or brandy may help to blunt or reduce attacks in a person with a severe form of Raynaud's disease.

One of the most important aspects in treating Raynaud's disease is some form of psychotherapy. Patients must be reassured that the disease, although it causes pain and temporary disability during the paroxysms of the attack, will not progress to loss of the fingers or even the limbs, as some patients have feared. In the milder cases or where there is little anxiety, reassurance and, if necessary, a mild tranquilizer will prove to be valuable therapeutic adjuncts.

In the small group of patients with progressive Raynaud's disease that results in skin ulceration or superficial gangrene of the tips of the digits, more aggressive measures are required. These include treatment of the lesions to prevent an infection from developing. The pain that is associated with the digital ulcer or tissue gangrene can often be very effectively controlled with the use of Serpasil, a drug containing reserpine. This drug can forestall the episodic attacks of spasm of the blood vessels, making it particularly useful in bringing about healing of ulcerated or gangrenous skin.

A new group of drugs holds promise in the treatment of functional vasospastic diseases such as Raynaud's disease. These agents, called calcium channel blockers, alter the action of calcium within the artery wall. Since calcium is a necessary ingredient for arterial tone (the ability of an artery to contract), when this functional activity is blocked, arterial tone is reduced and the artery dilates.

For patients with progressive Raynaud's disease associated with skin damage, surgical intervention in the form of an operation called a sympathectomy often produces beneficial effects. This surgery eliminates the control of the sympathetic nervous system over the small arteries in the digits. The sympathetic nervous system functions mainly to regulate the automatic, involuntary responses of the body to daily physiological events. After sympathectomy the arteries of the fingers become more or less permanently dilated and are much less responsive to external stimuli. The use of sympathectomy for treatment of Raynaud's disease should be limited to those patients in whom progression of the skin changes in the digits is apparent even under intensive medical therapy, or if the periodic episodic attacks continue to worsen before the tissue changes come about. Sympathectomy has produced excellent therapeutic results, with healing of tissue ulcers and relief of pain that previously seemed resistant to therapy.

—Howard C. Baron, M.D.

Hypertension in Children

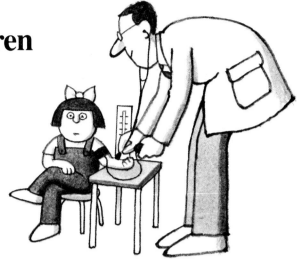

In recent years there has been an increasing awareness of the problem of hypertension in children and adolescents. Before 1970 high blood pressure was considered a rare occurrence in children, but during the past decade a great body of evidence has accumulated pointing to the fact that hypertension in this age group is relatively common. Although many cases of high blood pressure in childhood are secondary to an underlying disorder of the kidneys or heart, primary, or essential, hypertension is now being diagnosed with increasing frequency. Based on data from adults, this type of hypertension tends to run in families and probably has its origins in early life. With this in mind, there are two important questions to be answered: First, is it possible to detect those children who are at high risk for later, sustained hypertension in adulthood? Second, if, in fact, such individuals can be identified, is it possible through various methods of treatment, including diet and weight control, to change the course of their disease? At the present time these questions remain basically unanswered.

Detecting children at risk

Routine blood pressure measurements are now being recommended for all children over three years of age during regular checkups. Blood pressure levels at different ages can be recorded, and their change over time can be noted in a manner similar to charting of height and weight so that upward trends of blood pressure can be detected as early as possible. It is obvious that the earlier the diagnosis of high blood pressure is made, the better the chances of preventing the child from ending up with hypertension as an adult, with all its associated risks.

According to figures obtained from the National Center for Health Statistics, over 20 million adults, or about one-eighth of the entire adult population of the U.S., suffer from hypertension. Of these 20 million hypertensive adults, the vast majority are believed to have the primary form. Since this type of hypertension is believed to begin in early life, the important question that is as yet unanswered is how many of these adults showed evidence of high blood pressure when they were children.

The actual incidence of hypertension in children and adolescents has not been established. In large-scale screening studies, incidence has ranged between 0.6 and 20.5%. This very wide variation can be attributed both to differences in the definition of hypertension and to the methodology of the study. One recent survey found a 1.2% prevalence, using as the criterion for hypertension any child found to have a sustained level above the 95th percentile of recorded levels. The pediatric hypertension group at New York Hospital in New York City has estimated that the true incidence of childhood hypertension is around 5%. With the measurement of blood pressure now becoming a routine procedure in childhood, more and more data are being pooled in order to arrive at a more accurate figure.

In 1977 the National Heart, Lung, and Blood Institute appointed a task force on blood pressure control in children to review the current state of knowledge, consult with various experts in the field, and develop specific recommendations for the evaluation and treatment of hypertension in children. The task force report was published in 1977 as a supplement to *Pediatrics,* the journal of the American Academy of Pediatrics (AAP). This report was distributed to all the members of the AAP as well as to other interested health care professionals to alert them to the problem and recommend treatment.

Accurate measurements

Among the recommendations of the task force report was that *all* children over three years of age routinely have their blood pressures taken at least annually as a regular part of the physical examination and as part of their continuing health care. This simple recommendation, however, creates some methodological problems for the physician because of the difficulty in obtaining an accurate blood pressure reading in a preschool-age youngster.

The reading obtained from an upset or crying child must be considered highly unreliable compared with

Hypertension in children

the accuracy of the blood pressure determination of a cooperative older child or adult who sits quietly at rest during the procedure. Because young children are less frightened in the doctor's office and feel in greater control of their environment when they are not lying down, measurements always should be performed with the child sitting. It is recommended that before the cuff is placed around the child's arm, he should be given time to relax, to become familiar with the blood pressure equipment, and to be reassured that the procedure will not hurt. Further, the blood pressure reading should be performed in as quiet a room as possible, because the sounds that the physician hears through his stethoscope are fainter in children than in adults.

The size of the blood pressure cuff that is used is very important to the accuracy of the measurement. The cuff should be comfortable, circle the girth of the arm, and the width should cover approximately two-thirds of the upper arm. If the wrong-sized cuff is used, the blood pressure measurement may be completely unreliable. Since it is well known that blood pressure readings in children are very changeable, repeated measurements over a period of time rather than a single isolated determination are required in order to establish consistent observations.

Establishing standards

Based on a number of screening surveys of blood pressure in children, grids have been developed showing blood pressure distributions in normal children of various ages, both in boys and in girls. These grids are based on more than 11,000 children from three studies conducted in Muscatine, Iowa; Rochester, Minn.; and Miami, Fla. (see Figure).

The curves on these charts represent systolic and diastolic blood pressure readings for boys and girls from ages 2 to 18. The 50th percentile curve is the average, and the 95th and 5th percentiles are the measurements representing 5% of the population. Any child falling above the 95th percentile definitely has hypertension. Any child whose blood pressure reading consistently remains above the 90th percentile must be considered at high risk. With these grids it is now possible to compare a child's blood pressure reading with the blood pressure range for normal children of the same sex and age.

In establishing these standards, the population between ages two and five years consisted of both black and white children. There were no statistically significant differences between blood pressures of white and black children, so their data were pooled for presenta-

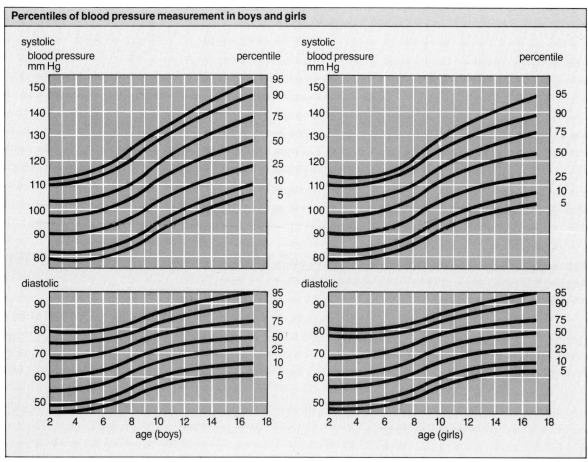

Percentiles of blood pressure measurement in boys and girls

Based on information from the National Institutes of Health, Bethesda, Md.

tion. (These data contrast with findings in adult blacks, who tend as a group to have higher blood pressure than whites.) There also was no significant difference between the blood pressures of boys and girls in this age group. However, the population used between the ages of 5 and 15 years was almost exclusively white. These grids lack information on childhood blood pressure levels in Native Americans, in Asian-Americans, in blacks, and in Hispanic-Americans, and thus may not accurately reflect the normal variance in these latter groups of children. Blood pressure levels for prepubertal black children may in fact be slightly higher than those of their Caucasian peers, but the data are too meager and unclear. The definite impression exists that, after puberty, blacks have significantly higher levels of blood pressure than Caucasians when matched for age and sex. Therefore, the present grids may turn out to have only limited value when assessing blood pressure levels in minority children.

For accurate comparison, when consulting these grids the blood pressure must be measured by the same method as used for the grids, using the right arm and the correct cuff size. Despite carefully following all these recommendations, the accuracy of a single blood pressure reading is always in doubt. Any child who is found to have a blood pressure that exceeds the 95th percentile should have the blood pressure measurement repeated at another examination before any workup is started to attempt to find the cause of the high blood pressure.

Unlike adults with hypertension, who often have associated symptoms, children with high blood pressure seldom show any symptoms or signs until the blood pressure becomes markedly elevated. Therefore, unless blood pressures in children are routinely taken, the diagnosis is usually entirely missed. A large study related to childhood hypertension was carried out in Europe, and results were published in 1979. Of the clinical symptoms in the 600 children studied, headache was by far the commonest symptom, found in 30% of the children, followed by nausea and vomiting in 13%.

Causes and controls

Primary, or essential, hypertension. It had long been held that essential hypertension was rare in children and that almost all children with high blood pressure had the secondary form that is associated with another disease. Some current data suggest, however, that occurrence of primary hypertension is seen more often than secondary hypertension, especially in the adolescent population.

Many epidemiologic surveys have focused on determining which factors have the greatest correlation with elevated blood pressure. Correlating the blood pressure levels of children with the blood pressure levels of their parents has demonstrated that inheritance is a significant factor. The strongest correlation exists be-

Adapted from *Jane Brody's Nutrition Book*, New York, W. W. Norton & Co., 1981

Table I: Sodium levels in processed foods

product	amount	sodium (mg)
Pepperidge Farm white bread	2 slices	234
Wonder enriched bread	2 slices	355
Hungry Jack Extra Lights pancakes	3 (4-inch)	1,150
Kellogg's corn flakes	1 ounce	320
Cheerios	1 ounce	330
Kellogg's Sugar Frosted Flakes	1 ounce	186
Campbell's tomato soup	10-ounce serving	1,050
Campbell's tomato juice	8 ounces	744
Milk	1 cup	130
Carnation's instant hot cocoa mix	1 packet (in water)	104
Lipton Vegetable Cup-a-Soup	8 ounces	1,058
Swanson fried chicken dinner	1 dinner	1,152
Swanson turkey dinner	1 dinner	1,735
Campbell's Beans & Franks	8 ounces	958
Chef Boyardee frozen cheese pizza	6.5 ounces	925
Oscar Mayer beef franks	1 frank	425
Oscar Mayer bologna	2 slices	450
Skippy creamy peanut butter	2 tablespoons	167
Jif creamy peanut butter	2 tablespoons	155
Chef Boyardee Beefaroni	7.5 ounces	1,186
McDonald's Big Mac	1	1,510
Burger King Whopper	1	909
Burger Chef hamburger	1	393
Arthur Treacher's fish sandwich	1	836
Kentucky Fried Chicken dinner; original recipe (3 pieces of chicken)	1	2,285
McDonald's Egg McMuffin	1	914
Dairy Queen Brazier Dog	1	868
McDonald's apple pie	1 pie	414
Burger King vanilla shake	1	159
McDonald's chocolate shake	1	329
Nabisco premium saltines	10 (1 ounce)	430
Ritz crackers	9 (1 ounce)	285
Lay's potato chips	14 (1 ounce)	230
Mister Salty very thin pretzel sticks	1 ounce	735
Planters cocktail peanuts	1 ounce	132
Heinz kosher dill pickles	1 large	1,137
Heinz mustard	1 tablespoon	212
Heinz tomato ketchup	1 tablespoon	154
Jell-O chocolate flavor instant pudding & pie filling	½ cup	480
Hostess Twinkies	1	190
Pillsbury sugar cookies	3	210
Pillsbury chocolate chip cookies	3	140
Pillsbury cinnamon raisin danish	1 serving (2 rolls)	540
Nabisco Oreo sandwich cookies	3	240

Based on analyses by Consumers Union, the Center for Science in the Public Interest, and manufacturers.

tween monozygotic (identical) twins, followed by dizygotic (fraternal) twins, and then full siblings. There is a weaker correlation between half-siblings and between parent and child. Researchers now acknowledge the genetic influence on the inheritance of blood pressure status but as yet do not know how this influence is exerted. It is not as yet known whether predictors of future high blood pressure can always be identified during childhood when there is a strong family history of high blood pressure. It is clear that those children with a strong history of hypertension are at greater risk and must be monitored very carefully.

There are a number of environmental, nongenetic factors that appear to correlate in varying degrees with high blood pressures of children. These factors are obesity, sodium intake, and psychological stress.

Physicians have known for many years that high blood pressure develops more frequently in overweight adults and often is related to the rate of increase of weight. Recently, similar trends have been noted in children and in adolescents. Some studies have demonstrated that the majority of children and adolescents found to have primary, or essential, hypertension are obese. Slowing the weight gain or losing some of the excessive poundage has been reported to lead to a prompt lowering of the blood pressure. Because of this and because overweight children and overweight teenagers tend to remain overweight as adults, the prevention and treatment of obesity in children is important. For an otherwise healthy but obese child who is found to have essential hypertension, the first order of business is to lose weight.

The role of sodium in relation to blood pressure levels in children and to the future development of adult hypertension has not been resolved. (Salt is a compound of 40% sodium and 60% chlorine; only about 25–30% of sodium consumed comes from a salt shaker. Much sodium is hidden in processed foods; it also is naturally present in some foods, such as celery, in relatively large quantities.) Many investigators stress the primary role of excess sodium intake in the development of hypertension, but this association has not been proved in the United States. However, studies on the Yanomano Indians in South America, who have a very low sodium intake, showed that blood pressure did not increase with age from infancy through the fifth decade and that adult hypertension does not exist among this group. It is true that these individuals may in fact be protected against hypertension by some as yet unidentified mechanism, but until this has been proved, the strong evidence for the critical role of excess salt ingestion in producing hypertension in genetically susceptible individuals appears clear. We also know that excessive salt intake can aggravate the course of hypertension. There is now general agreement that hypertensive children as well as children with strong family histories of hypertension should reduce their salt intake. The average American takes in between 10 and 20 g (2 to 4 tsp) of sodium per day—the recommended daily requirement is about 3 to 8 g of sodium. While the recommended sodium intake for children is lower than that for adults, infants and toddlers in the U.S. con-

sume as much as or more salt proportional to body weight than most adults. Aside from obviously salt-laden foods such as pretzels, potato chips, and salted nuts, other high sodium foods that must be avoided are catsup, relish, pickles, most canned soups, frankfurters, and pizza. Many children found to have essential hypertension can reduce their blood pressure levels to normal simply by reducing their daily salt intake.

The role of stress in the development of hypertension is very poorly understood. Elevations of blood pressures certainly occur during periods of emotional stress and strain. However, there is no evidence that a temporary rise initiated by emotion leads to sustained and fixed high blood pressure. It is not clear whether even prolonged stress or tension can produce chronic high blood pressure. Certain personality traits have been associated with high blood pressure in adults, but there has been as yet no similar correlation demonstrated in children or adolescents.

In the great majority of cases, childhood essential hypertension can be controlled by reducing the weight and the daily consumption of salt. For those children who do not respond to this regimen, specific antihypertensive medication may be indicated.

Secondary hypertension. There are many causes of secondary high blood pressure in children. The high blood pressure may be caused by various kidney diseases, coarctation (a congenital narrowing) of the aorta, or diseases involving the adrenal glands. The diagnosis of secondary hypertension requires a careful history and physical examination by the child's physician as well as certain laboratory tests, including urinalysis, kidney function, chest X-ray, and electrocardiogram. Occasionally a more extensive workup is necessary in order to arrive at the specific cause of the secondary hypertension. Treatment in such cases must be directed at not only reducing the blood pressure levels but also at appropriately treating the cause of the hypertension.

For both secondary and primary hypertension, the earlier the diagnosis is made, the better the prognosis. Early intervention may well prevent the serious consequences of adult fixed hypertension, including kidney damage and stroke. In most cases of childhood hypertension, the treatment is simple and effective. Parents should insist that their child's physician incorporate blood pressure testing as part of the regular checkup. This procedure is easy and painless, and the yield from the blood pressure determination is significant. Those children with family histories of high blood pressure should be watched carefully. This high-risk group should not be allowed to become obese and should be taught to eat a relatively low-salt diet.

—Alvin N. Eden, M.D.

Hysterectomy

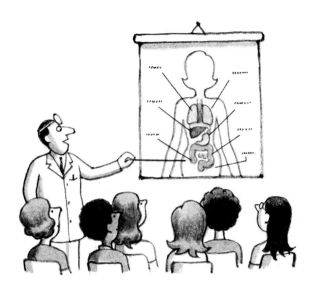

Modern abdominal surgery had its beginning with the skillful removal without anesthesia of a large ovarian tumor from Jane Crawford by Ephraim McDowell in 1809. The operation was performed on a kitchen table in backwoods Kentucky, and the patient lived on in health for 32 years. Hysterectomy through the abdominal wall was first attempted by Charles Clay of Manchester, England, in 1843; his patient did not survive. In 1853 Walter Burnham performed the first successful abdominal removal of a uterus in Massachusetts, but of his next 15 patients only 3 survived. References to removal of the uterus through the vagina, with rare survival of the patients, appear in ancient writings in the Hebrew Talmud and in early obstetric texts by Soranus of Ephesus (2nd century AD) and Aetius (6th century). Since these courageous beginnings, hysterectomy has become commonplace.

The reproductive function of the uterus and its symbolic significance make its removal an emotionally charged event. Often patients facing hysterectomy feel more anxious than they would over some other comparable type of surgery. Being aware of some of the basic physical, sexual, and emotional aspects of hysterectomy can help the patient face her surgery with greater equanimity.

Reproductive organs and their functions

Some knowledge of anatomy and physiology and the related medical terminology is essential to an understanding of hysterectomy and its effects. The ovaries produce in monthly cycles the two female hormones estrogen and progesterone, which are responsible for maintenance of sexual characteristics and prepare the uterus to receive a fertilized ovum (egg). In each cycle one ovary releases an ovum, which passes into a fallopian tube for transport to the uterus.

The uterus has a single major function, containing and then delivering the fetus and its placenta. It also serves as a conduit for sperm as they pass from the vagina to the fallopian tube, where the ovum is fertilized. Should fertilization not occur, the endometrium (tissue lining the uterus) is shed at menstruation. The cervix (neck) is the lowest portion of the uterus, protruding slightly into the vagina. The vagina serves as a receptacle for semen deposited during sexual intercourse; it is important to understand that coitus takes place in the vagina only. The uterus plays no part in the mechanics of coitus.

Types of hysterectomy

Depending on the condition that the hysterectomy is intended to treat, the surgeon may remove all or part of the uterus, the ovaries, and the fallopian tubes. For some malignant conditions, adjacent tissues may also be removed. These are the common types of hysterectomy:

Total hysterectomy (panhysterectomy): removal of the uterus and cervix. In this procedure the ovaries and fallopian tubes are retained.

Subtotal or partial hysterectomy: removal of the upper portion of the uterus, leaving the cervix in position. (This operation is performed infrequently in modern practice.)

Total hysterectomy and salpingo-oophorectomy: removal of the uterus, cervix, and one or both fallopian tubes and ovaries.

Wertheim's radical hysterectomy: removal of the uterus, cervix, both fallopian tubes, both ovaries, the upper portion of the vagina, and the lymph nodes in the pelvic area. (Radical hysterectomy is performed only for certain types of uterine cancer.)

The various operations (with the exception of subtotal hysterectomy and Wertheim's hysterectomy) can be performed through a vertical or horizontal abdominal incision below the navel or through the vagina. When performed through the vagina, the hysterectomy can be combined with repair of a prolapsed bladder or rectum that has sagged into the vagina from its usual position as the supporting tissues became stretched and weakened (often as a result of childbirth). Both approaches to the surgery work equally well, but discomfort is usually less after the vaginal approach, so most surgeons prefer to use this route, if possible. This route also spares the patient an abdominal scar. Contraindications for vaginal hysterectomy include too large a uterus, previous pelvic surgery causing possible adhesions (bands of fibrous tissue), the presence of other pelvic abnormalities such as endometriosis, virginity, or the necessity of exploring the rest of the abdomen or removing other structures.

Prior to the surgery tests routinely performed often include an X-ray examination of the kidneys, ureters, and bladder (IVP, or intravenous pyelogram) and a lower bowel X-ray examination (barium enema). Ultrasound examination of the pelvic area is also often done. Anesthesia for hysterectomy is usually general, but spinal anesthesia may be preferable in some instances. Most surgeons also prescribe an antibiotic that is given intravenously just before and for a short time after surgery to prevent infection.

Reasons for hysterectomy

The most common indications for hysterectomy are listed below, and a brief explanation of each disease or condition is given.

Precancerous and cancerous conditions. *Dysplasia of the cervix* (precancer of the cervix) *and carcinoma in situ of the cervix* (noninvasive or surface cancer of the cervix; also called *stage 0 carcinoma of the cervix*): These conditions are usually detected by a routine Pap smear. A biopsy of the cervix removes small portions of tissue for further examination to confirm the diagnosis. The early stage of the disease, called dysplasia, is sometimes a reason to advise hysterectomy, but this condition may also be treated by freezing, cauterization, or excision of a portion of the cervix, particularly when the patient wants to preserve her childbearing capacity. In carcinoma *in situ* of the cervix the cancer cells are confined to the lining of the cervix only and do not penetrate into the underlying tissues. When hysterectomy is done for this condition, only the cervix and uterus are removed, usually by the vaginal route. If future pregnancies are desired, part of the cervix may be removed as treatment, but usually with the advice that hysterectomy should be performed after childbearing is completed.

Carcinoma of the cervix (cancer of the neck of the uterus): In this disease the cancer cells have invaded underlying or surrounding tissues and may even have spread to distant sites in the body. The extent of spread is graded one to four. Only stages one and early stage two can be treated by Wertheim's hysterectomy (later stages are treated by X-ray radiation).

Atypical adenomatous hyperplasia of the endometrium (precancerous thickening of the lining of the uterus): This condition is generally discovered when a dilation and curettage of the uterus (D & C) is done because of heavy or irregular bleeding before the menopause or because of bleeding after the menopause. The hyperplasia (overgrowth) proceeds slowly and does not always progress to true cancer, but most authorities believe the risk to be great enough to advise hysterectomy (usually by the vaginal route). This condition should be distinguished from *cystic* hyperplasia of

the endometrium, which very rarely progresses to cancer and is often cured by D & C. Hormone therapy (usually some form of progesterone) can also be used.

Carcinoma of the endometrium (cancer of the lining of the uterus): This condition is more frequent after 50 years of age and is more common in women who are obese, diabetic, or hypertensive or have been taking estrogen medication for long periods after menopause. Most cases are treated by hysterectomy and removal of both fallopian tubes and ovaries. When spread of the cancer is suspected, the surrounding lymph nodes may also be biopsied or removed. In certain cases radiation treatment before or after surgery is called for; the rate of cure is high (generally over 75%).

Carcinoma of the ovaries and fallopian tubes: Ovarian cancer is more common than cancer of the fallopian tubes. Depending on the type of tumor and whether it has spread, the uterus may be removed as well as the ovaries and tubes to be sure of complete removal of cancerous tissue.

Other malignant conditions: Another type of malignant disease, sarcoma of the uterus, which may occur within fibroid tumors, also necessitates hysterectomy. In addition, for some cases of cancer of the rectum or urinary bladder, removal of the adjacent uterus, tubes, and ovaries is done to ensure complete removal of malignant tissue.

Nonmalignant (benign) conditions. *Uterine tumors:* Probably the most common indication for hysterectomy is the presence of *uterine leiomyomas* (fibroids), which are spherical tumors composed of connective tissue and muscle fibers that grow in the wall of the uterus. They can be single or multiple and may bulge inward or outward from the uterine wall. About 20% of all women over age 35 have leiomyomas. Small fibroids usually cause no symptoms and, as they very rarely become malignant, need no treatment if the uterus remains smaller than the size of a three-month pregnancy. If they cause the uterus to grow larger than this, or induce symptoms such as excessive bleeding with menstrual periods, pain, or pressure on the urinary bladder, these tumors are best removed. Surgery can usually be delayed until childbearing is completed; if surgery is imperative, removal of the fibroids only (myomectomy) can be attempted, but recurrence of tumors is quite common after this procedure. The better treatment is total hysterectomy. It can be done vaginally if the tumors are not too large. When the uterus is larger than the size of a 10- to 12-week pregnancy, the abdominal approach is preferred. The ovaries are usually conserved, but when the patient is past the menopause (and the ovaries have ceased functioning) or close to menopause, many surgeons will suggest their removal to prevent the possible later development of cancer of the ovaries.

Endometriosis and adenomyosis: Endometriosis is a condition in which the type of tissue lining the uterus (the endometrium) grows outside the cavity of the uterus and, still remaining sensitive to the action of the ovarian hormones, sheds and bleeds at each menstrual period. However, this blood and tissue cannot escape through the cervix but is trapped within the body cavities, where it causes irritation, swelling, and, later, scarring and adhesions as it is slowly reabsorbed. The condition may start as early as the late teens. It may be very slight or extensive and severe; it may grow slowly or rapidly; and it may cause no symptoms or severe symptoms. There may be pain with menstrual periods, an increase in the amount of bleeding at periods, pain during sexual intercourse, or increasing difficulty in achieving pregnancy. Treatment is often complex. In early stages endometriosis is treated by hormone therapy or surgical removal of the patches of endometriosis only. When childbearing is completed and symptoms are severe, the correct treatment is by hysterectomy, with removal of the ovaries. In younger women sometimes the ovaries may be conserved, but this can lead to recurrence of the condition.

In adenomyosis the endometrial tissue grows into the muscular wall of the uterus from within, causing enlargement and tenderness of the uterus and, often, increased menstrual bleeding with cramps. If it causes severe symptoms, hysterectomy may be warranted.

Pelvic infections: Most acute infections of the reproductive organs can be successfully treated with antibiotics. However, sometimes these infections become chronic or recurrent. This may result in the fallopian tubes becoming blocked and greatly distended by pus, with development of adhesions. In turn this may lead to severe chronic pain and infertility. If all other therapy fails and symptoms are persistent, the treatment of last resort would be removal of the swollen tubes and the uterus. In premenopausal women an attempt would be made to conserve the ovaries, but this might be impossible if the ovaries were severely involved in the infective process.

Disorders of uterine function: Hysterectomy is sometimes suggested when all other treatments have failed to relieve repeated and persistent excessive bleeding from the uterus, or when pain with the menstrual periods (dysmenorrhea) is severe, intractable, and persistent and is interfering with the patient's normal functioning. Such dysmenorrhea may occur when no demonstrable disease process can be found. In the case of excessive bleeding the physician will have tried one or more D & C operations and hormone therapy before recommending hysterectomy. For dysmenorrhea either pain medications or hormone therapy will have been persistently used.

A rare but lifesaving indication for hysterectomy is severe, uncontrollable bleeding occurring after childbirth, which is resistant to the usually effective treatments for this disorder.

Uterine and pelvic organ prolapse: Another quite common indication for hysterectomy is prolapse of the uterus, vagina, bladder, or rectum. These abnormalities usually occur as a result of stretching of the supporting structures during childbirth and become obvious near or after menopause. The main symptoms are of a mass protruding from the vaginal opening and of a dragging lower abdominal sensation. Even more distressing is the inability to hold urine when straining, running, jumping, laughing, coughing, or sneezing. This type of incontinence is cured by the surgery. Bladder and rectal prolapse can be repaired without removing the uterus, but there is no doubt that functional results are better and longer lasting if the uterus is also removed at the same time as the repairs are performed. The whole operation is done through the vagina; bladder and rectum are not entered or incised in any way.

Sterilization: When a woman desires permanent, surgical sterilization, the usual method is to close the fallopian tubes by the relatively simple operations of tying off and severing the tubes or by using heat or bands to block the tubes. There are, however, many physicians who believe it is justifiable to offer to the patient the alternative of vaginal hysterectomy. This has the advantage of ending monthly menstruation and of preventing all possible future diseases of the uterus. This solution would obviously be more attractive to the patient whose periods are heavy or painful. However, the risks and costs of this operation are higher than those of tubal closure, which is often done by means of a laparoscope through a tiny incision.

Aftereffects of hysterectomy

There has been a steady trend in modern surgery, as techniques and results have improved, to shorten the length of hospitalization. For otherwise healthy patients, an uncomplicated vaginal or abdominal hysterectomy requires a postoperative hospital stay of four to six days. When a vaginal repair has also been done for prolapse, the stay will usually be between five and ten days, not because of greater discomfort but because a bladder catheter is usually left in position for four or five days and resumption of comfortable, complete urination takes a variable number of days thereafter. After more extensive operations for cancer, the stay may be ten days or longer depending on speed of recovery.

After return home, physical activity should be resumed gradually. For the first week, only restricted activity should be undertaken; thereafter, light household tasks could be resumed. Usually the patient should not drive a car for two weeks. Vigorous activity, such as heavy housework, carrying a heavy package upstairs, or sports such as tennis, will be safe after six weeks, provided they are resumed gradually. If the hysterectomy was done through the abdominal approach, the recovery period will be slightly longer while the abdominal muscles knit back together. It may take several weeks before full strength and muscle tone return. The surgeon will give advice on when it is safe to begin exercises to tone up the abdomen.

All forms of hysterectomy result in permanent sterilization and cessation of menstrual flow. Sexual function, however, is usually unaffected. Sensory stimulation in coitus arises largely from the vulva, clitoris, and lower vagina, and hysterectomy does not interfere with this function. The vagina is not shortened by surgery and can still distend to accommodate the erect penis without difficulty. While it is true that the uterus contracts rhythmically at orgasm, the vast majority of patients are unable to detect any lessening of pleasure during orgasm. In fact, many patients describe enhanced pleasure because they no longer are worried about pregnancy, menstruation no longer interferes with sexual activity, and, if pain was caused by pressure on the cervix and uterus, this discomfort is removed.

If one or both ovaries are preserved, sexual desire (libido) is likewise unaffected. The patient will usually be aware of the continued cyclical production of estrogen and progesterone in that breast changes (which usually are apparent in the second half of each cycle) will continue to be felt. Premenstrual mood changes are also usually still present but to a lesser degree than before the surgery. These hormones are also responsible for maintaining the elasticity and thickness of the vaginal lining and for the production of a lubricating fluid by the lining during sexual stimulation. After hysterectomy hormone production usually continues until the time of natural menopause, when the ovaries normally cease functioning.

When both ovaries are removed, however, an immediate cessation of hormone production results in menopausal symptoms. Most, but not all, patients will experience hot flashes of variable frequency and duration. Also, over the course of months or years, vaginal elasticity and lubrication will slowly be reduced. A more delayed effect is decalcification and softening of bone. All these effects of reduced hormones can be reversed or prevented by the administration of estrogen in tablet form. There is a known link between estrogens and cancer of the endometrium, but of course this is not a concern of a woman who has had a hysterectomy. Estrogen replacement is generally advised unless other clear contraindications exist.

When repair of a prolapsed bladder or rectum has been done with the hysterectomy, it is quite usual to experience some tightness and discomfort upon resumption of coitus. Unless the tightening of the vagina has been excessive, it soon adjusts to sexual activity, and many patients (and their partners) report enhanced sexual pleasure. If the vagina remains uncomfortably tight, a minor operation can be done to adjust this. When a Wertheim's hysterectomy for cancer of the cervix has been performed, the vagina may be significantly shortened, and this can result in sexual

difficulty. Gentle persistence will often slowly increase the capacity of the vagina. When radiation therapy either precedes or follows this operation, the vagina may be constricted and more tender during coitus. Sometimes this effect of radiation may be permanent and, rarely, may be severe enough to prevent comfortable sexual intercourse.

There are no known effects of hysterectomy on the body chemistry as a whole except that removal of the uterus removes the source of prostaglandins during menstruation. This group of chemicals plays a large part in the cause of menstrual cramps, diarrhea, nausea, faintness, and headache at menstruation. Folklore has associated hysterectomy with weight gain after surgery, but there is no scientific basis for the connection. If a woman gains weight after surgery, it is because she has begun to eat more and exercise less.

The emotional effects of hysterectomy, however, can be harder to deal with. The well-informed woman who is emotionally stable and whose life circumstances are pleasant should suffer no untoward emotional effects from hysterectomy. On the contrary, removal of a diseased organ and its unpleasant effects gives a sense of well-being and relief. Women very frequently describe surprise at their sense of improved health after hysterectomy.

Temporary feelings of loss or mild depression sometimes occur soon after surgery as the woman adjusts to her loss of reproductive ability and makes unconscious adjustments in her body image. If a woman has identified her worth with her childbearing capacity, she will have a harder time coming to terms with her new circumstances. In emotionally unstable patients, particularly if preoperative counseling is inadequate, hysterectomy may trigger emotional disturbances of various types. In predisposed patients any operation may have this result. The alert physician will undertake psychological counseling or refer the patient to an appropriate therapist. The woman who is fully informed about her choices for treatment and who undergoes surgery knowing in advance what consequences to anticipate will be less apprehensive. The understanding and help of a supportive spouse and family can be powerful factors in emotional adjustment.

The question is sometimes raised whether hysterectomy is performed too often or unnecessarily. While there is no doubt that sometimes the operation is done when it could have been avoided, the vast majority of these operations improve the health of patients who are suffering from significant illnesses, with consequent improvement in the quality of their lives. Often the operation is manifestly lifesaving. When hysterectomy is offered to a patient, she should question her medical adviser about alternative treatments and should feel free to seek the reassurance and advice of another gynecologist to help in her decision.

—Lionel J. Schewitz, M.D.

Common Foot Problems

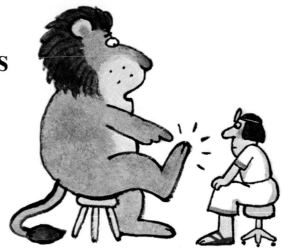

"To him whose feet hurt, everything hurts." This statement has been attributed to Socrates, who lived more than 2,300 years ago. Indeed, the foot often does mirror diseases that affect other parts of the body. For example, of nearly four million diabetics in the U.S. in 1973, 54% had related foot problems, including ingrown nails, ulcerations, infections, hammer toes, and other deformities, according to the Centers for Disease Control in Atlanta, Ga. Diabetic patients have 61% of all foot amputations. Many Americans suffer from arteriosclerosis, varicose veins, blood pressure abnormalities, and other circulatory diseases. Of these patients 18% have such related foot problems as ulcers, peripheral vascular disease, and forefoot and nail complaints. Of every 1,000 persons in the U.S., 117 are afflicted with arthritis. Sixteen percent of rheumatoid arthritic disease processes begin in the foot, and 85% of arthritics eventually experience foot involvement.

According to one estimate more than 40% of the American population have foot disorders. Between 15 and 20% of industrial injuries, sports injuries, and orthopedic operations involve the foot and ankle. Two percent of all visits to doctors each year are for foot problems, and foot problems are the primary reason for 500,000 hospital admissions annually. In the U.S. the cost of foot treatment exceeds $1 billion, and 4% of workmen's compensation payments are made for foot-related injuries.

The majority of persons with foot disorders suffer from one or more common problems. They include corns, neuromas, calluses, plantar warts, bunions, heel spurs, ingrown toenails, blisters, athlete's foot, and foot odor.

Corns

These abnormalities are found on the toes wherever there is an underlying bone prominence upon which the shoe exerts pressure. A bone prominence arises from a functional tendon imbalance, which causes a toe to assume a deformed position. This deformed position may be a hammer toe or a mallet toe. A hammer toe occurs when the first joint becomes prominent and begins to rub against the inner surface of the shoe. A mallet toe occurs when the tip of the toe assumes a downward position, with irritation against the sole of the shoe. Intermittent pressure caused by this contact elicits a localized skin response, which results in a buildup of thickened tissue that may develop its own blood and nerve supply. If tissue buildup is excessive,

the involved area becomes extremely painful to the touch and makes the wearing of shoes difficult.

Hammer toe formation is most common in the top of the second toe. It may result from a bunion, which is discussed below. Hammer toes can also appear in the tops and outer surfaces of the fourth and fifth toes, which develop corns when they rub the inner surface of the shoe. Ill-fitting shoes are definitely a causative factor. Corns at the tips of mallet toes usually occur on the third and fourth toes. When bone prominences form between toes, the corn they produce is termed a soft corn because the increased moisture between the toes causes softening of the thickened tissue.

Another type of corn-causing deformity, called claw toes, involves hammer formation in all digits, usually secondary to an underlying disease that affects the nerves and muscles. Examples are poliomyelitis, brain or spinal cord injuries, and muscular dystrophy.

Treatment of corns ranges from application of nonprescription remedies to surgical procedures in which the affected joint is realigned. Medications for self-treatment include corn pads with or without salicylic acid. Salicylic acid, a softening agent, should not be used by persons with vascular disorders associated with such diseases as diabetes or arteriosclerosis (hardening of the arteries) or with such vein disorders as thrombophlebitis. The chemical's skin-eroding action can cause ulcerations and infection in these individuals that eventually may require amputation. Salicylic acid should not be used for soft corns because its combination with the high moisture content of the corn may lead to severe inflammation. Other nonsurgical procedures include periodic corn trimming and padding, carried out in a podiatrist's office. Wearing longer and wider shoes helps to relieve the pressure on the tops and tips of the toes.

If pain and deformity persist after conservative treatment, surgery must be considered. The operation usually involves removal of the bony prominence, with re-

339

alignment of the toe. In most cases it can be done on an outpatient basis by a physician who specializes in foot surgery or a podiatrist.

Neuromas

Neuroma is a common problem that affects the forepart of the foot, usually between the third and fourth toes. This affliction, which usually takes about a year or two to develop, is noted as a sharp, shooting, cramping, or burning pain that is difficult to localize but seems to be centered between the involved toes. The pain is intermittent and usually arises when shoes are worn. Because neuroma affects 20 times more women than men, narrow, high-heeled shoes are likely a contributing factor. The condition is brought on by recurrent injury to the nerve branch between the third and fourth toes. The injury causes disorientation of the nerve fibers and enlargement of the nerve to several times its normal size. Tight or short shoes compress the enlarged nerve and thus elicit the symptoms.

For any nonsurgical treatment to work, the patient must avoid wearing high-heeled or narrow shoes to eliminate compression of the damaged nerve. Raising the area just behind the involved digits with a metatarsal pad under the ball of the foot brings relief in three out of ten cases. Sometimes injections of a local anesthetic and cortisone also help. If the neuroma persists, surgical removal of the enlarged nerve segment through the top of the foot is the procedure of choice. This surgery, which is done on an outpatient basis, relieves the symptoms in 95% of cases.

Calluses

Calluses may be found on any portion of the forefoot that is subjected to long periods of pressure or friction. The skin builds up thickened tissue as a defense mechanism to protect itself from further injury. Calluses are medically termed plantar keratoses, not to be confused with so-called plantar warts. Calluses occur chiefly in adults over 20 years of age and appear on the weight-bearing areas of the foot, notably on the inside and bottom of the big toe, the bottom of the ball of the foot, and the region below the heads of the five metatarsal bones, just behind the toes. The callus can be diffuse or deep-seated and quite painful. A callus below the first metatarsal head usually is associated with a high-arched or a flat foot.

The increased pressure and friction that produce calluses have a variety of causes, including elongated metatarsal bones, short metatarsal bones, a depressed metatarsal head, and abnormal foot function. (Abnormal foot function is recognizable by uneven shoe wear.) Overly loose- or tight-fitting shoes are also responsible.

A wide variety of nonprescription and physician-prescribed measures to treat calluses exist. Over-the-counter devices include callus pads with or without

salicylic acid. Frequent, gentle use of an abrasive stone or pad to reduce the thickness of the callus, followed by application of a skin-softening lotion, often brings relief. High-heeled shoes should be avoided, whereas shoes with soft soles of crepe or sponge, which decrease the pressure on the bottom of the foot, can be of great help.

If these measures do not relieve the problem, a podiatrist or physician should be consulted. The doctor may elect to remove the callus gently and to pad the area. If this is temporarily effective, he or she may decide to fabricate a customized foot support (orthosis), which relieves the areas of increased pressure. Such treatment works well in 60% of cases. Persistent calluses, particularly those below the metatarsal heads, may need surgery. The procedure of choice is elevation of the metatarsal head: the bone is cut through just behind the metatarsal head and allowed to heal in an elevated position. This procedure is successful in 70% of cases, but complications sometimes arise, such as transfer of the callus to an adjacent metatarsal head or recurrence at the original site.

Plantar warts

Plantar warts, or verrucae plantaris, which occur on the sole of the foot, differ in their origin from calluses. They are caused by a virus, the human papillomavirus, which is thought to enter the sole through a cut in the skin or a puncture caused by stepping on some sharp object. Because of pressure on the sole, these warts tend to grow inward, sometimes causing discomfort. Plantar warts may appear in just one small area or may be widespread (mosaic); they may disappear spontaneously or spread. They are common in persons between 3 and 20 years old but can occur at any age.

Nonprescription medications that contain salicylic acid are usually effective against plantar warts. If such treatment does not succeed over a two-month trial period, a podiatrist or dermatologist should be consulted. The simplest and best treatment usually consists of repeated applications of 40–60% salicylic acid, with tissue removal at two-week intervals. In stubborn cases surgery may be necessary. The wart is removed with an electric needle, frozen with liquid nitrogen, or simply cut away.

Bunions and hallux valgus

A bunion is defined as a swelling of the bursa (a fluid-filled sac) that overlies the inside and top of the first joint of the big toe. With continued shoe pressure this area may become inflamed and very tender and make walking difficult. Bunions have a variety of causes, including arthritis, cysts, injury, or an enlarged joint. The most common cause is hallux valgus, the angulation of the big toe toward the other toes. The terms bunion and hallux valgus are sometimes used synonymously, but this is incorrect.

Hallux valgus is one of the most common afflictions of the adult foot. The deformity may appear at any age but becomes more prevalent after age 30, when it occurs in one of every six white and one of three black persons. It also affects four times as many females as males. There are many causes of hallux valgus, some of which tend to be hereditary; they include flat feet, a long big toe, laxity of ligaments, muscle imbalance, and such underlying diseases as arthritis, osteoarthritis, and gout. Ill-fitting shoes have been implicated in the past, but according to several studies, tight or narrow shoes aggravate the condition rather than cause it. Persons who have never worn shoes may develop hallux valgus, indicating a cause other than shoes.

In the formation of hallux valgus the big toe deviates inward toward the smaller toes, and the inner bone (first metatarsal) gradually moves toward the inside border of the shoe. This change is accompanied by deviation or, in severe cases, dislocation of the joint complex and resulting imbalance of the small muscles in the region. Although not all individuals with hallux valgus have pain, progressive deformity of the big toe may cause misalignment and deformities, such as hammer toe, of the other toes and the formation of calluses.

Proper treatment of hallux valgus will alleviate bunion formation. Nonsurgical methods include the use of wide and low-heeled shoes, arch-support devices, over-the-counter bunion splints, and padding to relieve the pressure areas. Surgical treatment depends on the type and severity of the deformity. More than 80 types of operations have been devised for this purpose; they range from simple bump removal (which may accomplish little) to complex bone realignment and implantation of artificial joints.

Because surgery for the treatment of hallux valgus is complex, it should be performed by a podiatrist or orthopedic surgeon who has had at least one year of training and is board-certified in foot surgery. Ill-advised procedures by a surgeon who performs an occasional hallux valgus operation can lead to disastrous results, including recurrence of the problem, overcorrection, infection, formation of adjacent calluses, and so-called surgical arthritis, which causes pain with movement of the joint. Depending on the procedure performed, full recovery from hallux valgus may take six months to a year. As in any surgical procedure the surgeon should thoroughly acquaint the patient with potential complications and expected recovery time.

Heel spurs

Two main types of spurs may develop on the heel. The first, most commonly seen in adults over 40 years old, is a bony outgrowth usually located on the bottom portion of the heel bone. The patient complains of an aching pain, especially after arising or after sitting for some time. The pain, which is localized in the involved portion of the heel bone, recedes to a dull ache after

10–15 minutes of walking. Although heel spurs can be caused by rheumatoid arthritis, gouty arthritis, gonorrhea, or some other underlying systemic disease, the most common cause is excessive stress at the interface between the bone and plantar fascia. The latter is a strong band of tissue that extends from the inner, bottom portion of the heel bone to the toes. The function of this band is to maintain the integrity of the arch and to protect the bony structures of the foot. If there is excessive pulling due to walking or running, inflammation sets in with eventual formation of a spur.

This condition is usually treated nonsurgically with pads for the heel and arch area or with arch supports, which can be purchased over the counter. If pain persists, a professional should be consulted. Cortisone injections and use of a specially constructed arch support and heel cushion give relief in 90–95% of cases. Surgery should be undertaken only if nonsurgical treatment has failed after a one-year trial period. Recovery from this type of surgery can be long and quite painful.

The second common type of spur is an enlargement of the upper and outer portion of the heel bone. Repeated irritation of this area by ill-fitting shoes can lead to abnormal formation of a bursa, with swelling and pain. This deformity, usually found in women, can be traced to high-heeled shoes. These spurs may occur from adolescence up to age 40, when common sense often overcomes the desire for style. A pad that elevates the heel plus properly fitting shoes make up the usual treatment. Occasionally, conservative therapy is unsuccessful, and a surgeon must remove the spur.

Ingrown toenails

Ingrown toenails are due to an abnormally high curvature of the nails, which makes cutting of their corner sections extremely difficult. Because of improper cutting techniques a portion of the nail border remains under the skin, and the skin becomes infected. If the infection is of long standing, an abnormal mass of tissue called granulation tissue is formed; this eventually leads to deformity of the nail lip if the problem is not corrected. The big toe is involved most frequently, but ingrown toenails can occur on other toes as well. Inflammation of the adjacent tissue occurs often in male and female adolescents and less frequently in the older population.

Ingrown toenails can be prevented with proper nail cutting. Highly curved nails should be cut straight across, without digging into corners. Sometimes, if the condition is caught early and shows no infection, it can be treated by wedging a tiny piece of sterile cotton under the corner of the nail with a dull toothpick. This procedure, which raises the nail corner out of the skin, is repeated once daily with a new piece of cotton until the edge of the growing nail clears the skin.

The presence of infection is indicated by redness, with or without pain, and the formation of pus and granulation tissue. The infection may be treated with luke-warm boric acid soaks and the application of a nonprescription topical antibiotic; this should be done once daily for seven to ten days. A persistent infection calls for professional attention. The podiatrist or physician will usually drain the pus and remove the ingrown portion of the nail border. After the infection has cleared, the nail borders may be removed permanently to give the nail a more normal shape. In 25% of the patients the deformity is so severe that the entire nail must be permanently removed. This can be done as an outpatient procedure and yields good results. Ingrown nails should be treated quickly to prevent deformation of the nail lip and the necessity of more complex reconstructive surgery at a later date.

Blisters

A blister is a localized collection of fluid in the skin that raises the outer layer of skin and thus separates it from the underlying layers. Blisters may be a result of friction and injury or may be secondary to various dermatologic conditions including fungus infections, allergic reactions, viral infections, and eczema. Blisters also may form after first- and second-degree burns. The fluid in a blister may be water, blood, or pus. Blisters most commonly seen on the foot are caused by friction between the foot and the shoe and are frequent after such athletic activities as basketball, racquetball, tennis, jogging, and other sports that require rapid movement.

Prevention of blisters requires reduction of friction between the shoe and the foot, best achieved by selection and proper fitting of a shoe that is appropriate for the sport. Additional measures include lubrication of problem areas with petroleum jelly or dusting with an absorbent powder like talc or baby powder. Moleskin applied to bone prominences will also decrease the likelihood of blister formation.

Once a blister has formed, it is necessary to drain the fluid. This is best done in a doctor's office so that infection can be prevented. It is important that the patient not use an unsterilized needle or other object to pop the blister; this practice may drain the fluid but introduce bacteria into the blister. If the blister ruptures spontaneously, the outer layer should be left intact to provide a protective covering until healing takes place. Foot blisters secondary to dermatologic disorders are common and usually require care by a podiatrist or dermatologist.

Athlete's foot

Athlete's foot, also called ringworm or tinea pedis, is a common superficial infection of the foot, caused by a fungus. This disorder is a penalty of civilization and the wearing of shoes, which produces the warm, humid environment ideal for fungal growth. Most adult males will acquire a fungal infection of the foot at one time or another, but it is uncommon in women and children.

The means by which the fungi reach the feet are not well understood, and many myths have arisen regarding transmission and reinfection with athlete's foot. Men that are susceptible to infection appear to acquire it regardless of any precautions related to athletic activities, including steps to prevent exposure in gyms, swimming pools, or shower stalls. In truth, it has been almost impossible to culture infective fungi from these areas. Fungi are occasionally recovered from foot gear, but only with difficulty. Once an individual acquires the disorder, he or she remains a carrier for life.

Athlete's foot occurs in three forms: inflammation between the toes; infection accompanied by blister formation; and dry, scaly inflammation. Their treatment is simple. The feet are kept as dry as possible, since excessive wetness prolongs an active infection. Wetness can be avoided by thoroughly drying the feet, avoiding shoes with rubber soles, and wearing cotton socks and changing them frequently. The toes and feet should be dusted lightly with an over-the-counter antifungal powder. Overuse of powder can cause caking and infection. If the infection results in blisters, soaks in a mild astringent (e.g., a 6% aluminum chlorohydrate solution) for 30–45 minutes daily are necessary, followed by application of an antifungal cream when the blisters have subsided. Chronic scaly forms of athlete's foot are best treated with antifungal ointments, which should be applied only at night so that moisture buildup in the shoes is avoided. If symptoms persist, a podiatrist or dermatologist should be consulted.

Foot odor

Foot odor results from the activity of bacteria that thrive on dead skin cells in the warm, moist world of the shoe-confined foot. For many people the condition is effectively prevented by a program of good foot hygiene that includes frequent washing, daily changes of socks, and the wearing of lightweight, comfortable shoes that allow foot perspiration to escape. Persistent foot odor, however, is likely to be caused by hyperhidrosis, an abnormal increase in the amount of sweat produced, which increases bacterial growth. Generalized hyperhidrosis may be caused by diabetes, dysfunction of the thyroid, pneumonia, tuberculosis, obesity, or gout. Localized hyperhidrosis of the armpits, palms, and soles of the feet can result from nervousness, anxiety, pain, and a variety of other factors. For treatment of hyperhidrosis and resulting foot odor, rubber-soled shoes and socks made of synthetic materials should be avoided. The feet must be bathed once or twice daily. Judicious use of drying foot powders is recommended, along with soaks in an over-the-counter astringent. If the problem is severe, professional help is necessary. Oral medication may be useful in the treatment of this disorder but should be taken only under order of a physician.

—*Charles J. Gudas, D.P.M.*

Vasectomy

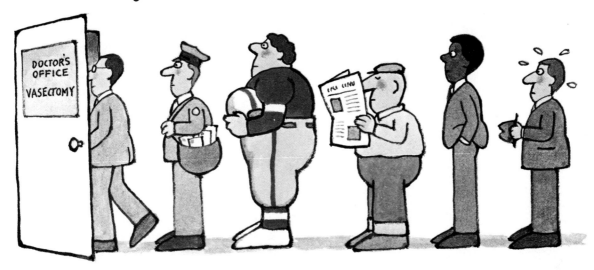

Vasectomy, a form of surgical sterilization of the male, is rapidly becoming one of the most popular methods of permanent contraception in many countries, including the United States. By 1982 approximately 6.5 million men in the U.S. had chosen this method of limiting family size, and about 500,000 more choose vasectomy each year. For these men and their wives this procedure offered a method of permanent contraception that was simple, safe, and effective. Although some research on animals has raised the possibility that vasectomy may have adverse long-term effects on health, all studies done on humans as of 1982 have given it a clean bill of health.

Surgical procedure

Vasectomies were not always so favorably received. Only after the 1920s, with the advent of safer anesthesia, improved surgical techniques, and antibiotics to combat infections, did such preventive surgical procedures as vasectomy become widely acceptable.

A vasectomy is now one of the simplest and safest of operations. It is usually done in a physician's office or in a clinic. Only a local anesthetic is used, and the entire procedure takes about a half hour. At least part of the cost of a vasectomy is covered by most private insurance plans and by Medicaid.

When performing a vasectomy, a surgeon makes two small incisions, one on either side of the scrotum, and then through them lifts out the vasa deferentia. These tiny tubes carry sperm from the testicles, where they are made, into the seminal vesicles, where they are stored until an orgasm occurs. The surgeon either cuts and ties or electrically seals (cauterizes) the ends of each vas deferens so that the sperm can no longer be transported through it.

After the operation there may be some soreness in the scrotal region, but this is usually not very bothersome after the first day. Many men have the operation on a Friday or Saturday and return to work on Monday. The physician may recommend that the man not undertake vigorous activity or heavy labor for about five days and that he also wear an athletic supporter during that time. In the vast majority of men the operation causes minimal inconvenience.

About one of every hundred men undergoing a vasectomy does develop a more serious complication. This may be an infection; sufficient bleeding to form a painful lump, called a hematoma; or inflammation of the epididymis, the small oblong body from which the vas deferens arises. These problems usually are resolved with little or no treatment and at their worst require an extra period of inactivity. No deaths from vasectomy have been reported in the United States.

The ease and safety of a vasectomy demonstrate why many couples decide to have the man sterilized rather than the woman. Even though newer procedures for female sterilization entail making only small incisions in a woman's abdomen, these operations still require hospitalization and more extensive anesthesia than does a vasectomy. In addition, because the incision in a woman is so small, there can be some difficulty in finding the woman's fallopian tubes, and there is a small chance of damaging a major blood vessel. The vas deferens, on the other hand, lies outside the abdomen and is easily accessible. Also, it is not near any large blood vessels.

Effectiveness

Several decades of experience have demonstrated that a properly performed vasectomy is one of the most

343

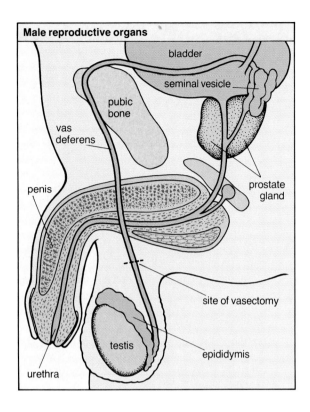

Male reproductive organs

bladder

seminal vesicle

pubic bone

vas deferens

penis

prostate gland

site of vasectomy

testis

epididymis

urethra

effective forms of contraception. Fewer than one in a hundred couples will experience a pregnancy following this procedure. This is much lower than the pregnancy rate when oral contraceptives are used, although it is not quite as safe as female sterilization.

When pregnancy does occur following a vasectomy, it can be due to faulty operative technique or spontaneous rejoining of the cut ends of one vas deferens. But it is more often due to failure to take appropriate contraceptive precautions in the first few months.

Another form of contraception is necessary for a time after a vasectomy because the operation prevents only the further entry of sperm from the testes into the vas deferens. It does not stop sperm already in those tubes or in the seminal vesicles from passing out through the urethra during subsequent orgasms. The quantity of sperm in the vas deferens varies, but best estimates are that between 10 and 20 orgasms are necessary to remove them all. In general physicians recommend using some supplementary form of birth control for about one to two months after vasectomy. Between four and six weeks after the procedure the physician examines a sample of the man's ejaculate to see whether all sperm are absent. Most experts recommend two such negative samples before a man is told he can dispense with other means of contraception.

Psychological and physical consequences

Over the years many fears have arisen about vasectomies. Men have always worried about whether it would affect their sex drive. One team of psychologists looked for evidence that vasectomized men would demand more frequent sex to assure themselves of their manliness and that this would cause marital problems. Other psychologists speculated that men who had a vasectomy would feel that their wives should in some way recompense them and that this expectation of a "payoff" would cause marital tensions. Some early investigations seemed to show that these fears were well-founded. But all carefully done studies in the last two decades have produced no evidence that a vasectomy jeopardizes a marriage. Researchers instead have found that a vasectomy often enhances a relationship between a man and a woman.

In several studies done in the late 1960s and 1970s psychologists asked vasectomized men whether they were satisfied with the operation and whether their sex life was more or less frequent and more or less satisfactory since the vasectomy. In all these recent studies between 95 and 99% of the men said that they were satisfied and would undergo the procedure again. In one survey 95% of the men said that they would recommend the surgery to other couples considering permanent birth control.

With regard to sexual activity, several studies discovered an increase in sexual intercourse following a vasectomy. This was not an attempt to compensate for a decreased feeling of masculinity, since in all studies 99% of the men said that their sex life was at least as enjoyable as it had been before the surgery. In 1975 one research group even found that the number of men considering separation or divorce decreased following vasectomy and that there also was an increase in communication between couples. In addition many women felt more free to initiate sex after their partners had had vasectomies.

Why did vasectomy get such a bad name several decades ago? It has been suggested that at that time vasectomy was associated with the sterilization of persons judged mentally or morally unfit, a practice that was common as recently as 1940. Vasectomies should be done only when men consent to them freely, or psychological problems may well arise.

The fears about harmful physical consequences from a vasectomy stem mostly from research on rats, rabbits, and monkeys. One of the earliest alarms was the possibility that a vasectomy would upset a man's hormonal balance and reduce his virility. Male sexual characteristics are due to the secretion of the hormone testosterone by the testes. Some physicians feared that a vasectomy would reduce the ability of the testes to produce this essential substance.

Again, early work on animals appeared to support this hypothesis. But many studies with humans have revealed that testosterone and other hormones vital to male sexual functioning remain normal following a vasectomy. These studies have included men who had

344

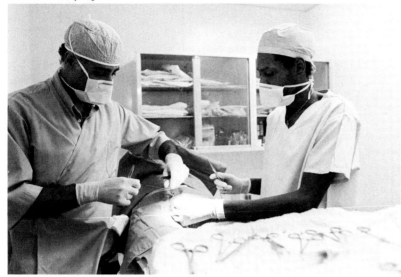

Vandell Cobb—*Ebony* Magazine

Vasectomy is frequently done in the doctor's office and does not require a hospital stay. It is gaining in popularity as a permanent form of contraception.

had a vasectomy as long as five years previously, and they have involved measurement of testosterone and two other vital sexual hormones, FSH (follicle-stimulating hormone) and LH (luteinizing hormone). (FSH controls sperm production by the testes, and LH regulates production of testosterone.) Although some researchers found changes in the levels of some of these hormones, the amounts were always within the normal range, and no changes in the men's behavior were detected.

Another fear that has been raised is the possibility that a vasectomy could upset the immune system, with ensuing damage to other organs in the body. Normally the body does not make antibodies to sperm because they are contained in the vas deferens and the immune cells are not exposed to them. But after a vasectomy sperm are free to leak from the ends of the vas deferens. In addition, because the testes continue making sperm, the sperm accumulate behind the sealed end of the vas deferens and sometimes rupture that tube and escape. As a result half or more vasectomized men have antibodies to sperm. (Such antibodies are also found in some men who have not had a vasectomy.)

Studies in experimental animals have produced indirect evidence that these antibodies to sperm may cause damage to the testes. But no such damage was found in biopsies from the testes of a group of men five years or longer after they had had vasectomies.

Research in monkeys also raised the possibility that the immune reaction to sperm could hasten atherosclerosis, the process that leads to heart disease and heart attacks. But recent studies of men who had had vasectomies several years earlier revealed no increase in heart disease. Studies of vasectomized men are continuing, but so far there is no evidence in humans that sperm antibodies following vasectomy are detrimental.

Best candidates for vasectomy

As mentioned above, one of the most important qualifications for a vasectomy is voluntary choice. If a man is under any pressure to undergo the surgery, he may feel resentment afterward.

Another major consideration is the consent of both members of the couple to the vasectomy. Some surveys have found increased marital discord when a couple has not discussed the decision adequately beforehand.

All workers in this field agree that the most important factor in deciding whether vasectomy is appropriate is an agreement by both the man and woman that their family is complete. Counseling for a couple considering vasectomy should stress that it is a form of birth control that is usually difficult to reverse; reversibility should not be considered a future option. In some cases it can be done, but even the surgeon who has been most successful in restoring male fertility states flatly that "We would not recommend vasectomy for a man who feels he may want to have more children." For this reason most surgeons are reluctant to perform the procedure on a young man who is unmarried or who is married but has only one child or no children at all.

In addition, couples should make sure that they do not expect the vasectomy to act as marital therapy. Although in some cases the operation enhances marital relations in a couple who are already well-adjusted, it cannot be expected to solve marital problems that stem from sources other than anxiety about becoming pregnant.

One final warning is that a vasectomy should not be considered a cure for impotence or a man's flagging libido. Despite one reputable physician's claim in 1936 that "The general [sexual] rejuvenating effect [of vasectomy] has been sufficiently observed in both animals and man by so many prominent men of science

345

as to remove any doubts about it," this claim has proved to be simply wishful thinking.

Reversibility of the procedure

Although most surgeons attempt to perform vasectomies only on men who say that they have completed their families, quite a few men at some later time desire to have their fertility restored. This may be due to remarriage and a desire to have children with a new wife, or it can be caused by the loss of children, for example, when the mother is awarded sole custody after a divorce. Some men who return within a short time to have the procedure reversed have suffered the death of a young baby.

Fortunately, for a man in such a situation, fertility can often be restored. During the first year after the operation successful reconnection of the ends of the vas deferens can be achieved in as many as 90% of all attempts. The success rate decreases with time after vasectomy and drops to about 50% after ten years.

The other important factor in determining successful restoration of fertility is the way in which the initial operation was performed. If electrical cauterization was used, reconnecting the ends of the vas deferens may be more difficult than if the tubes were cut and tied. If a large segment of the vas deferens was removed after it was severed, the reconnection will be still more difficult. (On the other hand, the incidence of spontaneous rejoining of the tubes appears to be lower following these two more extreme procedures.)

Even under the best of circumstances restoration of fertility is not routinely available. It was only with the introduction of microsurgery—operating while observing the vas deferens through a special microscope—that successful reversal of vasectomy became possible in more than 20 to 40% of cases. But not all surgeons perform microsurgical reconnection. As a result, success rates vary between practitioners.

It is this uncertainty about reversibility that prompts workers in the field to recommend some other method of birth control for any couple who think that there is even a slight chance that they might want more children. Some men have had samples of their sperm frozen before their vasectomies with the expectation that these sperm could be thawed and used to impregnate their wives should they later decide to have more children. Unfortunately, sperm banking has not fulfilled the hopes that many people had for it in the early 1970s. The reason is that conception rates with frozen sperm average only about 50%. It is only in the first four to six months after freezing that success rates with frozen sperm are as high as 80 to 90%.

Couples who want more information about vasectomy can contact the Association for Voluntary Sterilization, 122 E. 42nd St., New York, N.Y., 10168. This group will provide information about both vasectomy and permanent female contraception. They can also refer interested couples to qualified surgeons.

—*William A. Check*

Infant Nutrition

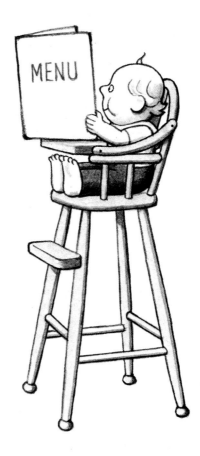

Optimal nutrition during the first year of life is very important for the future physical, emotional, and intellectual development of the child. Yet, despite what is now known about nutrition, many parents are not following the accepted recommendations about how to feed their babies. Among the major mistakes that they make are starting solid foods too soon, switching to regular cow's milk too soon, and overfeeding.

Breast-feeding is best

The ideal way to feed an infant during the first six months and beyond is to breast-feed. Human milk has been shown to be ideally suited to the infant's nutritional needs during the entire first year of life. Furthermore, there is strong evidence that, in addition to being nutritionally perfect, breast milk contains antibodies that protect the baby against certain viral and bacterial infections, especially those involving the gastrointestinal tract. Some preliminary results of large-scale investigations support the theory that breast-fed babies may be better able to handle cholesterol in later life than those who were bottle-fed. Breast-feeding is also easy, economical, and hygienic. It is ideal from the emotional and psychological points of view as well.

When breast-feeding is unsuccessful, inappropriate because of life-style, stopped after a few weeks, or simply if the choice is made to bottle-feed, there is no reason to feel guilty. The commercially available formulas today provide the most rational and desirable alternative to breast milk for meeting the infant's nutritional needs. Although not identical, they are quite similar to breast milk in their nutrient mix. In addition to being very close to breast milk in the amounts of carbohydrate, fat, and protein they contain, commercial formulas also have comparable concentrations of minerals and vitamins. Babies do very well on these formulas.

For the bottle-fed infant, the Committee on Nutrition of the American Academy of Pediatrics (AAP) recommends that an iron-fortified formula be used from the start. The rationale for this recommendation is that it prevents iron-deficiency anemia. Some pediatricians advise that a multiple vitamin (in liquid form, administered as "drops") be given to the infant daily, beginning at two weeks of age.

Avoid overfeeding

Whether you breast-feed or bottle-feed, the important point to remember is not to overfeed your baby. If you avoid overfeeding from the very beginning, you have a better chance of sparing your child all the unpleasantness and health hazards of growing up fat. An infant can be overfed by not allowing him to decide when the feeding is over. This occurs more often among bottle-feeding mothers than among the breast-feeding group. The bottle-feeding mother knows exactly how many ounces of formula she started with, and she will tend to make every effort to see to it that every last drop goes down the baby's throat. On the other hand, the breast-feeding mother has no way of knowing exactly how many ounces her baby has consumed on any one occasion, so the feeding usually stops when the baby is satisfied.

The facts are very clear. Fat babies have a greater chance of ending up as fat adults than do normal-weight or thin babies. If you notice that your baby has been gaining weight too rapidly, it is important that you discuss this with your doctor. There are a number of methods of determining if a baby is fat, including comparison with standard weight and age charts and measurement of skin folds with special calipers. The best method of all is just to look at your baby. Rolls of fat and extra chins are not difficult to notice. One rule of thumb you can use is that a baby should double the birth weight by five months of age and triple it by one year of age. For example, a baby with a birth weight of 6 lb should weigh around 12 lb at five months and 18 lb at a year. If your baby gains weight much more rapidly than this, you should alert your doctor about it.

Leave cow's milk to calves

Another current recommendation of the AAP's Committee on Nutrition is that an infant be kept on a diet of breast milk or commercially available iron-fortified formula for at least the first 12 months of life. It is not uncommon for many mothers to switch their babies to regular cow's milk during this period. This mistake should be avoided. Cow's milk may be ideal for calves, but it never was designed for human babies. More and more evidence has accumulated during recent years pointing to the potential dangers of feeding cow's milk to infants younger than one year of age.

Cow's milk contains too much salt and too much protein, much more than in either breast milk or commercially prepared formula. This excessive quantity of salt and protein requires a great deal of body water for proper elimination of the waste. Diarrhea is a common problem in infants, and the infant with diarrhea who is fed cow's milk is much more likely to develop dangerous dehydration than one who is fed breast milk or formula. There is yet another problem with feeding a baby cow's milk at this age. A certain percentage of infants below one year of age who drink cow's milk bleed into their gastrointestinal tracts, which can lead to iron-deficiency anemia. Finally, regular cow's milk contains no iron, and daily intake of iron is essential to prevent anemia. Despite all these potential dangers, many mothers still switch to cow's milk before the baby is 12 months of age.

Skim milk should never be used during the first year of life. Many parents become concerned about childhood obesity and automatically assume that they should switch to skim milk if their baby is gaining weight too rapidly. The fact is that there is even more sodium in skim milk than in regular cow's milk, far more than is healthy for an infant to ingest. Furthermore, many studies have shown that skim milk does not satisfy the basic energy requirements of infants. It has no place at all in the diet of any baby below one year of age.

Delay introducing solid food

The age at which solid foods should be introduced into the infant's diet is extremely important in terms of optimal infant nutrition. The current recommendations of the AAP's Committee on Nutrition is to withhold all solid food until the baby is at least four months of age. Most infant nutrition authorities agree, although there are varying opinions about the exact age to start solid foods. The consensus, however, is that solid foods can safely be introduced between four months and six months of age.

These current recommendations are a drastic change from those of ten years ago. At that time it was customary to start some solid food when the infant was three or four weeks of age. There are three basic reasons for this change in the approach to feeding the infant.

First, although there are no hard statistical data as yet, many authorities believe that before four months of age the added calories provided by the solid foods not only are unnecessary but probably contribute to excessive weight gain. These extra calories cause fat cells to multiply too rapidly; this factor plus the overfeeding result in a baby who is already started on the road to obesity. Strictly from the nutritional point of view, we now know that during the first four to six months of life an infant needs only breast milk or an iron-fortified formula and nothing more.

Second, there is presumptive evidence that starting an infant on solid foods too early will cause food allergies and perhaps even respiratory allergies such as bronchial asthma later in life. This association has not been proved as yet, but it is sensible not to take the risk.

Third, as Samuel Fomon, one of the foremost authorities on infant nutrition, has pointed out, a baby younger than five months of age usually has little or no control over his head and neck muscles. Therefore, any baby who is fed solid foods before this age is unable to turn away from the feeding when satiated. In such a case the mother is the one who decides how much food goes down the baby's throat. More often than not the amount is greater than the baby requires or wants. This results in overfeeding. By four or five months of age most infants have achieved fairly good control over the muscles of their head and neck and so are able to turn away when satisfied. This allows the baby and not the mother to decide when the feeding should stop.

One of the reasons so many parents are anxious to introduce solid foods is their belief that this will help the baby sleep through the night. But there is no proof of this. However, even if it were true, it is not a good enough reason to introduce solid foods too early. If the withholding of solids causes the inconvenience of getting up more often for a night feeding, it is well worth the extra effort.

A number of recent surveys have shown that the too early introduction of solid foods into the infant's diet remains one of the major faulty feeding practices in the United States. According to one study reported by Myron Winick, director of the Institute of Human Nutrition at Columbia University College of Physicians and Surgeons, 67% of infants in the United States are given solids by one month of age and 96% are eating solid foods by two months of age. And by two months of age, the average baby is consuming 135% of the recommended daily allowance for calories because of this too early introduction of solids.

The message about delaying the introduction of solid

Solid foods in the infant's diet		
age in months	type of food	time
4–5	precooked baby cereals,* 2 times a day	morning and evening
5–6	strained single fruits,† 2 times a day	morning and evening
6–7	strained vegetables†	lunch
7–8	strained meats	lunch
	plain yogurt	snack
	baby juices, no sugar added	between meals
8–9	egg yolk, strained, commercial or home-cooked	morning (every other day)
10–12	cottage cheese, toast, teething biscuits, pieces of banana, and other finger foods	
* Cereals are mixed with formula. † Fruits and vegetables are fed without formula.		

foods is beginning to have an effect on current feeding practices, but there is still a long way to go. Studies involving breast-feeding mothers have shown a significant change during the past few years. In 1976, for example, 76% of breast-fed infants were fed cereal at two months of age; in 1978 the number had dropped to 64%; and in 1980 the number dropped further to 54%. Similarly, in 1976, 64% of two-month-old infants who were being breast-fed also were being given commercially prepared baby food from a jar. In 1978, 43% ate commercially prepared baby food, and in 1980 the figure was reduced to 37%.

Based on the current state of knowledge, most pediatricians recommend that solid foods can be started at around four months of age. The schedule must be individualized since some babies have greater appetites than others. An infant who consumes over a quart of formula each day and continually cries between feedings for more milk obviously will need solid food earlier than a baby who is drinking less than a quart a day and is content between feedings. On the average, breast-feeding mothers are less eager to start solid foods than bottle-feeding mothers.

Offer new foods gradually

Foods should be introduced one at a time so that if the infant reacts adversely, the particular offending food can readily be identified and eliminated from the diet. Each new food should be started by giving the baby one teaspoon the first day and gradually increasing the amount each day. It is a good practice to wait at least three to four days between new foods to make certain that the baby tolerates that particular food. The usual signs of food intolerance are vomiting, rashes, gasiness, and excessive crankiness. The chart gives an average schedule for the introduction of solid foods.

It usually takes the baby a few days of practice to learn to swallow from a spoon. Infant cereals are introduced first because they are all fortified with iron in a form that is easily and readily digested and absorbed. Breast-fed babies need extra iron at around four to five months of age, as do infants who are fed formulas that

are not iron-fortified. The reason is that by four to five months of age, most infants have nearly depleted the iron supplies they received from their mothers before birth. Therefore, iron must be added to the diet of breast-fed babies or they will become iron-deficient.

It is important not to add sugar or salt to a baby's food. The baby food manufacturers have recently removed added salt from all their products and added sugar from most of them; the amount that remains is naturally occurring and is more than adequate for the baby's nutritional needs. Parents should not season their baby's foods based on their own food taste preferences. No baby is born craving salt or sugar, but he or she can easily learn to. A baby given drinks or solid foods with added sugar very soon becomes addicted to the extra sugar and will continue to demand sugar-laden foods as he grows older. These same rules apply to any baby foods prepared at home; controlling the amount of salt and sugar that is added may help prevent such subsequent health problems for your baby as tooth decay, high blood pressure, and obesity.

When your baby is around six or seven months of age, sips of water can be offered from a cup, followed shortly by juice in a cup. With the introduction of fruit juices, a word of caution about so-called nursing bottle syndrome is in order. It has been proved that babies who use the bottle as a pacifier and suck on the bottle containing juice (or milk for that matter) while lying down for extended periods of time destroy their teeth. Because of this, many pediatricians recommend that fruit juice should be fed only by cup. If your baby is fed milk or juice in a bottle, the important thing to remember is that he should drink it only while in an upright position. If your baby requires a bottle in order to fall asleep, make sure that it contains only water without any sugar added. This approach will prevent a great deal of tooth decay. (Treating decayed teeth in a two-year-old may require general anesthesia.)

Another effective measure that has been proved to reduce dental decay is the use of fluoride. Fluoride administration in childhood means a dramatic decrease in the incidence of tooth decay—and a reduction of family dental expenses as well. The AAP's Committee on Nutrition recently published new recommendations regarding fluoride supplementation for infants and children. It recommends fluoride supplementation in very early infancy, starting at two weeks and continuing until 16 years of age, with the amount of supplemental fluoride dependent on the fluoride content of the drinking water in the community. The status of the water supply in a community with regard to its fluoride concentration can be checked by calling the department of health. If you find that your water supply does not contain sufficient fluoride, your infant will require supplementation. This can be given in the form of fluoride drops or in combination with a multivitamin preparation. The daily dose will be determined by the level of fluoride in the water supply; this holds true for both breast-fed and formula-fed babies. The baby's physician should be able to tell you if extra fluoride is necessary and what the proper dose for your infant is.

Most babies rapidly learn to hold and handle a cup by themselves at about seven months, and this is good preparation for weaning later on. As you may notice from the chart shown previously, juices are not started until seven or eight months of age. It is unnecessary earlier because they receive all the vitamin C required in the daily multiple vitamin drop preparation. Furthermore, many infants do not like the taste of the juice and may spit it up, and some babies develop rashes. Plain yogurt is added to the baby's diet because it is well tolerated, easily digested, and of a consistency that is easy to swallow. Yogurt should be considered a substitute for part of the milk intake rather than part of the solid food diet.

Between 9 and 12 months of age the baby should be introduced to a variety of nutritious foods one by one. At this age most babies may be offered three well-balanced meals each day. This is a diet that contains daily servings from each of the four basic food groups:

1. Meat: includes meat, poultry, and fish with alternatives of eggs, dried beans, and soybeans.

2. Vegetable and fruit: includes all fruits and vegetables.

3. Milk: includes milk, cheese, yogurt, and various milk products.

4. Breads and cereals: includes breads and cereals that are whole-grained or enriched; also includes rice and pasta.

Many babies are introduced to regular table foods during this period, while still others prefer strained or junior foods. In either case, as stated earlier, do not add extra salt or sugar to your baby's food.

There is one aspect of feeding the infant that frequently upsets parents. At about 9 to 12 months many babies suddenly rebel against food. Mothers try everything in their power to force the food down the baby's throat. The baby in turn does everything in its power to refuse to eat, spitting the food out or pushing it away. It is normal and usual for many 9- to 12-month-olds to show a marked decrease in their appetites. Growth slows at this age and less food is required. A baby should never be forced to eat when not hungry. Allow the baby to eat as much or as little as he or she wants rather than as much as you think he or she needs.

The 9- to 12-month-old period is notorious for the start of iron deficiency anemia. Along with a natural decrease in appetite, many babies at this age are switched to regular cow's milk, which contains no iron. Many of these babies at this age prefer a great deal of regular cow's milk and take in very little solid food. This combination rapidly leads to iron deficiency and iron deficiency anemia. Since iron deficiency anemia may be associated with increased irritability and fatigue, growth retardation, decreased resistance to infection, and learning disabilities later on, it is essential that you prevent it from happening. The 9- to 12-month-old baby who is not continuing to drink iron-fortified formula should be fed infant cereals, green vegetables, meats, and eggs—all foods that contain iron. If your child is drinking regular milk at this age, make certain that it is not over one quart per day so that there will be enough appetite left to eat iron-containing solid foods. If your baby's solid food intake is minimal, supplemental iron can easily be given, either incorporated in the multivitamin preparation or separately. This should be discussed with the pediatrician.

If you follow these suggestions, your infant will receive a well-balanced and nutritionally sound diet. The right attitude about feeding is also very important. It is rarely necessary to coax a baby to eat. Mealtime should never become a contest between parent and baby; rather, it should be relaxed and pleasant. If your baby refuses to eat, he is simply not hungry. He will not starve by skipping a meal. Appetite should be the only factor in determining the amount of food consumed. Toward the end of the first year, when activity increases (crawling and standing), appetite will usually improve. But extra weight does not mean extra health. A fat baby is not a healthy baby. If you allow your baby to grow and gain at his or her own pace, under your doctor's supervision, you will not go wrong.

—Alvin N. Eden, M.D.

Breast-feeding

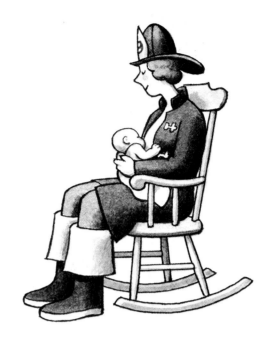

Breast-feeding is the ideal way to nourish the newborn infant. It is a process that brings both physical and emotional benefits to mother and baby. With rare exceptions, any new mother can do it. If, after a few days or weeks, she chooses to switch to bottle-feeding, the transition is easy and absolutely safe. She has made no financial investment, taken no risk, and caused no damage to herself or her infant.

Information confirmed by the U.S. National Center for Health Statistics and published by the American Academy of Pediatrics indicates that the incidence of breast-feeding has doubled in the past decade among women of all social and economic backgrounds. One survey by an infant-formula producer found that the percentage of infants who were breast-fed rose from 24.7 in 1971 to 55.3 in 1980; about a fourth of these infants were nursed for more than four months. Other estimates were lower: 25% was the estimate for mothers who tried breast-feeding and less than 10% for those who continued four months or more.

As late as 1900, virtually all women in the U.S. nursed their babies. Outside the industrialized, developed nations of the world, the vast majority still do, as they have done from time immemorial. But most of today's new mothers grew up in an era when breast-feeding was uncommon. The use of prepared formulas and the development of safe techniques of home sterilization created a revolution in baby-feeding in the mid-20th century, freeing mothers' time and giving them a greater degree of independence. In time, breast-feeding came to be considered somewhat primitive, and a false modesty developed about exposing the breast even within the family circle. The breast came to have only sexual connotations, to the extent that some men were uncomfortable about their wives' intention to breast-feed. As fewer and fewer women breast-fed, hospital routine became organized around bottle-feeding, and obstetricians themselves had little cause to encourage any change in established practice. The pattern of mother teaching daughter was broken, and without firsthand experience to draw on, the woman contemplating breast-feeding was likely to get more misinformation and discouragement than help. Today, happily, this situation is changing.

All that it takes to successfully breast-feed an infant are a few skills, support from the obstetrician and pediatrician, and a little determination. Encouragement and practical help are available from other women who have nursed, many excellent books, free government pamphlets, and groups such as La Leche League International and the Human Lactation Center. A knowledge of the lactation process also helps.

Lactation

Changes in the breasts begin to occur six to eight weeks after conception. The blood supply is increased, the breasts grow larger, and the areola (pigmented area around the nipple) grows darker. The infant's instinct to suck is strong and present so early that fetuses have been viewed sucking their thumbs in the womb. When the infant begins to nurse at his mother's breast soon after birth, the action not only satisfies the baby but also sets in motion a cascade of hormonal events known collectively as lactation.

After delivery the levels of the major female sex hormones, estrogen and progesterone, drop, and another hormone, prolactin, is secreted by the pituitary, the body's master gland at the base of the brain. Normally, the only time prolactin is released into the bloodstream is after birth and for the period of nursing.

Prolactin is what causes the mammary glands to produce milk, and it operates whether the breasts are big or small, thin or fat, upright or pendulous. Breast size and shape are determined by the age of a woman, heredity, and the amount of fat around and in them. The milk production center is a network of blood vessels, sacs, and ducts. Raw materials are brought by the bloodstream to milk-producing cells deep in the breast. Pools of fluid then flow through tiny streams in the breast to storage reservoirs to await release.

When the infant sucks, the action stimulates nerves

that send chemical messengers to the pituitary, which responds by releasing another hormone, oxytocin, into the bloodstream. Oxytocin is the same hormone that produces uterine contractions during labor. Within a few seconds of its release, oxytocin stimulates the mammary cells to contract and release milk. This "let-down," or ejection, reflex propels milk out of the nipples and in some cases is strong enough to produce a continuous stream that travels several feet. Many women report they know when let-down has occurred because their breasts begin to tingle. When nursing first begins, it may take several seconds to several minutes to experience let-down. After the milk supply is established, it may take only a baby's cry of hunger to produce it instantly.

It takes two to four days before the milk supply comes in completely. Average milk production on the second day after delivery is about 120 ml; this doubles by the fourth day and eventually reaches about 300 ml per day. Milk production is controlled by demand. Suckling or mechanically expressing the milk will keep it flowing; it soon ceases if nursing stops.

Another effect of prolactin is that as long as the baby suckles, prolactin suppresses the release of eggs from the mother's ovaries. Breast-feeding thus also functions as a form of contraception, but it is not reliable enough to be employed as the only means.

There are several factors vital to the success of nursing, including the length of the nipple and the duration of sucking. A nipple that is stubby or too short cannot reach the roof of the baby's mouth and the throat area, which must be stimulated to begin the nursing process. Nipple shields and extenders are available to solve the problem. If the nipple is too long, the baby may choke, a problem easily corrected by keeping some of the nipple out of the baby's mouth.

Because the sucking reflex keeps the whole lactation system going, it is important to empty the breasts, or nearly empty them, several times a day. If for some reason the baby cannot nurse around the clock, especially in the early stages of breast-feeding, the mother can use a manual or electric breast pump to empty the breasts and ensure continuation of the milk supply. A complete cessation of suckling will stop the process and dry up the milk.

Characteristics of breast milk

The first liquid a newborn gets from the breast is not actually milk but a "premilk" called colostrum. This somewhat sticky, sweetish, clear or yellow fluid is an ideal first food for a baby, higher in protein, minerals, and vitamins, and lower in fats and sugars than true milk, and easier to digest. All the components of colostrum have not yet been identified, but colostrum is known to contain antibodies to some infectious diseases, lysozymes (which break down bacteria), and immunoglobulins (proteins that are important agents in the immune system); all help protect the newborn from infection. True milk generally comes in within a few days of the colostrum.

Many women complain that their milk is "thin and bluish" and believe that means it is not "rich" enough to nourish an infant. In fact, that is the way mother's milk is supposed to look. A lifetime of looking at the white creaminess of cow's milk has misled women about what the appearance means nutritionally.

Both cow's and human milk contain proteins, sugars, minerals, and vitamins, but in different proportions and forms. Neither contains adequate amounts of vitamin D, vitamin A, or iron, so these are usually given to all babies as supplements. Cow's milk contains twice as much protein as human milk, but in a form the baby uses less efficiently. Human milk contains more essential amino acids, the building blocks of protein, so that the infant's body can produce the proteins it needs more efficiently. Breast milk also contains twice the amount of sugar of cow's milk, but again in a form that makes the baby's intestinal tract less susceptible to bacterial problems. The fat content of the milk is about the same, but in an unsaturated, therefore more healthful, form in breast milk.

Many mothers notice that their breast-fed infants have fewer, looser, and less odorous bowel movements. In addition, they may notice that breast-fed infants gain weight less rapidly than bottle-fed infants. Studies suggest that is because the cow's milk or other infant formulas contain elements that increase a baby's thirst, encouraging him to drink more. It is also true that bottle-fed infants tend to be given solid foods earlier than breast-fed babies. In addition, bottle-fed infants may be encouraged to finish emptying the bottle even after they have been satisfied. Some research has suggested that rapid weight gain in the first months of life triggers the production of larger numbers of permanent fat cells, increasing the child's risk of obesity later in life. Breast-feeding may help protect against this too-rapid gain.

Although most bottle-fed infants thrive and may be just as healthy as their breast-fed cribmates, some infants are sensitive to cow's milk and cannot digest it properly. Allergies, indigestion, cramps, diarrhea, and other symptoms may result.

Advice for the beginner

Once the decision has been made to breast-feed your newborn, it is essential to let everyone connected with the baby's care know about it. Doctors and nurses should be reminded that you plan to breast-feed and that they should avoid giving you any drugs that will adversely affect the infant or dry up the milk supply. Many obstetricians routinely order injections of drugs that dry up the milk to prevent discomfort in women who do not plan to nurse. A "stop" order must often be written for women who want to nurse.

If you are in a hospital that does not house new mothers and infants in the same room, you should remind the nurses and aides to bring you the infant for every feeding, including those at 2 AM and 6 AM. Many hospitals prefer to feed the infants in the nursery at those times for convenience, but new mothers need the suckling stimulation to get their milk supply established.

Do not be shy about asking for help. The first feedings are almost always awkward, but keep in mind that every skill must be taught. You are sharing an experience that every woman who has nursed for the first time has gone through.

Nurses' aides, volunteers (who are often grandmotherly veterans of breast-feeding), midwives, and roommates who have successfully breast-fed are often good sources of information, practical tips, and encouragement. A certain amount of aggressiveness is needed to ask for their guidance, but they are almost always delighted to teach. If you are embarrassed about nursing in public, ask for a screen. All hospitals have them.

A newborn may not be terribly enthusiastic about the first feeding or two. He may be sleepy, especially if you received anesthesia or painkillers during labor or birth. As many as 40% of all infants, studies show, need a little encouragement to begin to suck.

There are numerous illustrated guides that can help a new mother find the best physical position for nursing—sitting, lying down, propped on pillows, or sitting in a rocking chair. Each mother finds hers, along with bras and equipment to make her nursing more comfortable and convenient.

To start the nursing process, take advantage of the infant's natural "rooting" behavior. If you place the baby next to your breasts, he will begin to search with his mouth for the nipple. It is important to make sure the infant takes both the nipple and the areola into his mouth. The areola contains glands that secrete a lubricant to keep the nipple pliable and prevent soreness. It is also necessary for the baby to compress the areola to squeeze the milk out of the nipple.

Let your baby take the nipple—do not force it in his mouth or push his head against the breast. Help him get hold of the nipple and areola by pulling back on the breast with two fingers to elongate the area slightly. It is also important to keep the bulk of the breast from pressing against the baby's nostrils. A nursing infant must breathe through his nose. Keeping a finger pressed against the breast to keep it away from the nostrils is all that is required. To remove the baby from the breast, gently break the seal by slipping a finger between the breast and his mouth.

Lactation specialists recommend that nursing mothers use both breasts for each feeding. This will help assure adequate milk supply and avoid soreness in the nipples. The usual tactic is to alternate breasts for the first "round" of each feeding: the last breast suckled is

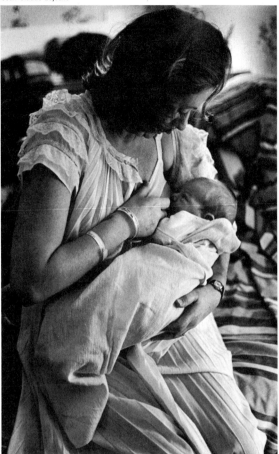

A bra with an opening in the front of the cup makes breast-feeding more convenient. Many authorities urge that nursing be continued for the full first year of life.

the first suckled at the next feeding. A recommended schedule to avoid soreness is three minutes at each breast the first day, adding about a minute a day, up to ten minutes at each breast.

Some new mothers worry that their babies are not getting enough to eat since they cannot see the amount drunk at each feeding. If the baby seems satisfied, sleeps well between feedings, and is gaining and developing normally, he is getting enough.

Care of the nursing mother

Through the centuries there has been much speculation about the nutritional needs of a nursing mother. The fact is that any reasonably well-nourished woman can deliver all the nutrients her infant requires and maintain her own health with just a few modest alterations in her diet. First, a new mother will need more liquid, because nursing is dehydrating. The liquid can include milk, water, juice, and even beer, wine, or liquor. Alcohol, however, should be consumed only in small amounts, since it can act as a diuretic and deplete the body of liquid—and it will be transferred to the infant.

The nursing mother also needs more calories—about 1,000 more than usual—to keep up with the energy demands of breast-feeding and milk production. But the wise mother can also lose her pregnancy fat while nursing if she is careful to make every calorie count and avoid empty calories. Nursing also stimulates the uterus to contract and helps eliminate the abdominal bulge that remains long after a baby has left the womb.

Any food that is safe for the mother is safe for the baby, although in a few cases a particular food will create digestive problems for him. If you suspect a food is causing problems, keep a diary of what you eat for a few days or a week to link the baby's symptoms with items on your menu. Then eliminate the suspicious foods and watch the results. A number of women report that foods such as cabbage, cucumbers, and spinach give their babies gas and that infants will stop nursing if the mother has eaten a lot of garlic.

Drugs taken by the mother may be transferred to the infant in breast milk. Because it is dangerous and unethical to test the effects of drugs on nursing infants, many effects are unknown. A good rule of thumb is to avoid all drugs—including the nicotine in cigarette smoke—unless prescribed by a physician, and to question the physician about the effects of all drugs that he or she prescribes.

Women who must take anticancer drugs, medicines to alter thyroid hormone levels, chloramphenicol (a potent antibiotic), and lithium (a psychoactive agent) should not breast-feed. Marijuana, barbiturates, sleeping pills, and "hard" drugs such as heroin will adversely affect the infant. Oral contraceptives are often cited as drugs to avoid. The evidence for the caution is still slim, and the American College of Obstetricians and Gynecologists recommends that physicians review individually each woman's case and need for contraception during nursing. Laxatives, diuretics, drugs to lower blood pressure, and some painkillers are risky. Always check with your physician if you take any over-the-counter medication. Take no prescription drugs without supervision.

Care of the breasts is simple. The nipple area should be cleaned with mild soap and water and rinsed before and after nursing. Exposing the nipples to the air is recommended to help the skin remain healthy and free from soreness. The nipples will probably be tender for the first few days. The most common complication is mastitis, an infection caused by the invasion of *Staphylococcus aureus* bacteria through a crack in the skin. Antibiotics usually clear up mastitis, but nursing must be discontinued while the drugs are taken.

Scheduling problems

For the modern woman considering breast-feeding there are problems of working breast-feeding into a life-style that may include an office or factory job, heavy family responsibilities, and the desire for time away from the infant.

There is no question that breast-feeding requires more or less regular and frequent feedings and limits a mother's freedom. Most women who successfully breast-feed do not find the restrictions overly severe or difficult to work around. They also note that within a month or two a well-fed breast-fed baby will accept feedings that are farther apart and will sleep through the 2 AM feeding. A few sips of water will also extend the periods between feedings so that a nursing mother can get away for more than two or three hours.

Once milk supply is well established, many nursing mothers find it easy to go out for an evening or a few hours during the day by leaving a supplemental bottle with a babysitter. The woman who must work a nine-to-five job, however, still has a hard time of it. Few companies sponsor day-care centers and nurseries for employees where a newborn can be nursed during the workday at lunch and coffee breaks.

If a part-time work schedule can be worked out during the nursing period, the new mother will find her life much simpler. If full-time work is a must, many women still manage it by feeding the baby in the morning before leaving for work, in the evening after arriving home, and at 10 or 11 PM. Some women also find it helpful to pump milk from the breast at midday. That relieves discomfort of overfullness and keeps the milk supply coming. If possible, the milk should be expressed into a sterilized bottle and refrigerated; the sitter can give the bottle to the baby for his next day's noon meal.

The American Academy of Pediatrics and other groups recommend up to six months of breast-feeding as the only or the primary source of an infant's food. In that amount of time, a newborn receives all of the benefits of nursing in terms of growth and health. Many women continue beyond that time period, and in some societies the newborn is nourished exclusively on breast milk for a year or more.

For further information

Further information on breast-feeding can be obtained from the following organizations: Human Lactation Center, 666 Sturges Highway, Westport, Conn. 06880, and La Leche League International, Inc., 9616 Minneapolis Ave., Franklin Park, Ill. 60131.

—Joann E. Rodgers

Varicose Veins

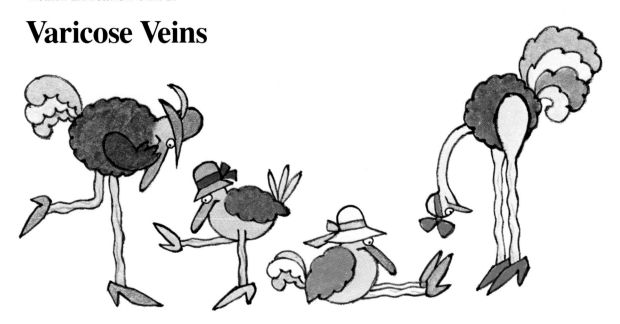

Varicose veins are one of the commonest ailments affecting the circulatory system. One in four women in the United States has varicose veins. Although it is often thought of as merely a nuisance disease, varicose veins can have serious complications. Blood clots can develop in the legs, and the important deep leg veins can become seriously affected. Although mankind has been troubled with varicose veins for thousands of years, the precise cause is not known.

What makes a vein "varicose"?

Most people think of varicose veins as the prominent bluish vessels that can be seen in the lower legs. All visible or prominent veins are not varicose, and many people have varicose veins that are not apparent at all. A varicose vein is one in which the vein walls have become stretched, so that the vein becomes dilated (and hence more visible). The veins most commonly affected are the superficial veins of the legs—the great, or long, saphenous vein and the small, or short, saphenous vein. Veins in the esophagus and genital area can become varicose; hemorrhoids are varicose veins in the rectum.

Inside each vein in the leg is a series of one-way valves that aid in moving the blood upward, against gravity, back to the heart and lungs. The veins with their valves can be compared to a canal with a series of locks; the blood moves into a vein segment, the valve closes behind it to prevent backflow, the next valve opens, and the blood moves on. In the legs there are both a superficial (close to the skin) and deeper system of veins, connected by communicating branches called perforator veins. If the valves of the veins do not function properly, the blood flow is subject to stasis, or slowing of flow, and may flow backward. In time the vein becomes stretched because of the pressure from

the blood and, in some cases, assumes a twisted, convoluted shape. The cause of valve malfunction has not yet been determined. In some individuals the valves are weak and prone to fail under stress conditions, and other persons are born with an insufficient number of valves for good functioning.

The absence of vein valves or the presence of weak or defective valves at birth suggests that a genetic defect plays a role in the development of varicose veins. In a number of studies it has been shown that as many as 70% of people with varicose veins have other members in their family with the same condition. A number of other theories as to the causes of varicose veins have been put forth. These include a prolonged low-fiber diet, constipation, prolonged sitting or standing, and pregnancy, all of which are associated with varicose veins. These factors may merely be accelerators of a preexisting defect occurring within the structure of the vein itself. Many women first develop symptoms of varicose veins during pregnancy, but pregnancy itself is not the cause.

Signs and symptoms

The appearance of a leg with varicose veins is variable. Ordinarily, when a person with a healthy leg stands, the lower-limb veins bulge slightly. This bulging disappears when the person lies down or elevates his legs. A varicose vein generally does not disappear when the leg is changed from the upright to the horizontal position. In women, in whom the fat layers just under the skin are usually much more abundant than in men, comparatively extensive varicosities often may lie hidden in the tissues just under the skin.

If there is a suspicion that bulging blue leg veins are varicose veins or if there is a family history of varicose veins, then an expert's advice should be sought. Physi-

355

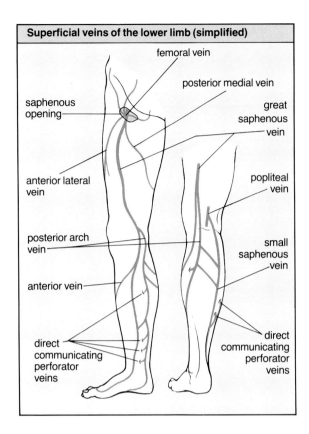

Superficial veins of the lower limb (simplified)

femoral vein

posterior medial vein

saphenous opening

great saphenous vein

anterior lateral vein

popliteal vein

posterior arch vein

small saphenous vein

anterior vein

direct communicating perforator veins

direct communicating perforator veins

cians specializing in vascular diseases, including qualified vascular surgeons, are most familiar with this disease and its treatment.

Most people with varicose veins make an appointment for a consultation because they have one or more symptoms or warning signs. The three most common symptoms are aching in the legs, swelling around the ankles, and the unsightliness of the swollen veins.

The most obvious sign of varicose veins, and therefore the one most people associate with this condition, is the disfiguring appearance of these tortuous veins. This is usually progressive, beginning in the small branches of the saphenous veins and continuing until eventually the entire saphenous system of veins is bunched, twisted, lumped, and contorted into what appears to be a bluish rope that bulges under the skin.

The aching from varicose veins is usually described as a feeling of heaviness or fullness in the legs, or a feeling of tiredness or fatigue. A dull aching sensation that occurs after prolonged standing in one place or prolonged sitting is very common. The ache can rarely be pinpointed, but when it is localized it is generally over a cluster of varicose veins. Aching is the most common reason a varicose vein sufferer will seek a doctor's help, and it is a symptom that is easy to relieve—at least temporarily. Walk, run, dance, and you will have no problem. But wait in line at the theater or supermarket, spend an evening at a stand-up cocktail party, or take a long plane trip, and you will probably suffer. A good rule of thumb is that any aching or a feeling of tiredness in the leg brought on by prolonged standing or prolonged sitting and relieved by leg elevation is due to varicose veins—unless proved otherwise.

When a person stands or sits for a long period of time, the blood pools in the saphenous veins as circulation fights against gravity. Walking, running, or any form of physical exercise makes the leg muscles contract, acting as an auxiliary pump that compresses the deep veins in the leg, aiding the return flow of blood to the heart. The superficial veins of the saphenous system drain into these veins through the series of perforator veins when venous flow is normal. The problem that causes the aching or the tiredness, namely stasis of the venous blood, is then eliminated.

The second symptom, swelling, or edema, of the ankles, legs, or feet, can be triggered by any number of things. For example, anyone who spends hours standing or sitting with the knees bent can develop swelling of the legs. Occasional swelling does not necessarily mean varicose veins. When varicose veins are a cause of edema, especially in people such as salesclerks, bartenders, security guards, dentists, and surgeons, who must stand for long periods, the ankle swelling usually appears toward the end of the day. A swollen leg can often be a challenge to the doctor, who must rule out a long list of other causes before he can attribute the swelling to varicose veins. The fact that there is a long list of causes should also serve as a warning that it is foolish and possibly dangerous to go without a medical explanation for a swollen ankle or leg.

Another frequent warning sign of varicose veins is night cramps, which can be very painful. The pain is triggered by unrelieved muscle spasms in the calf muscles of the leg and occurs most frequently at night. Some patients complain of night cramps as an early

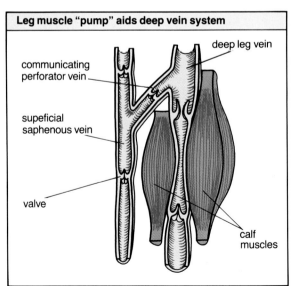

Leg muscle "pump" aids deep vein system

deep leg vein

communicating perforator vein

supeficial saphenous vein

valve

calf muscles

From *Pathologic Basis of Disease*, Stanley L. Robbins, M.D., and Ramzi S. Cotran, M.D., 2nd ed., Philadelphia, W. B. Saunders Co., 1979

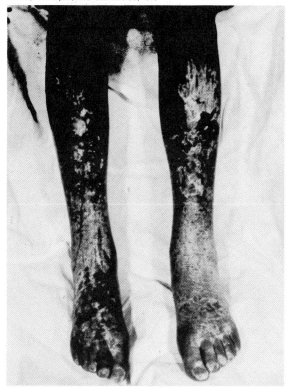

Although most people think of varicose veins as only a cosmetic problem, the impaired circulation they cause can lead to conditions such as stasis dermatitis (above).

symptom of varicose veins, while others, even with advanced varicose veins, have never experienced a leg cramp. Generally, massage followed by walking will bring relief. Sometimes Quinamm, a drug containing quinine sulfate, is effective in preventing and treating night cramps.

A woman with slender legs is more likely to notice the appearance of the first small blue lines than is a woman with heavier legs. Not infrequently, obese women or women with unusually heavy legs may have a fairly advanced case of varicose veins with nothing at all visible. Often, however, when a few small varicosities begin to show, it turns out to be a minor problem. Patients in this group are relieved to learn that surgery is not indicated.

Treatment and management

The goal of the treatment of varicose veins is both to alleviate the symptoms and, equally important, to prevent the development of serious complications, some of which may have fatal consequences. And since legs are often highly visible (witness the ever increasing number of male and female joggers, walkers, swimmers, bicyclists, and tennis players of all ages who wear shorts), correcting any cosmetic disfigurement becomes an additional goal.

The consensus among vascular specialists is that surgery is the most effective means of treating varicose veins and should be performed on most individuals who suffer from symptoms of their varicose veins. Surgery should be performed early, before symptoms worsen or before serious complications occur.

Injection therapy and elastic stockings also have a place in the management of individuals with varicose veins. However, both these methods have some serious shortcomings when used as the only method of treatment.

Injection therapy, also called sclerotherapy, has been used to close off the affected veins. Their blood load is diverted to the deeper vein system that is still functioning properly. A chemical is injected into the vein to induce a blood clot to form which blocks the vein and causes it to wither away. This technique does not always work and sometimes leaves unsightly discolorations on the skin, a poor trade-off if appearance was the main reason for having the procedure done. Furthermore, the clots sometimes extend into and destroy nearby normal veins.

After the injection of a chemical, the leg is bound tightly with elastic bandages for six weeks, to ensure that the vein remains collapsed. This technique is now used mainly for smaller veins and for malfunctioning perforator veins.

Elastic stockings are useful when surgery either is out of the question, is a poor choice, or must be postponed; for instance, during pregnancy or in a person with a chronic disabling disease such as a kidney or heart disorder. To be most effective, elastic stockings should be custom fitted. They should be replaced whenever they begin to stretch out of shape. Varicose veins, once they develop, are progressive and remain for the rest of a person's life. If a person chooses elastic stockings as the main treatment, he should remember that generally he will have to put them on each morning, probably for the rest of his life.

Surgery is the preferred method of treatment because it is effective, safe, and offers a good cosmetic result. The aim of the operation is to remove the faulty connections between the two systems of veins in the legs that allow the backward or wrong-way flow of venous blood. In the operation the vascular surgeon removes, or strips, the superficial varicose veins from the legs and ties off any malfunctioning perforator veins. The entire great saphenous vein, which runs from the groin to the ankle on the inside of the leg, is often removed. The small saphenous vein, running down the back of the leg from knee to ankle, may also be stripped. The stripping operation requires no more than a day or so of hospitalization, and one can return to regular activities within a week. Elastic bandages must be worn to support the legs for several weeks after the operation.

357

Varicose veins

Possible complications

One of the most common of complications of varicose veins is phlebitis or thrombophlebitis; the terms are used interchangeably but often improperly. Phlebitis itself is an inflammation of the vein wall; it is often shortly followed by the formation of a thrombus, or blood clot, within the vein, a condition called thrombophlebitis. The cause for concern is that the thrombus occasionally breaks loose (it is then called an embolus) and travels through the circulatory system. This migrating embolus can lodge in the lung, in which case it is called a pulmonary embolus, or blood clot in the lung. This is a dangerous situation that can lead to death.

Treating thrombophlebitis aggressively with rest and medication soon after the onset may prevent further growth of the thrombus and can convert what could be a long serious illness to a short benign one. Thrombophlebitis may precede yet another more serious condition: involvement of the deep veins of the leg in the inflammatory process and the development of a blood clot within the deep veins. This condition, referred to as deep vein thrombosis, often leaves the patient with a permanently swollen leg and can progress to a blood clot in the lung. Occasionally deep vein thrombosis may result in the formation of a varicose, or stasis, ulcer, probably the most debilitating complication of varicose veins. These ulcers can be quite large. They tend to recur until the underlying problem is solved. Bed rest with the leg elevated above the level of the heart may be necessary for healing.

Occasionally a varicose vein may rupture either spontaneously or following some trivial injury. Sometimes it can cause extensive and frightening hemorrhage. Fortunately, this occurs comparatively rarely, but it can be quite alarming. The best immediate treatment is to lie flat and elevate the leg about 24 inches above the rest of the body. This effectively lowers the pressure in the leg veins. Leg elevation plus a pressure dressing over the site should control the bleeding until medical attention can be sought. Never apply a tourniquet above the bleeding point, as this may actually increase bleeding. It may also damage leg tissues, especially in an older patient with fragile arterial circulation.

Prevention

Anything that causes undue pressure on the leg veins can accelerate the formation of varicose veins. Anything that helps the veins to function properly can postpone the appearance of varicose veins and may even prevent most of the serious complications.

Whenever possible, avoid prolonged periods of standing or sitting. If you must stand in line or sit for a long period of time, make a conscious effort to flex the muscles of the leg. Move your toes frequently; raise and lower yourself on the balls of your feet. It is a good idea to break up the inactivity of a long trip by walking for several minutes every hour or so. If you are on a long plane or train ride, walk up and down the aisle at least once an hour. Crossing the legs at the knee is a habit that should be broken, since it places added pressure on the leg veins.

The rule on clothing is simple. Any clothing that tends to constrict the flow of blood in the veins just beneath the skin can be hazardous. Avoid tight calf-length boots, pantyhose that are overly tight at the groin, and tight girdles that "strangle" the upper thigh.

Any person with decreased circulation should take meticulous care of the legs and feet. No injury or infection, however minor it may seem, should be left untreated. Itchy, scaly patches sometimes develop on the legs in patients with varicose veins. Care must be taken not to injure the skin from scratching, because any skin injury may progress to an ulcer.

If you have an inherited tendency to varicose veins or if you have suspicious blue bulges in your legs, these important measures may help to prevent symptoms or complications. At least once a day lie flat on your back and elevate your legs with the help of several pillows placed under them, above heart level, for about an hour. Exercise in any form is good prevention; walk, run, jog, or dance. Do anything but stand or sit still.

—Howard C. Baron, M.D.

Phlebitis

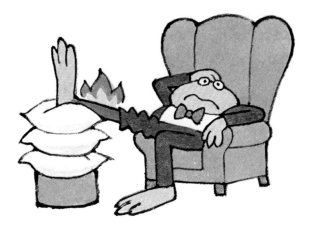

Phlebitis and thrombophlebitis are common problems affecting the veins, most often the veins of the legs. Phlebitis is an inflammation of the vein wall. When the inflammation is followed by the formation of a thrombus, or blood clot, as is often the case, the disease is termed thrombophlebitis. These problems can occur in either the superficial veins just under the skin or the deep veins surrounded by the leg muscles. Deep vein thrombosis, or clot formation, is a much more serious problem, as this can lead to a pulmonary embolus, or blood clot in the lung. About 150,000 persons die of pulmonary embolism each year in the U.S.; at least 5% of deaths from complications of surgery are due to pulmonary embolism.

Superficial thrombophlebitis

Acute local thrombophlebitis occurs frequently in patients with varicose veins; *i.e.,* veins that are abnormally dilated. Also termed varicose thrombosis, it occurs in patients who are otherwise well and in whom no precipitating factor other than varicose veins appears to be present. In a very small percentage of cases this condition may be brought on by injury.

The veins that are most commonly involved lie in the tissues just under the skin of the legs. There are two major superficial veins in the legs, with their interconnecting system of tributaries. The larger of the two, the great, or long, saphenous vein, runs up the inner portion of the calf and thigh, ending in the femoral vein in the groin; the small, or short, saphenous vein runs along the outer area of the ankle and passes up the back of the leg, terminating in the vein behind the knee, the popliteal vein.

Normally these veins carry a steady flow of venous blood back to the heart. This well-regulated system breaks down when one of the veins, generally varicosed, develops phlebitis. Very soon thereafter a thrombus, or blood clot, forms within the lumen (the hollow interior) of the inflamed vein. Adhering to the inner wall of the vein, the clot interferes with blood flow by obstructing the lumen. The inflamed vein is soon transformed into a tender cord, easily felt and often visible as a red line just under the skin.

In order to maintain normal circulation, blood should not clot within the blood vessels. When a blood vessel is injured, however, platelets, tiny blood cells that mediate normal clotting, help form a latticelike net of fibrin at the site of vein-wall injury. The web then enmeshes

blood corpuscles to form a plug known as a blood clot. This also happens when venous blood flow stagnates, as it often does in cases with varicose veins.

The body possesses a unique counterdefense against clot formation within the blood vessels. Both the platelets and the inner lining of the blood vessels are equipped with a negative electrical charge. Identical electrical charges, like identical magnetic poles, repel each other, whereas dissimilar charges attract each other. Therefore, platelets normally do not cling to the blood vessel lining nor to each other. But diseased veins often seem to lose their negative charge and no longer repel the platelets. Soon these cells accumulate on a vein valve leaflet, and a tiny blood clot forms.

The newly formed blood clot clings tenaciously to the vein wall, but as it grows, a portion of the clot may extend into other nearby veins or into the main veins in the leg, which are termed the deep veins. Sometimes a piece of the clot breaks loose from a deep vein and travels through the circulatory system. This migrating clot, called an embolus, can lodge in the lung and block off the important circulation there.

Incidence and causes. The occurrence of a pulmonary embolus in a patient with superficial thrombophlebitis transforms this condition into a potentially fatal disease. The incidence may be as high as 10% in patients who have been hospitalized for treatment of their phlebitis.

Except when the illness of a celebrity makes headlines (former president Richard Nixon is a case in point), few outside the medical community realize the high incidence of phlebitis and thrombophlebitis and the extent of the distress and discomfort they cause. As many as 40% of patients may develop thrombophlebitis following certain types of surgery. The presence of varicose veins prior to surgery is more than likely a major factor in most of the cases.

359

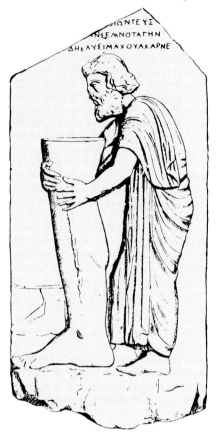

Ancient Greek physicians were aware of the problems associated with phlebitis. This votive tablet from the temple of Asclepius depicts the cure of phlebitis.

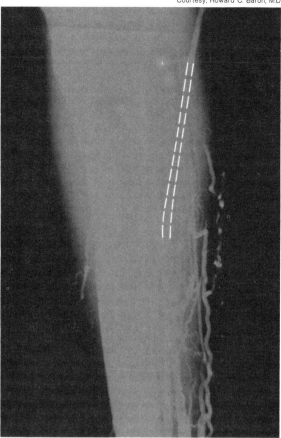

The dotted lines on this X-ray indicate the portion of the calf vein in which blood flow has been blocked off by the formation of a blood clot.

The varicose vein-phlebitis relationship has certain factors that can be identified as aggravators or precipitating causes: (1) injury to the leg; (2) certain types of surgery, especially those of long duration; (3) pregnancy; (4) insect bite on the leg; (5) athlete's foot; (6) previous episodes of thrombophlebitis in the leg; (7) prolonged bed rest, such as is required in cases of chronic disease; (8) obesity; and (9) stasis (stagnation) of blood in the legs following prolonged sitting. (This can occur following a long plane flight if the passenger remains seated throughout the trip.)

The etiology, or cause, of phlebitis was suspected as early as the last century. Rudolf Virchow, a German pathologist of the mid-1800s, first recognized the association of three general factors as a prelude to vascular thrombosis: "injury to the vessel wall, stasis, and increased coagulability of the blood." A major cause of stasis of venous blood flow is, of course, varicose veins with its accompanying valvular failure.

Symptoms. In general, anyone with varicose veins should be aware of the symptoms of phlebitis and thrombophlebitis. Usually, the first warning of the presence of superficial phlebitis is pain, sometimes accompanied by a *slight* swelling of the lower leg or ankle and an area of tenderness to touch over the course of the involved vein. When the patient touches the area with the inflamed segment of the vein, he can often locate the clot, which feels very much like a small cluster of grapes just under the skin. The skin is often warm and the onset sudden. Pain over the involved vein may be mild or severe. Often the patient experiences a feeling of weakness, accompanied by fever, chills, and loss of appetite. The involved portion of the vein is very often limited to an area easily covered by one hand. This is typical localized thrombophlebitis. In the subsiding stage the inflammation gradually recedes, often leaving a brownish patch on the skin over the site of the clot.

Treatment. When the phlebitis is localized and involves only a short segment of a superficial vein, surgery is not necessary. The patient can continue to go about his daily business. Exercise in the form of walking is especially encouraged. Wearing an elastic support stocking as part of the treatment is important to help correct the stasis of blood flow. The patient's normal routine should be interspersed with a period of

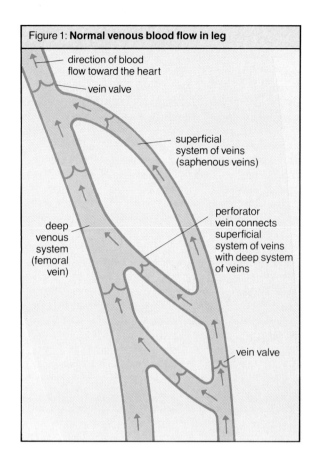

Figure 1: **Normal venous blood flow in leg**

direction of blood flow toward the heart

vein valve

superficial system of veins (saphenous veins)

perforator vein connects superficial system of veins with deep system of veins

deep venous system (femoral vein)

vein valve

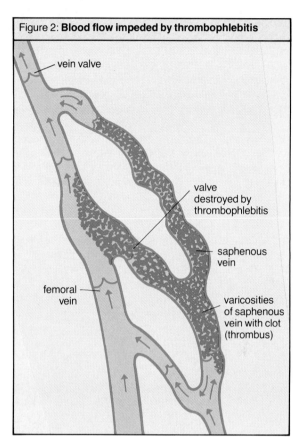

Figure 2: **Blood flow impeded by thrombophlebitis**

vein valve

valve destroyed by thrombophlebitis

saphenous vein

femoral vein

varicosities of saphenous vein with clot (thrombus)

The venous blood circulation in the legs is carried out by a system of superficial and deep veins that are connected by perforator veins. It is the superficial system that lies just under the skin that is most likely to develop varicose veins, phlebitis, and thrombophlebitis (blood clots).

lower-limb drainage. This can be accomplished by lying down with the legs elevated on several pillows above the level of the heart for about an hour every day. The patient should never be sent to bed as part of the therapy; this will only slow the blood flow in the legs. In most cases the patient's discomfort runs its course, and the localized area of superficial phlebitis subsides in a few days to several weeks.

Aspirin is usually prescribed, not so much for its analgesic effect but for its effect as an antiblood-clotting agent. Aspirin prevents platelets from functioning in the clotting process.

Occasionally, a more severe form of thrombophlebitis develops that involves much longer segments of the superficial veins in the leg. This generalized form requires an aggressive approach to therapy. Generalized thrombophlebitis of the superficial leg veins responds very well to surgery. Not only does surgery relieve the existing problem, removing both the clot and the diseased veins, but removal of the diseased veins can prevent even more serious complications from developing in the future. The period of disability is also shortened.

Deep vein thrombosis

Phlebitis and thrombophlebitis may precede a more serious condition, deep vein thrombosis—the involvement of the deep veins of the leg in the inflammatory process and the development of a large blood clot in the deep veins. After an attack of superficial phlebitis, the deep venous system becomes involved in the phlebitic process in as many as a third of patients. When this occurs the consequences are far from trivial. The patient may be left with a permanently swollen leg, a varicose ulcer, chronic dermatitis, brownish pigmentation about the lower leg, or even a lethal blood clot in the lung.

The real danger lies in the fact that this spread may take place without the patient's awareness. A group of varicose veins may show obvious thrombophlebitis, indicated by pain over the area, tenderness when the area is touched, and redness of the skin along the course of the vein. At the same time, a silent clot may also be growing in the saphenous vein, moving toward its junction with the femoral vein in the groin or extending through the veins in the leg that communicate directly with the deep system of veins.

361

Phlebitis

The deep veins of the lower limb are quite literally deep, protected by layers of tissue and surrounded by muscle. The muscle layers also serve as part of the pump mechanism for moving the blood uphill against gravity back to the heart. The deep veins of the legs possess probably the greatest number of valves of all the veins in the body. This is part of the problem; there are more valves that may be damaged and rendered incompetent by the inflammatory process.

Diagnosis. The commonest site in the deep veins for the development of thrombophlebitis is in the veins of the calf, especially those in the soleus muscle, one of the larger muscles of the calf of the leg. Swelling of the leg and tenderness when the calf muscles are squeezed are two of the cardinal warnings of the presence of deep vein thrombosis. But signs and symptoms can differ, depending on the veins involved.

A number of sophisticated diagnostic techniques are available to aid in detecting the presence of clots in the deep leg veins. These include phlebography (X-ray studies to visualize the veins of the limb) and ultrasound, which can pinpoint by an echoing process the location of a blood clot in a vein. The latter test is usually the most accurate in determining the presence of deep vein thrombosis.

Treatment. When nonoperative therapy is selected or when it is not possible or feasible to operate, after an initial short period of bed rest the treatment is composed of daily walking and bandaging the leg with an elastic support or a well-fitting elastic stocking. Aspirin or one of the antiblood-clotting agents such as heparin or coumarin are also administered. Agents such as streptokinase are sometimes administered to accelerate the dissolving of the clot by the body's own mecha-

nisms. Both of these types of drugs act on the entire bloodstream, so the patient must be carefully monitored while drugs are being taken. The form of treatment that is chosen depends upon various factors including the severity and extent of the condition, the amount of debility, the general state of the patient's health, and other factors such as pregnancy.

Treating thrombophlebitis aggressively by surgery soon after onset may prevent spread of the inflammation in the vein and its accompanying clot formation. It can also convert a long, incapacitating illness into a short and comparatively benign one.

Therapy has two basic goals. The first is alleviation of the cause of the disease, specifically the stagnation in venous blood flow. The second is prevention of the serious complications. The use of anticlotting agents such as heparin or the coumarin group of drugs serves the latter purpose but falls short of the first objective. These agents also have several important disadvantages. Their use requires a protracted period of hospitalization and extended and carefully supervised therapy ranging from six weeks to many months. In addition, this form of treatment does not remove or alter the underlying cause of the problem—the presence of varicose veins—which subjects the individual to recurring attacks of thrombophlebitis. As many as 25% of patients experience recurrence once therapy is stopped.

Surgery removes the underlying cause, thereby eliminating the source of repeated episodes of phlebitis and thrombophlebitis. It also shortens the recuperation time and has a lower incidence of progression to fatal complications.

—Howard C. Baron, M.D.

Irritable Bowel Syndrome

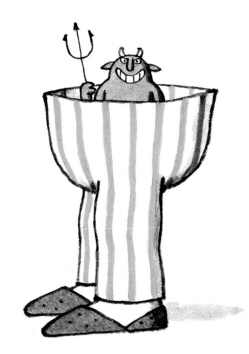

Irritable bowel syndrome is a disorder of the digestive system. The chief symptoms include lower abdominal pain and some disturbance in bowel habit, which may be constipation, diarrhea, or some combination of the two. The clinical diagnosis of irritable bowel syndrome depends upon the careful exclusion of all diseases that cause similar symptoms.

Irritable bowel syndrome has been called by many other names, including colitis, mucous colitis, spastic colitis, spastic bowel, and functional bowel disease. Many of these terms are unfortunate choices since the word colitis means inflammation of the colon, a finding that is not present in this disease. It must be stressed that there is no inflammation in irritable bowel syndrome and that the disorder should not be confused with the more serious ulcerative colitis. The term functional bowel syndrome is a broad classification of all gastrointestinal ailments in which there is impaired function but no organic inflammation or malignancy. Irritable bowel syndrome is one type of functional bowel disorder.

Symptoms

Irritable bowel syndrome is a common disorder. Many people have a mild form of this condition and do not seek medical help. It may take the form of severe diarrhea preceding an examination in school or an anticipated stressful interview. It may also manifest itself as occasional abdominal cramps. When the symptoms become persistent, many people consult their physicians. Irritable bowel syndrome is one of the most common disorders for which medical care is sought.

Normal bowel habit is a function that is difficult to define. In Western civilization normal bowel function averages at least three bowel movements per week. These normal movements are formed without blood and passed without cramps or pain. By contrast, people suffering from irritable bowel syndrome most commonly have some combination of pain, constipation, and diarrhea. Most have periodic episodes of lower abdominal crampy pain associated with prolonged periods of constipation, followed by episodes of severe diarrhea. Others may have considerable pain and only mild constipation. The rarest form of the disorder is severe painless diarrhea. A person suffering from this type may have eight to ten watery bowel movements after breakfast followed by other episodes of diarrhea after meals; this may occur following stressful events or just unex-

pectedly. Individuals with predominant constipation may resort to taking large quantities of laxatives or enemas, while others may have to depend upon frequent doses of antidiarrheal medication to control their symptoms.

It is important to emphasize that although irritable bowel syndrome is usually a mild annoyance for most people, it can be a severe disabling problem for some. Those in the latter group may be afraid to go to dinner parties, seek employment, or travel on public transportation.

Diagnosis

Irritable bowel syndrome is a diagnosis based on clinical symptoms along with the exclusion of serious organic bowel problems. The exclusion of other bowel disorders requires several tests and a physical examination. These tests are done for the sole purpose of exclusion and not to find any specific hallmark of irritable bowel disease.

The medical examination consists of a history, physical examination, and laboratory tests. The history focuses on the symptoms of irritable bowel syndrome and the degree of discomfort caused by this condition. Specific historical features will also be sought. Chief among these is the first appearance of symptoms. Irritable bowel syndrome is a chronic disorder beginning early in life, usually childhood, and does not have an abrupt onset. The appearance of symptoms late in life or symptoms beginning abruptly in an otherwise asymptomatic individual should raise suspicion of another problem. Other symptoms that are not part of the irritable bowel include rectal bleeding, continuous

363

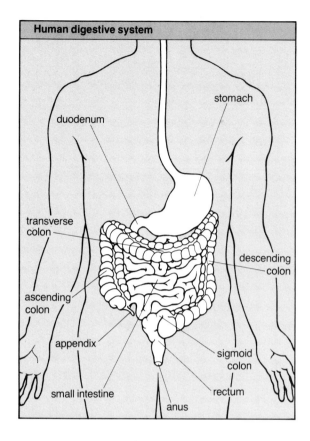

Human digestive system

stomach

duodenum

transverse colon

descending colon

ascending colon

appendix

small intestine

sigmoid colon

rectum

anus

to the naked eye and many times requires specific tests in order to identify it. It may be a sign of a malignancy, ulcerative colitis, or some infectious agent.

The stool specimen may also be subjected to a bacterial culture and a microscopic examination. The culture may reveal bacteria that cause abdominal pain, fever, and diarrhea. Microscopic examination may detect certain parasites that cause diarrhea or abdominal pain. The microscopic examination may also reveal large amounts of fat in the stool if special stains are used. Fat in large quantities is a sign of diseases causing malabsorption, a serious condition leading to diarrhea and weight loss.

The physician usually will perform a sigmoidoscopy in patients with altered bowel function. The sigmoidoscope, or proctoscope, is an instrument that is passed into the lower bowel through the anus. Either a rigid tube 25 cm (10 in) in length or a flexible fiber-optic instrument 60 cm (23 in) in length, it allows clinical and visual observation of the bowel lining (mucosa). The physician inspects for tumors, polyps, or mucosal inflammation, which makes its presence known by bleeding, swelling, or ulceration.

Radiographic studies of the intestinal tract may also be performed. A barium enema allows visualization of the entire colon or large bowel, whereas an upper gastrointestinal X-ray allows viewing of the esophagus, stomach, and small bowel. These studies are done to exclude other diseases and are normal in diagnosis of irritable bowel syndrome.

In summary, then, a complete history, physical examination, and specific laboratory studies allow the physician to diagnose other bowel disorders that may mimic irritable bowel syndrome. Such a procedure is required on at least one occasion but need not be repeated unless symptoms change. A person with irritable bowel syndrome should recognize the need for undergoing this examination in order to exclude other causes of bowel symptoms.

Causes of the syndrome

Despite many studies the cause of irritable bowel syndrome remains unknown. However, recent research has determined the causes of many of the symptoms.

Most symptoms are related to an abnormal pattern of motion (motility) of the large intestine (colon). The colon is the area of bowel approximately 1.5 m (5 ft) in length between the small intestine and the anus. Its major functions are the absorption of water and electrolytes (salts) from the digestive products entering from the small intestine and the storage of this fecal residue until defecation. Large quantities of liquid material enter the colon at its initial point, the cecum. This matter may remain there for several days, during which most of it is absorbed into the body. The fecal material passes through the colon by means of a delicately integrated process of motility. When this motility pat-

(noncrampy or nonepisodic) pain, weight loss, fever, and nocturnal discomfort. It is important to determine whether there is a family history of ulcerative colitis or Crohn's disease (regional enteritis) because some of these serious conditions tend to be clustered in families. Also, a recent history of foreign travel or drinking from a stream may lead to a diagnosis of an infectious cause of diarrhea.

During the physical examination the physician will look for evidence of some organic disease leading to diarrhea. The presence of an abdominal mass, an area of severe abdominal tenderness, blood in the rectum, or abnormal openings (fistulas) near the anal region will lead the physician to a diagnosis of other causes of abnormal bowel function. On occasion, changes in skin pigmentation, rashes, or skin bruises will also lead to a diagnosis of conditions other than the irritable bowel syndrome.

A thorough medical examination will also include several laboratory tests. Routine blood studies such as a blood count should be entirely normal. Anemia may be present in diseases in which gastrointestinal blood loss or the failure to absorb certain nutrients may also cause disordered bowel function. The stool in irritable bowel syndrome should be normal, with no blood present. Blood in the stool is a serious finding and may indicate other causes of abdominal pain or altered bowel function. Blood in the stool may not be apparent

tern is upset, cramps, constipation, or diarrhea may ensue. The motility of the colon is controlled by nerve and hormone activity upon the smooth muscle of the colon.

The normal pattern of motility is further controlled by changes in the electric potential of the colon muscle. These changes serve as a pacemaker similar to one controlling heart function. The colon propels the fecal residue slowly back and forth but mainly forward toward the rectum, the end part of the large intestine. The colon also has periodic segmental contractions that help to remove water from the feces.

In patients with irritable bowel syndrome the muscle of the lower portion of the colon undergoes abnormal types of contractions or spasms. These abnormal motions, which are exaggerations of the normal segmental contractions, are powerful spasms that are closely correlated with the episodic cramps or abdominal pain experienced in this disorder. They cause marked delay in passage of the fecal material, leading to prolonged mucosal contact and further absorption of water. The end result of this process is constipation with firm stools. In some patients abnormal patterns of contraction lead to rapid passage of feces and impaired water absorption, resulting in diarrhea.

The cause of abnormal colon motility in patients with irritable bowel syndrome is believed to be abnormal electrical activity in the large intestine. This abnormality is always present, but symptoms occur only when the bowel muscle is excited to contract. In this latter statement lies the explanation of the fluctuating symptoms of this disease. The bowel disorder is always present, but its potential for causing spasm or pain requires some inciting factor—usually diet or emotional stress. Most individuals relate that their symptoms follow a meal or occur when they are under stress.

Eating causes contraction of the colon by a response known as the gastrocolic reflex, which occurs by virtue of the actions of both nerves and hormones on the colon muscle. Normally this reflex provides the urge to have a bowel movement within 30 to 60 minutes after a meal. In patients with irritable bowel syndrome the gastrocolic reflex following a meal leads to cramps and possibly diarrhea. The magnitude of this response is directly related to the caloric content of the meal, especially the fat content. Fat in the form of oils, animal fat, or butter is the most important stimulus to colonic contraction. By contrast, sugars and dietary protein have minimal effect on the colon. Stress also stimulates abnormal colonic contractions in irritable bowel syndrome because the colon is controlled by neural elements influenced by the brain.

The recent progress in understanding irritable bowel syndrome has focused on the colon motility disorder rather than the psychological component of this condition. However, it must be understood that some patients with irritable bowel syndrome have psychological

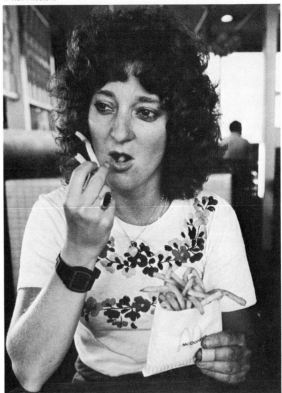

Sufferers of irritable bowel syndrome soon learn which foods are likely to precipitate an episode. Especially suspect are greasy fried foods.

problems and that treating those disorders may improve bowel symptoms.

Treatment

The treatment of irritable bowel syndrome may proceed in a logical and successful manner if the disorder is understood. Failure to understand it may lead to continued discomfort and frustration.

First, it must be realized that the irritable bowel syndrome is a chronic disorder marked by remissions and flare-ups. Its treatment is directed at symptom prevention and control. Presently cure is not possible. Thus, symptoms of irritable bowel syndrome may recur over a lifetime. Those suffering from the disorder must understand the nature of their illness and not continuously seek some simple cure. A sympathetic and knowledgeable physician should be consulted. In follow-up care other possible disorders superimposed upon irritable bowel syndrome must not be missed. If the nature of the abdominal pain should worsen or if bowel symptoms should change, medical help should be sought. New symptoms such as rectal bleeding, weight loss, fever, or weakness must be evaluated and not attributed to irritable bowel syndrome.

Victims of irritable bowel syndrome should not depend upon laxatives or enemas to treat constipation or antidiarrheals for diarrhea. Many individuals have become dependent upon laxatives and after many years of use have lost all normal bowel function and sensation. Long-term use of laxatives may also damage the nerves of the colon, leading to a condition called cathartic colon.

Since most symptoms are related to diet and emotional stress, these factors should be controlled as well as possible. Any specific dietary ingredient that an individual believes causes symptoms should be avoided if possible. Milk products, for example, may contribute to irritable bowel syndrome in persons with lactose intolerance. In this condition lactose in milk is not digested in the small bowel, causing gas to be formed in the colon. Large meals may induce attacks of pain and diarrhea and should be avoided. A diet low in fat, fried foods, or oils would be helpful in reducing the gastrocolic response. Small feedings of protein and carbohydrate are best for the person with irritable bowel syndrome.

Dietary bulk in the form of bran, fruits, vegetables, and cereals has been helpful in alleviating symptoms. Bulk diets keep the colon mildly distended, thus preventing pockets of high pressure that cause spasm from developing. Bulk also keeps water in the feces and prevents hard stools from forming. The amount of dietary bulk should be regulated to allow for a soft, easily passed stool without associated cramps. Many patients with irritable bowel syndrome do remarkably well when they follow this type of diet.

Stressful situations can trigger attacks of pain and diarrhea. However, avoidance of stress is difficult for most people. Recognition of the relationship between stressful events and the onset of bowel symptoms has been helpful in some cases in which the environment can be controlled to eliminate the stressful factors. For some persons with stress-related bowel symptoms tranquilizers have been used. Although they have been helpful in many cases, it must be recognized that a chronic disorder such as irritable bowel syndrome may lead to drug abuse.

Because the symptoms of irritable bowel syndrome are due to abnormal contractions of the colon, antispasmodic drugs are often used. These drugs do not remove the factor that causes the bowel spasm but simply reduce the force of the spasm. Sometimes the antispasmodic and tranquilizer agents are combined in one tablet. In general, it would be best to treat the irritable bowel syndrome with education, diet restrictions, and bulk materials before using either antispasmodic drugs or tranquilizers. In some cases, however, drugs must be used to control symptoms.

Complications

Irritable bowel syndrome usually has no serious complications. Some physicians believe that it leads to colonic diverticulosis (small outpouchings of the bowel wall) later in life, but this association has not been proved. Irritable bowel syndrome does not lead to cancer of the bowel or inflammatory bowel disorders such as ulcerative colitis.

The major complications associated with this condition relate to social problems and drug overuse. Many sufferers become fearful of travel or social events because of possible diarrhea or pain. Others may become dependent on laxatives or tranquilizers.

In conclusion, irritable bowel syndrome is a common condition presenting symptoms of abdominal pain and altered bowel function. Its diagnosis depends upon the exclusion of other conditions that may cause similar symptoms. In general, it is a benign but chronic disorder that leads to no serious complications. Treatment of the syndrome depends mostly on an understanding of the nature of the illness. Satisfactory control of symptoms can be achieved with some dietary restrictions, the use of high-bulk food, and, in some cases, the proper prescription of drugs.

—Sidney Cohen, M.D.

Labor

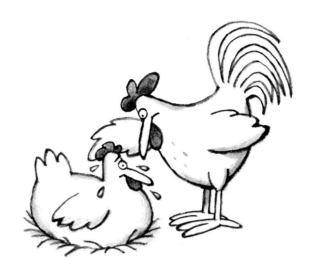

Pregnancy and the prospect of motherhood are positive, joyful experiences for most women. Yet few events in a woman's life subject her to more emotional and physical stress than the labor of giving birth. Part of this paradox rests on conflicting views of the events that end pregnancy and begin parenthood, collectively known as parturition. Some cultures glorify the laboring woman who remains stoic and isolated; others expect her to be active and vocal. Some religions and moral traditions describe the process as a punishment without meaning if unaccompanied by pain and fear. And in modern times, of course, the "rituals" of birth reflect the technological age. The process has been "medicalized," sterilized, and institutionalized. The other part of the paradox rests in reality. Labor and birth *are* stressful and carry intrinsic danger. There is pain involved, and labor requires strength-sapping hard work.

Advances in prenatal care, anesthesia, surgery, antibiotics, X-rays, sanitation, and nutrition have, of course, reduced the risks of childbirth. Fifty years ago 67 of every 10,000 mothers in the U.S. died in childbirth. Today the figure is fewer than 10 per 100,000, according to the National Center for Health Statistics.

There is no question that childbirth produces anxiety for millions of women. The usual hospital birth experience, especially for the first-time mother, found the woman in labor separated from her family and husband and overwhelmed by an unfamiliar and sterile atmosphere. She was overtaken by a series of events that she neither anticipated nor understood, fearful for her health and the welfare of her child.

Although childbearing is an almost universal female experience, each woman experiences it individually. Because individuals differ in their needs, there is no single "formula" for a perfect birth experience. What each woman can do to make the birth of her child joyful and fulfilling is to learn all she can about the events that are about to take place and how she can control the atmosphere and the sequence of events.

Preparing for childbirth

An estimated 30% of all pregnant women in the U.S. now take classes that offer detailed information, exercises, and instruction about parturition. Sometimes called psychoprophylaxis, prepared childbirth, natural childbirth, or Lamaze method, these childbirth education programs have also changed the way hospitals, nurses, and physicians care for women in labor. More

attention is being paid to the psychological needs of mother, father, and newborn.

Today, training for childbirth calls for exercises to tone abdominal and pelvic floor muscles, along with breathing and relaxation techniques that adjust the mother's physical and emotional activities during the stages of labor. Elisabeth Bing, a founder of the American Society for Psychoprophylaxis in Obstetrics, has taught prenatal exercises to thousands of women. She explains that the focus on breathing teaches the mother to "synchronize . . . respiration to the signals that you receive from the uterus. The strenuous activity will create a new center of concentration in the brain, thereby causing the painful sensations during labor to become peripheral, to reduce their intensity. The breathing will not only serve . . . as a focal point. It will, at the same time, bring a good deal of oxygen to the baby who needs this . . . as it is being squeezed and oxygen supply is diminished while the uterus is contracting. Furthermore, the uterine muscles need added amounts of oxygen in order to work efficiently."

In the 1930s Grantly Dick-Read, a British physician, was the first to widely publicize the idea that the pain encountered in labor was caused mostly by fear. His well-known book *Childbirth Without Fear*, first published in the U.S. in 1947, introduced thousands of prospective parents to the concept of prepared birth. Fernand Lamaze and others advanced the idea, and few in the medical profession now dispute its wisdom.

Basic good health, physical fitness, a positive attitude, emotional support, and breathing and relaxation skills cannot entirely eliminate the pain or risks of labor. Studies suggest, however, that there is less risk of birth injury, premature delivery, prolonged labor, and excessive bleeding with prepared childbirth.

The stages of labor

Data collected from studies of thousands of births have indicated that for a first baby labor usually takes between 8 and 12 hours, and about half that time for subsequent babies. Rapid labors, those under two hours, are rare and are more likely to tear tissues in the birth canal. A gradual, progressive labor is easier on both mother and child.

What triggers labor is still imperfectly understood, but sometime between the 38th and 40th weeks of pregnancy, oxytocin and other hormones set off the process by which the muscular uterus contracts and propels the baby out through the vagina. Some women about to go into labor discharge from the cervix a mucus plug, a clear watery material, or a small amount of reddish discharge known as "show." This indicates that the membranes surrounding the fetus are about to rupture. Nine out of ten women go into labor within 24 hours of the rupture of the membranes. These membranes are the amniotic sac that surrounds and contains the amniotic fluid; the rupture is sometimes referred to as "breaking the bag of waters." In some labors the membranes remain intact until the labor is well advanced, while in others the rupture takes place several days prematurely.

Labor is divided into three stages or phases. During the first stage the uterus begins to contract on its own and pull at its cervix, the "bottleneck" end of the organ which leads into the vagina. In order for the baby to pass out of the uterus, the cervix must become soft, thinned out, and flat, a process known as effacement. This process may begin a few weeks before the onset of true labor with painless, occasional contractions called Braxton Hicks contractions, or Hicks's sign (named for the English gynecologist who first described them).

After the effacement the first-time mother may experience "lightening." As the baby's head moves down in the pelvis against the cervix (a movement known as "engagement"), more room is left in the abdomen for the pregnant woman to breathe. There is less sense of fullness and a "lighter," less pregnant feeling. The new position of the fetus's head, however, puts pressure on the bladder, so the woman feels the need to urinate more frequently.

As the true first stage of labor gets under way, labor pains will be felt. These are caused by forceful contractions of the uterus that dilate, or open, the cervix to approximately ten centimeters in diameter (four to five inches) to let the baby's head go through.

The contractions of actual labor generally start 20 to 30 minutes apart, becoming stronger and closer together. Exercises that let the laboring woman relax all of her voluntary muscles may help if begun while the contraction builds to a peak and then drops off. False labor does sometimes occur, with contractions seeming to become more intense. A good way to distinguish them from the real thing is to move around or change activity. Real labor will progress in such a case, while false labor will stop.

As the fully active phase of labor gets under way (at about the time the cervix is three centimeters dilated), contractions are intense enough and close enough together so that the woman can no longer walk around or talk comfortably through them. Unless a home birth has been planned, this is usually the time to go to the hospital. It is not the best time to move around for the laboring woman, and labor may actually stop during travel, admission, and examinations. The prospective parents should prepare for the stress and plan ahead to cope with it. They should take pillows to prop and support the abdomen and legs during the trip, have the hospital bag packed, and arrangements for such things as the care of older children or pets in order.

Throughout the labor the mother's blood pressure, pulse, and temperature will be monitored. Nurses or physicians listen to fetal heart sounds and check the mother's abdomen. Periodic internal examinations via the vagina and rectum will monitor the progress of the labor. Many hospitals routinely attach an electronic monitor to the fetus's scalp through the vagina to constantly assess heart rate, respiration, and general status. In the first stage the baby's head has moved down into the pelvis. Late in this stage, when the cervix is fully dilated, the mother can begin to help push the baby out.

Contractions during the first stage slowly accelerate from mild to moderate (about 20 seconds in length and 5 to 20 minutes apart) to those lasting 40 to 50 seconds and occurring two to four minutes apart. In 20% of all births the amniotic membranes break in this stage of labor. If by the time the cervix is well dilated the membranes are still intact, the physician can easily and painlessly break them to improve the quality of contractions and shorten labor. Toward the end of the first stage, a period known as transition, the contractions may last up to 90 seconds and occur 30 to 90 seconds apart. During this time the cervix is dilating to its maximum.

The slow wave of a contraction now becomes long and strong, with several peaks. For most women, this is the toughest part of labor and the most uncomfortable. But it is also, for most women, the shortest, usually lasting less than an hour.

The second stage of labor begins when the cervical dilation is complete and the baby's head begins to enter the vaginal canal. This stage may last from one half hour up to two hours. The work of the uterus is now aided by the mother's voluntary efforts to contract the muscles in her lower abdomen and "bear down" or push. At the same time, the uterus pushes against the baby's buttocks with each contraction and helps move the baby down and out.

As soon as the head becomes visible in the vaginal opening, the baby has "crowned." At this time the physician may make a small cut, or episiotomy, under local anesthetic to enlarge the opening to help the baby pass through without tearing the vaginal walls. The doctor may also help rotate the baby's shoulders through the birth canal, after which the rest of the body slips out easily. Later a few stitches repair the cut, which heals quickly and without jagged edges. The second stage of labor ends when the newborn baby has been separated from the umbilical cord.

In the third stage the placenta and the fetal membranes are expelled. This so-called afterbirth is "born" the same way as the baby, as the uterus contracts to expel it. Rarely does the third stage last more than ten minutes. If the placenta has not been delivered within half an hour, the physician usually removes it manually after the mother is anesthetized. The uterus will continue to contract occasionally after delivery, sometimes for several hours or days.

Options for delivery

For women at high risk of complications during labor, regional or urban medical centers today have advanced technological obstetrical facilities. These services have been a tremendous boon to very young women, older women, women who expect multiple infants, women in premature labor (babies born too early are at higher risk for respiratory and central nervous system disorders), and women with diabetes, hypertension, or toxemia. The latter is a condition in which blood pressure skyrockets and threatens the blood and oxygen supply of the infant.

Research supporting the safety and benefits of less "medicalized" childbirth has led some women to choose to give birth in alternative birth centers in hospitals, and some opt for planned home births. In response to the demand by women for more personal, comfortable, and natural labor, hospital maternity units began several years ago to set aside special birthing rooms or suites. No electronic monitors, enemas, forceps, routine episiotomies, intravenous solutions, isolation, or other intrusions into the labor process are introduced unless there is clear medical need.

Many of these units have special beds that allow a woman to remain upright or semiupright during labor and delivery, positions that are often more comfortable and safer for both mother and child. Others have trained nurse-midwives on staff, homelike rooms with meal service, television sets, and curtained windows. The laboring mother can be attended by husband, parents, friends, and even older children.

Prospective parents should know that while such services are growing in the United States, they are by no means universal, nor are they meant for everyone. By some estimates only a third of women qualify, for medical or emotional reasons, for alternative birth center care. Other women are fearful and feel more secure with monitoring and more intensive hospital care. Some obstetricians have neither interest in nor training for alternative birth care. Without properly trained health personnel, alternative birth care can be risky.

The American College of Obstetricians and Gynecologists (ACOG) vigorously opposes home deliveries, despite a growing movement in favor of them. Their opposition is based on the possibility of the sudden development of life-threatening complications for mother or fetus. Home births are possible in some areas, attended by nurse-midwives or physicians. Only low-risk, well-prepared women are considered good candidates for home deliveries.

Analgesics and anesthesia

Perhaps no subject is of more interest to the woman about to have a baby than labor pain. A generation ago, women in labor often routinely received drugs, sometimes to the extent that they were unable to participate in or even remember the experience. Some obstetricians encouraged the heavy use of drugs and anesthetics because they believed it was easier on the mother and child. But recent research has confirmed that all drugs given during labor and delivery may be risky to the fetus or the mother or both.

There are times when anesthetics and analgesics are both appropriate and reasonably safe. If a woman is in serious pain, or fears that she will be, she should not feel guilty or ashamed to ask for and even demand sedation or anesthesia. Not all women—or all pain thresholds—are alike. The rule of thumb, however, is that the less anesthesia (which causes loss of consciousness) or analgesia (which causes pain relief) used during labor and birth, the better.

Narcotics or tranquilizers in the first stage of labor can help a mother relax and rest between contractions. Too much, however, can prolong the labor, and narcotics may depress the baby's bodily functions.

During the most active stages of labor, women may receive an epidural or caudal anesthetic. A needle is inserted into the back near the spinal canal (not in it), and a drug is injected that numbs the area from the waist down. Epidurals and caudals generally eliminate all pain. But they do have drawbacks. First, their administration requires highly skilled practitioners, preferably anesthesiologists, to assure safety. Some women are allergic to the drugs used, so the doctor should be informed about sensitivity to novocaine or similar medications. The numbing may also decrease blood pressure, requiring intravenous fluids to maintain blood volume in the vessels. Finally, these anesthetics frequently make a forceps delivery and episiotomies necessary, because the inability to feel makes pushing harder. Forceps deliveries, in which an instrument with curved blades is inserted into the birth canal to pull the baby down and out, are often lifesaving and necessary to prevent complications. But their use carries risk of bruising and damage to the infant's head and brain and to the mother's vaginal canal.

Other means of pain relief include a "saddle block"

(injection of anesthetic into the spinal canal, which numbs the area that on a horseback rider makes contact with the saddle), nitrous oxide gas (light doses lessen pain but do not put the patient totally to sleep), pudendal block (a deadening of the nerves in the area around the vagina just before delivery, especially if episiotomy and forceps are used), and paracervical block (injection of anesthetic into the tissues adjacent to the cervix). Paracervical blocks are no longer used widely, as the drug can be absorbed by the fetus.

Possible complications

Despite every precaution, problems and unexpected procedures can occur during labor and delivery. Parents-to-be are likely to hear most about the following:

Placenta previa. In this condition the placenta is between the cervix and fetus, covering the cervix and increasing the risk of severe, sometimes fatal, bleeding before birth. Painless vaginal bleeding during the last weeks of pregnancy is often a symptom.

Abruptio placentae. This condition occurs when the placenta begins to pull away from the uterus before delivery. It may cause heavy bleeding and severe pain. Half of all patients who develop abruptio placentae have high blood pressure. Sometimes the condition requires the induction of labor if the pregnancy is at term. If symptoms are severe, cesarean section is often necessary to save the baby.

Incompetent cervix. This condition simply refers to the inability of the cervix to stay tightly shut until just before birth. If it loses strength and opens, labor may begin prematurely. Early diagnosis and treatment (usually bed rest and the insertion of stitches to tighten the opening) can avert early labor in most cases.

Premature labor and delivery. If labor begins before the baby has matured, there is increased likelihood that the baby will be born with physical and mental handicaps. Sometimes these are minor, but at times the lungs are so immature that the brain is damaged seriously by lack of oxygen. Although infants born before 36 weeks of pregnancy make up fewer than 10% of all babies born in the U.S., they account for 75% of newborn deaths and 50% of all brain-damaged infants. Good prenatal care is the best way to prevent premature labor, since medical conditions associated with it can often be detected early enough for intervention.

Cesarean section. This involves surgically cutting through the abdomen to remove a baby from the womb. It is called for if the baby's head fails to engage after a reasonable time, if the head is too large to get through the pelvic opening, if there is a breech (feet or buttocks first) presentation, if the baby's heart rate is severely depressed or irregular, if the mother is sick, or if the uterus has been damaged by surgery or disease.

Induction of labor. Occasionally, as in the case of abruptio placentae, doctors must begin the process of labor in order to protect the baby and the mother. In the past many doctors induced labor with injections of oxytocin, which stimulates contractions, or by breaking the bag of waters. This was done primarily so that the doctor and the mother could schedule the birth at a convenient time. Research now confirms that induction of labor is at best a very risky procedure, to be done only for medical, and not "convenience," reasons.

Some common misinformation

Preparation for childbirth will dispel many myths and misconceptions, but old wives' tales seem to persist with a life of their own. Still widely held is the belief that once a woman has had a cesarean section, all of her subsequent children must be born that way. The ACOG, supported by several studies, has stated that many women may have normal vaginal deliveries after one or even multiple cesareans.

Another common misconception is that there are some drugs used in obstetrics that never reach the fetus. There is no such drug. All drugs, including those used for epidurals, cross the placenta. Behavior tests on newborns have found that these drugs decrease responsiveness in a baby for up to a week after birth.

Contrary to wide belief, forceps delivery is not always preferable to cesarean section. Many obstetricians agree surgery is preferable to high forceps delivery—applied before the cervix is fully dilated—to prevent prolonged force on the baby's head. Mid-forceps deliveries are falling out of favor for similar reasons.

Cesarean sections are also the subject of misinformation. They have become so common that the impression exists that they are no more dangerous than an appendectomy. The fact is that these operations cause infections in about half of all instances, including cystitis and abscesses. They are often accompanied by serious bleeding, adhesions from scar tissue, blood transfusion complications, heart complications, and even death. For the infant, cesarean sections may bring on jaundice, lung problems, and complications from anesthesia. Cesareans can be lifesaving for both mother and baby, but they are a major surgery and require a prolonged period of recuperation.

Resources for information

The following organizations can provide helpful information about prepared childbirth:

American Society for Psychoprophylaxis in Obstetrics, 1411 K St. NW, Suite 200 Washington, D.C. 20005.

International Childbirth Education Association, P.O. Box 20048, Minneapolis, Minn. 55420.

American College of Nurse-Midwives, 1522 K St. NW, Suite 1120, Washington, D.C. 20005.

Childbirth Without Pain Education Association, 20134 Snowden, Detroit, Mich. 48235.

—Joann E. Rodgers

Motion Sickness

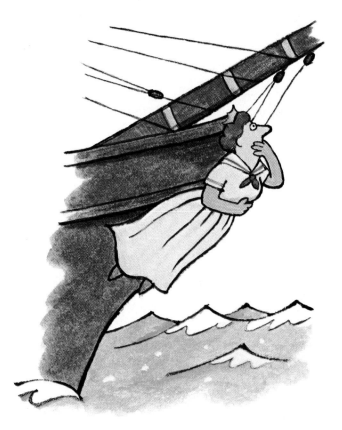

Nearly everyone has experienced, at least once, some or all of the symptoms of dizziness, perspiration, nausea, vomiting, increased salivation, yawning, and generalized malaise that make up the syndrome called motion sickness. Although a great deal of variation exists among individuals in their susceptibility to this affliction, nearly everyone will develop symptoms with the appropriate stimulation. Much of our knowledge about motion sickness is a by-product of the space program and the need to understand the reaction of the human body to weightlessness and the forces of acceleration. Concern with motion sickness, however, extends far back before the space age to man's first experience with an environment of motion. Seasickness, airsickness, and carsickness are all forms of motion sickness.

Motion sickness not only ruins vacation cruises and Sunday drives but has far more serious consequences as well. For example, a commander waiting with his troops in a small landing craft before a beach assault knows that some of his men will be incapacitated by motion sickness and contribute to the casualty rate. At its worst, prolonged, untreated motion sickness can drain the body of fluids and electrolytes and lead to prostration and death. Even experienced flyers and sailors are not immune. During the Apollo missions to the Moon astronauts experienced symptoms ranging from stomach awareness to vomiting and, more recently, crew members on the first space shuttle flights were similarly afflicted. It is reputed that the renowned British naval commander Lord Nelson was frequently plagued by seasickness, that Julius Caesar refused to travel by ship, and that Lawrence of Arabia got sick riding a camel.

Causes

Although the precise cause of motion sickness remains a mystery, a good deal is known about the body's response to motion and about those parts that are critical to the development or avoidance of motion sickness. In the 19th century it was thought that the stomach was the source of the malady, a logical idea since nausea and vomiting are among the most distressing symptoms. It is now recognized that the inner ear is the culprit.

The human inner ear has two anatomical and functional divisions. The cochlear portion is responsible for hearing, and the vestibular portion is responsible for balance or equilibrium. The vestibular portion consists of three semicircular canals, each in a plane at right angles to the planes of the other two canals. These canals are tubular, fluid-filled structures about one centimeter across and as thin as a pencil lead. In addition to the fluid, each canal contains a specialized nerve structure designed to perceive motion of the fluid. That motion results from the inertia of the fluid: as the head rotates in a plane of a canal, the fluid within lags behind. In addition to the semicircular canals two other structures in each ear are sensitive to linear motion, the utricle and the saccule, which are sometimes termed gravity receptors. Signals from the vestibular part of each ear are sent to the brain, where they are integrated with signals from the eyes and from special nerves that end in the joints of the neck, arms, and legs and other places where bones meet. All of these impulses are put together to give the body a feeling of where it is at any given moment with respect to the environment and to gravity in particular.

Vision, proprioception (the sensations coming from the joints), and the vestibular portion of the inner ear all contribute information, but it is the inner ear that is most important. Although nearly everyone will develop symptoms of motion sickness with the appropriate stimulus, one noticeable exception is the individual

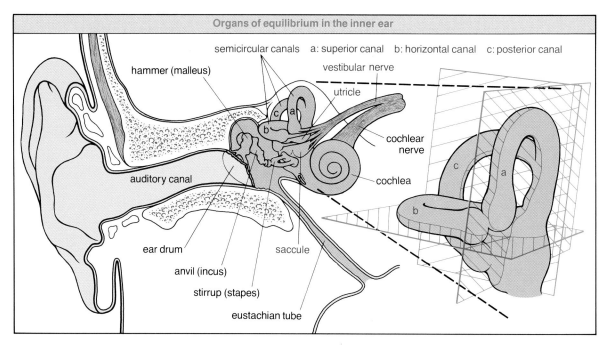

semicircular canals   a: superior canal   b: horizontal canal   c: posterior canal

hammer (malleus)

vestibular nerve

utricle

cochlear nerve

cochlea

auditory canal

ear drum

anvil (incus)

saccule

stirrup (stapes)

eustachian tube

The semicircular canals of the inner ear, three tiny, fluid-filled, tubular structures that lie at right angles to each other, are responsible for the maintenance of balance. This enables a person to maintain his equilibrium even with his eyes closed. One theory is that overstimulation of the nerves serving this area causes motion sickness.

born with a congenital absence or malformation of the inner ear. Congenitally deaf individuals have been shown to be immune to motion sickness.

Two theories try to explain motion sickness. The first uses the idea of overstimulation of the vestibular system, while the second involves the concept of conflicting information being sent to the brain from the eyes, ears, and joints. Neither theory is completely successful, but they do help people understand what situations are particularly likely to produce motion sickness and what can be done to avoid it. How these theories and other findings may apply can be illustrated in seasickness. On the ocean or any large body of water the movement of a floating object such as a boat is complex, with vertical, fore-and-aft, and side-to-side motion often occurring simultaneously. Such action stimulates all six semicircular canals (three per ear); the joints undergo constant change as muscles adjust to maintain stable body position; and the eyes look for a plane of reference. A person is more likely to become seasick below deck with no stable reference such as the horizon. On deck, a sailor with the stable horizon in view is able to see the rise and fall of the boat as well as feel it, and the messages received by the brain from all three systems agree. Unfortunately, if the motion stimulus is great enough, seasickness may still prevail.

The nausea and vomiting that are so distressing result from stimulation of the digestive tract by the autonomic nervous system and are due in part to the nearness in the brain stem of the nuclei (clusters of nerve

cell bodies) of the vestibular and vagus nerves. The vestibular nerve carries impulses from the vestibular part of the inner ear to the brain, while the vagus nerve supplies nerve fibers to many organs in the body, including the stomach and gut. In the brain stem, where nerve signals are integrated, signals from the vestibular nuclei are thought to "spill over" to the vagal nuclei, stimulating the vagus nerve and thus leading to nausea and vomiting. That these symptoms seem to have no survival role or other benefit to the individual supports the idea that the vagal stimulation is a spillover effect rather than a direct neural pathway.

Some people become motion sick through visual stimulation alone; for example, from watching a movie filmed from an airplane or a roller coaster. It is significant that even in visually induced attacks the ears must be functioning normally for sickness to occur, a requirement that suggests the existence of complex interconnections of the nervous system. In another category is the individual who becomes nauseated merely at the sight of a ship and within whom psychological factors are assumed to be influential.

Prevention and treatment

The best treatment for motion sickness is to escape the motion. If that is impossible or not practical, several other measures can be taken. Lying on the back has been shown to cut the incidence of motion sickness to 20% of that in the sitting position. This measure is particularly effective on ships, trains, and vehicles with

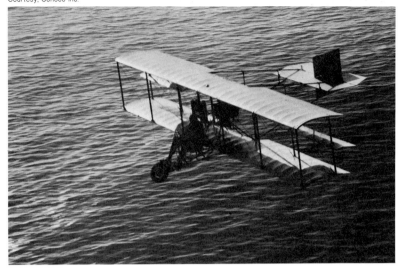

Some people can feel symptoms of motion sickness merely through watching a motion picture of a symptom-inducing situation. The movie To Fly, *shown at the Smithsonian Institution's Air and Space Museum in Washington, D.C., has made many viewers queasy.*

a swinging, side-to-side motion. Immobilizing the head to restrict its movement with respect to the vehicle can further aid in decreasing symptoms in those situations where a view of a stable reference is not possible. When such a reference as the horizon or the road ahead is visible, restricting head movement is not as beneficial. Vision can be a powerful suppressor of motion sickness when it is able to supply stabilizing information, but it is better to close the eyes if the inner ear and eyes are sending conflicting information to the brain. Studies have shown that mental alertness and activity suppress motion sickness in individuals given a mental challenge, while the feeling of sickness is aggravated in individuals asked to concentrate on their perception of motion.

In practical terms these findings mean that a seasick-prone person on a small pleasure boat should stay on deck rather than below and take an active part in sailing or operating the boat. If feasible, the ideal spot

is at the controls, where the helmsman must observe the craft's course, be aware of other boats or obstacles, and be attentive to the operation of the boat. On a large cruise ship, of course, this is not possible, and when conditions may not permit a view of the horizon, it is best to lie quietly on the back with the head still and the eyes closed. Carsickness is least likely for the individual in the front seat looking ahead, down the road, and mentally alert; a driver, in fact, is rarely carsick. On the other hand, a passenger in the back seat with his or her head down and reading may be inviting trouble.

Most people will gradually adapt to prolonged exposure to motion, particularly if the motion is not initially strong. The cerebellum of the brain seems to play a very important role in such adaptation. Laboratory animals experimentally deprived of the cerebellum are unable to adapt. A normal individual who has adapted to one type and intensity of stimulation may still become sick if exposed to a different or more intense

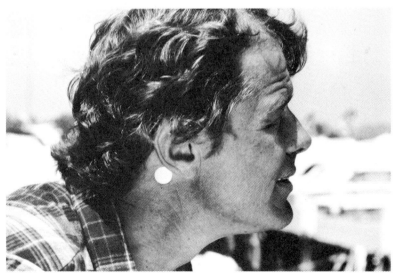

A new pharmaceutical approach to preventing motion sickness makes use of a small patch placed behind the ear. Called the Transderm-Scōp scopolamine therapeutic system, the patch delivers the drug through the skin for up to three days.

stimulation. Hence, travelers who have adjusted well to a sea cruise may still experience an attack if the liner becomes storm tossed or once they take a car trip on land. Unfortunately, for reasons not yet understood some individuals are never able to adapt.

Diet may influence the likelihood of becoming motion sick, but the mechanism is unknown and reports are largely anecdotal. Avoiding heavy, rich, and particularly greasy foods and emphasizing light meals of fruit and vegetables may be helpful. For people planning a sea cruise, this kind of diet should be kept up for a few days before as well as during the trip.

Used properly, drugs are often quite useful in preventing or treating motion sickness. They are generally felt to work best when taken preventively, but even when used optimally they may be less effective than the preventive measures discussed above. Recent research by the U.S. Navy and the National Aeronautics and Space Administration confirmed the effectiveness of some drugs and drug combinations in reducing susceptibility to motion sickness. Two categories of drugs were found useful.

The first includes drugs with antihistamine characteristics and anticholinergic drugs, which affect the central nervous system's response to acetylcholine (an important substance for transmitting nerve signals). The antihistamines in this group include such popular medications as dimenhydrinate (Dramamine), cyclizine (Marezine), meclizine (Bonine, Antivert), and promethazine (Phenergan). Scopolamine, an effective anticholinergic drug that is believed to work on both the inner ear and the vomiting reflex, is not as widely used as the antihistamines because at standard oral doses (0.6 mg), its side effects of drowsiness, dry mouth, and blurred vision are more bothersome. A high percentage of individuals, however, may respond very well to doses of 0.1–0.2 mg and avoid the untoward effects. Dimenhydrinate, cyclizine, and meclizine are all available in over-the-counter remedies for motion sickness.

A second group of medications shown to be effective are those that enhance the activity in the central nervous system of another important nervous system transmitter, norepinephrine. These drugs include dextroamphetamine sulfate (Dexedrine) and ephedrine. Dextroamphetamine, however, is a powerful stimulant and has the potential for abuse, which may limit its use.

For severe conditions either of two combinations of drugs is quite effective, but their relative proportions must be tailored to the individual by a physician. Scopolamine plus dextroamphetamine sulfate or promethazine plus ephedrine will protect most individuals. For moderate conditions dimenhydrinate appears useful based on controlled studies, and such mild conditions as carsickness may respond well to cyclizine or meclizine. As an alternative to oral administration, scopolamine is now available by prescription in the form of a small self-adhesive plastic patch (Transderm-Scōp) that allows the drug to be absorbed continuously and directly through the skin. Studies have indicated that transdermal scopolamine may produce fewer side effects than its oral form, although it apparently is not much more effective against motion sickness than oral dimenhydrinate.

To be effective all medications should be taken at least an hour before exposure to motion and typically must be taken repeatedly every few hours as long as the stimulus persists. Transdermal scopolamine needs 4–16 hours to reach peak effectiveness, but each patch works for about three days. Certain medical conditions may preclude use of one or more of these drugs, making it advisable to seek a physician's advice regarding their use.

Drugs intended to stave off motion sickness frequently are not very effective once an attack has begun, although their sedative side effects can be of some benefit. Medications intended for indigestion or stomach upset are also of little use since gastrointestinal distress is merely a by-product of the real problem.

Currently biofeedback is being explored as an alternative to preventive drug treatment, and some medical investigators view it as a promising long-range answer. Biofeedback, which requires special training, would allow patients control over many of their symptoms by giving them the ability to regulate heartbeat, muscle tension, blood pressure, and other ordinarily involuntary physical phenomena. This approach is still experimental, however, and its usefulness to the general public remains to be demonstrated.

— Rolf F. Ulvestad, M.D.

Hernias

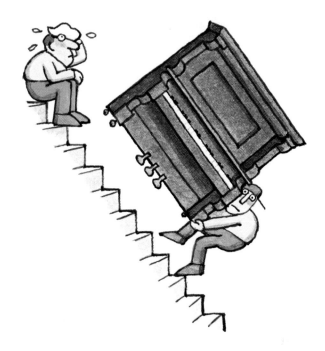

The term hernia is used to describe a weakness or an opening in a layer of tissue that encloses a body cavity. Although there are many types of hernias that affect all parts of the body, most hernias occur in the abdominal wall surrounding the peritoneal cavity. Herniorrhaphy, or surgical hernia repair, is performed on more than 750,000 patients a year in the U.S., making it one of the most common of all surgical procedures.

There are several factors that cause a hernia to appear. Some hernias are congenital, caused by a developmental failure before birth, when tissues that should fuse or narrow fail to close properly. With age, tissues may become weakened or stretched, so that heavy lifting or straining causes the weak area to give way. Other factors that increase the pressure within the abdominal cavity are chronic coughing, straining to defecate (caused by constipation), and straining to urinate (seen especially in older men with enlarged prostates).

The weakened and stretched tissue protruding into the opening is referred to as the hernial sac, which some envision as having ruptured, hence the commonly used (and inaccurate) term rupture. The sac is a stretched portion of the peritoneum, the thin tissue that lines the abdominal cavity. The contents of the hernial sac most commonly are intestines, which produce the characteristic bulge under the skin. If the contents of the sac can be pushed back into the abdominal cavity where they belong, the hernia is referred to as reducible. On the other hand, if the contents become trapped in the sac and cannot be reduced, the hernia is referred to as an incarcerated hernia.

If the contents are twisted or squeezed so tightly that their blood supply is interrupted, the hernia becomes strangulated. Strangulation may lead to gangrene of the sac and its contents. The consequences of a strangulated hernia can be most serious, even fatal; this condition requires a major operation for removal of the dead portion of the intestine and treatment for any infection of the peritoneal cavity. Frequently this operation must be performed as an emergency when the patient is not in optimal physical condition. In addition, because the tissue in the area may be swollen or infected, the likelihood of wound infection increases, and the repair itself cannot be totally secure, with a consequent higher incidence of recurrence of the hernia.

Avoiding this type of emergency operation is the most compelling reason for advocating repair of a hernia at the time it is found, before it becomes incarcerated or strangulated. Such an elective operation certainly carries a smaller risk for the patient. Despite the possibility of significant complications, generally only a small percentage of hernias develop complications. Most patients seek repair of their hernias not because of the risk involved but because hernias produce an annoying dull ache or discomfort or even severe pain. They also may be unsightly. To some patients even a small bulge is unacceptable, while others can tolerate even a swollen hernia that can be seen distorting the trousers.

Inguinal hernia

About 75% of all hernias occur in the inguinal (groin) area. There are several reasons why hernias occur in a particular area of the body. The vulnerability of the groin is due to a combination of several embryologic processes that take place in the fetus plus some inherent anatomic weaknesses of this area, especially in the male, in whom 86% of inguinal hernias are found.

In the male fetus the testicles lie inside the abdomen close to the kidneys. Several months before birth, the testicles begin descending to their position in the scrotum and finally reach this location shortly before birth. As the testicle and its blood vessels, along with the spermatic cord (the tube that carries the sperm), move through the peritoneum and the muscles of the abdominal wall itself to reach the scrotum, they create a tract along their path. This tract, called the inguinal canal, narrows to a tiny diameter or may seal completely just before birth. In a small percentage of infants the canal remains wide open with intestines inside it, so that the child is born with a hernia already present. As many as 10% of these infants have clinically evident hernias on both sides of the groin. Even with a tract that has

375

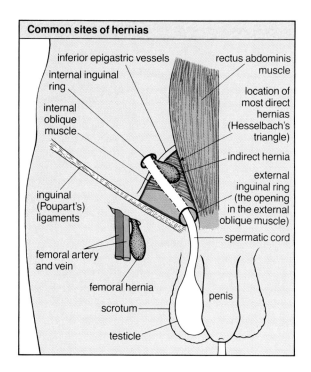

Common sites of hernias

- inferior epigastric vessels
- internal inguinal ring
- internal oblique muscle
- inguinal (Poupart's) ligaments
- femoral artery and vein
- femoral hernia
- scrotum
- testicle
- rectus abdominis muscle
- location of most direct hernias (Hesselbach's triangle)
- indirect hernia
- external inguinal ring (the opening in the external oblique muscle)
- spermatic cord
- penis

sealed, an actual or potential weakness remains which can later reopen as a hernia. In most instances, when the canal does reopen, it is for no apparent reason.

The reopening of the inguinal canal into a hernia may be simply a small bulge in the groin, but sometimes the tract reopens all the way into the scrotum. This type of hernia does not open straight out but finds its way out first through the "internal" inguinal ring of the peritoneum (the opening that allows the spermatic cord to pass through), then takes a slightly zigzag course downward for about two inches between the layers of the abdominal wall and then out again through the "external" inguinal ring, where the spermatic cord descends to the scrotum. From this point it can continue down into the scrotum. This is the reason why, when a physician examines for a hernia, he places a finger on the scrotum and the external ring and gently moves it upward, feeling for the bulge of the hernial sac descending from the internal ring. Asking the patient to cough helps expand a sac that may be empty and collapsed at that moment. Because of the path it takes, this type of hernia is called an indirect hernia. When it reaches all the way into the scrotum, some refer to it as a scrotal hernia. The indirect type of hernia is found most commonly in infants, children, and young adults.

There is another type of inguinal hernia that is encouraged by the anatomic weakness inherent in the way the layers of the abdominal wall in this area are arranged. While the abdominal wall is composed of a number of layers, some of these layers are missing in the inguinal region or put together in such a way that this area is relatively weak and subject to being

stretched out into a hernial sac. Such is the case with an area known as Hesselbach's triangle. One side of this triangle is the rectus abdominis muscle that runs up and down the front of the abdomen; the lower side is the inguinal ligament; and the upper border is made up of the inferior epigastric blood vessels supplying the middle of the abdomen. The internal inguinal ring is found just above these vessels. There is a variable lack of muscle layers in this triangle, making it more vulnerable to a direct outward bulge without any zigzag course, hence the term direct hernia for this type.

Direct hernias almost always occur in older people whose tissue has become more relaxed with age. Because this type of hernia does not have the same embryologic origin as the indirect type, it rarely goes down all the way into the scrotal sac. And because the direct type is more likely a bulging of the abdominal wall rather than a zigzag path along a tubular tract, intestines are less likely to be incarcerated or strangulated within such a hernia.

Surgical repair of inguinal hernia

Herniorrhaphy, or surgical hernia repair, is one of the most common operations performed by general surgeons and accounts for many admissions to children's hospitals. The preferred operation for infants and children is to expose the hernial sac, replace any viscera that may have protruded into the sac, then to tie off the sac at its base and remove it. This is done under general anesthesia, sometimes on an outpatient basis.

The best way to repair groin hernias in adults has not been definitively determined, although numerous operations have been devised, each with its strong advocates. The least that is necessary for the repair of an indirect hernia is for the sac to be excised and its neck tied flush with the abdominal wall.

For the direct type, where the neck is unusually broad and shallow, the hernial sac is not tied off but is inverted back into place. Something in addition must be done to strengthen Hesselbach's triangle, the tissue of which has already stretched to cause the hernia in the first place. Even in most adults with an indirect hernia, the tissue in Hesselbach's triangle is sufficiently weak that it needs to be strengthened to prevent a later herniation of the direct type. In such patients most surgeons try to be prudent about how extensive these preventive steps should be.

The Bassini herniorrhaphy is one of the most common operations to strengthen Hesselbach's triangle. In this procedure the sac of the indirect hernia is tied at its neck and the excess tissue discarded. The weak Hesselbach's triangle is obliterated by pulling some strong connective tissue (the conjoined tendon and transversalis fascia) down to the groin crease itself (Poupart's ligament) and anchoring it to this strong tissue. The spermatic cord is then placed in its normal position, and the strong outermost layer of the abdomen (aponeurosis of the external oblique muscle) is closed over this, followed by closure of the skin.

In a direct hernia there is usually a broad-based bulge, and many surgeons believe that the Bassini repair is not appropriate. An older and still very commonly used operation for this type of hernia is the Halsted repair. Here the initial step is the same as for the Bassini, but the aponeurosis of the external oblique muscle is overlapped (imbricated) very much like the front of a double-breasted jacket, so that it is a double layer of tissue covering and supporting the repaired Hesselbach's triangle. The spermatic cord then lies over the repair, in the fat just under the skin.

There are many surgeons who believe that the repair by the principle of multiple layers of tissue is not as good as the repair effected by attaching the conjoined tendon and transversalis fascia to the stronger iliopubic ligament (referred to as Cooper's ligament). Still others believe that all of the above described operations are either simply excessive or that a basic anatomic defect in Hesselbach's triangle cannot adequately be corrected by putting together tissue that never was meant to be so aligned in the first place. This has given rise to the increasing practice of using mesh to repair Hesselbach's triangle.

At the time of this operation the hernial sac itself is repaired as described above. Then the mesh, which is a pliable, strong, extremely inert plastic, can be fashioned to fit the shape of the triangle and then laid over this area. This mesh is like a coarse screen, and the tissue grows into it to produce a strong sheet of tissue.

Quite clearly, it is difficult to arrive at a consensus on the best operation for inguinal hernias if for no other reason than that these hernias are so variable that one treatment cannot be expected to be optimal for all types. Most surgeons have developed one or two of these operations to a high degree of reliability and can achieve results equal to those by other techniques.

A more recent trend is to repair inguinal hernias under local anesthesia, with a very short hospital stay. The ability of patients to return to their usual occupation varies widely with the individual, the type of work performed, and the type of hernia repaired. Generally speaking, however, those with repair of indirect hernias who have sedentary occupations can return to non-stressful work soonest.

Inguinal hernias are found much less commonly in women than in men. In women they can be repaired more easily and successfully because the local anatomy is less complicated.

Femoral hernia

A groin hernia that is distinctly more common in women is the femoral hernia, which accounts for about 33% of groin hernias in women and 2% in men. This type of hernia occurs in the inner thigh just immediately below the groin area and makes its exit through the same opening as the femoral artery, nerve, and vein. Sometimes patients mistake such hernias for swollen lymph nodes. Femoral hernias do not become large but often become incarcerated. They can be repaired with a good rate of success by an operation through an inci-

The latest tendency in surgical repair of hernia is to minimize the procedure, using local anesthetics if this is feasible and a short stay of only a day or so in the hospital. Patients are encouraged to exercise almost immediately after the operation.

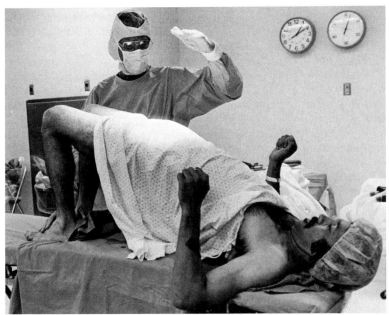

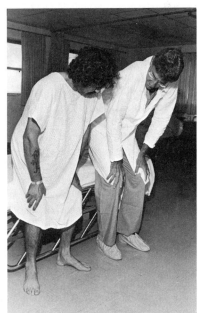

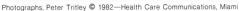

Photographs, Peter Tritley © 1982—Health Care Communications, Miami

sion in the groin. The recovery period is similar to that for inguinal hernias.

Umbilical hernia

Another group of hernias are those found around the umbilicus (navel). Umbilical hernias occur most commonly in infants or in older women, especially those who have borne children or who are overweight. Those in infants resolve spontaneously within six months in the great majority of cases. If they remain after a six-month period, umbilical hernias are not likely to regress and can be repaired safely, easily, and with a very low recurrence rate.

Those occurring in adults need to be repaired since they do not resolve spontaneously and often cause symptoms and, more important, they constantly pose the threat of incarceration and strangulation. In the repair of umbilical hernias in adults, an attempt is made to imbricate the tissue in the "vest-over-pants" technique to give it greater strength. The incision usually is made in a crosswise fashion, and the imbrication takes place from above downward so that the upper sheet of tissue (vest) lies over the lower tissue (pants).

Incisional hernia

Another type of hernia occurs in the incision from a previous operation and is called an incisional hernia. Since it is in the front (or ventral) part of the abdomen, it may be referred to as a ventral hernia. These hernias are the result, from a variety of causes, of a breakdown of the healing or the nonhealing of an incision. One cause is infection in the wound after surgery; instead of normal tissue healing to normal tissue, there is an excessive amount of weak scar tissue that becomes a part of the abdominal wall. Another cause is excessive strain on the operative incision as from a distended abdomen or excessive, unrestrained coughing after surgery. Incisional hernia may be initiated or aggravated by heavy lifting too soon after an abdominal operation. The resultant hernia can be variable in size and shape, ranging from gigantic and involving the entire abdominal wall to as small as the tip of the finger. Accordingly, the symptoms incisional hernias produce can vary widely—from almost minimal discomfort for any sized hernia, to severe pain in a hernia of modest size, to incarceration and even strangulation of long lengths of intestine. These hernias more commonly are repaired to alleviate the symptoms they produce, yet the more important reason is the risk of incarceration and strangulation. In time these hernias become larger and more difficult to repair.

Small and most medium-sized incisional hernias can be repaired by approximating the tissue to itself, preferably by imbrication. In many of the larger ones, the operation involves opening up the hernia, defining the margins, and discarding the excess tissue. The defect is then repaired, laying a sheet of mesh across the defect and stitching it to the margins. Over the mesh is laid the fatty layer of the abdominal wall that has been turned back. This tissue grows into the mesh to become incorporated as a strong new abdominal wall.

Hiatus hernia

The diaphragm is a sheet of muscle that divides the chest from the abdomen. Esophageal hiatus hernia occurs in the opening of the diaphragm through which the esophagus (about the width of a broomstick) passes just before it joins the stomach. Normally, the size of the stomach prevents it from moving through this opening and into the chest.

Factors that keep food from regurgitating from the stomach into the esophagus are the position of the stomach within the abdominal cavity, the difference in pressure between the abdominal and chest cavities, the somewhat oblique angle of the esophagus as it joins the stomach, and, finally, some sphincter action where the two join.

If, however, the esophageal hiatus (opening) is abnormally large and part of the stomach migrates intermittently or permanently into the chest, then the stage is set for stomach contents to regurgitate up into the esophagus. These contents include food, but the dominant symptoms of this condition are caused by stomach acid or the alkaline secretions from the duodenum, which may irritate the esophagus mildly or severely enough to produce ulcers, bleeding, and scarring. The symptoms can be simple regurgitation, a burning sensation in the stomach or esophagus, and even a severe burning under the sternum. These symptons occur most commonly after eating or when lying down (especially following meals). The symptoms can be relieved by drinking water to wash away the irritating secretions or by taking antacids. Clinical trials are under way to test the efficacy of drugs that strengthen the sphincter between the stomach and esophagus. If a hiatus hernia becomes very large or causes chronic bleeding, it can be repaired surgically by returning the stomach to its proper position and reducing the opening in the diaphragm to fit snugly around the esophagus.

The most important illness with which the symptoms of this condition can be confused is a heart attack. Sustained burning, pain, or pressure under the sternum must not be assumed to be caused by a hiatal hernia unless this diagnosis has been established and has produced these symptoms in the past. To avoid symptoms the hiatus hernia sufferer should avoid eating soon before bedtime. He should sleep on two or three pillows, so that the head and chest are higher than the abdomen, and raise the head of the bed by about six inches. Reduction of obesity and avoiding constrictive clothing help, too, because both tend to push the stomach into the chest.

—Steven G. Economou, M.D.

Health Education Unit 16

Hangover

On the morning after the night before, Norwegians say, "Jeg har tømmermenn." This expression, meaning "I have carpenters in my head," graphically describes the pounding headache that frequently accompanies a hangover. Other common consequences of occasional overindulgence in alcohol include nausea, heartburn, thirst, tremor, disturbance of equilibrium, fatigue, generalized aches and pains, dullness, depression, and irritability. Indeed, some 30 hangover symptoms have been identified; they reflect disturbances in the body's gastrointestinal, neurologic, and metabolic systems. Some people experience most of the symptoms, while others have only a few. Symptoms may vary greatly in intensity between individuals and in the same person from one time to the next.

Hangovers, dubbed by one wit "the wrath of grapes," easily are recognized for what they are. People rarely need to call a doctor, nor in fact is there much help a doctor can offer. Folk and patent remedies often are utilized in the hope of easing the discomfort. While a way to vanquish hangovers has yet to be found, fortunately, no matter how miserable a person feels, the hangover usually disappears completely within a few hours.

Although the impact of a hangover often is viewed primarily in terms of individual discomfort, hangovers also may exact an economic toll as a result of days lost from work. According to the *Fourth Special Report to Congress on Alcohol and Health,* issued in January 1981 by the Department of Health and Human Services, two out of every three adults in the United States consume alcohol and, hence, may be viewed as potentially at risk for at least an occasional hangover. Americans aged 14 and older on average consume more than 2.7 gal of alcohol per year; on a daily basis that is the equivalent of either 2.5 oz of whiskey, two cocktails, two glasses of wine, or two cans of beer. To scientists, hangovers are not a trivial concern; study of the phenomenon may have implications for increasing understanding of the alcohol withdrawal syndrome in alcoholics and for shedding light on a number of patterns of social behavior.

What triggers hangovers?

The archaeological records of the oldest civilizations and the most primitive peoples show use of alcohol. This product of natural fermentation has long been known to alter mood, producing feelings of pleasure or relief from tension and inhibition. These effects occur

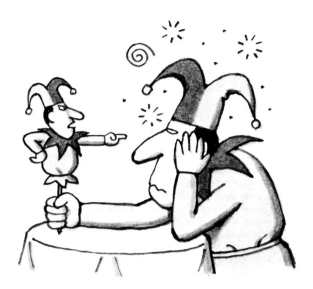

not, as often is mistakenly thought, because alcohol is a stimulant but rather because it is a depressant drug; *i.e.,* one that slows the activity of the brain.

"Alcohol does the most for you when you choose the time, place, and circumstances of drinking rather carefully," Morris Chafetz, who was founding director of the National Institute on Alcohol Abuse and Alcoholism (NIAAA), said in the book *Why Drinking Can Be Good for You.* He adds, "If you're going to be sharing a meal or enjoying human interchange, just sitting around in a relaxed way, then alcohol can be a terrific adjunct to the essential human experience of socializing. It's then that alcohol is at its best, a true servant of man."

Scientists have long tried to clarify the relative importance of various factors in producing the nasty constellation symptoms that make up the hangover. Numerous studies have focused on the quantity of alcohol or components of alcohol, the speed of drinking, the individual's weight and rate of metabolism, previous experiences with drinking, foods eaten before, during, and after drinking, dehydration, late hours, loss of sleep, exciting company, and even remorse. Such studies provide information on how alcohol works in body and brain and suggest ways a person may be able to avoid or at least minimize the unpleasant "morning after" consequences.

Can hangovers be avoided?

The first piece of practical advice is *Don't drink too fast or too much.* Alcohol enters the bloodstream within minutes of being consumed. Until recently it was thought that, on average, a person burned alcohol at the rate of one "typical drink," containing one-half ounce of alcohol, per hour. Today it is known that the process takes approximately twice that long. The NIAAA considers the following to be examples of a typical drink: a shot of spirits (1$\frac{1}{2}$ oz of 40% alcohol—80-proof whiskey or vodka), a glass of fortified wine

379

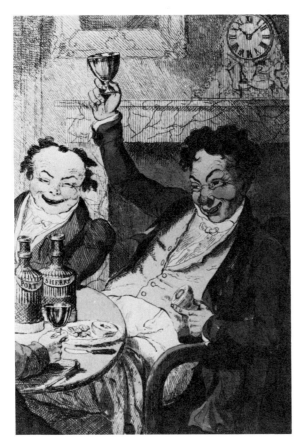
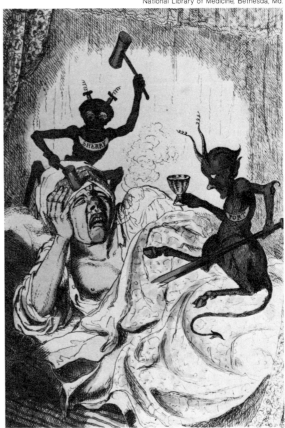

"Night" and *"Morning,"* two etchings by George Cruikshank from the early 19th century, luridly illustrate the major symptoms of a hangover, a pounding headache and a devil of a stomachache.

such as sherry (3 oz of 20% alcohol), a larger glass of table wine (5 oz of 12% alcohol), or a can of beer (12 oz of 4½% alcohol).

During ordinary social drinking, the body burns alcohol at a fairly constant rate; when alcohol is consumed faster than it is burned, it accumulates in the body and can be measured as progressively higher levels of alcohol in the blood. Since it is the liver that metabolizes at least 95% of alcohol consumed and since women tend to have smaller livers than men, women metabolize alcohol more slowly. Women also seem to absorb alcohol more quickly; their rates of absorption are even higher just prior to ovulation and menstruation. Women who are taking oral contraceptives metabolize alcohol more slowly than women who are not using them, according to studies at the Research Institute on Alcoholism of Buffalo, N.Y.

In a laboratory setting volunteers have consumed more pure alcohol than they would in an ordinary social situation without suffering hangovers the next day. However, according to a report in the *Quarterly Journal of Studies on Alcohol* (May 1970), most occasional and moderate drinkers can expect to suffer a hangover if they consume 1.5 ml of alcohol per kg of body weight over a six-hour period; for a 160-lb man, that amounts to about seven typical drinks. Some people will develop a hangover on less; others may not on more. A hangover begins when the concentration of alcohol in the blood begins to decrease; the most intensive hangover symptoms tend to occur approximately 14 hours after the start of a three-hour period of alcohol drinking.

Pay attention to what you drink. Constituents of alcoholic beverages known as congeners are thought to figure in the production of hangovers. Some of these nonalcoholic chemicals are constituents of the original raw materials of the liquor or are by-products of the fermenting, distilling, or aging of liquors and wines. Others are added for flavor and color.

Congeners may directly affect the body or alter the rates of absorption of alcohol into the body. Some congeners, in large quantities, are toxic. Drinks rich in congeners, including bourbon, brandy, rum, and red wine, are reputed to cause more severe hangovers than drinks low in congeners, such as gin and vodka. However, the total congener content in most alcoholic beverages consumed in the United States is low. Hence, many scientists feel that while congeners may modify the intensity of a hangover, they are not the primary cause.

Eat before and while drinking. Food sponges up alcohol and slows its absorption. Milk consumed during the hour before drinking will provide a coating for the stomach. Foods containing fat, such as cheese, buttered bread, or chicken livers, have "staying power"; eating a substantial meal while drinking is even better. Salty foods, such as peanuts, potato chips, and pretzels, are best limited because alcohol makes the body retain salt, and excess salt in turn contributes to morning-after thirst, aches, and malaise. Salty foods also may make a person thirsty while drinking, so that he drinks more.

While alcohol itself is highly caloric, it contains no vitamins, proteins, or other nutritious elements. A cocktail of alcohol mixed with orange juice, tomato juice, or eggnog may seem less potent than a straight drink, but the critical factor is the actual amount of alcohol consumed; by diluting the alcohol such mixers may, however, effectively lengthen the time a person takes to consume the drink. Diluting alcohol with water will slow its absorption. On the other hand, mixing it with carbonated beverages speeds absorption, because the gas creates pressure that speeds the passage of alcohol through the wall of the stomach and into the bloodstream. This fact explains the quick sensation of giddiness triggered by drinking champagne. Beer followed by whiskey is said to have a less explosive effect than the same combination taken the other way around because the alcohol content in beer is not only low but diluted, while that in whiskey is high and it usually is taken in less diluted form. Mixing types of alcoholic drinks does not, by itself, produce a hangover; however, some people find the practice unpalatable.

Consider the effect of your attitudes toward drinking. Chafetz has noted: "Study after study has shown that people in the United States are very uncomfortable about drinking. We're so ambivalent and guilt-ridden about it that one can only conclude that we feel there's something deeply wrong with taking alcohol." Beliefs about how people are supposed to act when drinking seem to influence an individual's reactions to alcohol. Psychologists at the University of Washington in Seattle documented the "think-drink" effect. They compared alcoholics and social drinkers in four drinking situations: expect alcohol/receive alcohol, expect alcohol/receive no alcohol, expect no alcohol/receive alcohol, and expect no alcohol/receive no alcohol. They found that people who expected to receive alcohol, whether they did or not, acted more relaxed and less self-conscious, whereas of those who did not expect to receive alcohol, only the people who actually received it were affected.

Negative attitudes toward drinking may make a hangover more likely. In a study of male alcoholics in a psychiatric ward at the Ann Arbor (Mich.) Veterans Administration Hospital, researchers found men labeling themselves light drinkers were as likely to report frequent hangovers as those calling themselves heavy drinkers. However, those who thought drinking was wrong reported having hangovers more often. This suggests, as the researchers stated, "the hangover itself might be thought of as a self-punitive response to drinking in violation of one's own beliefs that alcohol is bad."

Know your limits. Although any two people may feel or act differently after drinking the same amount of alcohol, experienced drinkers develop tolerance for alcohol and require more to get "high" than inexperienced drinkers. Yet even a person who seems to be "handling" his liquor well may suffer a hangover the next morning.

Can drugs prevent hangovers?

Scientists have yet to produce a "sobering pill." Numerous compounds, however, have been tested for their efficacy in blocking or neutralizing the effect of alcohol on the brain.

An independent advisory panel for the Food and Drug Administration (FDA) has been engaged for nearly the past decade in a review of all drugs sold over the counter in the United States with regard to their safety, effectiveness, and labeling. The review of drug products marketed to prevent inebriation or to minimize a hangover is still under way. However, a progress report from the panel indicates that activated charcoal is the only ingredient being reviewed that may be able to help prevent or minimize hangover symptoms. The ability of activated charcoal to adsorb, or collect, congeners in alcoholic beverages in laboratory test tubes—and in liquor manufacture—has been demonstrated. But, as previously mentioned, the role of congeners in producing a hangover is not established.

The only active ingredient reviewed by the panel thus far with the claim of preventing alcoholic intoxication is fructose, a form of sugar. While studies have shown that fructose will lower blood alcohol, the question remains whether this reduction is of practical significance under ordinary circumstances in which drinks are consumed.

How are hangovers best treated?

Some 2,500 years ago a Hindu medical writer described the hangover as feeling "as if one were wrapped in a sheet." Pulling the sheets over one's head and spending the day in bed is, indeed, a time-honored way to cope with a hangover. Over the years innumerable remedies have been proposed, from the medieval suggestion to slip a live eel into one's ale, to snorting oxygen, rolling in the snow, engaging in vigorous exercise, or rubbing a cut lemon in the armpits.

Still, proof is lacking that anything will make a hangover go away faster. Further, a hangover usually affects the entire body, while most remedies are targeted toward relieving specific symptoms. That does not mean that one must simply suffer through a hangover; rather, one should concentrate on the most troublesome problems.

The hangover headache that throbs or intensifies with each heartbeat and gets worse as a result of sudden head movements comes from dilation or expansion of the cranial blood vessels. Coffee may help, since caffeine constricts blood vessels. Aspirin or acetaminophen also may relieve headache pain. Some people feel better after a hot shower, with water running directly on the head, or after applying towels soaked in hot water to the forehead. Keep in mind that, in some instances, remedies that relieve one hangover symptom may worsen another; a person who has a churning stomach along with a headache would want to forgo both coffee and aspirin.

Because alcohol may irritate the lining of the stomach and intestines, nausea and queasiness are frequent symptoms. The best approach to handling them is to eat lightly, sticking to bland, easily digested foods such as toast and soft-boiled eggs. Some people find antacids helpful.

Thirst occurs because alcohol upsets the body's fluid balance. Alcohol shuts off the flow of antidiuretic hormone; hence, a person feels the need to empty the bladder more frequently and loses more water than usual through urination. Salt is lost along with water. As the alcohol level in the blood drops, the flow of antidiuretic hormone restarts and there is a rebound effect, causing a relative increase in water and salt. As a result, a person may feel both bloated and thirsty. The remedy is a double-pronged approach that helps adjust the fluid balance; one should consume slightly salty liquids. The standard panacea is chicken soup. Salt tablets are not recommended; their salt content is too high for this use.

Fatigue and general aches the next morning may in part be a response to stresses imposed the night before, by meeting new people, working hard at being entertaining, or dancing, for example. Late hours may be a factor; further, alcohol disrupts sleep, causing more frequent awakenings. Some people find coffee or hot or cold showers help revive them.

The notion that help can be gotten from "the hair of the dog that bit you" comes from a folk belief that the bite of a mad dog could be cured by the quick application of a hair from the dog. This belief had become associated with alcohol by 1546, when it appeared in John Heywood's *Proverbes,* a collection of English colloquial sayings: "I pray thee let me and my fellow have a haire of the dog that bit us last night." Scientists have demonstrated that alcohol the morning after can

slow an overactive stomach and take the edge off feelings of tension, making it possible to ignore hangover symptoms. The danger, of course, is that today's cure may become tomorrow's hangover.

Massive doses of vitamins, orange juice, oysters, chili pepper, and the like are lauded by various individuals as pet remedies. Although often lacking scientific basis, they may be effective as psychological boosters, since they may give the sense that one is "doing something."

The FDA advisory review panel has noted that over the years people have found it convenient to treat their generalized hangover symptoms with internal analgesics for headache, antacids for gastric distress, and caffeine for the fatigue or dullness. Hence, a preparation intended as a hangover remedy appropriately might contain a combination of analgesics, antacids, and stimulants.

Responsible drinking

No one denies that the most reliable ounce of prevention for a hangover is the ounce (or more) of alcohol that is not consumed. Public education programs stress responsible drinking. The Texas Commission on Alcoholism emphasizes "responsible hosting," encouraging partygivers to watch out for the welfare of their guests. Fruit juices, soft drinks, and other nonalcoholic beverages should be readily available for guests who choose not to drink or who feel that they have reached their limit. Most general purpose cookbooks give recipes for nonalcoholic drinks and punches. Hosts should not feel hesitant to suggest these alternatives.

Numerous bartender training programs have been launched across the U.S.; bartenders learn how to recognize people with problems and to be better listeners as well as where to refer customers who need professional help. Under so-called dram shop acts, now laws in several states, a person who serves alcoholic beverages to persons who actually or apparently are intoxicated may be liable for damages subsequently caused by the intoxicated person to property, self, or others. The impact of such laws is to discourage excessive drinking. There has been a trend since the mid-1970s to raise the minimum drinking age for distilled spirits; by 1982, 25 U.S. states had set that age at 21. Other approaches to reducing excessive drinking at bars include the establishment of facilities for serving free or low-cost food or nonalcoholic beverages, providing entertainment to encourage another focus of attention other than drinking, and setting house limits on the number of drinks allowed in a given period.

— Lynne Lamberg

Health Education Unit 17

Coping with Mastectomy

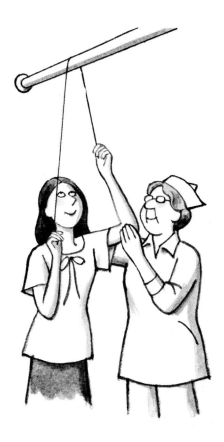

Ask any woman which disease she dreads most, and she will probably say "breast cancer." Mammary carcinoma is now almost epidemic in the U.S.: the American Cancer Society (ACS) and the National Cancer Institute (NCI) predict that about 112,000 new cases will be discovered in 1982. This means one of every 11 American women can expect to develop breast cancer, which accounts for 28% of all cancers in women. And mammary carcinoma is a lethal disease. An estimated 37,300 women, whose disease was detected in previous years, will die of breast cancer in 1982.

Why mastectomy?

Physicians and surgeons from the time of Hippocrates and Galen through the early 1800s treated mammary carcinoma by cutting off the afflicted breast as swiftly as possible; the wound was seared shut by fire cautery. Without the blessing of anesthesia, these primitive mastectomies were agonizing torture, and many women survived amputation only to die afterward from hemorrhage and infection.

In 1846 the introduction of ether revolutionized the practice of medicine. In breast cancer treatment the ability to anesthetize patients meant that surgeons could take the time to preserve tissues that had been removed unnecessarily in earlier centuries, when surgery had to be as rapid as possible. More time also meant they could probe and follow the spread of the cancer to the adjacent chest musculature and axilla (underarm area). In 1889 William Stewart Halsted, probably the foremost pioneer of modern surgery, perfected his radical mastectomy, in which the breast, both pectoral (chest) muscles, the underlying membranes, and all of the lymph nodes of the axilla were removed *en bloc,* in one continuous segment. He—like most of his medical and surgical contemporaries—believed that breast cancer spread like an infection from tissue to tissue or by way of lymph nodes and vessels. Thus, it seemed logical that excising the cancer plus as much of the surrounding flesh as possible would prevent its spread.

Women who survived Halsted radical mastectomies were left with deep holes in their chests and underarms and with long, ugly scars. Excision of all underarm nodes and vessels inevitably resulted in lymphedema (also known as "milk arm")—painful and unsightly swelling caused by trapped fluids whose escape routes had been removed. But for the first time in medical his-

tory, there were survivors. The Halsted radical mastectomy was saving women's lives.

Mastectomy today

Great progress and change occurred in all areas of surgery during the first half of the 20th century, but somehow the Halsted radical mastectomy continued to be performed. Not until the 1970s was enough known about the biology of the disease to convince most doctors that such extensive surgery was unnecessary. In June 1979 the National Cancer Institute formally issued a recommendation that "total mastectomy with axillary dissection" (also known as modified radical mastectomy) replace the 90-year-old Halsted as "standard treatment" for breast cancer in the United States.

The most important difference between the modified radical and the Halsted is that the pectoral muscles are saved, leaving patients with padding between their skin and the bones of their ribs. Because the *en bloc,* one-segment removal of the tissue is no longer considered necessary, the incision can usually be hidden by an ordinary brassiere or bathing suit. Mastectomees today can also wear sleeveless clothing and low necklines and no longer have to worry about hiding chest-wall dips and depressions; they can wear sweaters, T-shirts, and close-fitting dresses.

Attitudes about breast cancer have also changed.

383

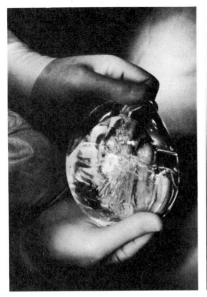
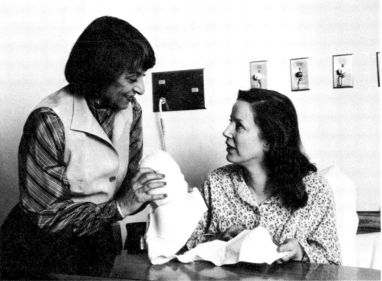

Two options are available to preserve normal appearance for a woman who has had a mastectomy. A plastic sac filled with silicone gel (left) can be surgically implanted under the skin, or a prosthesis (right) that matches the size and shape of the remaining breast can be worn externally.

There are now more than 100 commercially manufactured artificial breasts available, and some are made of fleshlike materials that feel like natural breasts. Manufacturers have developed ingenious tricks to prevent the prostheses from shifting, even during strenuous activities, and the prostheses are also available in varying colors to match women's skin tones. Some even have sculpted nipples, so if they choose mastectomees can go stylishly braless.

But losing one or both breasts is still traumatic. Even a modified radical mastectomy causes considerable physical pain, and thousands of women develop serious psychological problems related to sexuality, body-image, sense of wholeness, and often to a loss of self-esteem.

Even those women who are in early stages and need no immediate drug or X-ray therapy require careful and frequent follow-up examinations. The reason is that there were probably microscopic clusters of breast cancer cells (micrometastases) elsewhere in their bodies at the time of diagnosis. If one of these begins to grow, treatment to eradicate it must begin as soon as possible. Postmastectomy examinations are also needed because women who have had one cancer have the greatest risk of developing one in the other breast as well.

Coping with fear of recurrence

Second cancers develop in the remaining breast only about 15% of the time, but most women believe it is the most common site of first recurrences. All mastectomees, therefore, cope with the fear that they will find another breast cancer. Unfortunately, since no one yet knows the cause of breast cancer, there is no way to prevent it from developing. All that can be done is to find it at as early a stage as possible. Mastectomees must practice regular breast self-examination and have frequent checkups by their doctors. Most oncologists (cancer specialists) recommend that a breast X-ray or mammogram be taken every year.

A cancer found in the second breast is usually a "second primary" and is *not* a sign that the disease has spread. Although it does mean the patient will have to cope with another mastectomy, she is exactly where she was after the first in terms of prognosis if no involvement of the axillary lymph nodes is found.

The importance of a local recurrence in or around the incision or on the chest wall is controversial. Some doctors believe these are insignificant and treat them locally with small doses of X-rays. However, most oncologists think these are signs that the disease has begun to spread, and they usually prescribe systemic chemotherapy to destroy cancer cells present throughout the body.

There is no question, however, that metastasis, or spread to another organ, is an unhappy diagnosis, because it means the disease cannot be cured by any treatment in use today. However, there are many ways to try to keep the cancer from spreading further, so the discovery of a metastasis does not mean death is imminent. There are thousands of women living "in remission" or with the disease kept under control in other organs. But because the presence of metastases affects women's survival, oncologists are trying to prevent metastases from developing by giving high-risk patients some kind of prophylactic (or adjuvant) treatment immediately after surgery.

Today, the only predictor of which mastectomees are more likely to develop metastases is the finding of cancerous axillary lymph nodes at the time of mastectomy. These patients are Stage II (Stage I means no disease was found in the lymph nodes), and most of them are given drug or hormone treatments or both for about a year postoperatively.

All mastectomees must be carefully followed for at least the first five postoperative years in order to detect possible metastases as early as possible. Even Stage I patients have a 25% risk of developing spread. The vast majority (80%) of all metastases appear first in bone, most often in the spine, ribs, breastbone, and pelvis. Breast cancer may also spread to the lungs, liver, colon and rectum, uterus, ovaries, and (rarely) to the brain. Until the last decade there was no reason to try to detect early metastases: there was little or no treatment available for them. Now, however, the arsenal of available therapies is large enough to make early detection of spread imperative, because all treatments are most effective if the number of cancer cells in the body is small.

Women whose operations were done by general surgeons should be sure their doctors have had training or experience in managing breast cancer *after* mastectomy. If not, the American Society of Clinical Oncology can give them names of cancer specialists near their homes. If a woman cannot be in the care of an oncologist, she should be sure her doctor does periodic nuclear scans or X-rays of her bones, chest X-rays, Pap tests, and the special blood and urine analyses aimed at finding early signs of spread. Between these examinations patients should be sure to note and report any new or unusual bone pain that may or may not be "a touch of arthritis." They should also inform their doctors of any persistent coughing or hoarseness and changes of menstrual and bowel patterns. More than three-fourths of all metastases appear within the first three years after mastectomy, and it is normal to become somewhat of a hypochondriac during this critical period.

A few words of caution about scans and X-rays are essential. Both expose patients to ionizing radiation and must be used with caution for either diagnosis or treatment. Because of their need for frequent followup, mastectomees must have such exposure regularly, since the benefit of detecting an early metastasis outweighs all fear of risk. But the examinations should be done only by trained and certified personnel who have modern and well-maintained equipment. While there are private radiologists who are trained to take and interpret X-rays, nuclear-medicine apparatus for scanning is so expensive that it is usually found only in large medical centers and teaching hospitals. In general, these institutions are most likely to have well-trained personnel and excellent equipment.

Coping with the physical pain

Some women, even those who had Halsted radical mastectomies, report that their operations were entirely painless. This is unlikely, because amputation of any organ means flesh is cut, nerves and blood vessels are severed, and muscles are pushed and pulled. Removal of axillary nodes involves delicate dissection around major nerve trunks that serve the chest, arm, and back. To control postoperative pain, women are usually given strong drugs for several days, and these potent medications can cause unpleasant side effects.

Most women are entirely numb for a time after mastectomy and feel only constriction, a feeling of tightness or intense pressure around their chests. Soon afterward, many begin to experience "pins and needles" and sudden, sharp stabs of pain that might last only a few moments. Because of the axillary surgery, the upper arm is exquisitely sensitive, and even a silken sleeve feels like sandpaper. Nodal dissection can also affect the shoulder joint, and moving it is essential to prevent the joint from "freezing."

As for the operative site itself, cutting the chest nerves prevents women from feeling immediate pain in this area, including in the incision. Of course, sensation returns after varying lengths of time. Women are encouraged to wear a brassiere as soon after surgery as possible for psychological reasons, but most surgeons permit only cotton balls, tissues, or a soft handkerchief to fill its empty cup.

After a Halsted, special exercises must be done to educate auxiliary arm muscles so the affected arm is not permanently disabled. The muscles of the chest are not excised in a modified radical mastectomy, but they are usually stretched and pulled during the operation. Therefore, women having this operation must also do some exercises.

As time passes, all postoperative pain should disappear, and numb spots will gradually regain sensation. (Trying to shave a numb underarm area is an experience most women do not forget!) But, unfortunately, there are women whose pain never leaves. They cannot wear even a loose brassiere; they cannot tolerate any prosthesis. To function they must rely on strong analgesics. Physical therapy, directed by someone trained to treat postmastectomy problems, may reduce or even eliminate their pain; elastic sleeves and body suits sometimes help. Some women have been relieved by acupuncture treatments.

Coping with lymphedema

Lymphedema was once an inevitable complication of the Halsted radical mastectomy, but it can result from any breast cancer treatment involving either surgery or radiation. It is caused by the loss (through surgery) or damage (by radiation) of the narrow vessels that connect lymph nodes. These vessels normally channel wastes from tissues for excretion from the body. But lymphatic fluid also carries vital, healing components of the immune system to organs that have been injured by, for example, a mastectomy.

Although it was once believed that removing lymph nodes made patients more vulnerable to infection, this is not so; scientists have proved that there are hundreds of nodes scattered throughout the body to compensate within a short time for the loss of local nodes. It is infection, triggering a flow of fluid to the arm, that causes lymphedema, not the operation itself.

Because the arms hang downward, the force of gravity makes it easy for lymphatic fluid to enter. But the loss of the axillary vessels makes it difficult for the fluid to return upward, back into the body's circulation. The result is a swollen arm.

Though sometimes limited to the area between the shoulder and the elbow, the swelling often reaches the fingers. It not only is disfiguring but can cause pain—pain that may be valuable, because it is a signal that something must be done immediately or the lymphedema will worsen. Women who have no pain often do not notice the swelling until they cannot button a blouse cuff or fasten their watchbands.

At this time lymphedema is incurable, although it can be relieved by elevating the arm and squeezing a ball to help pump the fluid out. Another helpful exercise is standing about a foot away from a wall and pressing the hand (held flat) against it with as much force as possible. In addition, a mechanical "milking" of the arm by pneumatic machine can be performed by a trained therapist. Similar, less powerful, apparatuses can be bought for home use to provide temporary relief.

Steps should be taken to keep the condition from getting worse by trying to avoid injury to the affected arm. If any part of it is scratched, cut, or burned, the wound must be treated immediately to prevent infection. In addition, the NCI recommends that the following measures be taken:

1. No injections, inoculations, or blood-pressure readings should involve the affected arm. Women who have had nodes removed from both axillae must insist that these procedures be done using a leg.

2. Thimbles and sturdy garden gloves should be used *always* to prevent even invisible punctures when sewing or gardening.

3. Manicures must be done carefully to avoid cutting the cuticle.

4. Every hangnail, scratch, or cut to the affected hand or arm should be treated with antibiotic ointment and covered with a sterile dressing immediately.

Coping with the psychological pain

Although much has been said and written about the psychological pain of breast amputation, the true ex-

tent of women's grief cannot be measured. Those most severely traumatized "drop out" of society entirely: they refuse to see the ACS's Reach to Recovery volunteer; they consult no psychiatrist, psychologist, or social worker; they join no self-help group; they buy no prostheses. There is no way to know the depth of their pain, because—except for doctors and hospital-records librarians—no one knows they exist. Thus, studying the psychological trauma of mastectomy can be based only on information from those patients well-adjusted enough to ask for help or to be interviewed.

In September 1975 the Breast Cancer Advisory Center (BCAC) was established in Maryland to provide a free telephone hotline and mail service for breast cancer patients. Since then about 12,000 women have contacted the BCAC, and all letters and details of telephone conversations have been kept. The following summary of patients' attitudes and feelings about mastectomy is based on the center's records.

Universally, the reaction to having breast cancer is rage, even before the surgery is performed. Like most people who must cope with tragedy, women faced with this diagnosis cry, "Why me?"

After mastectomy, feelings and attitudes vary. Many women—especially those who had seen mothers, sisters, and friends die of breast cancer—feel relief and gratitude that the cancerous organ is gone. "Is it all out?" is their main concern.

They, however, are in the minority. Women who thought they were to have only a biopsy and awaken hours later to learn a breast was removed are furious. "Something was put over on me while I was unconscious," is usually their reaction. While they were asleep, a precious organ was amputated without their permission or participation. This outrage often remains with them forever. The anger seems to be directed first at their families or spouses for permitting it to happen; only rarely is there anger that is directed toward their doctors. But when women discover that there were available treatment options other than mastectomy, their rage is frequently turned inward. "Why did I panic? Why didn't I know better?" are common questions these women ask themselves.

Many women also feel guilt, certain that they did something wrong in the past to deserve the disease and it is their just punishment. Sexual behavior like masturbation, premarital or extramarital affairs, or even flirting with a friend's husband may be blamed. Learning about the familial nature of breast cancer makes many women feel guilty of passing a "bad seed" on to their daughters.

Virtually all women search for a cause; a bump or bruise is the most common, but drinking too much coffee, standing close to a microwave oven, vigorous lovemaking, or nursing infants are also suspected. (None of these is known to cause breast cancer.)

Although few of the women who contacted the

BCAC were rejected by husbands or lovers, many mastectomees believed this did or will happen. But often, conversation reveals that patients drive their partners away. For example, it is not uncommon for women to feel so mutilated and ugly that they refuse to resume their sex lives or even to be seen nude. (Indeed, some women cannot bear to look at their own incisions.) Because the affected arm is tender and sore for a time after mastectomy, women frequently ask partners to keep their distance; some are moved "temporarily" to spare rooms—never to be invited back. Some women who never enjoyed lovemaking use the mastectomy as an excuse for terminating sexual intercourse altogether. Their partners are then susceptible to advances from other women, but patients will insist it was the lost breast that drove them away. BCAC records show that the reverse is usually the case: where the marriage or relationship was strong, the tragedy actually brings the couple closer together and adds a dimension of love and togetherness that was not there before.

Stage II women who are given adjuvant therapy to prevent metastases have an added psychological burden to bear. Almost every combination of anticancer drugs causes alopecia, or hair loss. After losing a breast, an organ charged with so much emotion, they must also lose a more visible symbol of femininity and sexuality: their crowning glory. These drugs may have other, far more serious side effects; nonetheless, it is the baldness, added to breast amputation, that causes the most grievous psychological pain.

This brief description of feelings and attitudes about breast loss does not include information collected since breast reconstruction (reconstructive mammoplasty) has become widely available. The impact of plastic surgery to replace breasts lost to cancer has not yet been assessed, but undoubtedly these procedures will prevent much of the emotional pain of mastectomy.

Coping with the cost

Statisticians have estimated that breast cancer costs the U.S. economy billions of dollars annually in terms of money spent on doctors, nurses, hospital fees, and medications as well as in time lost at work. Breast cancer can be a personal financial catastrophe. *No* insurance company (including Medicare) pays for screening—periodic examinations to see if there are changes in the breast—even though the ACS and the NCI recommend that all women older than 50 have annual mammograms. So unless a symptom of breast cancer is found, high-risk women must spend at least $100 each year (usually much more) to follow the advice of the ACS and the NCI.

There are also instances where the cost of the mastectomy is not fully covered. For example, most insurance companies use a formula, the CRVS (California Relative Value Scale), to determine appropriate fees for specific surgical procedures. If a woman wants to

From *Textbook of Surgery*, David C. Sabiston, Jr., M.D., Philadephia, W. B. Saunders Co., 1981

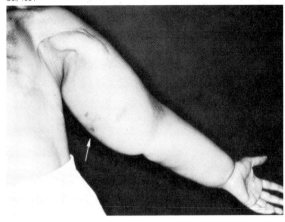

Physical therapy can relieve the discomfort of lymphedema, which results from the loss of the normal lymph drainage system in the arm especially after radical mastectomy.

go to a breast cancer specialist whose fee is higher than the CRVS authorizes for her part of the country, she must pay the difference herself. Many insurance companies do not cover outpatient X-ray treatments, should these be needed.

Even the best medical insurance coverage does not cover the costs of travel to a specialized cancer center for better treatment than is offered in smaller community hospitals. Nor are housekeepers and babysitters included, even though all patients need such help before and after surgery and during some phases of chemotherapy.

Although inexpensive kapok- or polyester-filled prostheses are available, well-fitting silicone breast forms are costly, ranging from about $125 for "AA cups" to $250 and more for larger sizes. Until recently, some insurance plans refused to pay for prostheses on the grounds that they were "cosmetic." Although all states have, by now, mandated these be covered as "rehabilitative appliances," mastectomees are not allowed to have a spare at the insurance company's expense. There is also a time interval required, usually five years, before a prosthesis can be replaced.

If a woman has malignant axillary nodes and needs adjuvant therapy, she may not be covered for any substances insurance companies consider "experimental." New agents are continually being developed, but their approval by the U.S. Food and Drug Administration (FDA) may take months or even years. Thus, it is often easy for third-party carriers to find loopholes that preclude payment.

An excellent example is tamoxifen citrate. This drug was shown to be effective as an adjuvant agent for postmenopausal estrogen-dependent breast cancer by July 1981. Results of a large-scale clinical trial were described in *The New England Journal of Medicine* by Bernard Fisher, chairman of the NCI's National Sur-

387

gical Adjuvant Breast Project. But because the FDA approval effective at that time applied only to tamoxifen's use for the treatment of advanced disease, many insurance companies refused to cover its high cost of $1.00 per tablet. Paying $60.00 each month for a single medication is prohibitive for many people, and some mastectomees "economized" by skipping days or by reducing the number of tablets prescribed.

Because most women suffer from drug toxicities for a few days of each treatment cycle, household help or babysitters are often needed during this time. Insurance does not pay for them, just as there is no reimbursement for transportation expenses and time lost from work.

Women with medical-surgical insurance must, therefore, cope with inadequate coverage. But a more serious problem, especially to younger patients, is not being able to obtain new health insurance policies (or life insurance) for ten years after the diagnosis of breast cancer. Older women are usually not as affected, because they or their husbands are not as likely to move to another area or to change jobs. Most people are covered by group insurance through places of employment, and third-party carriers must pay all costs of a disease contracted by clients while insured. None, however, is required to sell a new individual policy to people at high risk. Cancer patients, even those at a statistically low risk of recurrence, are in this category.

Of course, all people who suffer from disease have such problems. What makes the financial burden of breast cancer unique is that it attacks more than tens of thousands of women each year and, unlike malignancies of children and old people, this disease strikes women during their prime, most productive years of life. And unlike lung cancer in men, which kills most of its victims in fewer than five years, breast cancer patients may live with active disease for a decade or even longer, receiving treatment continually. Therefore, the total financial expense of the loss of these women's health to their families, to their employers, and to society is incalculable.

Women who have a mastectomy for breast cancer must cope first with fears of recurrence and the loss of a precious breast and with feelings of lost femininity and sexuality. They suffer from guilt, feeling that they did something wrong to cause them to be punished by cancer and by guilt that they may pass the disease to a daughter. Finally, women who need adjuvant therapy must cope with the toxic effects of anticancer drugs—especially baldness. These women must also cope with the knowledge that money needed to raise and educate children is instead being spent to treat their disease. Yet in spite of these problems, women do it. There are now more than one million women in the United States alone who have had one or two mastectomies, who have coped . . . and conquered.

—*Rose Kushner*

Sources of help for breast cancer patients

American Society of Clinical Oncology
435 North Michigan Avenue, Suite 1717
Chicago, Illinois 60611
(312) 644-0828

American Society of Plastic and Reconstructive Surgeons
233 North Michigan Avenue, Suite 1900
Chicago, Illinois 60601
(312) 856-1818

Association of Community Cancer Centers
11600 Nebel Street, Suite 201
Rockville, Maryland 20852
(301) 984-9496

Breast Cancer Advisory Center
11426 Rockville Pike, Suite 203
Rockville, Maryland 20850
(301) 984-1020

National Cancer Institute
Cancer Information Service
Bethesda, Maryland 20205
(800) 638-6694

National Cancer Institute's Diagnostic Lump Clinic
Radiation Oncology
Building 10, National Institutes of Health
Bethesda, Maryland 20205
(301) 496-5457

National Cancer Institute
Public Inquiries
Office of Cancer Communications
Building 31, National Institutes of Health
Bethesda, Maryland 20205
(301) 496-5583

National Surgical Adjuvant Breast Project
University of Pittsburgh School of Medicine
Pittsburgh, Pennsylvania 15261
(412) 624-2671

Reach to Recovery
American Cancer Society
777 Third Avenue
New York, New York 10017
(212) 371-2900
            or
the local unit or chapter of ACS
throughout the United States

SHARE
34 Gramercy Park
New York, New York 10003

Genital Herpes

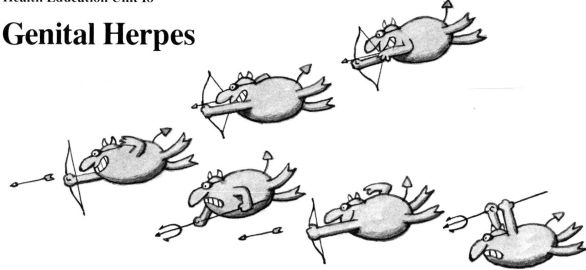

Millions of people are familiar with "cold sores" or "fever blisters," the most common form of infection caused by the herpes simplex virus. Recently, however, it has been the genital form of this viral assault that has captured the public's attention, and for good reason. From 1966 to 1979 there was a tenfold increase in patients conferring with physicians for treatment of genital herpes infection.

According to the U.S. Centers for Disease Control (CDC) in Atlanta, Ga., genital (type II) herpes afflicts as many as 15 million Americans—a figure that approximates the yearly total of all other forms of venereal disease. About 500,000 new cases are reported to the CDC each year. Some estimates double both of these figures, and herpes type II is now generally acknowledged as the most prevalent venereal skin infection in the United States. Indeed, a special report from the U.S. Public Health Service in 1980 called genital herpes "the most prominent sexually transmitted disease" of the decade, causing "chronic recurrent infection with frequent complications in perhaps 20 percent of sexually active adults."

For most people herpes simplex infections of either kind are unpleasant and unattractive but neither dangerous nor anguishing. In fact, in many persons there may be no symptoms at all. Antibodies against herpes simplex viruses—a sure sign of exposure—have been found in the blood of up to 95% of those tested, yet there are many people who cannot recall ever suffering the typical sores, blisters, pain, and itch the organisms cause. Their immune systems are probably able to keep the virus at bay.

Herpes infections were recognized for thousands of years before the viral culprit was identified. The name is from the Greek word meaning "to creep," describing the way the lesions seemed to move over the skin surface. There are at least 70 varieties of herpes viruses affecting the animal kingdom, and most biologists now believe that they originated as part of normal cells before they somehow acquired a form of semi-independence.

In addition to herpes simplex three other types affect man: varicella-zoster, responsible for chickenpox and shingles; Epstein-Barr, which causes both an unusual tumor of the jaw, especially among Africans, and most cases of infectious mononucleosis; and cytomegalovirus, a common cause of infections in fetuses which may produce mental retardation and a cause of infections in adults with faulty immune systems.

But genital herpes, commonly referred to simply as "herpes," has emerged as the sharpest focus of public fears about this group of viruses. Victims often express anguish and consider their herpes affliction a personal tragedy; a few have been driven to suicide.

Characteristics of genital herpes infection

The reason for all the current attention is that herpes has some unusual characteristics, often misunderstood, that make it anything but an ordinary health problem. Unlike other major sexually transmitted diseases (gonorrhea, for example), herpes is incurable. Once the virus invades the body it is there for life, unmoved by penicillin or any of the other drugs that work against common microbial infections.

Unlike many other infectious viral diseases such as colds and influenza, herpes can live and spread only by direct and intimate contact. The virus probably invades the body through the soft tissues and mucous membranes of the mouth and genitals or through breaks in the skin. In the case of herpes simplex type I, the cause of cold sores, spread is easily accomplished by kissing. This disease is often caught in childhood from close

389

family members. Type I can on occasion infect the genitals and type II on occasion the mouth and lips. The virus can also be transmitted to the eyes by rubbing them after touching an infected skin area. But in the vast majority of type II cases, spread requires genital or oral-genital sexual contact.

Herpes is a recurrent infection. A victim's initial infection usually appears one to four days after exposure to a fresh sore. Often the first hint of trouble is a tingling, itching, or burning sensation near the site of a coming infection. Within hours (or at most a few days) the skin becomes reddened and sensitive to touch. The lesions usually appear on the genitals, buttocks, or thighs. They can also be present in the rectum. Soon small red blisters appear, watery fluid at their center, accompanied by swelling, inflammation, and burning, sometimes severe, pain. Many people also get swollen glands, aches, a general sick feeling, and fever.

Most herpes lesions soon form oozy crusts, then scabs, and completely disappear from the skin within two weeks. However, the virus itself remains. Recent research confirms that herpesvirus becomes "latent," migrating to groups of nerve cells, called ganglia, located near the brain or spine. There the virus lies dormant for months, years, or even decades without causing a moment's trouble. Then, for reasons only partly understood (but not, as many believe, entirely at random), it reappears, creeping back along the nerve pathways to a point identical to or very near the skin area it originally infected. Recurrences are like the first infection, marked by blisters and crusty sores, but often are less severe. An estimated one-third of herpes victims experience at least one recurrence, and another third have frequent recurrences. These may happen regularly each month or each season for years or with confounding new patterns throughout life.

Herpes can be deceptive, especially in women, becoming active without displaying any symptoms even if symptoms were present during other bouts. This means that sexual partners of an infected person may be at risk of contracting the infection without warning.

Worse, it can mean brain damage or death to an infant born to an asymptomatically infected woman, because herpes can be transmitted to an infant as it passes through the birth canal. If the mother knows she is having a herpes flare-up or suspects she could have one, her doctor can monitor the pregnancy and perform a cesarean delivery. But without warning symptoms these devastating infections of infants can seem to come from nowhere. One study of herpes-infected babies showed that 70% of the mothers had no symptoms of herpes.

Associated problems

Women may also be at special risk from herpes for another reason. Many studies have linked type II infections to later development of cervical cancer. Several investigators have gone so far as to suggest that cervical cancer is a "venereal" disease. This may be a dramatic overstatement, but the links are undeniable.

Researcher Andre J. Nahmias of Emory University School of Medicine, Atlanta, found genital herpes three times as common among women with cervical cancer as in matched controls. Further tests in Baltimore, Boston, Chicago, and other cities yielded similar results. Studies of nuns and prostitutes show that cervical cancer is most prevalent among the latter and almost nonexistent in the former. In another investigation Irving Kessler of the University of Maryland School of Medicine studied several thousand women and found cervical cancer to be three to four times as prevalent among women who were married to men whose former wives had cervical cancer as among women married to either previously unmarried men or men whose former wives were free of cervical cancer. Virologist Fred Rapp and his colleagues at the Hershey Medical Center of Pennsylvania State University have demonstrated that herpes viruses can transform normal cells into cancerous cells.

Although there is as yet no scientifically acceptable proof that cervical cancer is a sexually transmitted disease caused by herpes, women who have once had genital herpes are advised to get a Pap smear to test for cancer cells in the cervix every six months, since this cancer is almost 100% curable in its early stages.

Herpes can also cause a potentially blinding condition known as herpes keratitis, an infection of the cornea of the eye. Autoinoculation, or self-transfer of the virus, is usually caused by touching a herpes sore and then rubbing the eye or even by using saliva to moisten contact lenses during an outbreak of oral herpes. The National Institute of Allergy and Infectious Diseases, a branch of the National Institutes of Health, estimated in 1979 that there are 500,000 cases of herpes keratitis in the U.S. each year.

Fortunately, two antiviral drugs, vidarabine and idoxuridine, are effective in treating herpes keratitis if the condition is caught early enough. Unfortunately, the drugs do not work on genital herpes.

Another group of people endangered by herpes are so-called immunosuppressed individuals, persons whose normal immune defense systems have been weakened or destroyed by drugs that they are taking to treat cancer or prevent rejection of a transplanted organ. The drugs may increase the patient's susceptibility to a first attack of herpes or encourage reactivation of a latent virus.

The psychological trauma

Another characteristic of this infection is that it causes great psychological trauma for many victims. In many, if not all, illnesses psychology plays some role in susceptibility, duration, and convalescence. Hormones and other biochemical substances influenced by stress

390

and emotional response are the probable mechanisms. In herpes the psychological factor seems to be especially significant.

Psychological factors may be important in both the resistance to genital herpes and in the adaptation made to having the disease. Sufferers face many coping problems owing to the nature of the disease—the fact that herpes is a recurrent disease that is transmitted sexually, that there is no known cure, that it tends to cause serious disturbances in physically intimate relationships, and that it attacks young people during vital periods of psychosexual development.

After the first shock of learning they have herpes, many patients respond by denying that the problem is serious. As recurrences appear, they feel isolated and frightened, angry at the person who infected them, and bitter at the thought of giving up dreams of sexual happiness, healthy children, and a loving relationship. They worry about developing cancer and about what to tell potential lovers or spouses. Men especially become anxious about their sexual performance. They begin to feel like social outcasts, wracked with guilt, shame, fear, and depression that increases with feelings of helplessness.

Not all patients experience such intense psychosocial problems. But because many do, it is important for any sexually active person of any age or socioeconomic status to learn the facts about causation, diagnosis, treatment, quackery, and successful ways of coping with the disease. With sound information and help from those who have dealt personally and professionally with herpes, no one need succumb to the kind of despair outlined above.

Diagnosis

Proper diagnosis of herpes is the first step. Since skin rashes and blisters can be a sign of hundreds of medical disorders, it takes an experienced physician to identify lesions of herpes. Most doctors can do this on the basis of the appearance of the lesions and information from a thorough medical history. If more evidence is needed, the best procedure is to collect cells from the lesions to "culture," or grow in a laboratory. Since the virus takes over its host cells in a characteristic way, microscopic examination of the culture can usually lead to a diagnosis within a few days. A second method of diagnosis, called a Tzanck smear, uses a special stain and is 60 to 80% effective in identifying herpes simplex virus.

With sophisticated tests it is possible to distinguish between type I and type II herpesviruses by sorting out genetic differences, but since these tests are difficult and expensive and of no real value at this time to the patient, they are rarely called for.

Some patients undergo a blood test that looks for the presence of antibodies to herpes, but the test is of absolute value only to rule out herpes. A negative result means that patient was never exposed to the virus. If the result is positive, however, it means only that at some time in the person's life he or she was exposed to the virus. That could have been years before and may not even have caused symptoms.

Finally, a Pap smear done by a gynecologist accurately diagnoses genital herpes in about two-thirds of all female cases. Many physicians will include a search for herpes when they routinely perform this test for early cervical cancer.

All in all, the diagnosis of genital herpes is not difficult to make in the vast majority of cases, provided the physician making it is familiar with the disease. Thus, gynecologists, dermatologists, urologists, general practitioners, and doctors who work in venereal disease clinics are the best choice if a herpes infection is suspected.

Treatment

In March 1982 acyclovir (Zovirax) was approved by the U.S. Food and Drug Administration for the management of genital herpes. Tests showed that acyclovir speeded the healing of herpes blisters and reduced growth of the virus. In clinical tests of 188 patients, acyclovir was shown to be of greatest worth in treating the initial outbreak of herpes lesions. This means a victim must recognize or suspect a herpes infection at the moment it emerges—a tricky and often impossible task. The drug had little effect on recurrent lesions in women but gave some relief in men. This drug also held great promise for ameliorating herpes infections in immunosuppressed cancer and transplant patients. It is the only approved drug for herpes genital infection.

Aspirin usually lessens pain and inflammation associated with herpes. But, contrary to widespread belief, over-the-counter cortisone creams, antibacterial ointments, and similar remedies may actually spread herpesvirus and delay healing. Herpes specialists recommend gentle soap and water cleansing of lesions and the use of drying agents such as epsom salts. If secondary bacterial infections occur because of the break in the skin, a physician can give advice on additional treatment. Keeping infected parts dry and clean not only helps relieve discomfort but reduces the risk of spreading infection to the eyes and mouth.

A proliferation of "cures"

Dozens of self-proclaimed cures for herpes tempt millions of herpes victims who are willing to try anything to get rid of the disease. About the only good many do is to the bank accounts of the promoters. Others may show promise but are unproven as either cures or aids to patients.

These include immune stimulators such as live-bacteria tuberculosis vaccine and other vaccines long known to mobilize the body's defense mechanisms. Trials have failed to demonstrate consistent results in herpes sufferers. Some doctors have tried zinc and vitamin C. Health food stores promote arginine and lysine—both amino acids. While there are some scientific underpinnings for choosing these agents—the amino acids, for example, inhibit virus replication in the laboratory—no proper studies have demonstrated any consistent positive effect of either of them.

Studies have, on the other hand, demonstrated the ineffectiveness of topical ether and the danger of so-called dye-light therapy. The latter involves applying a red, light-sensitive dye to the lesions, then shining a light on them. The theory was that the light would inactivate the viruses, which are also light sensitive. But virologists have found that such a breakdown of the virus made it better able to transform normal cells into cancerous cells in animals.

About the only unproven but popular treatment that might help and probably does not hurt is ice therapy. In this treatment ice cubes are placed on the lesions continuously for up to two hours. Not only does this numb the pain, burn, and itch but, according to some patients, if applied within 24 hours of a lesion's appearance, it speeds disappearance of the blister.

This and many other unproved treatments may work, in part, because of the victim's belief that he or she *can* do something to control the disease (the placebo effect). Less questionable are the interventions that have been shown to work to prevent initial infection, recurrences, and complications.

Prevention

Many herpes specialists believe that as many as 75% of herpes recurrences can be traced to environmental or emotional triggers. A major factor is trauma to the skin from sexual intercourse, massages, kissing, shaving, sunburn, dental work, the use of perfumes, and other infections. Menstruation and associated hormonal changes, colds, influenza, fever, and emotional stress are also triggers, as is exposure to the sun. General health and emotional state are also involved in the onset and recurrence of herpes

Avoiding the initial infection is, of course, the ideal. But a person who has already contracted herpes can help lessen recurrences by anticipating, as much as possible, the triggering causes. Some of these can be avoided completely, others minimized. There are several points to keep in mind.

1. Good nutritional status and a general state of good health make it less likely that the body will suffer any kind of microbial or viral assault.

2. Sexual promiscuity—having a multitude of sexual partners, often encountered under emotionally upsetting conditions—enhances the risk of contracting herpes both because of the chance of encountering a carrier and because stress increases susceptibility.

3. Contraceptives such as birth control pills and the diaphragm do nothing to prevent herpes. Condoms are of dubious value since the viruses can pass through the pores of the condom, but they may provide some protection. The only sure way to outwit herpes is to practice sexual abstinence. The next safest course is to exercise extreme caution in the selection of sexual partners.

4. Stress and emotional upsets can sabotage immune competence, bringing on a recurrence. It is wise to pay attention to one's health at these times and stay clear of high-risk contacts.

5. Such environmental conditions as weather changes, extreme conditions of wind, humidity, or dryness can trigger herpes recurrences by stressing the body. Clothing also plays a part—tight-fitting underwear and pantyhose have been implicated in bringing on recurrences.

A major concern of herpes patients is to avoid passing on the infection. There is no sure way to prevent the spread of herpes, but there are established strategies. From the time a herpes patient recognizes the earliest tingle or ache until sores are completely healed, he must take great care to avoid infecting others and spreading the infection to his eyes or mouth. Personal hygiene must be meticulous. During an outbreak it is essential to totally abstain from sexual intercourse or any kind of sex play that could bring skin in contact with the lesions. The use of a condom *between* recurrences helps protect the partner but will not be effective during an outbreak. And though it may be difficult, any new sex partner should be asked if he or she has genital herpes.

Today, research is rapidly advancing toward control of herpes infections by developing effective antiviral agents. Investigations into the genetic operation of herpesvirus may give scientists strategies for getting to it in its neural hiding places and so eradicating it from the body.

Experts agree, however, that for now, the best way to control herpes is with self-care and good sense. Cautious sexual relations, Pap smears for cancer detection, and cesarean sections to prevent infection of newborns can prevent herpes from ruining lives.

Group support is also a help. The American Social Health Association operates a national organization called the Herpes Resource Center (formerly known as Herpetics Engaged in Living Productively, or HELP). The 25,000 members sponsor and support information hotlines, seminars, clinics, and distribution of an up-to-date and well-produced quarterly publication, *The Helper*. For information write Herpes Resource Center, P.O. Box 100, Palo Alto, Calif. 94302.

—Joann E. Rodgers

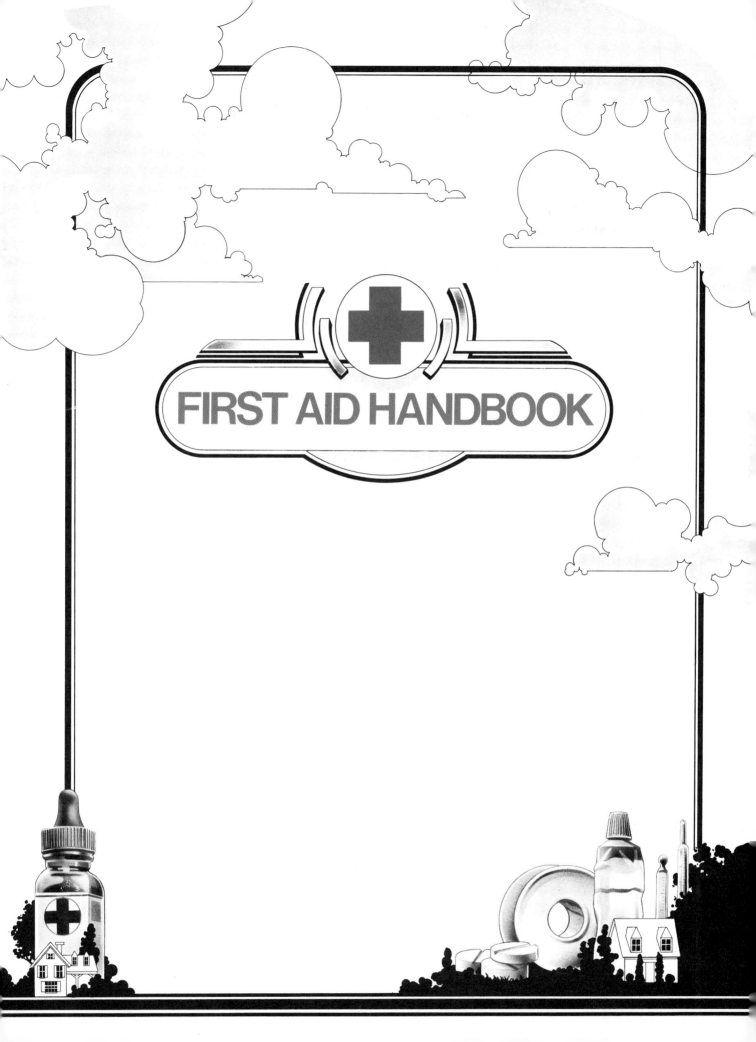

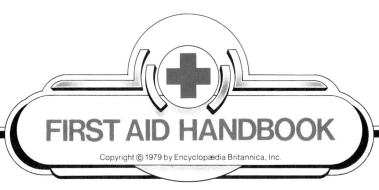

FIRST AID HANDBOOK

Produced in cooperation with the Educational Materials Committee
of the American College of Emergency Physicians,
G. Richard Braen, M.D., Chairman.

Authors

Roy D. Beebe, M.D., and G. Richard Braen, M.D.

ACEP Educational Materials Committee

Roy D. Beebe, M.D.
Michael L. Callaham, M.D.
Desmond P. Colohan, M.D.
Rodney D. Edwards, Jr., M.D.
Robert G. Haining, M.D.
Joel B. Hellmann, M.D.

Contents

Illustrations by John Youssi

Emergency Care and First Aid

Properly administered first aid can make the difference between life and death, between temporary and permanent disability, or between rapid recovery and long hospitalization. First aid is most frequently employed to help a family member, a close friend, or an associate, and everyone should be familiar with first aid techniques and should know how best to use the emergency care system.

Public education and public awareness of potential roles in first aid have lagged behind the development of the emergency care system, which includes emergency medicine as a special area of medicine, better equipped and better staffed emergency facilities, paramedical care, communications, and transportation. The concept of first aid as simply the immediate care of the injured person is obsolete. Today a person administering first aid must be able to establish priorities in care and must understand and implement *basic life support* in an attempt to maintain vital functions. Education will reduce the chances of error and the possibly harmful results of well-meant but misdirected efforts.

Accidents are the leading cause of death among persons one to 38 years of age. In addition, over 800,000 Americans die annually of heart attacks, and a great majority of these die before they reach a hospital. The annual cost of medical attention and loss of earning ability amounts to billions of dollars, not to mention the toll in pain, suffering, disability, and personal tragedy. Thus, the delivery of quality emergency care and public education in basic life support and first aid must be accorded a high priority.

Use of This Handbook

The purpose of this handbook is both to educate and to serve as resource material for commonly encountered emergencies. It is arranged in three sections. The first deals with basic life support and the treatment of immediately life-threatening emergencies. One must understand these concepts *before* an emergency arises, since the necessary techniques must be employed immediately, almost by reflex, if the victim is to be saved.

The second section deals with emergencies that are not immediately life-threatening. It covers the common emergencies in alphabetical order.

The final section covers prevention, preparation, and use of the emergency care system. Prevention is still the least expensive medicine, and several of its most important principles will be discussed. Each home should be prepared for an emergency by having a readily accessible first aid kit, appropriate telephone numbers, etc. This section also discusses what to do and what to expect at the emergency department.

Section One:
Basic Life Support—Treatment of Immediately Life-Threatening Emergencies

Cardiopulmonary Arrest (Heart and Respiratory Failure)

Cardiac arrest is the most life-threatening of all emergencies. If circulation and breathing are not reestablished within minutes, the brain will suffer irreparable damage. Cardiopulmonary resuscitation (CPR), or basic life support, if begun early enough, can be lifesaving. This very simple procedure requires no special equipment and can be begun by *any person* who has taken the time to receive appropriate instruction. Before attempting to utilize this procedure, one would be well advised, in addition to reading the description of basic life support that follows, to undertake formal certification in CPR. Such instruction is readily available through the American Heart Association or the Red Cross.

What Is Cardiopulmonary Arrest?

There are two absolutely vital systems in the body that must function if life is to continue: the *respiratory* system (lungs and respiratory tree) and the *circulatory* system (heart and blood vessels). The overall function of these two systems is to get oxygen into the blood and then to all parts of the body.

0-4 MIN.	CLINICAL DEATH	BRAIN DAMAGE not likely
4-6 MIN.		BRAIN DAMAGE probable
6-10 MIN.	BIOLOGICAL DEATH	BRAIN DAMAGE probable
OVER 10 MIN.		BRAIN DAMAGE almost certain

Phases of brain damage and death following cardiac arrest.

395

If either of these systems fails, or "arrests," death occurs very quickly unless the function is restored by CPR.

Respiratory or breathing failure has two basic causes: 1) obstruction of the intake of air or exchange of oxygen into the blood, and 2) impairment of the part of the brain (respiratory center) that controls the rate and depth of breathing. Obstruction can result from several factors, including the presence of large pieces of foreign material (such as food) in the upper airway, swelling and closure of the airway (as in severe acute allergic reactions), and damage to the oxygen-exchanging membranes in the lung (from drowning and smoke inhalation). By far the most common cause of upper airway obstruction that occurs in the patient who has been rendered unconscious is the flaccid tongue that falls backward against the back of the throat and obstructs the airway. The respiratory center may be suppressed by drugs (narcotics, sedatives, alcohol), and carbon monoxide, electric shock, and an interrupted supply of oxygen to the brain, as when the heart has stopped.

If the heart stops pumping, or arrests, the tissues of the body do not receive the blood and oxygen they need. When this happens to the brain, there is an almost immediate loss of consciousness and breathing stops.

What To Look For

If a cardiopulmonary arrest has occurred, the victim *always:* is unconscious; has no pulse in the neck (carotid pulse); is not breathing. The carotid pulse can be checked by feeling with the thumb and middle finger on either side of the windpipe (trachea). If a pulse is present, it will be felt here.

What To Consider

Any person who suddenly collapses (becomes unconscious), has no detectable pulse in the neck, and is not breathing has suffered a cardiopulmonary arrest. (A person who collapses while eating and is unable to breathe may well have a large piece of food caught in his windpipe. This is not literally a cardiac arrest,

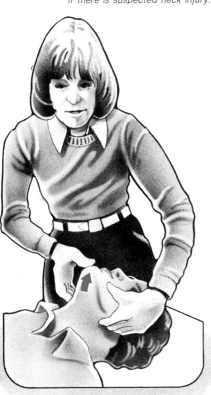

Lifting the jaw forward will help to open the airway. This is the preferred technique if there is suspected neck injury.

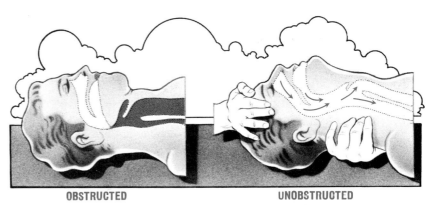

OBSTRUCTED　　　　　　　　　**UNOBSTRUCTED**

The back of the tongue may obstruct the airway. Lifting the victim's neck and tilting the head backward will open the airway. This method should not be used if there is any suspicion of neck injury.

but has been called a "café coronary" and will be discussed below.)

What To Do: The ABC's of CPR

If a person suddenly collapses and loses consciousness, it must be decided immediately whether a cardiopulmonary arrest has occurred. Any delay can result in permanent brain damage or death. Try to awaken the victim. If he cannot be awakened and if there are no palpable pulses (carotid) in the neck, begin the ABC's of cardiopulmonary resuscitation.

(A) Airway. **The first requirement is to assure a clear, unobstructed airway.**

 1. Place the victim on his back.
 2. Hyperextend the neck (lift the victim's neck and tilt his head backward as shown in the illustrations) and then lift the victim's chin forward; this lifts the tongue away from the back of the throat and helps to enlarge the airway. (Hyperextending the neck should not be done if there is any suspicion of neck injury.)

3. Listen for breathing by placing your ear near the victim's mouth, and watch the victim's chest for signs of breathing.

4. If there is no evidence of breathing, open the victim's mouth and remove any obvious foreign materials—false teeth, food, vomitus.

(B) Breathing (Mouth-to-Mouth Resuscitation). If opening and clearing the airway do not produce spontaneous breathing, it will be necessary to breathe for the victim.

1. With the victim's head in the hyperextended position, pinch his nostrils closed, take a deep breath, and place your mouth tightly over his mouth.

2. Exhale quickly and deeply, four times in rapid succession, each time removing your mouth and letting air escape passively from the victim's mouth.

3. If there is great resistance to your breath, no rise in the victim's chest, and no escape of air from his mouth, the airway may still be obstructed.

   a) Further hyperextend the victim's neck and lift his jaw.

   b) Look again for foreign objects in the mouth and throat.

   c) If none are found, you will have to try a different approach. Roll the victim on his side toward you and deliver four firm slaps between the shoulder blades. With the victim on his back, place your fist just above his navel and forcefully push once. Combined, these may force air out of his lungs and dislodge any foreign body that is trapped deeper in the airway; if so, the material should be removed from the victim's mouth.

4. If the mouth cannot be opened or is severely damaged, mouth-to-nose resuscitation may be used.

(C) Chest Compression. After assuring an open airway and delivering four breaths, check for carotid pulse in the neck, on either side of the windpipe. If there is no pulse, perform chest compression, or external cardiac massage.

1. Kneel beside the victim.

2. Place the heel of your hand just below the middle of the victim's breastbone and your other hand on top of the first. Do not let your fingers touch the victim's ribs or you may compress the wrong part of the chest.

3. Leaning directly over the patient, give a firm thrust straight downward. Let the weight of your shoulders do the work.

4. The breastbone should be pushed downward about two inches in the adult, and the compressions should be repeated 60 to 80 times each minute. (Note: Use of this procedure may crack some of the victim's ribs; proceed carefully, but do not stop CPR, since the alternative is death.)

5. CHEST COMPRESSION (EXTERNAL CARDIAC MASSAGE) SHOULD ALWAYS BE ACCOMPANIED BY ARTIFICIAL RESPIRATION!

   a) If there are *two rescuers:* one ventilation should be interposed between every five compressions at a compression rate of 60 per minute.

   b) If there is only *one rescuer:* two ventilations should be interposed between every 15 compressions at a compression rate of 80 per minute.

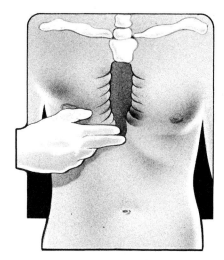

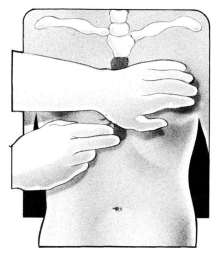

Find the tip of the sternum. The correct hand position for cardiac compression is two finger breadths above the tip of the sternum.

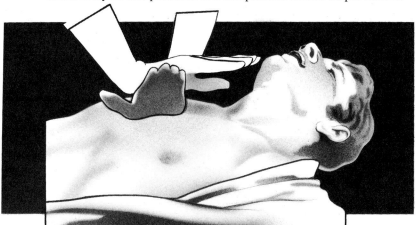

Place the heel of one hand on the sternum, and the heel of the other hand on the back of the first. Compressions of the chest should be done without placing the fingers on the chest wall.

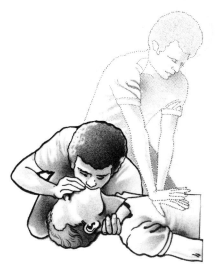

In "one-man" resuscitation, give two breaths between compressions at the rate of two breaths for every fifteen compressions.

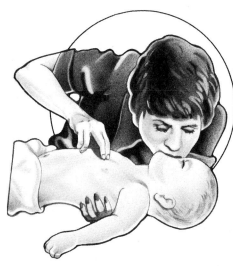

One person can resuscitate an infant by giving quick breaths while compressing the chest with the fingers of one hand.

6. If the victim is a child, the ABC's of CPR are the same except:
   a) Foreign bodies are more common in the airway.
   b) The person administering CPR puts his mouth over both the mouth and the nose of the victim.
   c) If an infant's head is flexed back too much, further obstruction of the airway can occur.
   d) Shallower breaths (puffs) should be used at 25 to 30 per minute.
   e) Exert pressure over the center of the breastbone, as the heart chambers (ventricles) to be compressed are higher in a child's body.
   f) Using only your fingertips, compress the chest ¾ to 1½ inches at a rate of 100 to 125 compressions each minute.

What Not To Do

1. Do not try to use CPR on any person who is alert and awake, or on any person who is unconscious but is breathing and has pulses.
2. Never compress the upper or lower ends of the breastbone; CPR is effective only when the flexible part of the breastbone that lies directly over the heart is compressed.
3. Do not interrupt CPR for more than 15 seconds, even to transport the victim.
4. Unless you are completely exhausted, do not stop CPR either until the victim is breathing adequately on his own and has a pulse, or until the care of the victim is taken over by more experienced medical personnel.
5. If the victim is revived, do not leave him unattended, because he may arrest again and require further CPR.

"Café Coronary" or Severe Choking While Eating

Anyone who collapses while eating may well have had a heart attack, but he may be choking on a large piece of food (usually meat). This most frequently occurs in older people, usually those who have poor teeth or false teeth, and frequently it is associated with some alcohol intake.

What To Look For

1. Before collapsing and losing consciousness, a victim who has been eating, possibly while also talking or laughing, may suddenly stand up and walk from the table, clutch his throat, or exhibit violent motions.
2. *He will not be able to talk.*
3. He may become blue.

What To Consider

The victim may be having a heart attack, but heart attack victims usually are able to talk prior to collapsing; they usually do not display quick violent motions, but collapse suddenly.

What To Do

The person will soon become unconscious and die if the obstructed airway is not cleared.

If the person is still standing:

1. Ask the victim to nod if he has food stuck in his throat.
2. Stand behind him and place one clenched fist in the middle, upper abdomen just below the ribs. Place your other hand on top of the first hand.
3. Give a very forceful pull of the clenched fist directly backward and upward under the rib cage (a bear hug from behind).
4. This will, ideally, act like a plunger and force the diaphragm upward, pushing any air left in the lungs out the windpipe and expelling or loosening the trapped object. The procedure may be repeated several times.
5. Once loosened, the foreign object can be pulled out.

If the victim has already collapsed:

1. Place him on his back, open his mouth and look for and remove any visible foreign material.
2. If none is seen, place the heel of your hand on the victim's mid-upper abdomen and give a forceful push.
3. This should dislodge the foreign material into the mouth, from which it can be removed. Repeat the procedure as often as necessary.

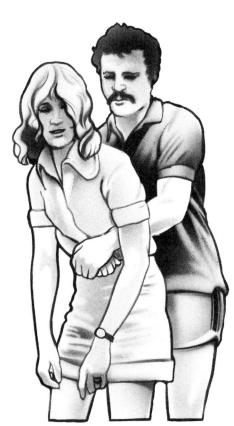

Food obstructing the airway in a "café coronary" may be loosened or expelled by an upper abdominal thrust or hug; using the fist of one hand placed in the abdomen just below the rib cage, give a forceful jerk upward.

4. If, after the object has been cleared, the victim still is not breathing, is unconscious, and is without a pulse, begin CPR.

What Not To Do

Do not stop CPR efforts until the victim revives or more experienced personnel arrive.

What To Expect

If the problem is noted early and foreign material is removed, the chances for the victim's survival are excellent.

Drowning

Fatal drowning and near drowning are common occurrences. Like cardiac arrest and "café coronary," drowning requires immediate action and basic life support.

What Is It?

Near or reversible drowning is much more common than fatal drowning. The near drowning victim may have no symptoms or he may need help because of severe respiratory distress and confusion. The drowned victim will be unconscious, will have no pulse, and will not be breathing.

What To Consider

1. The water may damage the lining of the lungs, resulting in a decreased ability to exchange oxygen from the air into the blood. Following a near

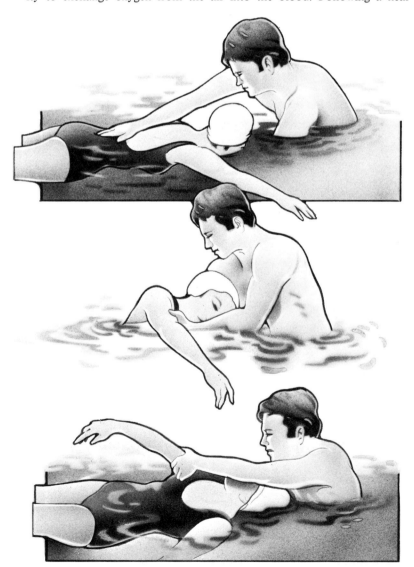

If there is a chance that a drowning victim has also injured his neck, particular care should be taken to protect the neck from further injury. The victim may be floated onto a board for removal from the water (see following page).

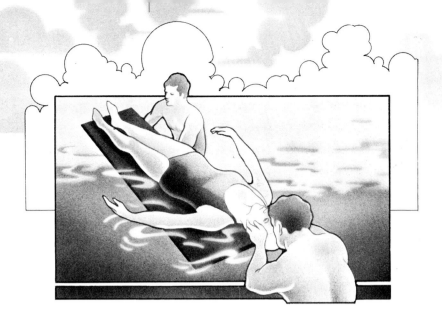

drowning the victim may suffer a cardiac arrest.

2. Always consider the possibility of an associated injury—for example, a broken neck, which is likely if the victim has dived into the water.

What To Do

1. Begin mouth-to-mouth resuscitation if the victim is unconscious and is not breathing, even while he is still in the water.
2. Give four quick breaths, followed by one breath every five seconds.
3. Remove the victim from the water without interrupting artificial respiration except for a few seconds (one minute at most). Once he is out of the water begin CPR.
4. If the victim has a suspected spinal injury, he should be placed on his back on a flat board for removal.
5. The victim of near drowning should be taken to the hospital *immediately*. If oxygen is available it should be used, and the victim should be watched closely for the possibility of cardiac arrest.
6. The distressed victim who has difficulty breathing, has blue color, and is semiconscious may require only artificial respiration, but be sure.

What Not To Do

1. Do not use the manual (arm lift) method of artificial respiration; it doesn't work.
2. Do not try to drain water from the victim's lungs.
3. Do not fail to take near drowning victims to the hospital immediately; such victims may quickly develop respiratory difficulty.
4. Do not stop CPR until more experienced medical personnel take over, or until you are completely exhausted.

Electric Shock

What Is It?

Even the relatively low voltages of electrical appliances that are used around the home can cause fatal electrocution. Death results from paralysis of the breathing center in the brain, from paralysis of the heart, or from uncontrolled, extremely rapid twitching (fibrillation) of the heart muscle.

What To Look For

1. The possibility of electrocution should be considered whenever an unconscious victim is found near an electric wire, a socket, or an appliance.
2. Electrical burns may or may not be apparent.

What To Consider

1. There are other possible reasons for unconsciousness, such as a head injury, seizure, or drug or alcohol ingestion.
2. Think of possible associated injuries (head injury, neck injury) before moving the victim.

400

What To Do

1. Disconnect the victim from the electrical source as quickly and safely as possible. This can be done by disconnecting the plug or appliance or by shutting off the main switch in the fuse box.
2. Alternately, use a dry, nonconductive, nonmetallic stick or pole to move the wire or victim. DO NOT TOUCH THE VICTIM UNTIL HE IS DISCONNECTED OR YOU MAY BECOME ANOTHER VICTIM.
3. If the victim remains unconscious and shows no pulse or respiration, begin CPR immediately. Continue until the victim revives or until more experienced medical personnel take over.
4. If there is an associated head, neck, or back injury, let trained medical personnel transport the victim.
5. Upon awakening, victims of electric shock often are confused and agitated, and, for a short time, they may need protection from falls and additional injuries.

What Not To Do

1. DO NOT TOUCH THE VICTIM UNTIL HE IS DISCONNECTED.
2. DO NOT MOVE THE VICTIM IF THERE IS A HEAD, NECK, OR BACK INJURY, EXCEPT TO REMOVE HIM FROM DANGER.

What To Expect

Even with adequate CPR the victim may need more advanced life support such as electric heart shock. However, he generally can be managed with basic CPR until more advanced life support becomes available.

Drug Overdose and Carbon Monoxide Poisoning

What Is It?

Although deaths from drug overdose and carbon monoxide poisoning may be associated with suicide attempts, such deaths do occur in other settings. An unsuspecting heroin addict may inject an exceptionally pure cut of the narcotic. A child may explore the medicine cabinet and ingest some sleeping pills, pain pills, or even antidiarrheal pills. Carbon monoxide poisoning occurs frequently in automobiles with faulty exhaust systems, in industry, and in burning buildings. These poisons all suppress the breathing center in the brain.

What To Do

1. If the person who has ingested pills is unconscious and without pulse or breathing, begin CPR.
2. If the victim is unconscious and is not breathing, but *has* pulses, perform mouth-to-mouth resuscitation only. Respiratory arrest is common in drug overdoses.
3. When transferring the victim to the hospital, take along any bottles and pills that may be associated with the poisoning.
4. Remove the victim from the carbon monoxide exposure and begin CPR.

What To Expect

Following a large drug overdose, even with adequate CPR the victim may not begin to breathe on his own or may not wake up for many hours, and he may need extended life support at the hospital in an intensive care unit.

Massive Hemorrhage (Bleeding)

Following the control of a victim's cardiorespiratory function, the next most urgent priority for the person giving first aid is to control hemorrhaging.

What Is It?

If major bleeding occurs, a large vessel (artery or vein) may be involved. Lacerated arteries tend to produce a pulsating stream of blood, signifying an injury that needs immediate first aid.

What To Consider

If the victim is bleeding massively, shock or inadequate blood circulation may develop and the victim may become unconscious or may have a cardiopulmonary arrest.

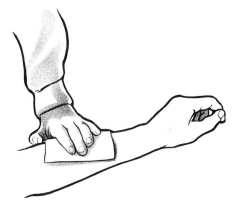

Direct, firm pressure is frequently the best way to stop bleeding.

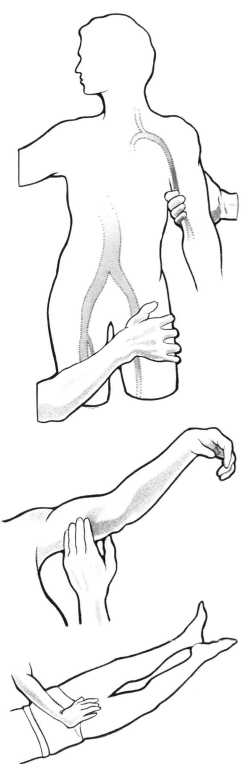

What To Do

1. Have the victim lie down to prevent fainting.
2. If he already has fainted, raise his feet higher than his head.
3. If the victim is unconscious, and there are no pulses or breathing, begin CPR.
4. With a clean cloth or sterile dressing, apply *direct pressure* over the wound to halt the bleeding. Most major bleeding (even arterial) will stop in a few minutes if this method is used.
5. Maintain the pressure until better trained medical personnel take over.
6. If severe bleeding of an arm or leg does not stop after several minutes of direct pressure, try to stop the circulation in the artery supplying the blood by pressing firmly against it with your hand or fingers. There are points (shown in the illustrations) on each side of the body where arterial pressure can be used to stop bleeding. (There are also pressure points in the head and neck, but they should *not* be used because of the danger of interrupting the supply of blood to the brain or the intake of air.)
7. When the bleeding stops, tie the dressing firmly in place.

What Not To Do

1. DO NOT TRY TO USE ARTERIAL PRESSURE POINTS IN THE HEAD OR NECK.
2. THE USE OF TOURNIQUETS SHOULD BE DISCOURAGED because they are often ineffective and do more harm than good.
3. If the injury has been caused by a large foreign object that is protruding from the victim's body, do not remove it, or you may further aggravate the injury.

What To Expect

1. Most bleeding can be controlled by direct pressure.
2. Lacerations of the scalp bleed profusely but are rarely associated with massive blood loss.
3. Lacerations of the torso may have penetrated into the chest or abdomen and must be evaluated by a physician.

Section Two:
Common, Not Immediately Life-Threatening Emergencies

Animal Bites

All animal bites (dog, cat, and wild animal, as well as human) are dangerous and need medical attention. In addition to the injury itself, there is a chance of infection, including tetanus and rabies.

Bites from wild animals, particularly skunks, foxes, raccoons, and bats, always should be evaluated by a physician.

What To Do

1. Thoroughly scrub the wound with soap and water to flush out the animal saliva. This should be done for at least ten minutes.
2. Cover the wound with a dry, clean cloth or dressing.
3. Consult a physician immediately for further cleansing, infection control, repair, and possibly for tetanus and rabies prevention.
4. If possible the animal should be caught or identified and reported to the local authorities for observation.

What Not To Do

Do not mutilate the animal, particularly its head. (If it is a wild animal and is killed, tests can be run by the local authorities to determine if it was rabid.)

Automobile Accidents

Even with the slower, safer speeds on U.S. highways, automobile accidents still account for the largest number of the nation's accidental deaths, as well as for numerous fatalities elsewhere. Automobile accidents may cause complex or multiple injuries, and priorities must be considered for the care of the injured.

If bleeding is too extensive to stop with direct pressure, locate the brachial or femoral arteries and apply pressure to stop bleeding distal to those points.

402

What To Do

1. Turn the car's engine off if it is still running.
2. Do as much first aid as possible *in* the car.
3. Move the victim only under the following circumstances.
   a) The car is on fire.
   b) Gasoline has spilled and there is a *danger* of fire.
   c) The area is congested, unsafe, and presents the danger of a second accident.
4. Check the patient for breathing and pulses.
5. Control any hemorrhaging.
6. If there is a head and neck injury or fracture of an extremity, wait for medical help before moving the victim, except to insure breathing or to stop significant bleeding.
7. If the victim must be moved to a medical facility, splint any fractures and support his head, neck, and spine on a backboard.
8. As soon as possible the accident should be reported to the appropriate authorities.

What Not To Do

Do not move unnecessarily a victim who is unconscious or who has a head or neck injury. It may be necessary to move a victim who has no pulse and is not breathing, or who is bleeding severely.

Backache, Acute

Most frequently, back pain is of recent onset and follows some type of acute exertion or unusual activity, such as lifting a heavy object. The pain usually results from muscular strain and may not become bothersome until hours after the exertion. Back pain that is associated with acute injury or with pain radiating down the legs may indicate a serious problem and demands immediate medical evaluation. In addition backache accompanied by blood in the urine might indicate injury to the kidney or the presence of a kidney stone, while backache with fever or urinary pain might signify the presence of a urinary tract infection.

What To Do

1. If a backache is nagging, mild, of recent onset, and is associated with recent activity, and if there is no pain radiating into the hip or leg, and if there is no bowel or urinary problem, it may be treated with:
   a) Absolute bed rest for 24–72 hours.
   b) A firm, nonsagging bed—a bed board might be used.
   c) Local heat or warm tub baths.
   d) Aspirin or an aspirin substitute might be helpful.
2. If the back pain is severe, with pain radiating into the hip or legs, or if it is associated with bowel or urinary problems, the victim should see a physician as soon as possible.
3. If the back pain follows an accident, it should be evaluated by a physician.
4. Back pain that does not improve within 48 hours should be evaluated by a physician.

Bleeding from the Rectum

The acute onset of bright red bleeding from the rectum may be caused by bleeding *hemorrhoidal* veins. The usual history includes constipation and straining to defecate, leading to bright red blood dripping into the toilet bowl and onto the toilet paper, frequently with associated rectal pain. The problem is common among pregnant women.

Rectal bleeding requires medical evaluation. If the stools are black and tarry, it is imperative to get a medical evaluation as soon as possible. The possibility that the bleeding originates higher in the intestinal tract must be considered, since bleeding within the rectum may be a sign of an ulcer, tumor, or inflammation.

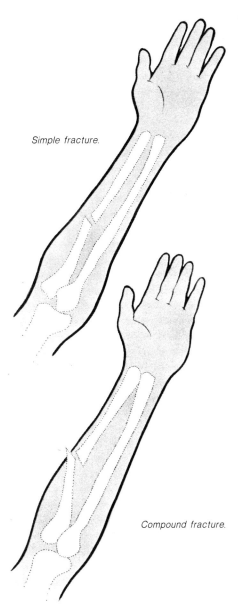

Simple fracture.

Compound fracture.

What To Do

1. If the bleeding is due to hemorrhoids:
    a) Warm tub baths three or four times daily may promote healing.
    b) Lubricating ointment such as petrolatum may decrease irritation to the hemorrhoids during bowel movements.
    c) Drinking plenty of fluids will soften the stool, as will bran cereals or stool softeners available from drug stores.
2. If bleeding persists, see a physician.
3. Get a physician's evaluation for black, tarry stools or for bright red rectal bleeding that is not known to be from hemorrhoids.

Blisters

Blisters are generally caused either by burns or by friction on the skin. Burn-related blisters can result from contact with flame or hot objects or with certain chemicals, and from severe sunburn or scalds. Blisters represent injuries to only a partial thickness of the skin. When a blister breaks, there is a loss of the natural protective insulation of the skin. Open, broken blisters are vulnerable to infection and tend to promote the loss of body fluids by evaporation. If blisters are very large, evaporation may be severe and may result in dehydration.

What To Do

1. Small blisters should not be opened. They should be protected with dry, soft dressings to prevent rupture.
2. Blisters resulting from contact with chemicals should be immediately and copiously washed with tap water to dilute the offending agent.
3. If a blister ruptures, the area should be washed gently but thoroughly with mild soap and water. The skin that covered the blister should be carefully removed, and the wound should be covered with a dry, sterile dressing.
4. Blisters of large areas of the body should be treated by a physician.

What To Expect

1. The pain from blisters usually subsides after one to two days.
2. Almost all blisters break and slough after four or five days, and the wound heals in about two weeks.
3. Ruptured blisters often become infected. Note any increased redness, pain, swelling, or heat about the wound, and be particularly aware of any red streaking up the extremity, pus from the wound, or fever.

Boils, Pimples, and Styes

When sweat glands of the skin become plugged, there may be bacterial growth and an accumulation of infected material (pus) inside the gland. Frequently, the accumulation of pus is absorbed by the body's natural defense processes. Occasionally, the area of infection expands, forming an abscess or boil (called a stye when on the eyelid). These are painful swellings that are red, warm, and can vary from less than a half inch to several inches in size. When these infections have reached this stage, the only way that the body can heal itself is to let the pus out through the skin.

What To Do

1. Apply warm, moist compresses as often as possible throughout the day (for 15 minutes every four hours).
2. When the boil or stye "points" and then ruptures, wipe the pus away gently with a dry, sterile cloth and cover it with a dressing. Continue to use warm, moist compresses.
3. If there are multiple boils or if the infection seems to be large, contact a physician.

What Not To Do

Do not attempt to squeeze or puncture boils, pimples, or styes. If hot compresses are used, early boils and styes may resolve. Most will "point" and rupture in two or three days and will then rapidly heal.

404

Broken Bones (Fractures)

A broken bone should be suspected whenever a person complains of pain with the loss of the normal use of an extremity. Fractures are seldom in and of themselves life-threatening emergencies, and one must make sure that the victim is safe from further harm and has good respiration and pulses before making any attempt to immobilize or move an injured person. Any victim suspected of having a broken neck or broken back should be handled in a special manner. (*See* Broken Neck or Back, below.)

There are two types of fractures that are important to recognize. Most fractures are "simple" or "closed," and the broken bone does not protrude through the skin. There are times, however, when the broken bone does pierce the skin; such breaks are known as "compound" or "open" fractures.

A word about sprains is in order here. Sprains may be managed at home if they are very mild. Aspirin, rest, elevation of the affected extremity, and local ice packs are the best treatment. If a sprain is severe, however, it should be treated like a fracture, and medical attention should be sought.

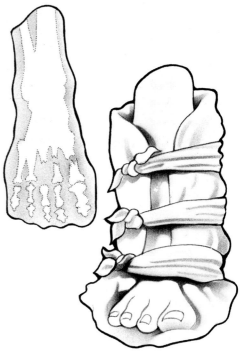

A simple splint for a broken ankle or foot may be made with a pillow or folded blanket or jacket and secured with roller bandages, tape, and so forth.

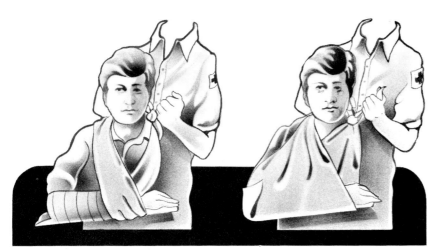

A broken forearm should be splinted and a sling should be applied. If a splint is not available, the sling itself will reduce the pain.

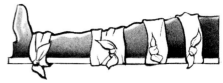

A broken bone in the lower leg should be splinted before transporting the victim.

What To Do

1. Make certain that the victim is breathing adequately and has pulses before even considering first aid for the fracture.
2. When there is reason to suspect multiple broken bones, or when the neck, back, pelvis, or thigh might be broken, it would be best to let trained emergency personnel transport the victim to the hospital.
3. If the broken bone protrudes through the skin, cover it with a dry sterile dressing, but do not try to push it back in. If there is excessive bleeding, use direct pressure to stop it. (*See* Massive Hemorrhage, above.)
4. If the victim must be moved, the fracture should be immobilized with splints to prevent further damage and to make the victim more comfortable (the pain of a fracture is caused by the two ends of the broken bone rubbing together). The basic principle of splinting is to immobilize the broken bone by securing the affected limb to some firm object (a piece of wood, broom handle, ski pole, several newspapers or magazines, or even an injured leg to the uninjured leg). Both ends of the splint must extend beyond the area of suspected fracture; the splint may be secured with bandages, belts, sheets, or neckties. Most injuries of the arm, wrist, or hand can be stabilized simply with a sling.

What Not To Do

1. Do not try to transport any accident victim who has an obviously unstable

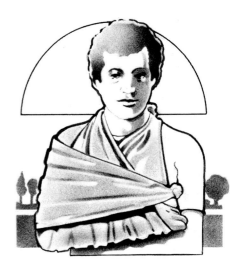

A broken collarbone can be splinted by first applying a sling to the arm, and then applying a wrap around the arm and chest, to reduce movement of the arm.

405

(floppy) extremity without stabilizing or splinting it first. Even though fractures can be disturbingly displaced, deformed, and very painful in themselves, they rarely represent life-threatening emergencies. If fractures are immobilized adequately, there frequently is a marked reduction in pain.

2. Do not attempt to move a victim with a suspected broken neck or back without trained medical personnel, unless it is absolutely necessary to do so.

Broken Neck or Back

The possibility of injury to the spine (neck and back) must be considered whenever a person is:

1. Involved in an accident of any type and subsequently complains of back or neck pain, has any degree of paralysis or weakness of an extremity, or has numbness or tingling of an extremity or part of his body.
2. Injured about the face or head in an accident, or is rendered unconscious.

What To Do

1. Make certain the victim is breathing and has pulses.
2. Unless it is absolutely necessary, do not move the victim, but let trained medical personnel do it.
3. Unless he is unconscious, the victim is safest on his back; avoid attempts to pick up his head or to move his neck.
4. If the victim is unconscious, convulsive, or vomiting, he should be rolled—carefully, and preferably by two people—onto his side, and his head should be supported very carefully on a pillow or coat.
5. If it is absolutely necessary to move the victim, he should be placed on a firm board. This should be done cautiously, with several people supporting the whole spine and the head. The neck or back should not be flexed (chin moved toward the chest or head dropped back).

What Not To Do

1. Do not allow any accident victim who complains of neck or back pain to sit or stand.
2. Do not give the victim anything to eat or drink.

Bruises and Black Eyes

Any direct trauma to the soft tissues (skin, muscles, etc.) of the body may injure the blood vessels as well. The damaged blood vessels then leak blood which, when it accumulates under the skin, at first looks black, in a few days looks yellow-brown, and then is reabsorbed. Also, direct trauma may cause swelling or fluid collection under the skin. The area about the eye, because of the loose tissue present, is particularly prone to this swelling, and when blood collects the result is a "black eye."

Bruises are frequent problems and are usually benign in that they represent minimal injury and get better by themselves. However, if the force is adequate, associated injuries can occur, including fractures, ruptured abdominal organs, collapsed lungs, and injuries to the eyeball. If there is an obvious deformity, severe pain, or impaired motion of an extremity, or if there is impaired vision, blindness, severe pain in the eye itself, or double vision, a physician should evaluate the injury.

What To Do

1. As soon as possible, place a cold compress or an ice bag (a towel soaked in ice water or a towel-covered plastic bag of ice) on the bruise. This will reduce the pain and swelling and should be continued for several hours.
2. Restrict any movement of the injured part, because the less it is used during the first few hours, the less it will swell. Elevation of the bruised part above the level of the heart also decreases swelling.

If the injury is only a bruise, the victim should be able to use the extremity. Most bruises and black eyes will enlarge and worsen in appearance for up to 48 hours after the injury, after which they will gradually shrink. The blue-black color becomes yellow-brown and then disappears in 10–14 days. If multiple bruises that are not associated with trauma appear over the body, a physician should be contacted, because this may indicate a blood clotting disorder.

Burns

The skin can be burned by flames, hot objects, hot liquids (scalds), excessive sun exposure, chemicals, and contact with electricity. There are three degrees or depths of burns:

First degree—reddened, hot, very painful, no blisters. Heals spontaneously.

Second degree—painful, red, blistered. Usually heals spontaneously.

Third degree—deep burns can be white or black and are always painless. These may require skin grafts.

Many burns that appear to be first degree may later develop blisters and may actually be second degree. Second-degree and third-degree burns frequently become infected and need more attention and care than do first-degree burns. Electrical burns frequently look small but may be much deeper than suspected. Burns in children and older people are more serious.

What To Do

1. For sunburn see below.
2. For flash burns, scalds, and small burns, towels or sheets soaked in cool water should be applied immediately for comfort.
3. If it is a chemical burn, the area should be washed copiously and continuously (under a running faucet if possible) for 15–30 minutes.
4. The burn should be dressed with sterile, dry, soft dressings.
5. If burns involve large areas of the hands or face, they should be examined by a physician.
6. Electrical burns should be treated by a physician.
7. Burns, like cuts, require tetanus prevention.

What Not To Do

1. Do not apply ointments, sprays, or greases to large wounds.
2. Never use butter on any burn.
3. Do not break blisters.
4. Do not pull off any clothing that adheres to the burn.

If a small burn becomes encrusted, has pus, or shows red streaking, it may be infected and should be seen by a physician. If large areas of the body have second- or third-degree burns, there may be an excessive water loss from the body with consequent shock. People with extensive burns, especially young children and old people, are very likely to go into shock, and they should be transported to a hospital emergency department as soon as possible. "Shock," in this case, refers to a low level of circulating bodily fluids, not to a psychological state.

Chest Pain

It is well established now that most heart attack deaths result from *treatable* disturbances of the heartbeat. The overall emphasis must be to get the person with a heart attack into an intensive care unit as soon as possible. To accomplish this there must be:

1. Equipped and staffed emergency departments.
2. Better prehospital care and transportation.
3. Public education on the signs and symptoms of a heart attack.
4. Public education on the techniques of basic life support—CPR. (*See* Cardiopulmonary Arrest, above.)

Denial of the pain and its significance, ascribing it to other causes (heartburn, gas, or pulled muscles), and trying different remedies (antacids or antiflatulence medications) often lead to fatal delays in proper medical treatment. Everyone must be aware of the significance of chest pain and heart attack.

Severe chest pain must always be considered a medical emergency. A correct diagnosis can only be made by a *physician*, using an appropriate medical history, an examination, and sometimes several laboratory tests—an electrocardiogram, chest X-ray, and blood tests.

There are several aspects of chest pain that are important. Heart attack pain is often described as a *dull* ache, tightness, squeezing, or as a heavy feeling that is usually diffusely located over the front of the chest. It is often associated with aching in the shoulders, neck, arms, or jaw. Many people become short of breath, sweaty, nauseated, and may vomit. If any of these symptoms occurs in an adult, he must be transported immediately to the nearest physician or emergency department.

What To Do

1. Chest pain, especially with the symptoms listed above, demands *immediate* medical attention. An ambulance should be called immediately.
2. While waiting, make the person comfortable and reassure him.
3. Do not give him anything by mouth except what a physician has prescribed.
4. Do not make him lie down if he is more comfortable sitting.
5. Do not leave him unattended. He may suffer a cardiac arrest and may require basic life support (CPR).

There are many other causes of chest pain that may need medical attention. Chest pain associated with fever and cough could be a symptom of pneumonia. Chest pain associated with coughing up blood or associated with thrombophlebitis (pain in the calf or thigh) might represent a blood clot in the lungs. A collapsed lung might cause chest pain and sudden shortness of breath.

There are numerous causes of chest pain, such as severe heartburn, viral pneumonia, inflammation of the cartilages of the ribs, and pulled muscles, that are not life-threatening, but a physician must make these diagnoses.

Childbirth, Emergency

Childbirth is a natural and normal phenomenon, and it rarely requires advanced medical training to carry out a safe delivery. For a variety of reasons (inadequate transportation, very short labor, etc.) many babies are born unexpectedly, outside of the hospital.

Labor is the cyclical contraction of the uterus (womb) which helps to open up the end of the uterus (cervix) to allow passage of the baby. These contractions usually are painful and occur with increasing frequency and duration until the delivery. The duration of labor is different for every woman. Frequently labor lasts for 12 or more hours for a first baby, but the time may be reduced to a few hours or less for the woman who has borne several children.

Delivery is the passage of the baby through the birth canal and the vagina. The mother will usually experience *rectal* pressure and will know that the child is being born. The reflex action is to push or "bear down." The child's head and hair will be visible at the opening of the vagina. If the woman is "pushing" and the infant is visible, the birth is imminent. If a foot, an arm, the buttocks, or the umbilical cord is first to appear, take the mother to a hospital immediately.

What To Do

1. Let nature take its course. Do not try to hurry the birth or interfere with it.
2. Wash your hands and keep the surroundings (sheets, etc.) as clean as possible. (Fresh newspaper is often sterile, if sheets or blankets are unavailable.)
3. Support the emerging baby and let it slide out.
4. Once the baby is delivered, support him with both hands, keeping his head lower than the rest of his body to allow the fluid to drain from his mouth.
5. Place the infant on a dry towel or sheet and cover him immediately. Heat loss is a problem for newborn babies.
6. Aluminum foil wrapped around the baby's body will retard heat loss.
7. If the baby is not breathing begin mouth-to-mouth resuscitation, very gently, using puffs of air from your cheeks.
8. It is not necessary to cut the umbilical cord, and one may choose to have this done at the hospital. If medical care will be significantly delayed, however, use the following procedure to cut the cord: using a clean (boiled) ribbon, cord, or string, tie the cord tightly at two points, one that is four inches from the baby and the other at least eight inches from the baby. Cut the cord with clean, boiled scissors between the two ties.
9. Do not wash the white material from the baby (this is protective).
10. Warmly wrap the infant and transport it to the hospital.
11. After the child has been delivered, knead the womb by applying firm pres-

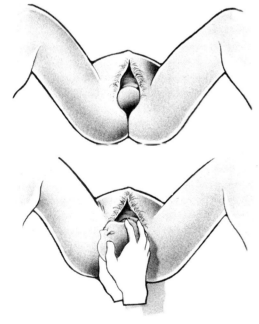

If childbirth is imminent, the top of the baby's head will begin to bulge through the mother's labia. Support the head with one hand on each side (not over the baby's face), and ease the shoulders out. The baby will be quite slippery, so be careful not to drop it.

sure to the lower abdomen.

12. The mother should remain lying down until the bleeding stops and the placenta (afterbirth) has been expelled.

13. When the placenta is expelled, minutes after the birth of the child, it should be retained and taken to the hospital for examination.

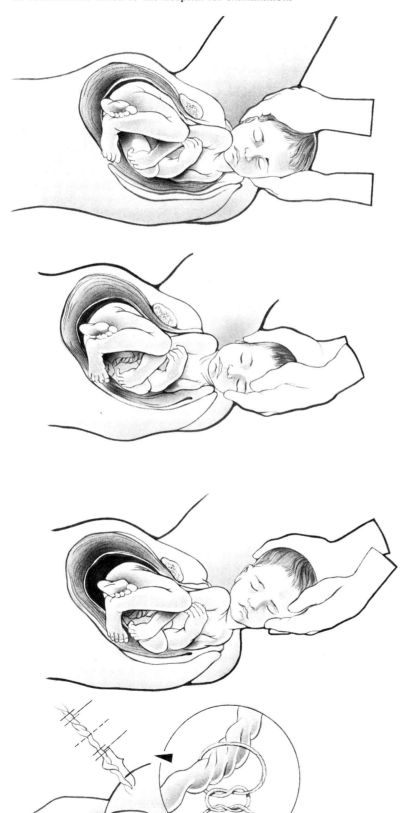

After delivery, the umbilical cord may be tied using a sterilized cord. Tie the cords at four and eight inches from the baby.

CORE TEMPERATURE	SYMPTOMS
94°	CONFUSION
90°	HEARTBEAT BECOMES IRREGULAR
86°	LOSS OF MUSCLE STRENGTH DROWSINESS AND UNCONSCIOUSNESS
77°	CARDIAC ARREST AND DEATH

As the body's core (central) temperature drops, the victim becomes confused and ultimately may die.

Cold, Overexposure, and Frostbite

Overexposure. Each year many people die from cold exposure resulting in *hypothermia*. The people who are particularly at risk include elderly persons with poor circulation, individuals who unpreparedly become exposed to low temperatures and high winds, and people who are intoxicated with alcohol. Poor circulation, poor protection from the elements, and alcohol dilate blood vessels in the skin and allow heat loss that lowers the body core (central) temperature. Malfunction of the brain, heart, and lungs may then occur.

What To Do

1. Remove the person from cold exposure and place him in the warmest place possible.
2. Cover the patient to prevent further loss of body heat.
3. If the victim is awake and able to swallow, give him *warm, nonalcoholic* drinks.
4. Watch for a cardiac arrest and be prepared to carry out CPR.

What Not To Do

1. Do not give alcoholic beverages.
2. Do not leave the person unattended.
3. Do not risk burning the person by the use of hot water bottles.

Frostbite. Frostbite is a common injury in winter weather, particularly when low temperatures are combined with wind. Exposed, small parts of the body are the most susceptible (nose, ears, fingers, toes, and face). Again, the elderly and the intoxicated are the most susceptible. Initially, the involved part begins to tingle and then becomes numb. Frozen tissue usually is dead white in color.

What To Do

1. Remove the person from the cold as soon as possible.
2. Every effort should be made to protect the frozen part. If there is a chance that the part might refreeze before reaching medical care, it may be more harmful to thaw it and let it refreeze than to await arrival at the treatment area for thawing.
3. Rapid rewarming is essential. Use lukewarm (not hot) water between 100° and 110° F (37–43° C) or use warmed blankets. Within about 30 minutes, sensation may return to the part, which may become red and swollen. At first the rewarmed part will tingle, but it will begin to be painful and tender to the touch.
4. When the part is warm, keep it *dry* and clean. If blisters appear, use sterile dressings.
5. See a physician as soon as possible.

What Not To Do

1. Do not give alcoholic beverages.
2. Take care not to burn the person by using water that is too hot.
3. Do not let the part refreeze.
4. Do not rub the injured part; friction may cause further damage.

Convulsions

Convulsions and epileptic attacks are frightening to watch. The victim's lips may become blue, he may make a crying noise, his eyes may roll back, and his body may be jerked by uncontrollable spasms. Many seizures occur in people with known seizure disorders who have forgotten their medications, in alcohol abusers who have recently stopped drinking, and in children with an acute febrile illness (febrile seizures or seizures associated with fever in children). *Febrile convulsions* are quite common among children aged six months to three years. They result from an abrupt rise in the child's temperature and are generally of short duration (usually ending by the time the victim arrives at the emergency department). The victim usually awakens soon after the seizure.

What To Do

1. Turn the victim onto his side so that saliva is able to drain out without being inhaled into the victim's lungs.

410

2. If it can be done safely, place a rolled handkerchief in the victim's mouth between his teeth to prevent him from biting his tongue. Do not force a spoon or other object into the victim's mouth.
3. Most people who have had a seizure need prompt medical attention at the nearest emergency department.
4. The child with febrile convulsions is treated by reducing the fever. Cool towels or sponge baths may help to lower the child's temperature.
5. If the victim has fallen or shows evidence of head trauma, he should be assumed to have a broken neck and should be treated accordingly. (*See* Broken Neck or Back, above.)

What Not To Do

1. Do not force objects into the mouth of the convulsing person.
2. Do not get bitten by the convulsing person.
3. Do not try to restrain the convulsive movements. Protect the victim from further injury.

Following the seizure (most last less than ten minutes) the person will usually fall asleep or will be confused.

Do not assume that the seizure is "just a seizure" in either a child or an adult, since seizures may be signs of other problems such as head injury, meningitis, or tumor.

Croup

What Is It?

In the fall and winter months, when houses are dry and warm, young children (usually younger than three years) may develop a "croupy," barking cough. This condition usually is caused by a viral inflammation of the trachea (windpipe) and of the larger airways, and the infection may cause severe respiratory distress.

What To Do

1. For mild cases (most cases), lowering the temperature in the room and using a humidifier will quickly help the croupy breathing. A bathroom filled with steam from a running shower may be helpful.
2. Aspirin and liquids may be used to combat low-grade fever.
3. If there is a high fever, difficulty in swallowing or talking, or respiratory distress, the child should be seen by a physician as soon as possible.

Most cases of croup are mild, and they will usually clear up after two or three days if corrective measures are taken.

Cuts, Scratches, Abrasions

Small cuts, abrasions, and scratches are common occurrences and generally require only thorough cleansing and bandaging for protection. Some cuts are larger and may require stitches for closure to minimize scarring, to reduce the chance of infection, and to restore function. Deeper cuts may involve blood vessels, and they may cause extensive bleeding or may damage muscles, tendons, or nerves.

What To Do

1. All minor wounds and abrasions should be *thoroughly* washed. There should be no dirt, glass, or foreign material left in the wound. Mild soap and water are all that are necessary.
2. Bleeding can be stopped by direct pressure that is applied over the wound with a sterile, dry dressing, and by elevating the injured part.
3. Most wounds should be covered with a dressing to protect them from further harm and contamination.
4. All bites (human or animal) should be treated by a physician because of the likelihood of infection. (*See* Animal Bites, above.)
5. If there is any question about the need for sutures, the wound should be examined by a physician.
6. If the wound is dirty or extensive, or if the victim's tetanus immunization is not up to date, there may be the need for a booster immunization.

7. Watch carefully for signs of infection (usually they do not appear for several days). The signs are:
   a) a reddened, hot, painful area surrounding the wound,
   b) red streaks radiating from the wound,
   c) swelling around the wound, with fever and chills.

   If an infection appears, see a doctor at once.

Diabetic Coma and Insulin Reaction

Diabetics have difficulty using the sugar in their blood. *Insulin* lowers the blood sugar level. As would be expected, it may be difficult to adjust the daily insulin requirement to the intake of sugar-containing foods and to the individual's activity level. Because of this, some diabetics occasionally suffer either from *insulin reaction* (which is a blood sugar level that is too low) or from *diabetic coma* (which can be thought of as a blood sugar level that is too high).

Insulin reaction, or acute hypoglycemia, may cause the person to become acutely confused, incoherent, sweaty, or shaky. Eventually, the person may lose consciousness.

What To Do

1. Determine if the victim is a diabetic.
2. If he is *conscious*, give him some form of sugar (a lump of sugar, candy, sweets, or soft drinks that are not artificially sweetened).
3. Even if recovery is prompt, all victims should be evaluated by a physician.

What Not To Do

Do not try to give sugar to someone who is unconscious.

Diabetic coma with hyperglycemia (a high blood sugar level) is quite different. The onset is more gradual, taking several hours or longer. The victim may have warm, flushed skin, with a very dry mouth and tongue. He frequently may be drowsy but rarely is unconscious. His breath may smell fruity (like nail polish remover), and he may be dehydrated.

What To Do

A person in a diabetic coma needs prompt treatment by a physician.

Diarrhea (in a small child)

Diarrhea may be caused by many factors, ranging from simple nondigestion of eaten foods to such conditions as bacterial or viral infections of the intestinal tract. In a small child, acute prolonged diarrhea may rapidly cause dehydration and death. The younger the child and the more prolonged the diarrhea, the more dangerous is the threat to health. Maintenance of adequate hydration is the main goal of therapy.

The signs of dehydration are: lethargy, dryness of the mouth and armpits, sunken eyes, weight loss, and the absence of urination. A child who continues regularly to wet his diapers generally is not dehydrated.

What To Do

1. Small children with acute diarrhea should be given water, liquid Jell-O, or pediatric salt solutions. Milk and whole foods should be withheld for the first 24 – 48 hours of the diarrhea. In acute diarrhea, the bowel is unable to digest and absorb some of the sugars in milk, which worsens the diarrhea.
2. If the diarrhea persists for more than 48 hours, a physician should be contacted.
3. If the diarrhea causes signs of dehydration, or if the child stops taking in fluids, a physician should be contacted immediately.
4. Almost all diarrheal states in children are well on the road to recovery within 48 hours. For the bottle-fed child, half-strength formula can be substituted for regular formula for one or two days before resuming full-strength formula. If the diarrhea persists, a physician should be consulted.

What Not To Do

1. Do not continue milk and whole food during an acute diarrheal state.
2. Do not use adult antidiarrheal medications for children.

412

Dislocated Joints

It is frequently impossible to tell the difference between dislocated joints and broken bones until X-rays have been taken.

What To Do

1. Probable dislocations in the hand, arm, shoulder, or jaw usually do not require an ambulance for transportation to the hospital. Victims should, however, be transported safely and comfortably.
2. If there is a dislocation of the hip or knee, ambulance transportation will be needed.
3. Slings or splints may be helpful. (*See* Broken Bones, above.)

What Not To Do

Do not attempt to move or manipulate the joint, or to set a dislocation yourself; the bone may be broken if these procedures are done improperly.

Eye Pain (something in the eye)

Even a small speck of dirt in the eye can cause intense pain. The covering of the eye is quite sensitive and, even after the foreign material is removed, there may be a feeling of irritation. Redness and tears are frequently present.

What To Do

1. Examine the eye by pulling the lower lid down while lifting the upper lid off the eyeball. Most specks will be visible.
2. Gently splash water from a faucet to attempt to remove the foreign material.
3. Gently attempt to wipe the speck off with a moistened corner of a clean cloth, handkerchief, or cotton swab.
4. If the speck does not come off *easily*, or if there is persistent discomfort, a physician should be seen as soon as possible.
5. If irritating liquids are splashed into the eye, irrigate the eye with cool tap water for 30 minutes and then seek medical attention.

Fainting—Dizziness

Fainting is a sudden but momentary loss of consciousness. There are a variety of causes for it, including fatigue, hunger, sudden emotional upset, poor ventilation, etc. The person who has fainted looks pale and limp but is breathing and has a normal pulse. Simple fainting is not associated with chest pain or seizures, and the unconsciousness does not last for more than one or two minutes.

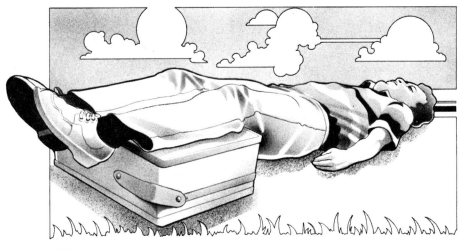

If a person faints, place him on his back or side and elevate the legs above the head.

What To Do

1. Place the victim on his back or side, with his legs higher than his head.
2. Check his airway, breathing, and pulses.
3. Apply cold compresses to the victim's forehead, and have him inhale aromatic spirits of ammonia.

4. If fainting is associated with chest pains, seizures, or severe headache, or if it lasts more than one or two minutes, the victim should be transported by ambulance to a physician.
5. If a person reports that he feels faint, have him sit with his face in his lap or stretch out on his back until he feels better.

Fainting is a relatively common problem and almost always quickly resolves in one or two minutes. Nevertheless, other causes should be considered—heart attack, stroke, internal bleeding, and insulin reaction.

Fever

Fever is an elevated oral temperature above 98.6° Fahrenheit or above 37° Celsius. Fever is a manifestation of the body's response to infection (viral or bacterial) or to foreign substances that the body is attempting to reject. People with fever frequently report muscle and bone pains, headaches, chills, and a hot feeling. Viral infections (colds, influenza, and even viral gastroenteritis) almost invariably are associated with low-grade fevers and are the most common causes of such fevers.

In susceptible children younger than three years of age, a *rapidly* rising fever may induce febrile seizures. (*See* Convulsions, above.)

What To Do—Adults

1. Aspirin and acetaminophen (aspirin substitute) are the two most effective antifever medicines available. If used appropriately, they not only effectively lower the temperature but also will provide some relief for the bone and muscle aches.
2. The person with fever should take a lot of fluids, as higher temperatures increase evaporation of water and thus accelerate dehydration.
3. Bed rest helps.
4. If the fever is very high (102° or more) and persistent (most fevers last less than 24 hours), a physician should be consulted.
5. Fever associated with chest pains, shortness of breath, cough, or with the production of sputum, or with confusion, headache, a stiff neck, abdominal pain, or earache should be evaluated by a physician as soon as possible.

What To Do—Children

1. Fever of 100° or more in an infant (less than 30 days old) is always an emergency, and the child should be seen immediately by a physician. Every household should have a thermometer for taking children's temperatures.
2. In addition to fluids and bed rest, children with temperatures over 100° may be given aspirin or acetaminophen (aspirin substitute) every four hours in doses of not more than 60 mg for each year of life.
3. The child *should not be* overly dressed but should be dressed lightly (T-shirt and diapers are enough).
4. If a child develops a temperature of 103° or more, and the fever does not respond to aspirin or acetaminophen, the child should be placed in a tub of lukewarm water (not cold) and should be sponged for at least 30 minutes.
5. If the fever still does not respond, a physician should be contacted.
6. Any child with a febrile seizure, lethargy, signs of dehydration, or excess irritability should be seen by a physician.

What Not To Do

Do not sponge a child with alcohol; it is potentially toxic and is flammable. The sudden cold is often frightening to a child.

Food Poisoning

Food poisoning is a term applied to the combination of nausea, vomiting, or diarrhea that is attributed to contaminated food. The symptoms may be identical to those of viral gastroenteritis (stomach flu), but with the lack of an associated fever. Some other causes of the same symptoms include emotional stress, viral infections, inorganic or organic poisons, or food intolerance. Food poisoning itself is caused by toxins produced by bacteria growing in the food. The most common organism causing food poisoning is the *Staphylococcus.* In

Staphylococcus food poisoning, vomiting and diarrhea generally develop within one to 18 hours following ingestion of the contaminated food.

What To Do

1. Generally, food poisoning resolves spontaneously within a few hours. Clear liquids should be offered as tolerated.
2. If vomiting or diarrhea is prolonged, dehydration may develop. In some cases, medical attention should be sought.

What Not To Do

1. Do not take antibiotics. They are useless in this type of poisoning.
2. Do not force the victim of food poisoning to drink fluids if he has any respiratory difficulty. Victims who develop respiratory difficulty should be seen immediately by a physician.

Foreign Objects in the Nose, Ear, Throat

Nose

1. If the object cannot be withdrawn or teased out easily, consult a physician at once.
2. Do not allow violent nose-blowing.
3. Do not deeply probe the nose yourself. You may push the object deeper into the nostril or you may cause harm to the nasal tissues.

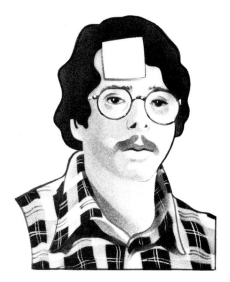

Ear

1. If the object cannot be withdrawn easily, consult a physician.
2. The tissues of the ear are very delicate and can easily be damaged. Pushing the object in further may even rupture the eardrum.

Throat

1. Large objects caught in the throat can cause severe difficulty in breathing (*see* Café Coronary, above). This requires immediate care.
2. Small objects can be swallowed—coins, fishbones, etc. Such smaller objects that get caught or that irritate the throat and that cause no difficulty in swallowing or breathing should be given a chance to pass. Drinks of water followed by eating soft foods—such as bread—may help. If the object remains caught or if irritation persists for more than two or three hours a physician should be notified.
3. Someone who has an irregular object—such as a pull tab from a beverage can, a piece of wire, or glass—caught in his throat needs immediate medical attention.

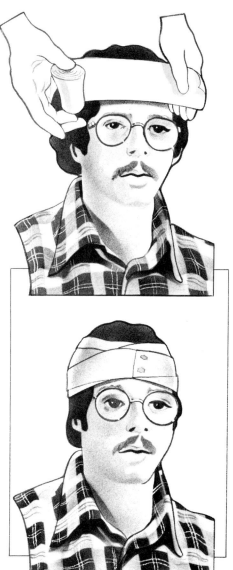

Head Injury

Injuries to the head may include lacerations and contusions of the scalp, fractures of the skull, or brain injuries. Whenever someone has suffered a serious injury to his head, one must always consider whether there might have been an associated injury to the neck. If there is a possibility of an associated neck injury, the victim should not be moved except by skilled personnel unless there is a chance that he might inhale secretions or vomitus. In that case, the victim may be very carefully rolled onto his side.

What To Do

1. Severe, deep lacerations should not be cleansed or irrigated. Instead, sterile dressings should be placed over the wound and should be secured snugly with a roller bandage. Heavy pressure should not be applied to severe lacerations because there may be an associated fracture of the skull and too much pressure may drive a fragment of bone into the brain.
2. Note any loss of consciousness or altered mental status. An examining physician will need this information.
3. Make sure that the victim's pulse and respiration are normal. If the victim might inhale his secretions or stomach contents, very carefully turn him onto his side. Note the size of the victim's pupils. If the victim is unconscious or confused and one of his pupils becomes larger than the other, this is a medical emergency and he should be seen immediately by a physician.

If there is an open head injury, apply a sterile dressing and secure it with a roller bandage. If there is significant bleeding, apply the roller bandage firmly.

415

4. Keep the victim lying down, but do not place a pillow under his head since doing so may cause further damage to the neck if it also has been injured.
5. Make sure that the victim's airway remains open. At times, CPR or artificial respiration (see above) may be needed.

Any head injury accompanied by a loss of consciousness should be evaluated by a physician as soon as possible. Even though the victim may regain consciousness, further brain damage may develop.

Heatstroke (sunstroke), Heat Exhaustion (heat prostration), and Heat Cramps

Heatstroke is a failure of the body's ability to keep itself cool and maintain a normal temperature. The first symptom is usually confusion, irrational behavior, passing out, or seizures. The patient has a fever, and the pulse is usually rapid and weak. Heatstroke generally affects the elderly, young infants, persons with heart disease, athletes or others doing hard work under hot conditions, and persons who have been drinking alcohol. This is a very serious condition, and immediate treatment is necessary.

What To Do

1. For heat exhaustion, move the victim to a cool place and elevate his legs. If he can take fluids by mouth, give him small amounts of water.
2. Heat cramps may also be treated with salt solutions taken orally (½ teaspoon of salt in a glass of water).
3. Heatstroke, manifested primarily by a very high temperature, should be treated by placing the patient in a cool place, by removing his clothing, and by applying cool water or ice packs to his body. The victim's extremities should be massaged vigorously to aid circulation, and immediate cooling is crucial.
4. If the victim has suffered from heatstroke, heat exhaustion, or prolonged heat cramps, medical attention should be sought.

What Not To Do

1. Avoid giving water without added salt, because this may further deplete the body's salt concentration.
2. Avoid the immediate reexposure of the victim to the heat, because he may be very sensitive to high temperatures for a time.

Nosebleeds

Nosebleeds are generally caused by trauma to the nose, which can result from nose-picking, from colds when there is hard nose-blowing, or from drying of the nasal mucosa. Most commonly, nosebleeds originate from the area of the nasal septum. Nosebleeds may also be associated with hypertension, bleeding disorders, or nasal tumors.

What To Do

1. To prevent the inhalation or swallowing of blood, have the person sit up and lean forward.
2. Gently squeeze the nose closed for 10 to 15 minutes by the clock.
3. If the bleeding stops have the victim rest quietly for a few hours. During this time there should be no stooping, lifting, or vigorous nose blowing. Seek medical attention if the nosebleed is profuse or prolonged. The blood loss from a nosebleed can be considerable, and some people even go into hemorrhagic shock following a nosebleed.

What Not To Do

Do not allow the victim to resume normal activities for a few hours after the nosebleed has subsided.

Poisoning

Poisoning is a common occurrence, particularly in households in which there are children. For the most part poisoning is accidental, but occasionally someone will ingest a poison during a suicide attempt. Households should be equipped to handle poisoning, and syrup of ipecac should be available.

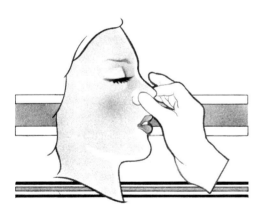

A nosebleed frequently can be stopped by firmly pinching the nose closed.

416

Generally there are five kinds of poisons that might be ingested: a) pesticides, b) drugs, c) strong alkalies and acids, d) petroleum products, e) poisonous plants.

Two of these, petroleum products and strong alkalies and acids, are worthy of special note, because vomiting should *never* be induced if they have been ingested. Examples of petroleum products include turpentine, paint thinner, furniture polish, gasoline, and liquid shoe polish. Examples of strong alkalies include drain cleaner, lye, and some bleaches. In the case of strong alkalies or other strong substances that may cause chemical burns, the mouth and esophagus are burned when the poison is swallowed. If the person is made to vomit, he will be burned a second time as the chemical is passed up the esophagus and out the mouth again. In the case of petroleum products, vomiting may lead to inhalation of the poison, with a resulting chemical pneumonia.

The best way to handle poisons is to take precautions against their ingestion, particularly when small children are present. Medicines, detergents, and cleaning products should all be placed on a high shelf, not under the sink where children can easily find them. In addition, poisons should be kept in appropriate containers. It is dangerous to keep gasoline or furniture polish in a soft drink bottle because a child may drink from that bottle, thinking that it contains a soft drink.

What To Do

1. Initially, give ½ glass of water or milk to anyone who has ingested a poison, unless the victim is *unconscious* or is having convulsions.
2. Decide whether or not to induce vomiting. Look in the victim's mouth for burns that might indicate the ingestion of an acid or alkali. Also, smell the victim's breath to see if it smells like a petroleum product. If either sign is present, do not induce vomiting. If the poisoning has been caused by pesticides, drugs, or poisonous plants, vomiting may be induced by putting one's fingers into the back of the victim's throat to induce gagging and vomiting, or by using syrup of ipecac. Children should be given approximately one teaspoon to one tablespoon of syrup of ipecac, and adults should be given two tablespoons. Vomiting should occur within 20 to 30 minutes.
3. Contact your local physician or emergency department for further instructions. A Poison Control Center may recommend specific antidotes. Antidotes that are listed on the packaging of poisonous products may not be correct or the procedure for their administration may be faulty. It may be better to contact a Poison Control Center for specific instructions.
4. If respiratory difficulty or shock develop, they should be treated appropriately.

What Not To Do

1. Do not allow poisons to be within the reach of children.
2. Do not induce vomiting if alkalies, acids, or petroleum products have been ingested.
3. If the victim is unconscious or is having convulsions, do not give him water, and do not induce vomiting.
4. Do not store poisonous materials in food bottles or jars.

Poison Ivy, Poison Oak, and Poison Sumac

Contact with poisonous plants such as poison ivy, oak, or sumac frequently produces local itching and redness in allergic individuals. In some people the rash that develops is characterized by vesicles (small blisters). More severe reactions include headache, fever, and malaise.

What To Do

1. Contaminated clothing should be removed and all exposed areas of the body should be washed with soap and water.
2. Once the rash has developed, soothing lotions may be applied to the skin. Many of these lotions are available without prescription at a pharmacy. Cool, moist compresses also are valuable for relieving itching.
3. If blisters appear and begin to ooze, they may be treated with wet dressings —sterile gauze pads saturated with a solution of baking soda and water

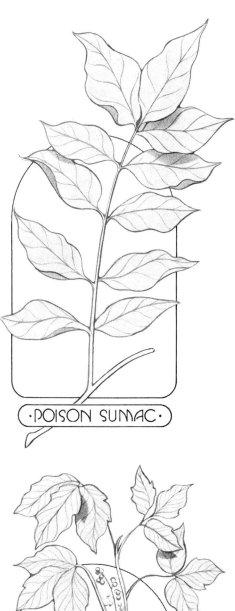

· POISON SUMAC ·

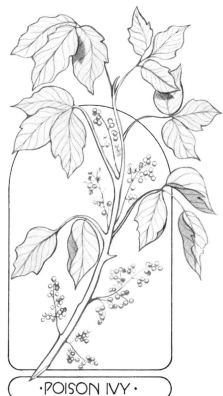

· POISON IVY ·

417

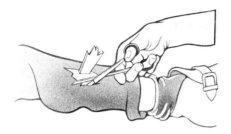

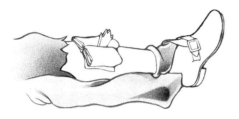

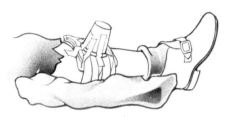

Objects stuck deep through the skin (or into the eye) should not be removed. If the object is too large to be secured in place by simply using a dressing, a paper cup taped over it may reduce further injury.

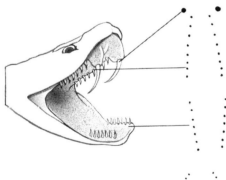

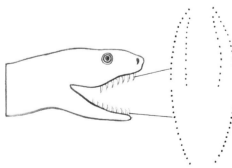

Pit vipers generally produce conspicuous fang marks. Nonpoisonous snakes and coral snakes will not leave fang marks.

(one tablespoon of baking soda to one pint of water).

4. If a severe reaction occurs, if there is a fever, or if a large area of the body is involved, seek medical advice.

Puncture Wounds

Puncture wounds are created by penetrating objects such as nails, knives, sticks, and needles. Puncture wounds do not bleed as readily as lacerations and thus there is less natural cleansing of the wound and a higher rate of infection.

What To Do

1. The site of the puncture wound should be cleansed with soap and water, after which a clean dressing should be applied.
2. For severe puncture wounds, seek medical attention to guard against tetanus infection and for consideration of antibiotic therapy.

What Not To Do

Do not remove any foreign object that is protruding from the wound. As moving the object may cause further damage, the physician should attend to such wounds.

Rape

Rape is the unlawful carnal knowledge of a woman by a man, forcibly and against the woman's will. In the United States, rape is common, and friends or relatives are frequently called on to render assistance to rape victims.

What To Do

1. The rape victim should be protected from further harm and should be assured that she is safe.
2. If she is injured and is bleeding, direct pressure should be applied to the bleeding points. Never, however, apply hard pressure to the rectal or vaginal areas.
3. If she has a broken extremity, it should be treated appropriately.
4. Always remember that a rape victim has an absolute right to refuse medical, legal, or psychological help; however, she should be encouraged to see a physician as soon as possible.

What Not To Do

1. Even though the victim may feel unclean, she should be advised not to bathe, douche, or urinate, because doing so may destroy some evidence needed by the medical examiner.
2. The scene of the crime should not be touched, because this may invalidate existing evidence that would lead to the conviction of the attacker.
3. The victim should be advised not to change her clothing until she has been examined medically, because some evidence may be lost.

The trauma of the rape victim does not end with the rape itself. She may develop psychological problems or have marital difficulties for days or even years following the incident. In many communities, counseling services have been established specifically for the benefit of these victims.

Snakebite

In the United States there are two groups of poisonous snakes: the coral snakes and the pit vipers. The coral snake is found from North Carolina to Florida, through Louisiana to central Texas. The Sonoran coral snake is found in Arizona and southwestern New Mexico. The pit vipers include the copperhead, water moccasin, and rattlesnake. Rattlesnakes and other pit vipers account for the greatest number of the venomous snakebites in the United States, while coral snakes account for a very small number. Coral snakes produce relatively inconspicuous fang marks. Pit vipers produce a more conspicuous injury, with fang marks surrounded by swelling and blood-filled blisters.

The effect of a poisonous snake's bite depends on the size of the victim, the location of the bite, the amount of venom injected, the speed of absorption of the venom into the victim's circulation, and the amount of time between the bite and the application of specific antivenom therapy.

418

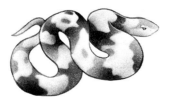

copperhead

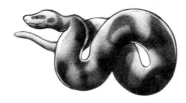

water moccasin

diamondback rattler

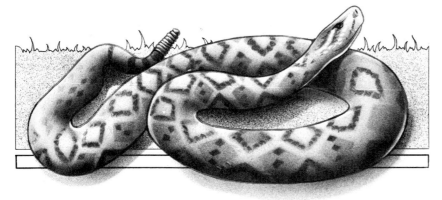

coral snake

What To Do

1. First aid begins with reassuring and calming the victim.
2. The victim should be transferred to a physician as soon as possible. Even if the bite was inflicted by a nonpoisonous snake, a physician may want to give tetanus prophylaxis and antibiotic therapy.
3. Immobilization of the bitten extremity will help retard absorption of the toxin.
4. A tourniquet applied above the bite may retard systemic absorption of the venom and may be useful when there is a delay in reaching an emergency department. The tourniquet should not be so tight as to cause disappearance of peripheral pulses in the foot or the hand.

What Not To Do

1. Incisions over the fang marks are not recommended.
2. Do not give the victim alcohol in any form because it may increase absorption from the skin.

Spider Bites and Scorpion Stings

The reaction to the toxins of spiders and scorpions varies from mild, with resulting local pain, redness, and swelling, to severe, with convulsion, nausea, vomiting, muscular pain, and even shock. In the United States the two spiders that are generally the most harmful are the black widow spider (*Latrodectus mactans*) and the brown recluse (*Loxosceles reclusa*).

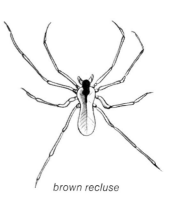

brown recluse

What To Do

1. Wash the wound with soap and water and apply a clean dressing.
2. A medication like aspirin may help relieve the pain.
3. For spider bites, scorpion bites, and any insect bite associated with intense pain, severe swelling, and discoloration, a physician's evaluation should be sought.
4. If the spider or scorpion has been killed, don't discard it. A physician may be able to further identify the species if he sees it.

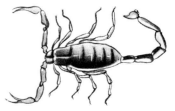

scorpion

The brown recluse spider is about one inch in length overall, including the legs; it has a dark, violin-shaped marking on its lighter back. Scorpions range from one-half to seven inches in length. The body of the female black widow spider is about one inch long, and there usually is a reddish, hourglass-shaped marking on the underside of the abdomen.

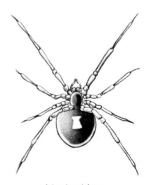

black widow

419

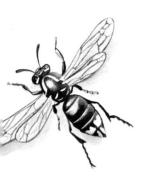

Stings (Wasp, Bee, Yellow Jacket, and Hornet)

The stings from these insects are relatively common, and they rarely cause death except in highly sensitive individuals. The sting may be painful, but the symptoms are usually mild and are of short duration.

Some people are highly sensitive to insect stings and may develop an allergic reaction, possibly with anaphylaxis (a massive allergic reaction) and subsequent death.

What To Do

1. Most people have no problem from an insect sting, and relief from the local discomfort can be obtained from various home remedies—local cool compresses or a solution of cool water and baking soda.
2. Aspirin or an aspirin substitute sometimes helps.
3. If the person is highly sensitive to insect bites and has developed allergic reactions in the past, seek *immediate* medical attention. If medical attention will be delayed more than a few minutes, attempt to remove and discard the stinger and attached venom sac (in the case of the honeybee) by carefully scooping it out with a fingernail. Ice should be applied to the area of the bite.

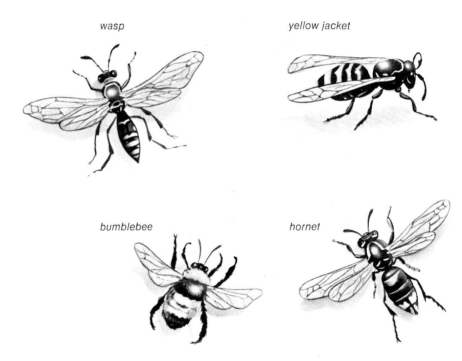

wasp

yellow jacket

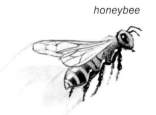

honeybee

bumblebee

hornet

Stroke

Strokes are often referred to as cerebral vascular accidents. "Cerebral vascular" refers to the blood vessels in the brain, which are affected either by a clot or by rupture with subsequent hemorrhage. Major strokes may be accompanied by facial weakness, an inability to talk, the slurring of speech, loss of bladder and bowel control, unconsciousness, paralysis or weakness (particularly on one side of the body), or difficulty in breathing and swallowing. Sometimes strokes are associated with vomiting, convulsions, or headaches.

The most important things to watch are breathing and vomiting. Recovery from strokes is quite variable.

What To Do

1. If the victim is having difficulty breathing, his airway should be opened. (*See* Cardiopulmonary Arrest, above.)
2. The victim should be positioned on his side so that his secretions will drain out of his mouth and not into his airway.

420

3. If vomiting occurs, the victim should be kept on his side and his mouth should be wiped clean of vomitus.
4. Get prompt medical attention for all stroke victims.

What Not To Do

1. Fluids should never be administered by mouth unless the victim is fully conscious.
2. The victim should not be left alone for any length of time because of the chance of his vomiting and then inhaling the vomitus.

Sunburn

Ordinary sunburn is caused by overexposure to the sun's ultraviolet rays. The initial symptoms may begin as early as one hour after exposure and are manifested in painful redness and swelling of the area, and, in more severe cases, in the formation of blisters over the sun-exposed areas. When very large areas of skin are involved, fever, gastrointestinal upset, and weakness may occur.

Fair-skinned people and people taking certain medications should avoid exposure to the sun. Even dark-skinned people should initially avoid being in the bright midday sun for longer than 30 minutes. For added protection there are many good sun-screening ointments, creams, and lotions available. The most common and most effective ingredient in these is para-aminobenzoic acid (PABA), which screens out the ultraviolet rays that cause sunburn.

What To Do

1. Mild sunburn can be treated at home with cool compresses.
2. If there is an accompanying fever, aspirin may help.
3. Commercially available lotions often have a soothing effect on the skin.
4. For more severe cases, it may be necessary to consult a physician.

What Not To Do

1. Avoid further exposure to the sun until the acute reactions have subsided.
2. Avoid greasy preparations.

Sunburns usually resolve themselves, but occasionally the blisters become infected. If much of the skin has peeled off, the underlying skin will be quite sensitive to reexposure to the sun for several days or weeks.

Unconsciousness

Unconsciousness is a sleeplike state from which one may or may not be arousable. A person in "stupor" may be aroused with stimulation and only then with difficulty, while a person in coma cannot be aroused even by the most powerful stimuli.

The most common causes of unconsciousness are fainting, intoxication with alcohol, head trauma, strokes, poisoning or drug overdoses, seizures, diabetic acidosis, hypoglycemia, various types of shock, and hypoxia. Elderly, poorly nourished, or otherwise debilitated people are more prone to unconsciousness regardless of the nature of their illness.

The cause of unconsciousness is often difficult for even a physician to diagnose, and laymen should be careful not to ascribe a patient's unconscious state to something like intoxication. Alcoholics are of course not immune to other more serious causes of unconsciousness.

What To Do

1. Any unconscious person should be checked for an open airway and for palpable carotid pulses (*see* Cardiopulmonary Arrest, above).
2. If the person is not arousable but is breathing well and has good carotid pulses, he should be placed on his side so that he will not inhale any stomach contents if he vomits.
3. Anyone who is comatose should be evaluated by a physician. If drug ingestion or poison is suspected, the containers from the suspected toxin should be brought to the emergency department. Observations made about the person before his lapse into unconsciousness also will be of great help to the examining physician.

What Not To Do

1. Unconscious persons should not be left alone for any length of time, except for summoning help.
2. Fluids should never be administered by mouth and vomiting should never be induced.
3. Do not unnecessarily move an unconscious person unless you are certain he does not have a neck injury.

If unconsciousness resulted from a fainting attack, the victim may awaken within a few minutes. If unconsciousness recurs or if the person remains unconscious for several minutes, an evaluation by a physician should be sought.

Vomiting

Vomiting is the action by which the stomach rids itself of its contents. Vomiting can be caused by disturbances in either the abdomen or the head.

Causes of vomiting arising in the abdomen include: irritation or mechanical obstruction at any level of the intestinal tract, or irritation of abdominal organs like the gallbladder.

Causes of vomiting that originates in the vomiting centers in the head include: emetics (drugs), various toxins (poisons), increased pressure inside the head, decreased oxygen content of the blood in the head, disturbances of the semicircular canals of the ear (as occurs with seasickness), and, occasionally, psychological factors.

Severe or prolonged vomiting may lead to dehydration. When vomiting is associated with respiratory difficulty it may indicate that some of the vomitus was inhaled, and this is a medical emergency.

Simple acute vomiting may be caused by the effects of alcohol on the stomach lining, by dietary indiscretions, by viral gastroenteritis, or by the morning sickness of pregnancy. Severe or prolonged vomiting may reflect more severe gastrointestinal or systemic disease.

What To Do

1. Care should be taken to turn bedridden people onto their sides, so that they do not inhale any vomited stomach contents.
2. If a comatose person vomits, he should be turned onto his side and the vomitus should be cleared from his mouth.
3. After the initial episode of vomiting, solid food should be withheld temporarily and clear liquids should be given. (A clear liquid is one through which it is possible to read a newspaper.)
4. If the person goes twelve hours without vomiting, solid foods may be resumed, beginning with dry foods such as crackers.
5. If vomiting is prolonged or associated with severe abdominal pain, seek medical attention.

What Not To Do

1. Milk or formula should not be given to infants until the vomiting has subsided.
2. Solid foods should not be given to adults and children until the vomiting has subsided.

Section Three:

The Emergency Care System

To be most effective, emergency care must begin as soon as possible at the scene of an accident. In the home—one of the most common accident sites—there are two important steps that should be taken *before* an accident occurs: prevention and preparation.

The cheapest and most effective medicine is prevention. Every attempt to make the home as safe as possible is mandatory. Accidents in the home may be prevented by keeping stairways well lit and entryways unobstructed, by the careful placement of loose rugs, by proper care and maintenance of electrical appliances and cords, and by the proper shielding and use of power tools.

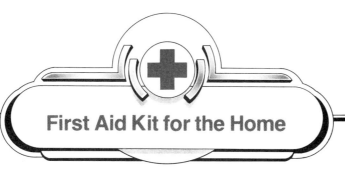

First Aid Kit for the Home

Every home should have a separate box (not just the medicine cabinet)
containing at least the following supplies

First Aid Tools
Thermometer, oral
Thermometer, rectal
Flashlight
Hot water bag
Pair of scissors
Pair of tweezers
Packet of needles
Safety matches
Ice bag

First Aid Material
Aspirin, adult
Aspirin, children's, or aspirin substitute
Bottle of ipecac syrup (2 to 3 oz)
Bottle of aromatic spirits of ammonia
Antiseptic cream for burns
Sunscreen medication (para-aminobenzoic acid)

First Aid Dressings
Sterile 4″ × 4″ dressings
Gauze (2″ wide) for bandaging
Box of assorted adhesive dressings
1″ adhesive tape

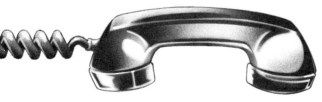

Appropriate List of Telephone Numbers
911 (the universal emergency call number in some communities)
Local hospital emergency department
Ambulance or rescue squad
Police department
Family physician
Poison Control Center (if one is available in the area)
Fire department

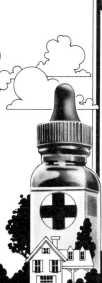

Particular care should be taken in the home to prevent poisoning. All prescription and over-the-counter drugs (including aspirin, cold remedies, and vitamins) should be stored in "child-proof" containers. In addition, old medications should be flushed down the toilet. The passage of time may cause drugs either to lose their potency or, through evaporation, to increase in potency. All medicine should be stored out of the sight and reach of children.

All cleaning solutions, drain and oven cleaners, solvents, and petroleum products (kerosene, gasoline, turpentine, charcoal lighter), insect spray, roach tablets and roach powder should be stored on high or locked shelves where children can't get at them. Never put any of these substances in a beverage or food container. Beverage bottles look particularly inviting to toddlers.

Prehospital Care

Whenever there is *anything but* the most simple injury or medical problem, it is best to call an experienced ambulance or rescue squad. It is always better to err on the side of calling EMS people rather than procrastinating at the victim's expense. Many services are upgrading their capabilities with better equipment and training. Most ambulance drivers and attendants are at least basic Emergency Medical Technicians (EMT's). The EMT's have received 81 hours of intensive first aid training, have passed a minimal proficiency test, and are certified by a state health agency. Many communities also have advanced EMT's (paramedics) available for emergency care. These individuals are basic EMT's but have had an additional 500 to 1,000 hours of intensive training in advanced life support (defibrillation, use of intravenous medications, advanced airway management, etc.). They generally function through radiocommunications with a hospital-based physician.

To Summon Emergency Aid

Have the telephone numbers of an ambulance service or, if none is available, the local police or fire department readily accessible. When you call, be as calm as possible. *Do not* hang up until all of the following information has been given: a) your name; b) your location (how to get there); c) your telephone number; d) the type of emergency (number of people involved, etc.).

The Emergency Department

The emergency department of the local hospital is the best facility to evaluate and treat true emergencies. Because many people may be seeking emergency care at the same time for different degrees of emergencies, the emergency department might seem to be a very confusing place. Most emergency departments, however, are organized to quickly establish priorities for care, and to provide appropriate treatment for each individual as soon as possible within the limits of those priorities.

The system starts with the nurse, who usually sees the victim first and, by means of a few basic medical questions or tests (temperature, blood pressure, pulse, etc.), attempts to determine the nature of the victim's problem. This nurse is trained to recognize life-threatening problems and to assure that they are seen and evaluated first. In an emergency department patients are not seen on a first-come, first-served basis. For example, a person with a sprained ankle would have to wait to be seen until a man with severe chest pains had been treated.

Better hospital emergency departments have physicians present around the clock to see and treat emergencies. These physicians are specialists in the treatment of emergency problems. Their availability in the hospital and their special training make them the physicians best suited to initially evaluate and stabilize any true emergency. The emergency physician's practice frequently is confined to the emergency department, and he should not be assumed to be in competition with one's regular physician.

Index

This is a three-year cumulative index. Index entries to *World of Medicine* articles in this and previous editions of the *Medical and Health Annual* are set in boldface type, *e.g.,* **Eye Diseases and Visual Disorders.** Entries to other subjects are set in lightface type, *e.g.,* hemodialysis. Additional information on any of these subjects is identified with a subheading and indented under the entry heading. The numbers following headings and subheadings indicate the year (boldface) of the edition and the page number (lightface) on which the information appears.

Eye Diseases and Visual Disorders
82–218; **81**–216
acute mountain sickness complications **82**–261
cancer **81**–226
diabetes complications **83**–251
first aid **83**–413; **82**–413; **81**–413
headache symptoms and effects **81**–27
infectious diseases and interferon's use **81**–259
microsurgery and treatment use **82**–312

All entry headings, whether consisting of a single word or more, are treated for the purpose of alphabetization as single complete headings and are alphabetized letter by letter up to the punctuation. The abbreviation ''il.'' indicates an illustration.

443

Now there's a way to identify all your fine books with flair and style. As part of our continuing service to you, Britannica Home Library Service, Inc. is proud to be able to offer you the fine quality item shown on the next page.

Booklovers will love the heavy-duty personalized **Ex Libris** embosser. Now you can personalize all your fine books with the mark of distinction, just the way all the fine libraries of the world do.

To order this item, please type or print your name, address and zip code on a plain sheet of paper. (Note special instructions for ordering the embosser). Please send a check or money order only (your money will be refunded in full if you are not delighted) for the full amount of purchase, including postage and handling, to:

Britannica Home Library Service, Inc.
Attn: Yearbook Department
Post Office Box 6137
Chicago, Illinois 60680

17 68

(Please make remittance payable to: Britannica Home Library Service, Inc.)

IN THE BRITANNICA TRADITION OF QUALITY...

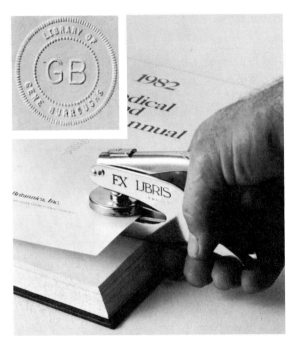

EX LIBRIS
PERSONAL EMBOSSER

A mark of distinction for your fine books. A book embosser just like the ones used in libraries. The 1½″ seal imprints "Library of _____" (with the name of your choice) and up to three centered initials. Please type or print clearly BOTH full name (up to 26 letters including spaces between names) and up to three initials.
Please allow six weeks for delivery.

Just $20.00

plus $2.00 shipping and handling

This offer available only in the United States.
Illinois residents please add sales tax

Britannica Home Library Service, Inc.